Bethesda Handbook
of Clinical Oncology

Bethesda Handbook
of Clinical Oncology

Second Edition

Editors

Jame Abraham, MD, FACP
Chief, Section of Hematology/Oncology
Associate Professor of Medicine
Medical Director, Mary Babb Randolph Cancer Center
West Virginia University
Morgantown, West Virginia

James L. Gulley, MD, PhD, FACP
Director, Clinical Immunotherapy Group, Laboratory of
Tumor Immunology and Biology, Center for Cancer Research,
National Cancer Institute, National Institutes of Health,
Bethesda, Maryland

Carmen J. Allegra, MD
Chief Medical Officer
Network for Medical Communication and Research
Atlanta, Georgia

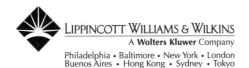
LIPPINCOTT WILLIAMS & WILKINS
A **Wolters Kluwer** Company
Philadelphia • Baltimore • New York • London
Buenos Aires • Hong Kong • Sydney • Tokyo

Acquisitions Editor: Jonathan W. Pine
Developmental Editor: Scott Scheidt/Louise Bierig
Project Manager: Bridgett Dougherty
Senior Manufacturing Manager: Ben Rivera
Marketing Manager: Adam Glazer
Design Coordinator: Terry Mallon
Production Services: Laserwords Private Limited
Printer: R.R.Donnelley Crawfordsville

2nd Edition
© 2005 by Lippincott Williams & Wilkins
530 Walnut Street
Philadelphia, PA 19106
www.lww.com

1/e published 2000

Library of Congress Cataloging-in-Publication Data
Bethesda handbook of clinical oncology / editors, Jame Abraham, James L. Gulley, Carmen J. Allegra.—2nd ed.
   p. ; cm.
  Includes bibliographical references and index.
  ISBN 0-7817-5116-0
  1. Cancer--Handbooks, manuals, etc. I. Title: Handbook of clinical oncology.
 II. Abraham, Jame. III. Gulley, James L. (James Leonard), 1964- IV. Allegra, Carmen J.
  [DNLM: 1. Neoplasms—therapy—Handbooks. QZ 39 B562 2005]
  RC262.5.B485 2005
  616.99'4--dc22
                                                        2005006353

---

                                                        10 9 8 7 6 5 4 3 2

*We dedicate this book to those whose lives are touched by cancer
and to the caregivers who spend endless hours taking care of them.*

"May I never forget that the patient is a fellow creature in pain.
May I never consider him merely a vessel of disease."
— Maimonides
(*12th century philosopher–physician*)

Contents

SECTION 9: HEMATOLOGIC MALIGNANCIES

SECTION 10: OTHER MALIGNANCIES

SECTION 11: SUPPORTIVE CARE

SECTION 12: TARGETED TREATMENTS AND COMPLIMENTARY AND ALTERNATIVE MEDICINE

SECTION 13: COMMON PROCEDURES AND CHEMOTHERAPY DRUGS

APPENDIX

Contributing Authors

Jame Abraham, MD, FACP *Chief, Department of Medicine, Associate Professor, Section of Hematology/Oncology, Medical Director, Mary Babb Randolph Cancer Center, West Virginia University, Morgantown, West Virginia*

Manish Agrawal, MD, MA, MSc *Staff Investigator, Medical Oncology Clinical Research Unit, National Cancer Institute, National Institutes of Health, Bethesda, Maryland*

Oncologist, Department of Oncology, Associates in Oncology and Hematology, Rockville, Maryland

Carmen J. Allegra, MD *Chief Medical Officer, Network for Medical Communication and Research, Atlanta, Georgia*

Ramin Altaha, MD *Assistant Professor, Section of Hematology/Oncology, Robert C. Byrd Health Sciences Center, West Virginia University, Morgantown, West Virginia*

Christina M. Annunziata *Clinical Fellow, Medical Oncology Clinical Research Unit, National Cancer Institute, National Institutes of Health, Bethesda, Maryland*

Philip M. Arlen, MD *Staff Clinician, Laboratory of Tumor Immunology and Biology, Center for Cancer Research, National Cancer Institute, National Institutes of Health, Bethesda, Maryland*

Susan Bates, MD *Senior Investigator, Cancer Therapeutics Branch, National Cancer Institute, National Institutes of Health, Bethesda, Maryland*

Jason R. Beckrow, DO *Oncology Fellow, Department of Internal Medicine, Michigan State University, East Lansing, Michigan*

Oncology Fellow, Breslin Cancer Center, Ingham Regional Medical Center, Lansing, Michigan

Michael J. Birrer, MD, PhD *Deputy Branch Chief, Department of Cell and Cancer Biology, National Cancer Institute, National Institutes of Health, Rockville, Maryland*

Marc R. Blackman, MD *Chief, Endocrine Section, Laboratory of Clinical Investigation, National Center for Complementary and Alternative Medicine, National Institutes of Health, Bethesda, Maryland*

Oscar S. Breathnach, MB, FRCPI *Clinical Instructor, Department of Medicine, University College Cork, Cork, Ireland*
Consultant Medical Oncologist, Department of Oncology, Cork University Hospital, Cork, Ireland

June Cai, MD *Assistant Professor of Psychiatry, Department of Psychiatry and Human Behavior, Brown University Medical School, Providence, Rhode Island*
Director, Division of Consulation-Liaison Psychiatry Service, Department of Psychiatry, The Miriam Hospital, Providence, Rhode Island

Jane Carter, RN, MSN *Research Nurse Specialist, National Cancer Institute, National Institutes of Health, Bethesda, Maryland*

Deborah Charest-Gutierrez, RN BSN *Clinical Manager, Department of Nursing, Procedure, Vascular Access, Conscious Sedation Service, National Institutes of Health, Bethesda, Maryland*

Richard W. Childs, MD *Senior Investigator, Tumor Immunology/Stem Cell Transplantation, Hematology Branch, National Heart, Lung, and Blood Institute, National Institutes of Health, Bethesda, Maryland*

Barbara A. Conley, MD *Professor and Chief, Section of Hematology/Oncology, Department of Medicine, Michigan State University, East Lansing, Michigan*

Jorge E. Cortes, MD *Professor, Deputy Chair and Chief, Chronic Myelogenous Leukemia Section, Department of Leukemia, M.D. Anderson Cancer Center, The University of Texas, Houston, Texas*

Michael Craig, MD *Fellow, Section of Hematology/Oncology, Department of Medicine, West Virginia University, Morgantown, West Virginia*

Gregory Curt, MD *Senior Medical Director, AstraZeneca Oncology, Garrett Park, Maryland*
Guest Researcher, Radiation Oncology Branch, National Institutes of Health Clinical Center, Bethesda, Maryland

William L. Dahut, MD *Chief, Genitourinary Clinical Research Section, Medical Oncology Clinical Research Unit, National Cancer Institute, National Institutes of Health, Bethesda, Maryland*

Suzanne G. Demko, PA-C *Physician Assistant, Chief, Office of Nurse Practitioners and Physician Assistants, Medical Oncology Clinical Research Unit, National Cancer Institute, National Institutes of Health, Bethesda, Maryland*

Neelima Denduluri, MD *Clinical Fellow, Medical Oncology, Clinical Research Unit, National Cancer Institute, National Institutes of Health, Bethesda, Maryland*

Marcel P. Devetten, MD *Assistant Professor, Department of Medicine, Director, Blood and Marrow Transplantation Program, University of Nebraska Medical Center, Omaha, Nebraska*

Marnie Dobbin, MS RD, CNSD *Clinical Research Dietitian, Department of Nutrition, National Institutes of Health Clinical Center, Bethesda, Maryland*

J. Paul Duic, MD *Resident, Department of Emergency Medicine, Johns Hopkins School of Medicine, Baltimore, Maryland*

Cynthia E. Dunbar, MD *Head, Molecular Hematopoiesis Section, Hematology Branch, National Heart, Lung, and Blood Institute, National Institutes of Health, Bethesda, Maryland*

Howard A. Fine, MD *Senior Investigator/Branch Chief, Neuro-Oncology Branch, National Cancer Institute and National Institute for Neurologic Disorders, National Institutes of Health, Bethesda, Maryland*

Tito Fojo, MD, PhD *Senior Investigator, Cancer Therapeutics Branch, National Cancer Institute, National Institutes of Health, Bethesda, Maryland*

Arlene A. Forastiere, MD *Professor of Oncology, Department of Oncology, Johns Hopkins University School of Medicine, Baltimore, Maryland*

Barry L. Gause, MD *Senior Investigator, Medical Oncology Clinical Research Unit, National Cancer Institute, National Institutes of Health, Bethesda, Maryland*

Juan C. Gea-Banacloche, MD *Staff Clinician, Experimental Transplantation and Immunology Branch, National Cancer Institute, National Institutes of Health, Bethesda, Maryland*

Head, Infectious Disease Consult Service, National Institutes of Health Clinical Center, Bethesda, Maryland

David Gius, MD, PhD *Chief, Molecular Radiation Oncology, Radiation Oncology Branch, Center for Cancer Research, National Cancer Institute, National Institutes of Health, Bethesda, Maryland*

Martin E. Gutierrez, MD *Head, Lung Cancer Clinical Research Section and Head, Office of Navy-Oncology, Medical Oncology Clinical Research Unit, National Cancer Institute, National Institutes of Health, Bethesda, Maryland*

James L. Gulley, MD, PhD, FACP *Director, Clinical Immunotherapy Group, Laboratory of Tumor Immunology and Biology, Center for Cancer Research, National Cancer Institute, National Institutes of Health, Bethesda, Maryland*

Upendra P. Hegde, MD *Assistant Professor of Medicine, Department of Internal Medicine, Division of Hematology and Oncology, University of Connecticut Health Center, John Dempsey Hospital, Farmington, Connecticut*

Lee J. Helman *Chief of Pediatric Oncology, Acting Scientific Director for Clinical Sciences, Center for Cancer Research, National Cancer Institute, National Institutes of Health, Bethesda, Maryland*

Anne M. Horgan *Clinical Instructor, Department of Medicine, University College Cork, Cork, Ireland*

Thomas E. Hughes, PharmD, BCOP *Clinical Pharmacy Specialist, Department of Pharmacy, National Institutes of Health Clinical Center, Bethesda, Maryland*

William R. Jarnagin, MD, FACS *Assistant Professor of Surgery, Department of Surgery, Weill Medical College of Cornell University, New York, New York*

Associate Attending Surgeon, Department of Surgery, Memorial Sloan-Kettering Cancer Center, New York, New York

Michael J. Keating, MD *Professor of Medicine, Department of Leukemia M.D. Anderson Cancer Center, The University of Texas, Houston, Texas*

David P. Kelsen, MD *Chief, Gastrointestinal Oncology Service, Edward S. Gorden Chair in Medical Oncology, Memorial Sloan-Kettering Cancer Center, New York, New York*

Hung T. Khong, MD *Assistant Professor, Departments of Medicine and Pharmacology, Head Clinical Immunotherapeutics Research Laboratory, USA Cancer Research Institute, University of South Alabama, Mobile, Alabama*

George P. Kim, MD *Assistant Professor, Division of Hematology/Oncology, Chief of Gastrointestinal Cancer Section, Mayo Clinic Cancer Center, Jacksonville, Florida*

Christopher Klebanoff *Emory School of Medicine, Atlanta, Georgia*

David R. Kohler, PharmD *Oncology Clinical Pharmacy Specialist, Pharmacy Department, National Institutes of Health Clinical Center, Bethesda, Maryland*

Herbert L. Kotz, MD *Consultant, Medical Oncology Clinical Research Unit, National Cancer Institute, National Institutes of Health, Bethesda, Maryland*

Barnett S. Kramer, MD, MPH *Associate Director for Disease Prevention, Office of Disease Prevention, National Institutes of Health, Bethesda, Maryland*
Editor-in-Chief, Journal of the National Cancer Institute, Bethesda, Maryland

Pallavi P. Kumar, MD *Clinical Fellow, HIV and AIDS Malignancy Branch, Center for Cancer Research, National Cancer Institute, National Institutes of Health, Bethesda, Maryland*

Gregory D. Leonard, MB, BCH, BAO, Bed Sci *The Royal College of Physicians, Dublin, Ireland*
Consultant Medical Oncologist, Old School of Nursing, Waterford Regional Hospital, Dunmore Road, Waterford, Ireland

Richard F. Little, MD *Senior Clinical Investigator, HIV and AIDS Malignancy Branch, Center for Cancer Research, National Cancer Institute, National Institutes of Health, Bethesda, Maryland*

Patrick J. Mansky, MD *Staff Clinician, National Center for Complementary and Alternative Medicine, National Institutes of Health, Bethesda, Maryland*

Michael E. Menefee, MD *Clinical Fellow, Medical Oncology Clinical Research Unit, National Cancer Institute, National Institutes of Health, Bethesda, Maryland*

Richard A. Messmann, MD, MHS, MSc *Assistant Professor, Department of Hematology/Oncology, Michigan State University, East Lansing, Michigan*
Director of Cancer Research, Great Lakes Cancer Institute, Lansing, Michigan

Hamid R. Mirshahidi, MD *Fellow, Section of Hematology/Oncology, Department of Medicine, West Virginia University, Morgantown, West Virginia*

Brian P. Monahan, MD, FACP *Chair and Associate Professor of Medicine, Department of Hematology and Medical Oncology, Uniformed Services, University of the Health Sciences, Bethesda, Maryland*
Program Director Hematology and Medical Oncology Division, National Naval Medical Center, Bethesda, Maryland

Manish Monga, MD *Staff, Department of Oncology, Wheeling Hospital, Wheeling, West Virginia*

Sattva S. Neelapu, MD *Assistant Professor, Department of Lymphoma and Myeloma, M.D. Anderson Cancer Center, University of Texas, Houston, Texas*

Naomi P. O'Grady, MD *Medical Director, Department of Critical Care Medicine, Procedures, Vascular Access and Conscious Sedation Services, National Institutes of Health, Bethesda, Maryland*

Eileen M. O'Reilly, MD *Assistant Attending/Assistant Professor of Medicine, Department of Medicine, Memorial Sloan-Kettering Cancer Center, New York, New York*

Maryland Pao, MD *Deputy Clinical Director, National Institute of Mental Health, National Institutes of Health, Bethesda, Maryland*

Edwin M. Posadas, MD *Clinical Fellow, Medical Oncology Clinical Research Unit, National Cancer Institute, National Institutes of Health, Bethesda, Maryland*

Muzaffar H. Qazilbash, MD *Assistant Professor, Department of Blood and Marrow Transplantation, M.D. Anderson Cancer Center, University of Texas, Houston, Texas*

Eddie Reed, MD *Director of Mary Babb Randolph Cancer Center, Laurence and Jean DeLynn Chair of Oncology at Robert C. Byrd Health Sciences Center, West Virginia University, Morgantown, West Virginia*

Avi S. Retter, MD *Clinical Fellow, Medical Oncology Clinical Research Unit, National Cancer Institute, National Institutes of Health, Bethesda, Maryland*

Donald L. Rosenstein, MD *Chief of Psychiatry Consultation-Liaison Service, Deputy Clinical Director at Office of the Clinical Director, National Institute of Mental Health, National Institutes of Health, Bethesda, Maryland*

Kerry Ryan, MPH, MSHS, PA-C *Physician Assistant, Medical Oncology Clinical Research Unit, National Cancer Institute, National Institutes of Health, Bethesda, Maryland*

M. Wasif Saif, MD, MBBS *Assistant Professor, Department of Medicine, Division of Hematology/Oncology and Department of Pharmacology/Toxicology, University of Alabama at Birmingham, Birmingham, Alabama*

Gisa Schun *Assistant Professor of Medicine, Section of Hematology/Oncology, West Virginia University, Morgantown, West Virginia*

Muhammad Kamran Siddique, MD *Fellow, Division of Hematology/ Oncology, Department of Medicine, Michigan State University, East Lansing, Michigan*

Fellow, Division of Hematology and Oncology, Department of Medicine, Breslin Cancer Center, Ingham Regional Center, Lansing Michigan

Chris H. Takimoto, MD, PhD *Director of Pharmacology, Institute for Drug Development, Cancer Therapy & Research Center, San Antonio, Texas*

Clinical Associate Professor of Medicine Division of Medical Oncology, University of Texas Health Science Center, San Antonio, Texas

Carter Van Waes, MD, PhD *Senior Investigator and Chief, Head and Neck Surgery Branch, National Institute on Deafness and Other Communication Disorders, Clinical Research Center, National Institutes of Health, Bethesda, Maryland*

Clinical Director National Institute on Deafness and Other Communication Disorders, Clinical Research Center, National Institutes of Health, Bethesda, Maryland

Dawn B. Wallerstedt, RN, CRNP *Nurse Practitioner, Research, National Center for Complementary and Alternative Medicine, National Institutes of Health, Bethesda, Maryland*

Wyndham H. Wilson, MD, PhD *Chief, Lymphoma Section, Experimental Transplantation and Immunology Branch, Center for Cancer Research, National Cancer Institute, National Institutes of Health, Bethesda, Maryland*

Sarah M. Wynne, MD *Clinical Fellow, Laboratory of Immunoregulation, National Institute of Allergy and Infectious Diseases, National Institutes of Health, Bethesda, Maryland*

Preface

The Bethesda Handbook of Clinical Oncology is a clear, concise, and comprehensive reference book for the busy clinician to use in his or her daily encounters with patients. The book has been compiled by clinicians who are working or are trained at the National Cancer Institute and National Institutes of Health as well as by scholars from MD Anderson Cancer Center, Memorial Sloan-Kettering Cancer Center, Johns Hopkins Oncology Center, and other academic institutions. To limit the size of the book, less space has been dedicated to etiology, pathophysiology, and epidemiology and greater emphasis has been placed on practical clinical information. For easy accessibility to the pertinent information, long descriptions are avoided, and more tables, pictures, algorithms, and phrases are included.

The Bethesda Handbook of Clinical Oncology is not intended as a substitute for the many excellent oncology reference textbooks essential for a more complete understanding of the pathophysiology and management of complicated oncology in patients. We hope that the reader-friendly format of this book, with its comprehensive review of the management of each disease and with treatment regimens including dosage and schedule, will make this book unique and useful for oncologists, oncology fellows, residents, students, oncology nurses, and allied health professionals. For the second edition, we have updated the sections and have added two relevant topics (on targeted therapy and on complementary and alternative medicine).

Acknowledgments

We thank all our friends and colleagues who worked hard to make this book possible. We thank Jane Carter, RN, who wrote the chapter on end-of-life care for the book and whose life is touched by cancer now.

This book would not have been possible without the strong and continued support of Jonathan Pine, the senior oncology editor at Lippincott Williams & Wilkins. We thank our wives, Shyla, Trenise, and Linda, for their encouragement and support in this endeavor.

SECTION 1

Head and Neck

1

Head and Neck Cancer

Barbara A. Conley*, Arlene A. Forastiere†, David Gius‡,
and Carter VanWaes§

*Department of Medicine, Michigan State University, East Lansing, Michigan;
†Department of Oncology, Johns Hopkins University School of Medicine, Baltimore,
Maryland; ‡Radiation Oncology Branch, Center for Cancer Research, National Cancer
Institute, National Institutes of Health, Bethesda, Maryland; and §Head and Neck Surgery
Branch, National Institute for Deafness and Other Communicative Disorders, National
Institutes of Health, Bethesda, Maryland

Tumors of the head and neck are the sixth most common malignancy in the United States, with a yearly incidence of 40,000 to 50,000 cases. Ninety percent of these cancers involve squamous cell histology. The most common sites are the oral cavity, pharynx, larynx, and hypopharynx. Nasal cavity and paranasal sinus cancers, salivary gland malignancies, and various sarcomas, lymphomas, and melanoma are less common.

EPIDEMIOLOGY

The worldwide incidence of head and neck squamous cancer is more than 500,000 cases per year, and in the United States, it comprises approximately 4% to 5% of all new cancers and 2% of all cancer deaths (11,000 per year) (1). Most patients are older than 50 years, and incidence increases with age; the male-to-female ratio is 2.5:1. The age-adjusted incidence is higher among black men, and, stage-for-stage, survival among African Americans is lower overall than in whites. Approximately 34% of oral and pharyngeal cancers present as localized disease, 46% present as locoregional (i.e., locally advanced or involving regional lymph nodes) disease, and 10% present as metastatic disease.

RISK FACTORS

Tobacco and alcohol use are major risk factors for developing cancer. Heavy alcohol consumption increases the risk twofold to sixfold, whereas smoking increases the risk fivefold to 25-fold, depending on gender, race, and the amount of smoking. Both factors together increase the risk 15-fold to 40-fold. Smokeless tobacco and snuff are associated with oral cavity cancers. Case–control studies show that the relative risk for developing erythroplasia cancer in tissues in contact with snuff powder (cheek and gum) is nearly 50-fold (2). In many parts of Asia and some parts of Africa, chewing betel with or without tobacco and slaked lime is associated with premalignant lesions and oral squamous cancers (3,4).

Alcohol and tobacco affect the entire respiratory mucosa, leading to multifocal mucosal abnormalities known as "field cancerization" (5). There is a 2% to 6% per year risk for a second head and neck, lung, or esophageal cancer in patients with a history of cancer in this area. Those who continue to smoke have the highest risk. Second primary cancers represent a major risk factor for death among survivors of an initial squamous carcinoma of the head and neck (6–8).

Epstein-Barr virus (EBV) has been detected in virtually all nonkeratinizing and undifferentiated nasopharyngeal cancers but less consistently in squamous nasopharyngeal cancers (reviewed in 9). Correlation has been observed between the presence of papillomavirus and oral and oropharynx cancers (10–12).

Other risk factors include sun exposure (lip cancer); occupational exposure to nickel (nose and ethmoids), radium (antrum), mustard gas (sphenoid), chromium (sinuses and nose), leather (ethmoids and nasal cavity), and wood dust (ethmoids and nasal cavity); radiation exposure (thyroid and salivary gland cancer); EBV exposure (nasopharyngeal cancer); and, possibly, vitamin A deficiency and marijuana. Disorders of DNA repair (e.g., Fanconi anemia) as well as organ transplantation with immunosuppression are associated with increased risk of squamous head and neck cancer.

PREVENTION AND CHEMOPREVENTION

The most important recommendation for prevention of head and neck cancer is to avoid smoking and to limit alcohol intake. Premalignant lesions occurring in the oral cavity, pharynx, and larynx manifest as leukoplakia (a white patch that does not scrape off and that has no other obvious cause) or erythroplakia (friable reddish or specked lesions) (see Table 1.1). The risk of leukoplakias without dysplasia progressing to cancer is about 4%. However, up to 40% of severe dysplasias or erythroplasias progress to cancer. Retinoids can reversibly improve premalignant histology. In a small randomized placebo-controlled trial in patients treated for a head and neck cancer, isotretinoin decreased the incidence of second primary tumors (13). A larger definitive randomized, placebo-controlled trial in patients with curatively treated stages I and II head and neck squamous cell carcinoma failed to find any benefit of 13-*cis*-retinoic acid in preventing

TABLE 1.1. *Premalignant lesions*

Premalignant lesions	Leukoplakia	Erythroplakia	Dysplasia
Clinical features	White patch or plaque occurring in surface of mucous membrane that does not rub off, once other oral diseases are ruled out	Bright red velvety plaques that cannot be characterized clinically or pathologically as being due to any other condition	Can present as leukoplakia, erythroplakia, or without obvious macroscopic findings
Probability of progression to malignant lesions	4%	15%–30% of dysplastic Lesions	15%–30%
Histopathology	Hyperkeratosis associated with variable histologic findings; rarely contain dysplasia or carcinoma. (Invasive or *in situ* carcinoma found in only 6% of cases)	Mild to moderate dysplasia in 10% of patients; severe dysplasia, *in situ* or invasive carcinoma in 90% of cases	True histologic diagnosis: pleomorphic changes, increased number of nucleoli, prominent nucleoli

From McFarland M, Abaza NA, El-Mofty S. In: Damjanov I, Linder J, eds. *Anderson's pathology.* St. Louis: Mosby, 1996, with permission.

second primary cancers or in survival (14). Euroscan, a large European chemoprevention trial that randomized patients with stage I to stage III non–small cell lung cancer or head and neck squamous cancer to either vitamin A (as retinyl palmitate) or *N*-acetylcysteine (a free radical scavenger), neither drug or both drugs, also failed to find preventive benefit (15).

Presently, there is no effective chemoprevention for patients at risk for head and neck squamous cancer. Chemoprevention outside a clinical trial is not recommended and is potentially harmful. Two large randomized chemoprevention trials for lung cancer demonstrated a worse outcome for those patients randomized to Vitamin A and β-carotene (CARET study) or to β-carotene alone (ATBC study) (16–19).

ANATOMY

A simplified depiction of extracranial head and neck anatomy is presented in Fig. 1.1.

The patterns of lymphatic drainage divide the neck into several levels (see Fig. 1.2). Level *I* comprises the submental or submandibular nodes; level *II* (upper jugular lymph nodes) extends from the skull base to the hyoid bone; level *III* (middle jugular lymph nodes) is the area between the hyoid bone and the lower border of the cricoid cartilage; level *IV* (lower jugular lymph nodes) is the area between the cricoid cartilage and the clavicle; level *V* is the posterior triangle; level *VI* is the anterior compartment from the hyoid bone to the suprasternal notch, bounded on each side by the medial carotid sheath; and level *VII* is the area of the superior mediastinum. Masses more than 3 cm in greatest dimension are generally groups of nodes or a single node, with the tumor extending into the soft tissues (20). Knowledge of the lymphatic

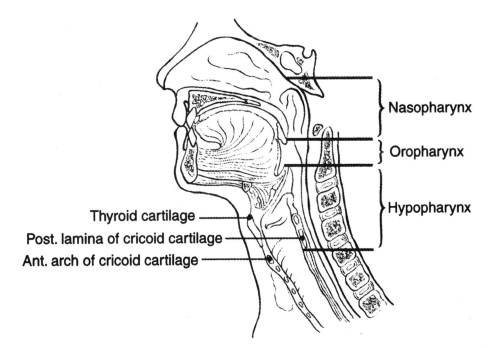

FIG. 1.1. Sagittal section of the upper aerodigestive tract. (Used with the permission of the American Joint Committee on Cancer (AJCC), Chicago, Illinois. The original source for this material is the *AJCC Cancer Staging Manual, Sixth Edition* (2002) published by Springer-Verlag New York, www.springer-ny.com.)

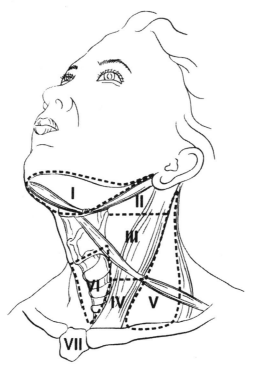

FIG. 1.2. Diagram of the neck showing levels of lymph nodes. Level *I*, submandibular; level *II*, high jugular; level *III*, midjugular; level *IV*, low jugular; level *V*, posterior jugular; level *VI*, tracheoesophageal; level *VIII* (superior mediastinal) is not shown. (Used with the permission of the American Joint Committee on Cancer (AJCC), Chicago, Illinois. The original source for this material is the *AJCC Cancer Staging Manual, Sixth Edition* (2002) published by Springer-Verlag New York, www.springer-ny.com.)

drainage of the neck assists the surgeon in planning the extent of neck resection and in locating a primary tumor when a palpable lymph node is the initial presentation.

STAGING SYSTEM

Staging is based on physical examination and imaging tests. The staging system put forth by the American Joint Committee for Cancer (AJCC) (see Table 1.2) and the Union Internationale Contre le Cancer (UICC) [tumor, node, metastasis (TNM)] is used. The AJCC classification (20) emphasizes resectability status by dividing advanced disease stages into stage IVA (resectable), stage IVB (unresectable), and stage IVC (distant metastatic disease).

The T classification indicates the extent of the primary tumor. It differs for each site. For primary tumors of the oral cavity, hypopharynx, and oropharynx, lesions greater than 4 cm are classified as T3. Vocal cord paralysis with a larynx or hypopharynx primary indicates at least T3. Lesions with local invasion of adjacent structures indicate T4.

The N classification is uniform for all primary sites, except nasopharynx. For all primary sites except nasopharynx, any clinical lymph node involvement indicates at least stage III, and nodes larger than a single 3-cm ipsilateral node are classified as stage IV regardless of T stage.

The presence of distant metastasis (M1) indicates stage IVC disease. Mediastinal lymph node involvement is considered distant metastasis.

Tumor grade has not shown significant association with outcome and is not considered when staging head and neck cancers.

TABLE 1.2. *TNM staging of head and neck tumors*

Definition of TNM
Primary Tumor (T)
- TX Primary tumor cannot be assessed
- T0 No evidence of primary tumor
- Tis Carcinoma *in situ*

Nasopharynx
- T1 Tumor confined to the nasopharynx
- T2 Tumor extends to soft tissue
- T2a Tumor extends to the oropharynx and/or nasal cavity without parapharyngeal extension[a]
- T2b Any tumor with parapharyngeal extension[a]
- T3 Tumor involves bony structures and/or paranasal sinuses
- T4 Tumor with intracanial extension and/or involvement of cranial nerves, infratemporal fossa, hypopharynx, orbit, or masticator space

Oropharynx
- T1 Tumor 2 cm or less in greatest dimension
- T2 Tumor more than 2 cm but not more than 4 cm in greatest dimension
- T3 Tumor more than 4 cm in greatest dimension
- T4a Tumor invades the larynx, deep/extrinsic muscle of tongue, medial pterygoid, hard palate, or mandible
- T4b Tumor invades lateral pterygoid muscle, pterygoid plates, lateral nasopharynx, or skull base or encases carotid artery

Hypopharynx
- T1 Tumor limited to one subsite of hypopharynx and 2 cm or less in greatest dimension
- T2 Tumor invades more than one subsite of hypopharynx or an adjacent site, or measures more than 2 cm but not more than 4 cm in greatest diameter without fixation of hemilarynx
- T3 Tumor more than 4 cm in greatest dimension or with fixation of hemilarynx
- T4a Tumor invades thyroid/cricoid cartilage, hyoid bone, thyroid gland, esophagus, or central compartment soft tissue[b]
- T4b Tumor invades prevertebral fascia, encases carotid artery, or involves mediastinal structures

Regional Lymph Nodes (N)
Nasopharynx
The distribution and the prognostic impact of regional lymph node spread from nasopharynx cancer, particularly of the undifferentiated type, are different from those of other head and neck mucosal cancers and justify the use of a different N classification scheme.
- NX Regional lymph nodes cannot be assessed
- N0 No regional lymph node metastasis
- N1 Unilateral metastasis in lymph node(s), 6 cm or less in greatest dimension, above the supraclavicular fossa[c]
- N2 Bilateral metastasis in lymph node(s), 6 cm or less in greatest dimension, above the supraclavicular fossa[c]
- N3 Metastasis in a lymph node(s)[c] >6 cm and/or to supraclavicular fossa
  - N3a Greater than 6 cm in dimension
  - N3b Extension to the supraclavicular fossa[d]

Oropharynx and Hypopharynx
- NX Regional lymph nodes cannot be assessed
- N0 No regional lymph node metastasis
- N1 Metastasis in a single ipsilateral lymph node, 3 cm or less in greatest dimension
- N2 Metastasis in a single ipsilateral lymph node, more than 3 cm but not more than 6 cm in greatest dimension, or in multiple ipsilateral lymph nodes, none more than 6 cm in greatest dimension, or in bilateral or contralateral lymph nodes, none more than 6 cm in greatest dimension.
  - N2a Metastasis in a single ipsilateral lymph node more than 3 cm but not more than 6 cm in greatest dimension
  - N2b Metastasis in multiple ipsilateral lymph nodes, none more than 6 cm in greatest dimension
  - N2c Metastasis in bilateral or contralateral lymph nodes, none more than 6 cm in greatest dimension
- N3 Metastasis in a lymph node more than 6 cm in greatest dimension

continued on next page

TABLE 1.2. *Continued*

Distant Metastasis (M)

MX   Distant metastasis cannot be assessed
M0   No distant metastasis
M1   Distant metastasis

Stage Grouping: Nasopharynx

Stage 0	Tis	N0	M0
Stage I	T1	N0	M0
Stage IIA	T2a	N0	M0
Stage IIB	T1	N1	M0
	T2	N1	M0
	T2a	N1	M0
	T2b	N0	M0
	T2b	N1	M0
Stage III	T1	N2	M0
	T2a	N2	M0
	T2b	N2	M0
	T3	N0	M0
	T3	N1	M0
	T3	N2	M0
Stage IVA	T4	N0	M0
	T4	N1	M0
	T4	N2	M0
Stage IVB	Any T	N3	M0
Stage IVC	Any T	Any N	M1

Stage Grouping: Oropharynx, Hypopharynx

Stage 0	Tis	N0	M0
Stage 1	T1	N0	M0
Stage II	T2	N0	M0
Stage III	T3	N0	M0
	T1	N1	M0
	T2	N1	M0
	T3	N1	M0
Stage IVA	T4a	N0	M0
	T4a	N1	M0
	T1	N2	M0
	T2	N2	M0
	T3	N2	M0
	T4a	N2	M0
Stage IVB	T4b	Any N	M0
	Any T	N3	M0
State IVC	Any T	Any N	M1

[a]Parapharyngeal extension denotes posterolateral infiltration of tumor beyond the pharyngobasilar fascia.

[b]Central compartment of soft tissues includes prelaryngeal strap muscles and subcutaneous fat.

[c]Midline nodes are considered ipsilateral nodes.

[d]Supraclavicular zone or fossa is relevant to the staging of nasopharyngeal carcinoma and is the triangular region originally described by Ho. It is defined by three points: (a) the superior margin of the sternal end of the clavicle, (b) the superior margin of the lateral end of the clavicle, (c) the point where the neck meets the shoulder. Note that this would include the caudal portions of levels IV and V. All cases with lymph nodes (whole or part) in the fossa are considered N3b.

Used with the permission of the American Joint Committee on Cancer (AJCC), Chicago, Illinois. The original source for this material is the *AJCC Cancer Staging Manual, Sixth Edition* (2002) published by Springer-Verlag New York, www.springer-ny.com.

TABLE 1.3. *Common presenting signs and symptoms of head and neck cancer*

Painless neck mass
Odynophagia
Dysphagia
Hoarseness
Hemoptysis
Trismus
Otalgia
Otitis media
Loose teeth
Ill-fitting dentures
Cranial nerve deficits
Nonhealing oral ulcers

PRESENTATION

Signs and symptoms are usually secondary to mass effect and/or pain from primary tumor or involved lymph nodes and invasion of adjacent structures or nerves (see Table 1.3). Adult patients with any of these symptoms for more than 4 weeks should be referred to an otolaryngologist. Delay in diagnosis is common: either patient delay or repeated courses of antibiotics for otitis media or sore throat, for example. A lateralized firm cervical mass in an elderly smoker is highly suggestive of squamous cell carcinoma. For nasopharyngeal cancers, the most common presenting symptom is a neck mass, sometimes in the posterior triangle. In advanced lesions, cranial nerve abnormalities may be present.

With the exception of hypopharyngeal and nasopharyngeal cancers, distant metastases are uncommon at presentation. The most common sites of distant metastases are lung and bone; liver involvement is less common.

DIAGNOSIS

The history should include:

a. tobacco exposure (pack-years, amount chewed, and duration of habit, current or former)
b. alcohol exposure (number of drinks per day)
c. other risk factors mentioned earlier
d. cancer history of family
e. signs and symptoms listed in Table 1.3
f. thorough review of systems.

The physical examination should include:

a. careful inspection of the scalp, ears, nose, and mouth;
b. palpation of the neck and mouth, assessment of tongue mobility, determination of restrictions in the ability to open the mouth (trismus), and bimanual palpation of the base of the tongue and floor of the mouth;
c. special attention should be given to the examination of cranial nerves.

Abnormalities are suggested by asymmetry in the physical examination. Referral for direct and indirect laryngoscopy should be strongly considered for symptoms of hoarseness or sore throat not cured by a single course of antibiotics.

Friability (easy bleeding), an indicator of an early malignant process and erythroplakia (Table 1.1), is frequently associated with severe dysplasia or carcinoma *in situ* and the site should be biopsied. When neck mass is the first presentation, the primary site can be located and biopsied in approximately 80% of cases. If no primary site is obvious, tissue diagnosis can be obtained by fine needle aspiration (FNA) biopsy of the node, with sensitivity and specificity approaching 99%. A nondiagnostic FNA does not rule out the presence of tumor.

Computerized tomography scan (CT scan) remains the primary imaging study for evaluation of metastatic adenopathy. Magnetic resonance imaging (MRI) may complement the CT scan. Positron emission tomography (PET) scans are being used more frequently to detect tumors that are not obvious on other scans, but this technique is still under evaluation (21,22).

Laryngoscopy and nasopharyngoscopy should be performed. With occult primary tumors, directed biopsies of the nasopharynx, tonsil, base of tongue, and pyriform sinus should be performed (see Fig. 1.3). Bilateral tonsillectomy will sometimes reveal the source of an occult cancer.

Surgical biopsy of a neck mass is contraindicated if a squamous cell carcinoma is suspected. Studies show that open biopsy may worsen local control, increase the rate of distant metastases, and decrease overall survival rate, possibly by spreading the disease at the time of the biopsy. Finally, an open biopsy does not provide any information additional to that obtained from FNA, and laryngoscopy is still necessary for treatment planning.

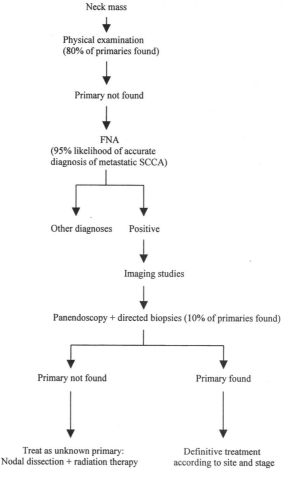

FIG. 1.3. Evaluation of cervical adenopathy when a primary cancer of the head and neck is suspected.

WORK-UP AND STAGING EVALUATION

After the diagnosis of cancer is established, the patient should be clinically staged by physical examination and radiologic studies, usually by CT scan and/or MRI of the primary tumor, neck, and chest. CT scan better defines the cortical bone and is better than MRI for evaluating metastatic adenopathy. MRI has superior soft tissue contrast, does not involve radiation, and may be better than CT scan for primary tumor staging. PET scanning is still undergoing evaluation for sensitivity and specificity (21,22). A chest radiograph or chest CT scan is indicated for all patients because of the risk of a second malignancy. Additional studies vary according to the clinical stage, symptoms, and primary site.

PROGNOSIS

The most important determinant of prognosis is stage at diagnosis. The 5-year survival for stage I patients exceeds 80% but is less than 40% in stage III and IV disease. Most patients have locally advanced disease involving one or several lymph nodes on one or both sides of the neck. The presence of a palpable lymph node in the neck generally decreases the survival rate by 50% compared to the same T stage without node involvement.

Most relapses occur locoregionally. Distant metastases are more commonly seen later in the course of the disease, or as part of relapse after successful initial treatment, and predominantly involve lung, bone, and liver. The lifetime risk of developing a new cancer for a patient with head and neck cancer is 20% to 40% (6,8). After 3 years, development of a new cancer represents the greatest survival risk (see Tables 1.4 to 1.6).

SCREENING

Careful examination of the head and neck is warranted in individuals with risk factors or suggestive symptoms. Mucosal abnormalities and palpable neck masses should be biopsied (see the section, Diagnosis).

The United States Preventive Task Force (http://www.ahcpr.gov/clinic/uspstfix.htm) does not recommend regular screening for oral cancer in the general population but recommends counseling for cessation of tobacco use and limitation of alcohol intake. The American Cancer Society (www.cancer.org) recommends oral examination or dental appointments. The oral examination should include inspection of all mucosal areas, assessment of range of motion of tongue, bimanual palpation of floor of mouth, palpation of the tongue, and assessment of dental health. Any of the complaints described earlier require evaluation, especially if symptoms persist for more than 4 weeks or after treatment for presumed infection.

TREATMENT

The management of patients with head and neck cancer is complex. The choice of treatment modality depends on the stage and site of disease. Patients with locally advanced disease should be evaluated (prosthodontics, nutrition, speech, and swallowing) by a multidisciplinary team including otolaryngologist or head and neck surgical oncologist, radiation oncologist, medical oncologist, dentist, and personnel involved in rehabilitation before treatment is initiated.

In general, either surgery or radiation is effective as single-modality therapy for patients with early-stage disease (stage I or II) for most sites. The choice of modality depends on local expertise, patient preference, and functional result. For the 60% of patients with locally advanced disease (stage III, IV, and M0), combined-modality therapy is indicated.

Surgery

The nature of the surgical procedure is determined primarily by the size of the tumor and the structures involved. Extensive surgeries and those involving function of the tongue

TABLE 1.4. *Head and neck cancer: Oral cavity*

Site	Epidemiology	Natural history and common presenting symptoms	Nodal involvement	Prognosis (5-yr survival)
Lip	Risk factors are sun exposure and tobacco; 3,600 new cases a year; 10 to 40 times more common in white men than in black men or women (black or white)	Exophytic mass or ulcerative lesion; more common in lower lip (92%); slow-growing tumors; pain and bleeding	5%–10% Midline tumors spread bilaterally Level I more common (submandibular and submental); upper lip lesions metastasize earlier: Level I and also preauricular 30% (70% if T4)	T1, 90% T2, 84% With Lymph node involvement, 50%
Alveolar ridge and retromolar trigone	10% of all oral cancers; M:F, 4:1	Exophytic mass or infiltrating tumor, may invade bone; bleeding, pain exacerbated by chewing, loose teeth, and ill-fitting dentures	Levels I and II more common	T1, 85% T2, 80% T3, 60% T4, 20%
Floor of mouth	10%–15% of oral cancers, (occurrence 0.6/100,000); M:F, 3:1; median age, 60 yr	Painful infiltrative lesions, may invade bone, muscles of floor of mouth and tongue	T1, 12%; T2, 30%; T3, 47%, and T4, 53% Levels I and II more common	By stage: I, 85%–90% II, 80% III, 66% IV, 32%
Tongue (anterior two thirds)	6,200 new cases/yr; median age, 60 yr; M:F, 3:1	Exophytic or infiltrative pain, occasional difficulty in speech and deglutition	Greatest propensity for lymph node metastasis of oral cavity sites; bilateral involvement, 25%; level II more common, followed by I, III, and IV	Early stage node negative, 74% Advanced stage, 30%
Hard palate	0.4 cases/100,000 (5% of oral cavity); M:F, 8:1; 50% cases squamous, 50% salivary glands	Deeply infiltrating or superficially spreading pain	Less frequently: 6%–29%	By stage: I, 75% II, 46% III, 36% IV, 11%
Buccal mucosa	8% of oral cavity cancers in United States; Women > men	Exophytic more often, silent presentation; pain, bleeding, difficulty in chewing	10% at diagnosis Levels I and II more common	18%–77% all Stages

M:F, male-to-female ratio.

TABLE 1.5. *Head and neck cancer: Oropharynx and larynx*

Site	Epidemiology	Natural history and common presenting symptoms	Nodal involvement	Prognosis (5-yr survival)
Base of tongue	4,000 new cases annually in the United States; M:F ratio, 3 to 5:1.	Advanced at presentation (silent location, aggressive behavior); Pain, dysphagia, weight loss, and otalgia(from cranial nerve involvement); Neck mass is a frequent presentation	All stages: 70% (T1) to 80% (T4); Level II and III more common, also IV, V, and VI	By stage: I, 60%; II, 40%; III, 30%; IV, 15%
Tonsil, tonsillar pillar, and soft palate	Tobacco and alcohol are the most significant risk factors	Tonsillar fossa: more advanced at presentation: 75% stage III or IV, pain, dysphagia, weight loss, and neck mass. Soft palate: More indolent, may present as erythroplakia	Tonsillar pillar T2, 38%; Tonsillar fossa T2, 68% (55% present with N2 or N3 disease)	Tonsillar fossa, 93% (stage I) to 17% (stage IV); Soft palate, 85% (stage I) to 21% (stage IV)
Posterior pharyngeal wall		Advanced at diagnosis (silent location); Pain, bleeding, and weight loss; Neck mass is common initial symptom	Clinically palpable nodes; T1, 25%; T2, 30%; T3, 66%; T4, 75%; Bilateral involvement is common	By stage: I, 75%; II, 70%; III, 42%; IV, 27%
Supraglottis	35% of laryngeal cancers	Most arise in epiglottis; early lymph node involvement due to extensive lymphatic drainage; two-thirds of patients have nodal metastases at diagnosis	Overall rate: T1, 63%; T2, 70%; T3, 79%; T4, 73%; Levels II, III, and IV more common	By stage: I, 70%–100%; II, 50%–90%; III, 45%–70%; IV, 20%–60%
Glottis	Most common laryngeal cancer	Most favorable prognosis; late lymph node involvement; usually well differentiated, but with infiltrative growth pattern; hoarseness is an early symptom, 70% have localized disease at diagnosis;	Sparse lymphatic drainage, early lesions rarely metastasize to lymph nodes. Clinically positive: T1, T2 < 2%; Levels II, III, and IV more common; T3, T4, 20%–25%	T1, 74%–86%; T2, 67%–75%; T3, 55%; T4, 50%
Subglottis	Rare, 1%–8% of laryngeal cancers	Poorly differentiated, infiltrative growth pattern unrestricted by tissue barriers; rarely causes hoarseness, may cause dyspnea from airway involvement; two-thirds of patients have metastatic disease at presentation	20%–30% overall; Pretracheal and paratracheal nodes more commonly involved	26% overall

M:F, male-to-female ratio.

TABLE 1.6. *Head and neck cancer: Hypopharynx, nasal cavity, paranasal sinuses, and nasopharynx*

Site	Epidemiology	Natural history and common presenting symptoms	Nodal involvement	Prognosis (5-yr survival)
Hypopharynx	2,500 new cases yearly in United States; etiology: tobacco, alcohol, and nutritional abnormalities	Aggressive, diffuse local spread, early lymph node involvement; occult metastases to thyroid and paratracheal node chain; pain, neck stiffness (retropharyngeal nodes), otalgia (cranial nerve X), irritation, and mucus retention 50% present as neck mass; high risk of distant metastases	Abundant lymphatic drainage Up to 60% have clinically positive lymph nodes at diagnosis	Survival varies between sites within hypopharynx T1, T2, 40% T3–T4, 16%–37%
Nasal cavity and paranasal sinuses	Rare, 0.75/100,000 occurrence in United States Nasal cavity and maxillary sinus, four-fifths of all cases M:F, 2:1 Increased risk with exposure to furniture, shoe, textile industries; nickel, chromium, mustard gas, isopropyl alcohol, and radium	Nonhealing ulcer, occasional bleeding, unilateral nasal obstruction, dental pain, loose teeth, ill-fitting dentures, trismus, diplopia, proptosis, epiphora, anosmia, and headache, depending of site of invasion Usually advanced at presentation	10%–20% clinically positive nodes Levels I and II more common	60% for all sites all stages, 30% for T4 Principal determinant for survival is local recurrence
Nasopharynx	Rare (< 1/100,000) except in North Africa, Southeast Asia, and China, far northern hemisphere Associated with EBV, diet, genetic factors	Most common initial presentation: neck mass Other presentations: otitis media, nasal obstruction, tinnitus, pain, and cranial nerve involvement	Clinically positive: WHO I, 60% WHO II and III, 80%–90%	T1, 37%–60% T2, 46%–68% T3, 16%–25% T4, 11%–40%

M:F, male-to-female ratio; EBV, Epstein–Barr virus.

frequently require myocutaneous flaps or microvascular free flaps to achieve a more functional reconstruction.

Resectability depends on the experience of the surgeon and the rehabilitation team. In general, a tumor is unresectable if the surgeon believes that all of the gross tumor cannot be removed or that local and distant control will not be achieved after surgery even with adjuvant radiation therapy. Generally, involvement of the skull base, pterygoid, and deep neck musculature, and of the major vessels portends a poor outcome with surgery as a primary modality.

Cervical lymph node dissections may be elective or therapeutic. Elective neck dissections are done at the time of surgery in patients with necks that are clinically negative when the risk of a positive lymph node is at least 30%. Therapeutic neck dissections are done for clinically obvious masses. Cervical lymph node dissections are classified as radical, modified radical, or selective. The radical dissection includes removal of all lymph nodes in the neck from levels *I* to *V* (Fig. 1.2), including removal of the internal jugular vein, spinal accessory nerve, and sternocleidomastoid muscle. This surgery is now rarely performed because of excessive morbidity, especially loss of shoulder function. The modified radical dissection preserves one or more of the nonlymphatic structures. In selective neck dissections, only certain levels of lymph nodes are removed on the basis of the specific lymphatic drainage from the primary site. With no palpable or CT scan evidence of clinical nodal involvement, nodal metastases will be present beyond the confines of an appropriate selective neck dissection less than 10% of the time. Sentinel lymph node dissection and PET scanning are currently being evaluated for use in diagnosing positive lymph nodes in patients with necks that are clinically negative.

Radiation Therapy

The use of radiation as a single therapy in early-stage tumors (i.e., T1 and T2) is as efficacious as surgery. The choice of therapy depends on expected quality of life, functional outcome, sequelae of therapy, and options for treatment in case of recurrence.

In locally advanced tumors (i.e., T3 and T4), radiation therapy is combined with surgery. In general, postoperative radiation is preferred over preoperative radiation according to the results of two randomized prospective studies that show superior local control and minimally increased survival in the postoperative radiation arm in hypopharyngeal cancer patients (23).

Postoperative radiotherapy is recommended for patients at high risk for local recurrence [i.e., T4 tumor, close or positive margins (<5 mm), perineural or perilymphatic or vascular invasion by the tumor, multiple or large positive nodes, and/or extracapsular invasion (23)].

The radiation type (i.e., dose, fractionation regimen, and indication for brachytherapy) varies for specific sites and for definitive versus adjuvant therapy. The standard fractionation regimen in the United States is 1.8 to 2.0 Gy once daily, 5 days per week. The total dose of irradiation for definitive treatment is in the range of 70 to 80 Gy depending on the treatment schedule given and on the ability to shield normal tissue. Recent large randomized trials of hyperfractionated accelerated radiation as the primary treatment modality in locally advanced disease have shown improved local control but no or minimally increased survival with b.i.d. or t.i.d. fractionation as well as with the "concomitant boost" technique, in which radiation is given daily early in the course, then twice daily at the end of the course, with the second treatment representing a "boost" volume (24,25). Most of these regimens result in increased acute toxicities but similar long-term toxicities compared to daily fractionation. Conformal and Intensity Modulated Radiation Therapy techniques are being used to conform and confine the radiation dose to the tumor while maximally sparing the normal tissue, particularly salivary glands (26,27).

Common severe acute radiation toxicity includes epidermitis, mucositis, loss of taste, xerostomia, dysphagia, and hair loss. Dental evaluation and necessary extractions should be performed before radiation because dental extractions in a radiated mandible can lead to osteonecrosis (28). Dentulous patients should be given prophylactic fluoride. Patients receiving radiation are at high risk for tooth decay due to the xerostomia caused by injury to the salivary glands as well as mucosal damage. The drug amifostine has been shown in a randomized trial to decrease the incidence of chronic severe radiation-induced xerostomia from 57% to 34% in patients receiving postoperative radiation (single agent) to a maximal dose of 60 cGy (29).

Brachytherapy can be used as a definitive treatment for early-stage tumors or combined with external beam radiation in more advanced lesions in selected tumors (e.g., tongue, floor of mouth, tonsil, and nasopharynx) with excellent results. Brachytherapy is an option for recurrent cancers of the head and neck, particularly in previously irradiated patients.

Chemotherapy

Until relatively recently, chemotherapy was used mainly for palliation of patients with locally recurrent or disseminated disease without proven survival advantage. Combination chemotherapy yields higher response rates but has increased toxicity and no proven survival advantage when compared with single agents. The choice of single-agent or combination chemotherapy depends on the patient's preference and performance status.

Single agents with more than 10% response activity are listed in Table 1.7 (30–50). Several combination regimens have been developed to improve response rates (see Table 1.8) (51–57). The combination of cisplatin and infusional 5-fluorouracil (5-FU) produces a 70% response rate and a 27% complete remission (CR) rate in chemotherapy-naive patients (58), but the response rate is 30% to 35% in patients who have relapsed after radiation therapy.

Platinum-based chemotherapeutic regimens and the single agent methotrexate are the most commonly used regimens for metastatic disease. Carboplatin may be slightly less active than cisplatin for head and neck squamous cancer, but carboplatin combinations with other chemotherapy agents are generally better tolerated than those with cisplatin. Carboplatin is preferred in patients at high risk for cisplatin toxicity, that is, those with renal dysfunction, neuropathy, or hearing loss (59).

Both docetaxel and paclitaxel have shown antitumor activity (39–44). Several dosing schedules for paclitaxel have been investigated. Three-hour infusions are probably the best balance between theoretically optimum exposure and tolerable toxicity (60). Docetaxel is usually administered at doses of 60 to 100 mg per m^2 every 3 to 4 weeks. Weekly schedules are being evaluated for both drugs. Taxane combinations, including paclitaxel with ifosfamide and cisplatin or carboplatin, and docetaxel with cisplatin and 5-FU (61) show promising response rates.

Prior to the use of taxane combinations, meta-analyses and randomized trials demonstrated improved response for cisplatin compared with methotrexate, improved response for cisplatin and 5-FU combination compared with single drugs, and improved response for cisplatin and 5-FU combination when compared with other regimens for treatment of recurrent or metastatic head and neck squamous cancer (62,63). In the metastatic or recurrent setting, the response rate of cisplatin and infusional 5-FU combination (Table 1.8) is approximately 30%, with less than 10% complete responses. A randomized trial of cisplatin and 5-FU versus carboplatin (300 mg per m^2) and 5-FU versus weekly methotrexate in patients with recurrent or metastatic head and neck squamous cancers demonstrated response rates of 32%, 21%, and 10%, respectively. Median survival was not improved by combination chemotherapy (6.6, 5.0, and 5.6 months, respectively) (51).

The role of chemotherapy has expanded significantly over the last decade because of the results of clinical trials incorporating chemotherapy in multimodality regimens for previously untreated disease.

Studies have evaluated the use of chemotherapy administered before (i.e., neoadjuvant or induction chemotherapy), during (i.e., concomitant chemotherapy), or after (i.e., adjuvant chemotherapy) radiation therapy or surgery.

Combined modality (chemoradiation) is indicated for patients with locally advanced disease that would require total laryngectomy if treated by surgery and who wish to preserve the larynx, for patients who are technically resectable but who are not medically fit enough for surgery, and for patients with technically unresectable locally advanced cancer. In the patient who presents with locally advanced tumor concomitant with distant metastasis, local control of the disease may prevent infectious and necrotic complications.

TABLE 1.7. *Active chemotherapeutic agents for squamous cell cancer of the head and neck*

Drug	Dose	Response rate	Median survival	Reference	Comments
Methotrexate	40–60 mg/m^2/wk	16%–23.5%	6 mo	30–32	Better response rates reported in patients not exposed to chemoradiation or platinum
Cisplatin	50 mg/m^2 d1–8 80–100 mg/m^2 q21–28d	8%–28.6%	6 mo	30–32	
Carboplatin	60–80 mg/m^2 qd × 5 q4–5wk or 400 mg/m^2 q4wk	24%–26%	26 wk	33,34	
Oxaliplatin	130 mg/m^2 q3wk	6%–13%	5 mo	35	
5-FU	1 g/m^2/24 h CI for 9–120 h q3wk	72%		36	8 of 11 patients, previously untreated
UFT/LV	300 mg/m^2/d and LV 90 mg 3 x daily for 28 d every 35 d 600 mg/d daily	21% 32.4%	8.7 mo	37,38	
Paclitaxel	250 mg/m^2 over 24 h, with G-CSF 80 mg/m^2/wk	36%–40% 9.3%	9.2 mo 235 d	39,40	
Docetaxel	80–100 mg/m^2 q21d	11%–42%		41–44	11% in platinum-refractory patients
	35–45 mg/m^2/wk	three of seven pretreated head/neck cancer patients	not reported for head and neck		
Pemetrexed (LY231514)	500 mg/m^2 q21d	26%	7.3 mo	45	
Irinotecan	75 mg/m^2/wk × 2 q3 wk or 75–125 mg/m2/wk × 4q5 wk	14.2% 26.3%	214 d	46	
Gemcitabine	800–1,250 mg/m^2 weekly × 3q4 wk	13%		47	
Vinorelbine	30 mg/m^2/wk	7.5%–16%	32 wk	48,49	
Gefitinib	500 mg/d	10.6%	8.1 mo	50	Prior systemic therapy allowed

5-FU, 5-fluorouracil; CI, continuous infusion; UFT, uracil/ftorafur; LV, leucovorin; G-CSF, granulocyte colony stimulating factor; MTA, multi-targeted antifolate.

TABLE 1.8. *Active combination chemotherapeutic regimens for squamous cell cancer of the head and neck*

Regimen	Response rate	Median survival	Reference	Comments
Phase III Cisplatin 100 mg/m² 5-FU 1,000 mg/m²/d CI × 96 h q21d	32%	6.6 mo	51	277 patients No prior chemotherapy Doses modified ≤ 25% toxicity or lack of toxicity
Carboplatin 300 mg/m² 5-FU 1,000 mg/m²/d CI × 96 h q28d Methotrexate 40 mg/m²/wk Cisplatin 80 mg/m² d 1 5-FU 600 mg/m² over 4 h d 2–5 Vinorelbine 25 mg/m² d 2, 8 q28d	21% 10% 55%	5 mo 5.6 mo 9.7+mo	52	80 patients No prior chemotherapy
Cisplatin 100 mg/m² Paclitaxel 175 mg/m² (3 h infusion) q21 d	28%	9 mo 30% 1 yr survival	53	No significant difference from cisplatin-5FU in efficacy or quality of life; cisplatin and paclitaxel may have fewer toxicities compared to cisplatin and 5-FU
Cisplatin 100 mg/m² 5-FU 1,000 mg/m²/d; CI × 96 h q21d	23%	8 mo 41% 1yr survival		
Paclitaxel 175 mg/m² (3 h infusion) Ifosfamide 1,000 mg/m² 2 h infusion d 1–3 Mesna 600 mg/m² d 1–3 Carboplatin AUC6 d 1 Or Cisplatin 60 mg/m² d 1 q21—28d	58–59%	8.8– 9.1 mo	54,55	Few patients had prior chemotherapy
Paclitaxel 135 mg/m² d 1; cisplatin 75 mg/m² d 2; 5-FU 1 g/m²/d on d 2–5 continuous infusion every 21 d	60%	6 mo (range 1–26 mo) 37% 1 yr survival	56	Phase I /II trial All had prior radiation, but were chemotherapy naive.
Docetaxel 80 mg/m² d 1, cisplatin 40 mg/m² d 2, 3 and 5-FU 1 g/m²/d continuous infusion d 1–3 q28 d	44%	11 mo (range 1–18 mo) 49% 1 yr survival	57	Most patients had prior radiation but not prior chemotherapy G-CSF needed-15% had febrile neutropenia

Induction Chemotherapy

Induction chemotherapy followed by definitive radiation therapy in patients responding to chemotherapy has been studied for organ preservation in patients with locally advanced cancers of the larynx and of the hypopharynx. No significant survival difference has been demonstrated for chemotherapy followed by radiotherapy compared to surgery followed by radiotherapy in these patients (64,65). Close follow-up is indicated in the event that salvage surgery is needed. For laryngeal cancer, concomitant cisplatin and radiation therapy leads to better local control and organ preservation than neoadjuvant chemotherapy and radiation or radiation alone (66). Induction chemotherapy followed by radiation did not show any benefit when compared to radiation alone.

Presently, induction chemotherapy followed by radiation therapy can be considered standard only for patients with previously untreated locally advanced squamous cancers in the hypopharynx. Cisplatin, 100 mg per m^2 IV, on day 1 and 5-FU, 1,000 mg per m^2 daily as continuous IV infusion, for 5 consecutive days (days 1 to 5), repeated every 3 weeks, followed by radiation therapy in patients who were complete responders exhibited equivalent survival rates in a phase III trial compared to surgery followed by radiation therapy (65). Induction chemotherapy does not increase surgical or radiation therapy complications. Prognostic factors for survival include performance status, tumor site, and stage.

CONCOMITANT CHEMORADIATION

The rationale for concomitant chemoradiation is based on experimental evidence of synergism between chemotherapy and radiation that is theoretically mediated by interference of chemotherapy with multiple intracellular radiation-induced stress-response pathways involved in apoptosis, proliferation, and DNA repair (67). The finding that certain chemotherapeutic agents (e.g., cisplatin, 5-FU, taxanes, and hydroxyurea) can induce radiosensitivity and increase log cell kill for radiation supports this treatment strategy. Cisplatin, the most extensively evaluated drug in recent large randomized trials, has the advantage of not having mucositis as toxicity, although as a radiation enhancer, it does increase radiation-induced mucositis.

Recent meta-analyses and randomized clinical trials published before 1994 show that for locally advanced head and neck squamous cell carcinoma, concomitant chemoradiation produces a small but significant survival advantage of about 8% compared to radiation therapy alone (68–70). The U.S. intergroup compared concomitant cisplatin and radiation to split-course radiation with cisplatin and 5-FU to standard radiation alone in patients with unresectable head and neck squamous cancer and showed that concurrent cisplatin at 100 mg per m^2 every 21 days with daily radiation significantly improved survival rates (71). A randomized trial of cisplatin and 5-FU followed by radiation versus concurrent cisplatin and 5-FU with radiation in patients with unresectable head and neck cancer showed similar survival rates but improved locoregional control for the concomitant arm. This early study highlighted the importance of aggressive supportive care for concomitant regimens, including adequate fluid and electrolyte support (72). Concomitant platinum-based chemoradiation has become standard therapy for patients with unresectable advanced head and neck cancer with good performance status.

Although no randomized phase III trial has been done, results using taxanes with 5-FU and/or cisplatin show promising results as do regimens containing 5-FU and hydroxyurea with concomitant twice-daily radiation, with both chemotherapy and radiation administered together every other week (73). A phase randomized II study compared three regimens of concurrent chemoradiation for stage III or IV head and neck squamous carcinoma in 241 patients: a continuous infusion of cisplatin (10 mg/m^2/day) and 5-FU (400 mg per m^2) daily for the final 10 days of once-daily radiation (chemotherapy boost), hydroxyurea (1 g every 12 hours) and 5-FU (800 mg/m^2/day) continuous infusion for 5 days with radiation (entire regimen given every other week), or paclitaxel (30 mg per m^2) and cisplatin (20 mg per m^2) given weekly with daily radiation. Grade 4 or greater toxicity occurred in 22%, 29%, and 23% of patients in each arm, respectively, although three deaths occurred in the chemotherapy boost arm. The estimated

2-year disease-free and overall survival rates were 38.2% and 57.4%, 48.6% and 69.4%, and 51.3% and 66.6%, respectively (74).

Current studies are evaluating the possibility that induction chemotherapy followed by chemoradiation and/or surgery can increase locoregional disease-free and overall survival rates for patients with locally advanced head and neck squamous cancer.

Agents that inhibit epidermal growth factor receptor (EGFR) signaling are being evaluated as radiation enhancers in head and neck squamous cancers. More than 90% of head and neck squamous cancers express EGFR (75), and increased expression has been correlated with poorer survival rates after radiation therapy (76,77). Upregulation of EGFR after radiation has been noted in cell lines (78). Blocking EGFR signals enhances radiosensitivity and chemotherapy effects in preclinical models (79). Clinical studies are ongoing with combinations of EGFR inhibitors with radiation and with standard chemotherapy agents. A recent phase III trial of cisplatin with either placebo or the EGFR antibody C225 in patients with metastatic or recurrent head and neck squamous cancer found no significant advantage in adding the EGFR inhibitor (80). Additional molecular alterations, in addition to expressing EGFR, are likely to be important for response to EGFR inhibitors.

Elective lymph node dissection is often carried out after chemoradiation in patients with N2, N3, or multiple nodes at diagnosis, regardless of nodal response to chemoradiation, when complete response is obtained at the primary site. N2 or greater nodes often (about 20%) harbor tumor even if a clinically complete response is obtained in the neck with chemoradiation (81). Surgical salvage may be attempted if complete control is not achieved at the primary or locoregional site. Major complications with surgical salvage are found in about 52% of patients previously treated with organ-preserving regimens (82).

As expected, concomitant regimens are associated with increased toxicity compared with sequential chemoradiation. Patients should be followed closely for dehydration, electrolyte abnormalities, and adequacy of nutritional intake. Most centers place enteral feeding tubes prophylactically prior to the start of treatment for patients undergoing concomitant chemoradiation because the incidence of grade 3 or greater mucositis is 70% to 80%.

Adjuvant Chemotherapy

A large randomized study in resected patients with stage III or IV disease compared adjuvant radiation therapy with adjuvant chemotherapy followed by radiation. This trial showed improved local control and overall survival rates approaching statistical significance for a subset of patients treated with chemotherapy who were at high risk for local recurrence. Patients with low-risk disease (negative resection margins, one or no positive nodes, and no extracapsular spread of tumor) did not benefit from adjuvant chemotherapy (83).

Adjuvant concomitant cisplatin and radiation in patients at high risk for recurrence after surgery has been studied both in Europe and in the United States. Both studies found a possible benefit in disease-free or overall survival for patients receiving concomitant cisplatin and radiation (84,85).

SITE-SPECIFIC HEAD AND NECK TUMORS

Oral Cavity

The oral cavity includes the lip, anterior two thirds of the tongue, floor of the mouth, buccal mucosa, gingiva, hard palate, and retromolar trigone. Approximately 20,000 new cases are diagnosed annually in the United States. Squamous cell carcinoma is the histologic type observed in most cases.

The epidemiology, natural history, common presenting symptoms, risk of nodal involvement, and prognosis for specific subsites are shown in Table 1.4. Early lesions (stages I and II) are treated with surgery or radiation therapy as single-modality therapy. For resectable locally advanced disease (stages III and IV, and M0), surgery followed by radiation therapy is indicated (see Fig. 1.4). Definitive radiation therapy with or without chemotherapy is an option for patients with resectable disease at any stage who have high medical or surgical risks, or according to patient preference (based on discussions about quality of life, functional outcome, and toxicity profile of each treatment). Treatment for locally advanced and metastatic disease is discussed in subsequent text.

Oropharynx

The oropharynx includes the base of the tongue, tonsils, posterior pharyngeal wall, and the soft palate.

The epidemiology, natural history, common presenting symptoms, risk of nodal involvement, and prognosis for specific subsites of the oropharynx are shown in Table 1.5. Treatment may include primary surgery and postoperative radiotherapy or primary radiation therapy, with chemotherapy if stage III or IV, thereby reserving surgery for management of regional node metastases or for salvage of persistent disease. Chemoradiation is an acceptable standard of care for treating locally advanced oropharyngeal cancer when organ preservation is desired. Randomized trials show that concurrent chemotherapy and radiotherapy significantly improve locoregional control and survival compared with radiotherapy (86). Increased complexity and toxicity of this combined-modality approach mandates that the patient has adequate performance status and psychosocial resources.

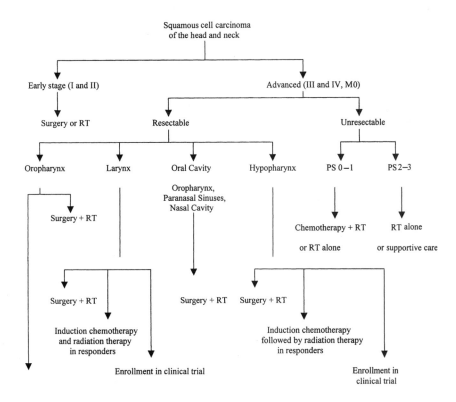

FIG. 1.4. Treatment for head and neck squamous cell carcinomas (M0).

Larynx

More than 9,500 cases of laryngeal cancer were diagnosed in the United States in 2003. Risk factors are a history of tobacco and/or alcohol intake. In addition, certain dietary factors and exposure to wood dust, nitrogen mustard, asbestos, and nickel have been implicated as etiologic factors. The male-to-female ratio for laryngeal cancer is 4.5:1, with a peak incidence in the sixth decade of life. This disease is 50% more common in African Americans than in whites and 100% more common in whites than in Hispanics and Asians. More than 95% of laryngeal cancers are squamous cell carcinomas.

Laryngeal cancers can be supraglottic, glottic, and/or subglottic. The epidemiology, natural history, common presenting symptoms, risk of nodal involvement, and prognosis for specific subsites of the larynx are shown in Table 1.5.

Early cancers not requiring laryngectomy (T1–T2 N0) are usually treated with radiation. If lymph nodes are involved, neck dissection and/or neck radiation is indicated. Locally advanced resectable tumors (T3–T4 or T2 N+) may be treated with surgery and adjuvant radiation if locoregional risk factors are present (i.e., close or positive margins, T4 tumor, lymphatic or vascular or perineural involvement, vascular invasion, multiple positive nodes, extracapsular invasion, subglottic extension, or prior tracheostomy). An alternative is the use of combined radiation and chemotherapy. In 1991, the Veterans Administration Laryngeal Study Group trial established (64) that sequential chemotherapy with cisplatin and infusional 5-FU followed by radiation therapy in highly responsive patients resulted in equivalent survival and a larynx preservation rate of about 66% compared to treatment with surgery followed by radiation. However, high volume T4 disease (with destruction of larynx or massive extension of supraglottic laryngeal cancer to the base of tongue) should be treated with surgery followed by radiation therapy rather than by organ preservation therapy, if possible.

A subsequent randomized phase III trial conducted in the United States comparing radiation therapy alone, sequential chemotherapy and radiation therapy, and concomitant cisplatin and radiation therapy for organ preservation in patients with locally advanced laryngeal cancer demonstrated that concurrent cisplatin (100 mg per m^2 on days 1, 22, and 43) and radiation therapy resulted in better laryngectomy-free survival, larynx preservation rate, and local–regional control rate than either sequential (induction) cisplatin and 5-FU followed by radiation therapy or radiation therapy alone. Induction chemotherapy followed by radiotherapy was shown to have no advantage over radiotherapy alone. Survival rate was not significantly different for the three treatments, in part reflecting the ability to surgically salvage laryngeal cancer patients treated for organ preservation. It is of interest to note that patients who received any chemotherapy regardless of receiving radiotherapy or not had a lower metastatic rate at 2 years than did patients who received radiation alone (66).

Speech rehabilitation is critically important for patients with advanced laryngeal cancer who are undergoing total laryngectomy. Phonation options include a mechanical electrolarynx, esophageal speech, and tracheoesophageal puncture. Most patients can obtain satisfactory communication through one of these techniques.

Patients whose lesions are unresectable or patients who are considered to have high surgical risks are candidates for definitive radiation therapy with chemotherapy if performance status is good. The treatment for a patient with metastatic disease is discussed later.

Hypopharynx

The epidemiology, natural history, common presenting symptoms, risk of nodal involvement, and prognosis for specific subsites of the hypopharynx are shown in Table 1.6.

Early cancers not requiring laryngectomy (most T1 N0–N1; small T2 N0) can be treated with surgery or radiation. Locally advanced resectable tumors (T3–T4 any N) may be treated with surgery followed by radiation or sequential or concomitant chemoradiation. In these cases, surgery involves total laryngectomy and partial or total pharyngectomy and neck dissection.

Even with this radical surgery and the consequent functional impairment of the tumor, the survival prognosis is poor.

Combined-modality treatment with chemotherapy and radiation allows organ function preservation with chances of survival being equivalent to that after surgery. Patients who achieve a CR at the primary site after two to three cycles of induction chemotherapy (Table 1.6) receive definitive radiation, whereas those achieving less than CR at the primary site undergo surgery. A large randomized trial is in progress comparing induction chemotherapy followed by radiation therapy to concomitant chemoradiation in patients with hypopharyngeal cancer. The outcome of this trial will provide more definitive information on the most efficacious therapy.

Patients who are prone to high surgical or medical risks can be treated with radiation. The management of metastatic disease is discussed later.

Nasal Cavity and Paranasal Sinuses

The epidemiology, natural history, common presenting symptoms, risk of nodal involvement, and prognosis for carcinomas of the nasal cavity and paranasal sinuses are shown in Table 1.6.

Most tumors are squamous cell carcinomas and are usually slow growing with low incidence of metastasis.

Carcinomas of the nasal cavity and paranasal sinuses are usually detected in patients in advanced stages because of the relatively silent tumor location. Treatment follows the same general guidelines as those for oral cancer. If feasible, surgery is the preferred primary management.

Nasopharynx

The epidemiology, natural history, common presenting symptoms, risk of nodal involvement, and prognosis for nasopharyngeal cancer are shown in Table 1.6. It is extremely rare in most parts of the world, with an incidence of less than 1 case per 100,000 population. However, it is endemic in certain areas, including North Africa, Southeast Asia, China, and the far northern hemisphere. EBV is strongly associated with nasopharyngeal carcinoma. This association has been demonstrated by serologic studies and by the detection of the viral genome in tumor samples. Diet (salt-cured fish and meat) and genetic susceptibility are other probable risk factors; tobacco and alcohol are not risk factors, except in a minority of cases.

The World Health Organization (WHO) classification divides nasopharyngeal carcinoma into three types: type I, keratinizing squamous cell carcinoma; type II, nonkeratinizing squamous cell carcinoma; and type III, undifferentiated carcinoma (20). Type II, the most common, is also sometimes referred to as *lymphoepithelioma* because of the characteristic exuberant lymphoid infiltrate accompanying malignant epithelial cells.

The most common initial presentation is a neck mass. Other presenting signs and symptoms are related to tumor growth, with resulting compression or infiltration of neighboring organs. These include serous otitis media, nasal obstruction, tinnitus, pain, and involvement of one or multiple cranial nerves.

Nasopharyngeal carcinoma has a high metastatic potential to regional nodes and distant sites. WHO type I has the greatest propensity for uncontrolled local tumor growth and the lowest propensity for metastatic spread (60% clinically positive nodes) compared with WHO type II and type III cancers (80% to 90% clinically positive nodes). Even though type I WHO cancer is associated with a lower incidence of lymphatic and distant metastases than are types II and III, its prognosis is worse because of a higher incidence of deaths from uncontrolled primary tumors and nodal metastases.

The prognoses for different stages of nasopharyngeal carcinoma are shown in Table 1.6.

General treatment guidelines are shown in Fig. 1.5. Surgery is usually not recommended because of anatomic considerations and the pattern of spread of the cancer via the retropharyngeal lymphatics. Radiation has been the standard treatment, with good results (local control

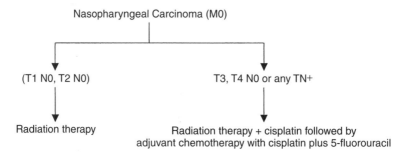

FIG. 1.5. Treatment of nasopharyngeal carcinoma (M0).

rates: T1–T2, 70% to 90%; T3–T4, 30% to 65%), and remains the standard of care for early (stages I and II) cancer.

In a randomized trial in the United States, concurrent cisplatin (cisplatin 100 mg per m^2 every 21 to 28 days) and daily radiation followed by three courses of adjuvant cisplatin and 5-FU was shown to improve overall survival (76% for concurrent chemoradiation versus 46% for radiation therapy alone) (87). On the basis of this study, concurrent chemoradiation followed by adjuvant chemotherapy is considered standard treatment for locally advanced nonmetastatic (stages III and IV) nasopharyngeal cancer in the United States. Other drugs, such as taxanes, appear to have activity but have not been evaluated extensively.

ADVANCED HEAD AND NECK TUMORS: UNRESECTABLE, RECURRENT, AND METASTATIC DISEASE

In patients with good performance status (ECOG 0-1), concurrent radiation and chemotherapy is considered standard treatment for patients with newly diagnosed locally advanced unresectable disease. In several recent trials, chemoradiation therapy was shown to improve the overall survival, disease-free survival, and/or local control when compared with radiation therapy alone. Several cisplatin- or carboplatin-containing regimens and several standard and altered fractionation-radiation regimens have been evaluated. In patients with poor performance status, radiation alone is a reasonable option.

Local or regional recurrences can sometimes be salvaged by radiation therapy or surgery. In patients unable to undergo resection, re-irradiation with a dose of 60 cGy with or without concomitant chemotherapy can achieve prolonged survivals in about 15% to 20% of highly selected patients (88). In nasopharyngeal carcinoma, a second course of radiation may be delivered. If salvage is not possible, palliative treatment will be guided by the performance status of the patient.

Single-agent or combination chemotherapy is indicated for palliation of patients with good performance status with local or distant recurrence and of those patients presenting with distant metastasis. Combination chemotherapy achieves higher response rates at the cost of increased toxicity when compared with single-agent chemotherapy. The most active agents are listed in Table 1.7. Cisplatin plus infusional 5-FU (Table 1.8) or cisplatin with a taxane are the most commonly used combination-chemotherapy regimens. Weekly methotrexate or taxanes have also shown some activity in patients with advanced head and neck tumors. Oral agents, such as gefitinib (Iressa) may have some palliative effect (30–32,50). The choice of single-agent or combination chemotherapy (61) depends on preference and performance status of patients. Patients with good performance status, no prior chemotherapy for treatment of recurrent disease, and minimal tumor burden may benefit most from combination chemotherapy. A small subset of these patients may achieve durable CR and prolonged survival. However, the median response duration to combination or single-agent chemotherapy is about 3 months.

The median survival for patients with locally recurrent or disseminated disease is 6 to 9 months, and only 20% to 30% are alive at 1 year. No therapy has been shown to affect survival rate. Therefore, whenever possible, patients should be encouraged to enroll in clinical trials that evaluate new agents or new combination regimens.

Cancer of Unknown Primary Site (of the Head and Neck)

The work-up of a patient with a neck mass is shown in Fig. 1.3. In 10% of cases, a primary tumor is not found, and the term "cancer of unknown primary site" is used.

Cervical lymph node involvement (except supraclavicular) by carcinoma indicates a head and neck primary tumor. Unknown primary tumors of the head and neck are usually treated with neck dissection and radiation. The prognosis is roughly equivalent to cancers with the same N (nodal) status. Five-year survival ranges from 30% to 50% in patients treated definitively.

A supraclavicular mass often represents spread from an infraclavicular (thoracic or abdominal) cancer, and the work-up and treatment of these cancers is beyond the scope of this chapter.

Salivary Gland Cancer

Salivary gland cancers make up about 3% of all head and neck cancers diagnosed in the United States yearly. Tobacco and alcohol consumption are not risk factors, except possibly in women. Ionizing radiation and certain occupational exposures (e.g., in workers in rubber and automotive industries, wood workers, and farm workers) have been associated with the development of salivary gland cancer.

The salivary glands are classified as major (parotid, submandibular, and sublingual) and minor (distributed along upper aerodigestive tract, predominantly in the oral and nasal cavities and the paranasal sinuses). Most of the salivary gland cancers arise from the parotid glands; sublingual and minor salivary gland cancers are rare.

Most salivary gland tumors are benign, and the most common histology is pleomorphic adenoma, which is characterized by slow growth and few symptoms, and is most frequently seen in the parotid gland. The most common presentation of benign salivary gland tumors is asymptomatic swelling of the lip, the parotid, or the submandibular or the sublingual glands. Persistent pain or neurologic involvement (mucosal or tongue numbness and facial nerve weakness) suggests malignant disease. The benign salivary gland tumors are listed in Table 1.9.

The clinical characteristics and prognosis of specific malignant salivary gland tumors are shown in Table 1.10.

Surgery is the mainstay of treatment for all localized stages of salivary gland tumors. Postoperative radiation is indicated for localized tumors of high-grade histology, that are large, with close or positive margins, and/or positive regional lymph nodes. Radiation is the primary treatment for unresectable tumors. The role of chemotherapy is limited to the management of locally recurrent, unresectable disease or distant metastatic disease. There is no established standard chemotherapy for salivary gland cancer. Regimens employing cisplatin, carboplatin, anthracyclines, taxanes, cyclophosphamide, and 5-FU result in transient responses in 14% to

TABLE 1.9. *Salivary gland benign tumors*

Pleomorphic adenoma (benign mixed tumor)
Warthin tumor (papillary cystadenoma lymphomatosum)
Monomorphic adenoma
Benign lymphoepithelial lesion
Oncocytoma
Ductal papilloma
Sebaceous lymphadenoma

TABLE 1.10. *Salivary gland malignant tumors: clinical characteristics and prognosis*

Histology	Clinical characteristics	Prognosis
Mucoepidermoid carcinoma	Most common malignant tumor in major salivary glands. Most common in parotid glands (32%) Low grade: Local problems, long history, cure with aggressive resection. Rarely metastasizes High grade: locally aggressive, invades nerves and vessels, and metastasizes early	Low grade: 76%–95% 5-yr survival High grade: 30%–50% 5-yr survival
Adenocarcinoma	16% of parotid and 9% of submandibular malignant tumors Grade correlates with survival	76%–85% 5-yr survival 34%–71% 10-yr survival
Squamous cell carcinoma	Uncommon: 7% of parotid gland and 10% of submandibular gland malignant tumors Grade correlates with survival Squamous cell carcinoma of temple, auricular, and facial skin can metastasize to parotid nodes and can be confused with primary parotid tumor	24% 5-yr survival 18% 10-yr survival
Acinic cell carcinoma	<10% of all salivary gland malignant tumors Low grade with slow growth, infrequent facial nerve involvement, infrequent and late metastases (lungs) Regional metastasis in 5%–10% of patients	82% 5-yr survival 68% 10-yr survival
Adenoid cystic carcinoma	Most common malignant tumor in submandibular gland (41%), 11% of parotid gland High incidence of nerve invasion, which compromises local control 40% of patients develop metastases. Most common site of metastases is the lung. Patients may live many years with lung metastasis, but visceral or bone metastases indicate poor prognosis	50%–90% 10 yr survival: 30%–67% 15 yr survival: 25%
Malignant mixed tumor	14% of parotid gland and 12% of submandibular gland cancers May originate in previous pleomorphic adenoma Lymph node involvement in 25% of cases 26%–32% of patients develop metastases	31%–65% 10 yr; 23%–30%

30% of patients with adenocarcinoma or mucoepidermoid carcinoma (89), but the effect on survival is unknown. Patients with good performance status should be encouraged to enter clinical trials.

Follow-up

Curative treatment of patients with head and neck cancer should be followed by a comprehensive head and neck physical examination every 1 to 3 months during the first year after treatment, every 2 to 4 months during the second year, every 3 to 6 months from years 3 to 5, and every 6 to 12 months after year 5. The thyroid-stimulating hormone (TSH) level should be checked every 3 to 6 months if the thyroid is irradiated. Generally, thyroid hormone replacement therapy should begin when, and if, TSH remains stably elevated, before symptoms of hypothyroidism appear. Up to 50% of patients will develop hypothyroidism by 5 years after radiation therapy to the head and neck. Patients with nasopharyngeal tumors who were treated with radiation are at risk for pituitary failure (90,91).

The highest risk of relapse is during the first 3 years after treatment. After 3 years, a second primary tumor in the lung or head and neck is the most important cause of morbidity or mortality. Because of this risk, a semiannual chest radiograph is recommended. Some recurrences, as well as second primaries, can be treated with curative intent.

OTHER HEAD AND NECK TUMORS

Sarcoma

Soft tissue sarcomas of the head and neck are relatively rare. Of head and neck sarcomas, 80% are seen in adults and 20% are in children. These tumors are heterogeneous and can present in any head and neck site, commonly as a submucosal or subcutaneous painless mass. In the hypopharynx and nasopharynx, the presenting symptoms may be cranial nerve abnormalities or airway or swallowing difficulties. As in sarcomas at other sites, grade is an important prognostic indicator. High-grade, aggressive tumors such as malignant fibrous histiocytoma, angiosarcoma, osteogenic sarcoma, neurofibrosarcoma, and soft part sarcomas tend to be locally aggressive and spread along neurovascular structures, fascia, and bone. In addition to aggressive local behavior, there is a high risk for metastatic disease, particularly in lung, bone, central nervous system, and liver. Metastatic disease may occur without local lymph node involvement. Sarcomas may arise after radiation therapy, but this is very uncommon in the head and neck region. The prognosis for these secondary sarcomas may be worse than for primary sarcomas.

Treatment depends on stage, age of the patient, tumor type, location, and size. Wide margin *en bloc* resection is the goal, but may not be possible because of the proximity of vital structures. Adjuvant postoperative radiation and/or brachytherapy can improve local control in aggressive sarcomas. The major indications for adjuvant radiation are high-grade sarcomas or positive margins, lesions greater than 5 cm, and recurrent sarcoma. Elective neck radiation is not necessary because the incidence of occult positive lymph nodes is low. Soft tissue and possibly osteogenic sarcomas may benefit from adjuvant or neoadjuvant chemoradiation. Such patients should be referred to clinical trials when possible. Overall survival rate approaches 60% for patients with sarcomas of the head and neck (92,93).

Melanoma

Mucosal melanomas represent less than 1.5% of all melanomas. About 50% of mucosal melanomas occur in the head and neck, and more than 20% of melanomas that occur in the head and neck region are mucosal. The age of diagnosis is 60 to 80 years. The hard palate is the most common site. Nearly one-third of these tumors are amelanotic. The proportion of mucosal melanomas is higher in African American and Hispanic populations than in white populations. Although rare in the United States, mucosal melanomas are more frequent in Japan and in some parts of Africa. Mucosal melanomas may be multiple, may have satellite lesions, may invade angiolymphatics, and can metastasize. They behave more aggressively than skin melanomas. Lymph node metastasis is observed at presentation in up to 48% of patients. Surgery is the mainstay of treatment for local or locoregional disease. Prophylactic lymph node dissection is not recommended. Radiation, when used, is usually employed adjuvantly for positive margins or used palliatively for local recurrence or unresectability. Adjuvant use of radiation has not been shown to improve survival. Prophylactic nodal radiation is not recommended. Chemotherapy and immunotherapy have been studied, but the effect of these interventions on survival when used as palliation or as adjuvant therapy has not been defined. Patients should be encouraged to enter clinical trials where available. Mean overall 5-year survival is 17% (range 0% to 48%) (94).

REFERENCES

1. Jemal A, Murray T, Samuels A, et al. Cancer Statistics, 2003. *CA Cancer J Clin* 2003;53:5–26.
2. Rodu B, Jansson C. Smokeless Tobacco and Oral cancer: a review of the risk and determinants. 2004 *Crit Rev Oral Bio Med* 15(5);252–263.
3. Norton SA. Betel: consumption and consequences. *J Am Acad Dermatol* 1998;38(1):81–88.
4. Sankaranarayanan R, Duffy SW, Day NE, et al. A case-control investigation of cancer of the oral tongue and the floor of the mouth in Southern India. *Int J Cancer* 1989;44(4):617–621.
5. Slaughter DL, Southwick HW, Smejkal W. Field cancerization in oral stratified squamous epithelium: clinical implications of multicentric origin. *Cancer* 1953;6:963–968.
6. Schwartz LH, Ozsahin M, Xhang GN, et al. Synchronous and metachronous head and neck carcinomas. *Cancer* 1994;74:1933–1938.
7. Laccourreye O, Veivers FD, Hans S et al. Metachronous second primary cancers after successful partial laryngectomy for invasive squamous cell carcinoma of the true vocal cord. *Ann Otol Rhino Laryngol* 2002;111:204–209.
8. Cooper JS, Pajak TF, Rubin P, et al. Second malignancies in patients who have head and neck cancer: incidence, effect on survival and implications based on the RTOG experience. *Int J Radiat Oncol Biol Phys* 1989;17:449–456.
9. Niedobitek G. Epstein-Barr virus infection in the pathogenesis of nasopharyngeal carcinoma. *J Clin Pathol: Mol Pathol* 2000;53:248–254.
10. Mellin H, Friesland S, Lewensohn R, et al. Human papillomavirus (HPV) DNA in tonsillar cancer: clinical correlates, risk of relapse, and survival. *Int J Cancer (Pred Oncol)* 2000;89:300–304.
11. McKaig RG, Baric RS, Olshan AF. Human papillomavirus and head and neck cancer: epidemiology and molecular biology. *Head & Neck* 1998;20:250–265.
12. Gillison ML, Koch WM, Capone RB, et al. Evidence for a causal association between human papillomavirus and a subset of head and neck cancers. *J Natl Cancer Inst* 2000;92:709–720.
13. Hong WK, Lippman SM, Hittelman WN, et al. Retinoid chemoprevention of aerodigestive cancer: from basic research to the clinic. *Clin Cancer Res* 1995;1:677–686.
14. Khuri F, Lee JJ, Lippman SM, et al. Isotretinoin effects on head and neck cancer recurrence and second primary tumors. *Proc Am Soc Clin Oncol* 2003;22:90a.
15. van Zandwijk N, Dalesio O, Pastorino U, et al. EUROSCAN, a randomized trial of vitamin A and N-acetylcysteine in patients with head and neck cancer or lung cancer. *J Natl Cancer Inst* 2000;92:977–986.
16. Omenn GS, Goodman GE, Thornquist MD, et al. Risk factors for lung cancer and for intervention effects in CARET, the BETA-CAROTENE and Retinol Efficacy Trial. *J Natl Cancer Inst* 1996; 88(21):1550–1559.
17. The Alpha-Tocopherol, Beta Carotene Cancer Prevention Study Group. The effect of vitamin E and beta carotene on the incidence of lung cancer and other cancers in male smokers. *N Engl J Med* 1994;330:1029–1035.
18. Albanes D, Heinonen OP, Taylor PR, et al. Alpha tocopherol and beta carotene supplements and lung cancer incidence in the alpha tocopherol, beta carotene cancer prevention study: effects of base-line characteristics and study compliance. *J Natl Cancer Inst* 1996;88(21):1560–1570.
19. Lippman SM, Lee JJ, Karp DD, et al. Randomized phase III intergroup trial of isotretinoin to prevent second primary tumors in stage I non-small cell lung cancer. *J Natl Cancer Inst* 2001;93(8):605–618.
20. Greene FL, Page DL, Fleming, ID, et al. *AJCC Cancer Staging Manual*, 6th ed. New York: Springer-Verlag, 2002.
21. Schechter NR, Gillenwater AM, Byers RM, et al. Can positron emission tomography improve the quality of care for head-and-neck cancer patients? *Int J Radiat Oncol Biol Phys* 2001;51(1):4–9.
22. Wong RJ, Lin DT, Schoder H, et al. Diagnostic and prognostic value of [^{18}F]fluorodeoxyglucose positron emission tomography for recurrent head and neck squamous cell carcinoma. *J Clin Oncol* 2002;20:4199–4208.
23. Cooper JS, Pajak TF, Forastiere A, et al. Precisely defining high-risk operable head and neck tumors based on RTOG #85-03 and #88-24: targets for postoperative radiochemotherapy? *Head Neck* 1998; 20:588–594.

24. Dische S, Saunders M, Barrett A, et al. A randomised multicentre trial of CHART versus conventional radiotherapy in head and neck cancer. *Radiother Oncol* 1997;44:123–136.
25. Fu KK, Pajak TF, Trotti A et al, RTOG. A Radiation Therapy Oncology Group (RTOG). Phase III randomized study to compare hyperfractionation and two variants of accelerated fractionation to standard fractionation radiotherapy for head and neck squamous cell carcinomas: first report of RTOG 9003. *Int J Radiat Oncol Biol Phys* 2000;48(1):7–16.
26. Amdur RJ, Parsons JT, Mendenhall WM, et al. Split-course versus continuous course irradiation in the postoperative setting for squamous cell carcinoma of the head and neck. *Int J Radiat Oncol Biol Phys* 1989;17(2):279–285.
27. Marcial VA, Amato DA, Pajak TF. Patterns of failure after treatment for cancer of upper respiratory and digestive tracts: a Radiation Therapy Oncology Group Report. *Cancer Treat Symp* 1983;2:33–40.
28. Vissink A, Burlage FR, Spijkervet FKL, et al. Prevention and treatment of the consequences of head and neck radiotherapy. *Crit Rev Oral Biol Med* 2003;14(3):213–225.
29. Brizel DM, Wasserman TH, Henke M, et al. Phase III randomized trial of amifostine as a radioprotector in head and neck cancer. *J Clin Oncol* 2000;18(19):3339–3345.
30. Hong WK, Schaefer S, Issell B, et al. Prospective randomized trial of methotrexate versus cisplatin in the treatment of recurrent squamous cell carcinoma of the head and neck. *Cancer* 1983; 52:206–210.
31. Schornagel JH, Verweij J, deMulder PHM, et al. Randomized phase III trial of edatrexate versus methotrexate in patients with metastatic and/or recurrent squamous cell carcinoma of the head and neck: A European Organization for Research and Treatment of Cancer Head and Neck Cancer Cooperative Group Study. *J Clin Oncol* 1995;13(7):1649–1655.
32. Grose WE, Lehane DE, Dixon DO, et al. Comparison of methotrexate and cisplatin for patients with advanced squamous cell carcinoma of the head and neck region : a Southwest Oncology Group Study. *Cancer Treat Rep* 1985;69(6):577–581.
33. Eisenberger M, Hornedo J, Silva H, et al. Carboplatin (NSC 241240): an active platinum analog for the treatment of squamous cell carcinoma of the head and neck. *J Clin Oncol* 1986;4(10):1506–1509.
34. Al Sarraf M, Metch B, Kish J, et al. Platinum analogs in recurrent and advanced head and neck cancer: a Southwest Oncology Group and Wayne State University Study. *Cancer Treat Rep* 1987;71(7-8): 723–726.
35. Degardin M, Cappelaere P, Krakowski I, et al. Phase II trial of oxaliplatin (L-OHP) in advanced, recurrent and/or metastatic squamous cell carcinoma of the head and neck. *Oral Oncol Eur J Cancer* 1996;32B(4):278–279.
36. Tapazoglou E, Kish J, Ensley J, et al. The activity of single-agent 5-fluorouracil infusion in advanced and recurrent head and neck cancer. *Cancer* 1986;57:1105–1109.
37. Colevas AD, Amrein PC, Gomolin H, et al. A phase II study of combined oral uracil and ftorafur with leucovorin for patients with squamous cell carcinoma of the head and neck. *Cancer* 2001; 92:326–331.
38. Tanaka J, Inuyama Y, fujii M, et al. Clinical Trials on UFT I the treatment of head and neck cancer. *Auris Nasus Larynx* 1985;12(Suppl. 2):S261–S266.
39. Smith RE, Thornton DE, Allen J. A phase II trial of paclitaxel in squamous cell carcinoma of the head and neck with correlative laboratory studies. *Semin Oncol* 1995;22(3 Suppl. 6):41–46.
40. Forastiere AA, Shank D, Neuberg D, et al. Final report of a phase II evaluation of paclitaxel in patients with advanced squamous cell carcinoma of the head and neck: an Eastern Cooperative Oncology Group Trial. *Cancer* 1998;82:2270–2274.
41. Numicot G, Merlano M. Second line treatment with docetaxel after failure of a platinum-based chemotherapy in squamous-cell head and neck cancer. *Ann Oncol* 2002;13:331–333.
42. Dreyfuss AI, Clark JR, Norris CM, et al. Docetaxel: an active drug for squamous cell carcinoma of the head and neck. *J Clin Oncol* 1996;14(5):1672–1678.
43. Briasoulis E, Karavasilis V, Anastasopoulos D, et al. Weekly docetaxel in minimally pretreated cancer patients: a dose-escalation study focused on feasibility and cumulative toxicity of long-term administration. *Ann Oncol* 1999;10:701–706.
44. Catimel G, Verweij J, Mattijssen V, et al. Docetaxel (Taxotere^R), an active drug for the treatment of patients with advanced squamous cell carcinoma of the head and neck. *Ann Oncol* 1994;5:533–537.
45. Pivot X, Raymond E, Laguerre B, et al. Pemetrexed disodium in recurrent locally advanced or metastatic squamous cell carcinoma of the head and neck. *Br J Cancer* 2001;85(5):649–655.
46. Murphy BA, Cmelak A, Burkey B, et al. The role of topoisomerases in head and neck cancer *Oncology (Huntington)* 2001;15(7 Suppl. 8):47–52.

47. Catimel G, Vermorken JB, Clavel M, et al. A Phase II study of Gemcitabine (LY 188011) in patients with advanced squamous cell carcinoma of the head and neck. *Ann Oncol* 1994;5:543–547.
48. Degardin M, Oliveira J, Geoffrois L, et al. An EORTC-ECSG phase II study of vinorelbine in patients with recurrent and/or metastatic squamous cell carcinoma of the head and neck. *Ann Oncol* 1998; 9:1103–1107.
49. Saxman S, Mann B, Canfield V, et al. A phase II trial of vinorelbine in patients with recurrent or metastatic squamous cell carcinoma of the head and neck. *Am J Clin Oncol* 1998;21(4):398–400.
50. Cohen EE, Rosen F, Stadler WM, et al. Phase II trial of ZD1839 in recurrent or metastatic squamous cell carcinoma of the head and neck. *J Clin Oncol* 2003;21(10):1980–1987.
51. Forastiere AA, Metch B, Schuller DE, et al. Randomized comparison of cisplatin plus fluorouracil and carboplatin plus fluorouracil versus methotrexate in advanced squamous cell carcinoma of the head and neck: a Southwest Oncology Group Study. *J Clin Oncol* 1992;10(8):1245–1251.
52. Gebbia V, Mantovani G, Agostara B, et al. Treatment of recurrent and/or metastatic squamous cell head and neck carcinoma with a combination of vinorelbine, cisplatin and 5-fluorouracil: a multi-center phase II trial. *Ann Oncol* 1995;6:987–991.
53. Murphy B, Li Y, Cella D, et al. Phase III study comparing cisplatin & 5 fluorouracil (F) versus cisplatin & paclitaxel in metastatic/recurrent head and neck cancer. *Proc Am Soc Clin Oncol* 2001;20:224a.
54. Shin DM, Khuri FR, Glisson BS, et al. Phase II study of paclitaxel, ifosfamide and carboplatin in patients with recurrent or metastatic head and neck squamous cell cancer. *Cancer* 2001;91:1316–1323.
55. Shin DM, Glisson BS, Khuri FR, et al. Phase II trial of paclitaxel, ifosfamide and cisplatin in patients with recurrent squamous cell carcinoma. *J Clin Oncol* 1998;16(4):1325–1330.
56. Hussain M, Gadgeel S, Kucuk O, et al. Paclitaxel, cisplatin and 5-fluorouracil for patients with advanced or recurrent squamous cell carcinoma of the head and neck. *Cancer* 1999;86:2364–2369.
57. Janinis J, Papadakou M, Zidakis E, et al. Combination chemotherapy with docetaxel, cisplatin and 5-fluorouracil in previously treated patients with advanced/recurrent head and neck cancer. *Am J Clin Oncol (CCT)* 2000;23(2):128–131.
58. Jacobs C, Lyman G, Velez-Garcia E, et al. A phase III randomized study comparing cisplatin and fluorouracil as single agents and in combination for advanced squamous cell carcinoma of the head and neck. *J Clin Oncol* 1992;10:257–263.
59. Forastiere AA. Overview of platinum chemotherapy in head and neck cancer. *Semin Oncol* 1994; 21(15 Suppl. 12):20–27.
60. Takimoto CH, Rowinsky EK. Dose-intense paclitaxel: Déjà vu all over again? *J Clin Oncol* 2003; 21(15):2810–2814.
61. Lamont EB, Vokes EE. Chemotherapy in the management of squamous-cell carcinoma of the head and neck. *The Lancet* 2001;2:261–269.
62. Browman GP, Cronin L. Standard chemotherapy in squamous cell head and neck cancer: what we have learned from randomized trials. *Semin Oncol* 1994;21:311–319.
63. Kish JA, Ensley JF, Jacobs J, et al. A randomized trial of cisplatin (CACP) + 5-fluorouracil (5-FU) infusion and CACP + 5-FU bolus for recurrent and advanced squamous cell carcinoma of the head and neck. *Cancer* 1985;56:2740–2744.
64. Department of Veterans Affairs Laryngeal Study Group. Induction chemotherapy plus radiation compared with advanced laryngeal cancer. *N Engl J Med* 1991;324:1685–1690.
65. Lefebvre JL, Chevalier D, Lubomski B, et al. Larynx preservation in hypopharynx and lateral epilarynx cancer: preliminary results of EORTC randomized phase III trial 24891. *J Natl Cancer Inst* 1996;88:890–899.
66. Forastiere AA, Goepfert H, Maor M, et al. Concurrent chemotherapy and radiotherapy for organ preservation in advanced laryngeal cancer. *N Engl J Med* 2003;349(22):2091–2098.
67. Dent P, Yacoub A, Contessa J, et al. Stress and radiation-induced activation of multiple intracellular signaling pathways. *Radiation Res* 2003;159:283–300.
68. Bourhis J, Pignon JP. Meta-analyses in head and neck squamous cell carcinoma: what is the role of chemotherapy? *Hematol Oncol Clin North Am* 1999;13(4):769–775.
69. El-Sayed S, Nelson N. Adjuvant and adjunctive chemotherapy in the management of squamous cell carcinoma of the head and neck region: a meta-analysis of prospective and randomized trials. *J Clin Oncol* 1996;14(3):838–847.
70. Pignon JP, Bourhis J, Domenge C, et al, on behalf of the MACH-NC Collaborative Group. Chemotherapy added to locoregional treatment for head and neck squamous-cell carcinoma: three meta-analyses of updated individual data. *The Lancet* 2000;355:949–955.
71. Adelstein DJ, Li Y, Adams GL, et al. An intergroup phase III comparison of standard radiation therapy and two schedules of concurrent chemoradiotherapy in patients with unresectable squamous cell head and neck cancer. *J Clin Oncol* 2003;21(1):92–98.

72. Taylor SG IV, Murthy AK, Vannetzel JM, et al. Comparison of neoadjuvant cisplatin and fluorouracil infusion followed by radiation versus concomitant treatment in advanced head and neck cancer. *J Clin Oncol* 1994:12(2):385–395.

73. Vokes EE, Stenson K, Rosen FR, et al. Weekly carboplatin and paclitaxel followed by concomitant paclitaxel, fluorouracil and hydroxyurea chemotherapy: curative and organ-preserving therapy for advanced head and neck cancer. *J Clin Oncol* 2003;21(2):320–326.

74. Garden AS, Harris J, Vokes EE, et al. Preliminary results of Radiation Therapy Oncology Group 97-03: a randomized phase II trial of concurrent radiation and chemotherapy for advanced squamous cell carcinomas of the head and neck. *J Clin Oncol* 2004;22(14):2856–2864.

75. Grandis JR, Melhem MF, Gooding WE, et al. Levels of TGF-alpha and EGFR protein in head and neck squamous cell carcinoma and patient survival. *J Natl Cancer Inst* 1998;90(11):824–832.

76. Ang KK, Berkey BA, Tu X, et al. Impact of epidermal growth factor receptor expression on survival and pattern of relapse in patients with advanced head and neck carcinoma. *Cancer Res* 2002; 62:7350–7356.

77. Dassonville O, Formento JL, Francoual M, et al. Expression of epidermal growth factor receptor and survival in upper aerodigestive tract cancer. *J Clin Oncol* 1993;10:1873–1878.

78. Schmidt-Ullrich RK, Valerie KC, Chan W, et al. Altered expression of epidermal growth factor receptor and estrogen receptor in MCF-7 cells after single and repeated radiation exposures. *Int J Radiat Oncol Biol Phys* 1994;29:813–819.

79. Huang SM, Harari PM. Modulation of radiation response after epidermal growth factor receptor blockade in squamous cell carcinomas: Inhibition of damage repair, cell cycle kinetics ad tumor angiogenesis. *Clin Cancer Res* 2000;6:2166–2174.

80. Burtness BA, Li Y, Flood W, et al. Phase III trial comparing cisplatin + placebo to cisplatin + anti-epidermal growth factor antibody (EGF-R)C225 in patients with metastatic/recurrent head and neck cancer. *Proc Am Soc Clin Oncol* 2002;21:226a.

81. Brizel DM, Albers ME, Fisher SR, et al. Hyperfractionated irradiation with or without concurrent chemotherapy for locally advanced head and neck cancer. *N Engl J Med* 1998;338:1798–1814.

82. Weber RS, Berkey MS, Forastiere A, et al. Outcome of salvage total laryngectomy following organ preservation therapy. *Arch Otolaryngol Head Neck Surg* 2003;129:44–49.

83. Laramore G, Scott C, Al-Sarraf M, et al. Adjuvant chemotherapy for resectable squamous cell carcinomas of the head and neck: report on intergroup study 0034. *Int J Radiat Oncol Biol Phys* 1992; 23:705–713.

84. Cooper JS, Pajak TJ, Forastiere AA, et al. Postoperative concurrent radiotherapy and chemotherapy for high risk squamous-cell carcinoma of the head and neck. *New Engl J Med* 2004; 350; 19: 1973–1944.

85. Bernier J, Domenge C, Ozsahin M, et al. Postoperative irradiation with or without concomitant chemotheraphy for locally advanced head and neck cancer. *New Engl J Med.* 2004; 350,19: 1945–52.

86. Calais G, Alfonsi M, Bardet E, et al. Randomized trial of radiation therapy versus concomitant chemotherapy and radiation therapy for advanced-stage oropharynx carcinoma. *J Natl Cancer Inst* 1999;91(24):2081–2086.

87. Al Sarraf M, LeBlanc M, Giri PGS, et al. Chemoradiotherapy versus radiotherapy in patients with advanced nasopharyngeal cancer: phase III randomized intergroup study 0099. *J Clin Oncol* 1998; 16(4):1310–1317.

88. Kao J, Garofalo MC, Milano MT, et al. Reirradiation of recurrent and second primary head and neck malignancies: a comprehensive review. *Cancer Treat Rev* 2003;29:21–30.

89. Forastiere A, Licitra L, Grandi C, et al. Major and minor salivary glands tumors. *Crit Rev Oncol Hematol* 2003;45:215–225.

90. Mercado G, Adelstein DJ, Saxton JP, et al. Hypothyroidism: a frequent event after radiotherapy and after radiotherapy with chemotherapy for patients with head and neck carcinoma. *Cancer* 2001; 92:2892–2897.

91. Colevas AD, Read R, Thornhill J, et al. Hypothyroidism incidence after multimodality treatment for stage III and IV squamous cell carcinomas of the head and neck. *Int J Radiat Oncol Biol Phys* 2001; 51(3):599–604.

92. Pellitteri PK, Ferlito A, Bradley PJ, et al. Management of sarcomas of the head and neck in adults. *Oral Oncol* 2003;39:2–12.

93. Patel SG, Meyers P, Huvos AG, et al. Improved outcomes in patients with osteogenic sarcoma of the head and neck. *Cancer* 2002;95:1495–1503.

94. Lengyel E, Gilde K, Remenar E, et al. Malignant mucosal melanoma of the head and neck – a review. *Pathol Oncol Res* 2003;9(1):7–12.

SECTION 2

Thorax

2

Non–Small Cell Lung Cancer

Anne M. Horgan and Oscar S. Breathnach

Department of Medicine, Cork University Hospital, Cork, Ireland

Primary carcinoma of the lung was an uncommon cancer until the 1930s. Since then, there has been a dramatic increase in the incidence of lung cancer that has not yet abated. Lung cancer is now the most common cause of cancer mortality in both men and women, having surpassed breast cancer as the leading cause of cancer deaths in women in the mid-1980s.

- In 2003, approximately 171,900 new cases were expected, with 157,200 resultant deaths.
- Only 13% of all patients with lung cancer are expected to live for 5 years.
- Survival rates have been stationary over the last two decades despite new therapeutic agents.
- The long period between the initial exposure to tobacco carcinogens and the development of clinical lung cancer suggests that multiple steps are required to express the malignant phenotype.
- Prevention of smoking will have the greatest impact on curbing lung cancer and on ensuring prolonged survival.

RISK FACTORS

- **Smoking:** As many as 90% of patients with lung cancer have a history of smoking. The epidemic of lung cancer in the 21st century reflects the birth cohort patterns of active cigarette smoking. However, among the general population of individuals as old as 74 years of age, the cumulative probability of developing lung cancer in those who smoke one or more packs of cigarettes per day is 10% to 15%. Ninety percent of regular smokers aged 30 to 39 years would have smoked their first cigarette before the age of 18, and 70% of them would have been regular smokers by 18 years. Almost none of the regular smokers would have started after the age of 20. Recent evidence suggests that children and young adults are more prone to DNA damage from smoke exposure than older adults are.

  The risk of lung cancer after smoking cessation appears to be related to the level of consumption. The risk in persons who had smoked 1 to 20 cigarettes per day falls by 1.6-fold after 16 years of smoking cessation. In those persons who had smoked 21 or more cigarettes per day, the risk of developing lung cancer after 16 years of smoking cessation remains four times greater than that of a person who has never smoked. Of concern is the fact that almost 50% of all high school children in the United States use some form of tobacco. National cigarette smoking rates for high school children have recently risen by 32% (from 1991 to 1997), with little change in the prevalence of smoking among adults (47 million people). New adolescent smokers are replacing those smokers who have died from cancer or other smoking-related causes, and those who have quit. These trends, if left unchecked, will increase the future occurrences of lung cancer.

35

According to the U.S. Environmental Protection Agency (EPA), approximately 3,000 nonsmoking adults die from lung cancer each year because of breathing the smoke of others' cigarettes. Analysis shows that sidestream smoke emitted from a smoldering cigarette between puffs contains virtually all the carcinogenic compounds that have been identified in the mainstream smoke that is inhaled by smokers. The risk of dying from lung cancer is 30% higher for a nonsmoker living with a smoker compared to a nonsmoker living with a nonsmoker.

- **Occupational:** Exposure to agents such as arsenic, asbestos, beryllium, chloromethylethers, chromium, hydrocarbons, mustard gas, nickel, and radiation (including radon) have been linked to the development of lung cancer. Asbestos exposure in smokers is associated with a synergistic risk for developing bronchogenic carcinoma. Radon exposure in underground mines with poor ventilation is associated with an increased risk for developing lung cancer.
- **Residential:** There is no conclusive evidence to state that residential radon exposure significantly contributes to lung cancer, although inferences from the studies on occupational exposure would suggest such a link. Case–control studies have yielded conflicting reports. The exact risk of indoor exposure to radon remains uncertain.

TABLE 2.1. *Suggested therapeutic chemotherapy regimens*

Regimen	Dose	Cycle duration
Carboplatin–Paclitaxel		
Carboplatin	AUC 5 i.v. d 1	q21d
Paclitaxel	175–225 mg/m^2 i.v. d 1	
Carboplatin–Docetaxel		
Carboplatin	AUC 5 i.v. d 1	q21d
Docetaxel	75 mg/m^2 i.v. d 1	
Gemcitabine–Carboplatin		
Gemcitabine	1,000 mg/m^2 i.v. d 1, 8	q21d
Carboplatin	AUC 5 i.v. d 1 only	
Vinorelbine–Cisplatin		
Vinorelbine	30 mg/m^2 i.v. d 1, 8	q21d
Cisplatin	80 mg/m^2 i.v. d 1 only	
Docetaxel	75 mg/m^2 i.v. d 1	q21d
Gemcitabine	1250 mg/m^2 i.v. d 1,8	q21d
Vinorelbine	30 mg/m^2 i.v. d 1,8	q21d
Genetic mutations in non–small cell lung cancers		
Recessive oncogene (tumor suppressor gene) and allelotype abnormalities	NSCLC	
Rb mutations (13q14)	~20%	
p16/CDKN2 mutations (9p21)	~50%	
p53 mutations (17p13)	>50%	
3p deletions	>80%	
Microsatellite alterations	Present	
Dominant oncogene abnormalities		
ras mutations	~30%	
Her-2/neu overexpression	~30%	
myc family amplification	>50%	
bcl-2 overexpression	>50%	
Telomerase expression	~90%	

AUC, area under the curve; i.v., intravenous.

- **Dietary:** Two recent studies have suggested an adverse effect of supplemental ß-carotene and retinol administration on the incidence of lung cancer and overall mortality in high-risk individuals.
- **Familial/genetic:** The contributions of hereditary factors to the development of lung cancer are probably less well understood than those of the common forms of solid tumors in humans. The proof that the familial occurrence of lung cancer has a genetic basis is complicated by the central role of cigarette smoking in causing this form of cancer. A large number of families will be required for nonclassical linkage analysis, such as segregation analyses and sib-pair linkage approaches, to define the acquired loci involved for inherited forms of lung cancer.

Histologically identifiable preneoplastic lesions found in the respiratory epithelium of lung cancer patients and smokers include hyperplasia, dysplasia, and carcinoma *in situ*. Loss of heterozygosity (LOH) is common in lung cancer. 3p loss has been shown to occur early in non–small cell lung cancer (NSCLC) and is detectable in hyperplastic, precancerous bronchial lesions. K-*ras* mutations are detectable in the later carcinoma *in situ* stage. There is conflicting evidence about the timed appearance of microsatellite deletions. Table 2.1 outlines a summary of these genetic changes in NSCLC.

PATHOLOGY

Table 2.2 outlines the World Health Organization WHO classification of NSCLC. Adenocarcinoma is the most frequently diagnosed form of NSCLC in both men and women, having replaced squamous cell carcinoma. The reason for this is unclear, but the following hypothesis has been proposed. Increased strength and frequency of inhalation is required to maintain nicotine levels in chronic smokers who smoke low-tar, filtered cigarettes. Low-tar cigarettes are less irritating to the proximal bronchial tree, thereby allowing deeper inhalation, which permits the carcinogens in the inhaled vapor to penetrate deeply.

Bronchioloalveolar carcinoma, although currently classified as a subtype of adenocarcinoma, demonstrates clinical features, suggesting that it represents a distinct histologic form of NSCLC. These features are manifested as a greater tendency for occurrence in women and nonsmokers; the development of bilateral, multifocal pulmonary involvement, with a lesser tendency for extrathoracic metastases; and a better survival rate than a similar stage of NSCLC.

TABLE 2.2. *WHO classification of non–small cell lung cancer*

Histologic types of NSCLC: Modified WHO classification
a. Squamous cell carcinoma
i. Epidermoid
ii. Spindle cell variant
b. Adenocarcinoma
i. Acinar
ii. Papillary
iii. Bronchioloalveolar
iv. Solid carcinoma with mucin
c. Large cell
i. Giant cell
ii. Clear cell
d. Adenosquamous

NSCLC, non–small cell lung cancer; WHO, World Health Organization.

SYMPTOMS AND SIGNS OF LUNG CANCER

- A minority of patients present with an asymptomatic lesion that is discovered incidentally on a chest radiograph.
- Most lung cancers are discovered because of the development of a new symptom or worsening of a clinical symptom or sign.
- No set of signs or symptoms are pathognomonic of lung cancer, and so the diagnosis is usually delayed.
- Clinical signs and symptoms of lung cancer may be divided into four categories: the symptoms (a) resulting from local tumor growth, (b) resulting from regional spread, (c) caused by distant metastases, and (d) related to paraneoplastic syndromes. Table 2.3 outlines the characteristic symptoms or signs.

TABLE 2.3. *Symptoms and signs of lung cancer*

- **Primary Disease**
    Central or endobronchial tumor growth
        Cough
        Sputum production
        Hemoptysis
        Dyspnea
        Wheeze (classically unilateral)
        Stridor
        Pneumonitis, with fever and productive cough (secondary to obstruction)
    Peripheral tumor growth
        Pain, from pleural or chest wall involvement
        Cough
        Dyspnea
        Pneumonitis
- **Regional involvement (either direct or metastatic spread)**
        Hoarseness (recurrent laryngeal nerve paralysis)
        Tracheal obstruction
        Dysphagia (esophageal compression)
        Dyspnea (pleural effusion, tracheal or bronchial obstruction, pericardial effusion, phrenic nerve palsy, lymphatic infiltration, and superior vena cava obstruction)
        Horner syndrome (sympathetic nerve palsy)
- **Metastatic involvement (common sites)**
    Bone involvement
        Pain, exacerbated by movement or weight bearing; often worse at night
        Fracture
    Liver metastases
        Right hypochondrial pain
        Icterus
        Altered mentation
    Brain metastases
        Altered mental status
        Seizures
        Motor and sensory deficits
- **Paraneoplastic syndromes**
        Clubbing
        Hypertrophic pulmonary osteoarthropathy
        Hypercalcemia
        Dermatomyositis
        Eaton-Lambert syndrome
        Hypercoagulable state
        Gynecomastia

MAKING THE DIAGNOSIS OR PLANNING THERAPY

- Once a suspected tumor is identified, it is then necessary to obtain a histologic diagnosis and accurately stage the tumor.
- The stage of the disease provides an index of the prognosis and allows selection of an appropriate therapeutic approach.
- In some cases, tissue diagnosis may not be established until the time of definitive surgical resection.
- Because 30% to 50% of patients have metastatic disease at the time of presentation, clues to the clinical stage will often be evident from the patient's clinical history and from his or her physical examination.
- Sputum cytology is the noninvasive technique used for the diagnosis of NSCLC. It is most sensitive for centrally located tumors.
- Other noninvasive methods of tumor evaluation include chest radiographs, computerized tomography scan (CT scan) of chest (including the liver and adrenals), magnetic resonance imaging (MRI) (particularly for superior sulcus tumors), and positron emission tomography (PET) scanning. To evaluate the potentially involved sites as directed by a patient's symptoms, plain radiographs, radionucleotide bone scans, and CT scan of the brain are often useful. Apart from sputum cytology, these tests can only infer the presence of cancer.
- Invasive techniques are usually required to obtain the tissue sample(s) to make a conclusive histologic diagnosis. These include bronchoscopy (with brushings and washings), transthoracic bronchial biopsy, CT scan–guided transthoracic biopsy, thoracocentesis (for pleural effusions), and mediastinoscopy with mediastinal node biopsy.
- CT scan and MRI can provide information about hilar and mediastinal nodal involvement of the tumor. Size is the criterion used to distinguish normal from abnormal nodes, with a short axis nodal diameter of 1 cm being typically used as the upper limit of normal. However, nodal enlargement may relate to hyperplastic reactive nodes, particularly in patients with postobstructive pneumonia. The accuracy of CT scan and MRI for detecting metastatic hilar (N1) or mediastinal disease is only 62% to 68% and 68% to 74%, respectively.
- Patients with clinical stage I to III disease with a central tumor or peripheral tumors greater than 2 cm should have a mediastinoscopy with mediastinal node biopsy, particularly if the nodes are greater than 1 cm in diameter on radiologic evaluation.
- Recent studies have shown that 2-[F-18] fluoro-D-glucose–positron emission tomography (FDG–PET) imaging is more accurate in detecting lymph node metastases. Combination chest CT scan and PET scan may replace the need for mediastinoscopy and help avoid unnecessary thoracotomies.
- Plain films, CT scan, and MRI findings are often suggestive of chest wall or mediastinal invasion but may not be definitive in confirming the same unless a chest wall mass, rib destruction, or gross encasement of the mediastinal structures is present. An advantage of MRI in evaluating chest invasion is its superior soft-tissue contrast resolution and multiplanar capability. The sensitivity (63% to 90%) and specificity (84% to 86%) of MRI in diagnosing chest wall invasion is similar to that of CT scan. However, MRI is the technique of choice in evaluating superior sulcus tumors, as CT scan is limited by axial plane and streak artifact from the shoulders.
- Common sites of metastatic disease from NSCLC are lymph nodes, brain, bone, liver, and adrenal glands. Routine radiologic evaluation of occult metastases in the absence of clinical or laboratory findings remains controversial and is not generally recommended. However, if a person with known NSCLC develops bone pain, it is most important to assess the weight-bearing bones to avoid the development of pathologic fractures.
- Persons with clinically apparent resectable disease commonly have a metastatic work-up, including CT scan of the brain and bone, to avoid potentially unnecessary surgical intervention (see Table 2.4).

TABLE 2.4. *Imaging options*

Local disease evaluation	Metastatic disease evaluation
Plain radiographs	Bone: plain films and bone scan
CT scan of chest (including adrenals and liver)	Brain: CT scan or MRI
MRI chest	Liver: CT scan (part of the CT scan of chest)
PET	Spinal cord: MRI
	PET: optional

CT scan, computerized tomography scan; MRI, magnetic resonance imaging; PET, positron emission tomography.

- The TNM staging system followed earlier was revised in June 1997 (see Table 2.5). The revised staging divides stage I and stage II into A and B categories and modifies stage IIIA to more accurately represent the prognostic implications of the anatomic extent of disease.
- The T1 N0 M0, T2 N0 M0, and T1 N1 M0 anatomic subsets are designated as separate entities and the T3 N0 M0 category is placed in stage IIB to more accurately reflect differences in clinical outcome.
- Stage IIIB and IV categories have remained unchanged, with two exceptions: satellite tumor nodule(s) in the primary-tumor lobe are designated T4, and separate metastatic tumor nodule(s) in the ipsilateral nonprimary-tumor lobe(s) of the lung are designated M1. However, it is still difficult to separate a single satellite or metastatic nodule in the non–tumor-bearing lobe from a synchronous primary lung cancer unless they are of different histologic type.
- Despite different clinical outcomes, no distinction has been made between stage IIIB disease with and without malignant effusion.
- Tables 2.5, 2.6, and 2.7 provide TNM descriptions and stages, the prognosis per clinical and pathologic stage, and the description of mediastinal nodal status, respectively.

Pretreatment Evaluation

It is important that all preexisting medical conditions are evaluated and the required therapeutic interventions instituted to improve the patient's condition. Through selecting appropriate operative candidates, the potential complications in the preoperative period are minimized.

Pulmonary function tests help determine the feasibility of resection and the extent of possible resection. A minimum preresection FEV_1 (forced expiratory volume in 1 second) of 2 L, 1 L, or 0.6 L is required before considering a pneumonectomy, lobectomy, or segmentectomy, respectively. The FVC (forced vital capacity) should be at least 1.7 to 2 L as a general cutoff for resection candidates. Cigarette smoke acts as an irritant to the bronchial tree, contributing to excess mucus secretion and airway hyperactivity. Patients should be encouraged to stop smoking at least 8 weeks prior to the surgical resection.

Prognostic Features

The patient's performance status (PS) is a key factor in predicting not only the patient's ability to receive therapy but also his or her prognosis. Recognized prognostic factors are

- **Performance status:** Patients with PS 3–4 are not considered appropriate candidates for either surgical resection or chemotherapy. Radiation therapy may be appropriate for specific issues, such as relief from bone pain secondary to bone metastases.

TABLE 2.5. *Staging system for non–small cell lung cancer*

Lung cancer staging: TNM classification

TX	Primary tumor cannot be assessed, or tumor is proven by the presence of malignant cells in sputum or bronchial washings but not visualized by imaging or bronchoscopy
T0	No evidence of primary tumor
Tis	Carcinoma *in situ*
T1	Primary tumor <3 cm in greatest dimension, surrounded by lung or visceral pleura, without bronchoscopic evidence of invasion more proximal than in the lobar bronchus (i.e., not in the main bronchus)
T2	Tumor with any of the following features:
	>3 cm in greatest dimension
	Involves main bronchus, ≥2 cm from carina
	Invades the visceral pleura
	Associated with atelectasis or obstructive pneumonitis that extends to the hilar region but does not involve the entire lung
T3	Tumor of any size that directly invades any of the following:
	Chest wall (including superior sulcus tumors)
	Diaphragm
	Mediastinal pleura
	Parietal pericardium
	Involves main bronchus <2 cm from the carina
	Associated atelectasis or obstructive pneumonitis of the whole lung
T4	Tumor of any size that directly invades the following:
	Mediastinum, trachea or carina, and esophagus
	Vertebral body, heart, and great vessels
	Malignant pleural or pericardial effusion
	Satellite tumor within the ipsilateral primary-tumor lobe of the lung
N1	Ipsilateral: peribronchial and/or hilar lymph nodes, intrapulmonary nodes by direct extension of primary tumor
N2	Ipsilateral: mediastinal and/or subcarinal lymph nodes
N3	Contralateral: mediastinal, hilar, scalene, and supraclavicular lymph nodes
	Ipsilateral: scalene and supraclavicular lymph nodes
M1	Presence of distant metastases.

Stage I	T1–T2	N0		M0
Stage II	T1–T2,	N1(T1–2)	T3 N0	M0
Stage IIIA	T3 N1 M0,	N2 (T1–T3)		M0
Stage IIIB	N3 (T1–T4)	T4 (N0–N3)		M0
Stage IV	Any T	Any N		M1

From Mountain CF. Revisions in the international system for staging lung cancer. Chest 1997; 111(6): 1710-1717, with permission.

- **Stage of disease:** The higher the stage, the worse the prognosis, as outlined in Table 2.6.
- **Weight loss:** A documented weight loss of 10% in the 6 months prior to the diagnosis is associated with a poor prognosis.
- **Presence of systemic symptoms:** These symptoms usually reflect advanced-stage disease.
- **Histology:** Patients with large cell carcinoma, followed by those with adenocarcinoma, are reported as having a poorer prognosis than those with either squamous cell or bronchioloalveolar carcinoma of lung.
- **Sex:** Women tend to have a better prognosis than men have.
- **Gene mutations:** p53 expression, K-*ras* mutations at codon 12, and lack of H-*ras* p21 expression are associated with a poor outcome.

TABLE 2.6. *Prognosis for clinical and pathologic stage of disease*

Stage		Clinical stage 5-year survival (%)	Pathologic stage 5-year survival (%)
T1 N0 M0	(IA)	61	67
T2 N0 M0	(IB)	38	57
T1 N1 M0	(IIA)	34	55
T2 N1 M0	(IIB)	24	39
T3 N0 M0	(IIB)	22	38
T3 N1 M0	(IIIA)	9	25
T1–3 N2 M0	(IIIA)	13	23
T4 N0–2 M0	(IIIB)	7	—
T1–4 N3 M0	(IIIB)	3	—
T1–4 N0–3 M1	(IV)	1	—

From Mountain CF. Revisions in the international system for staging lung cancer. Chest 1997; 111(6): 1710-1717, with permission.

TABLE 2.7. *Nodal stations for intrapulmonary, hilar, and mediastinal adenopathy*

N2 nodes (lie within the mediastinal pleural envelope)
Superior mediastinum
    a. Highest mediastinal nodes
    b. Upper paratracheal nodes
    c. Prevascular/Retrotracheal nodes
    d. Lower paratracheal nodes
Aortic nodes
    e. Subaortic nodes (aortopulmonary window)
    f. Para-aortic nodes (ascending aorta or phrenic)
Inferior mediastinum
    g. Subcarinal nodes
    h. Paraesophageal nodes (below carina)
    i. Pulmonary ligament nodes
N1 nodes (lie distal to the mediastinal pleural reflection and within the visceral pleura)
    j. Hilar nodes
    k. Interlobar nodes
    l. Lobar nodes
    m. Segmental nodes
    n. Subsegmental nodes

From Mountain CF. Revisions in the international system for staging lung cancer. Chest 1997; 111(6): 1710-1717, with permission.

MANAGEMENT

Early stage disease (Stages I and II)

Surgical resection is the treatment of choice in patients with stage I or stage II NSCLC, provided they are medically fit for the procedure. For patients who are medically unfit for surgery, radiation therapy is the treatment of choice. Although no randomized trial has compared these approaches, results from retrospective comparisons favor surgery in terms of long-term survival. However, one must remember that patients who are unfit for surgery, and hence receiving radiation therapy, are also more likely to do less favorably.

A lobectomy is currently the operation of choice in patients with adequate pulmonary reserves, based on results of the Lung Cancer Study Group (LCSG).

The LCSG performed a randomized controlled trial comparing lobectomy to wedge resection in patients with T1 N0 M0 NSCLC.

TABLE 2.8. *Summary of recurrence rates following surgical resection in patients with early stage non–small cell lung cancer*

		Anatomic failure rates following surgery alone		
Author	Stage	No.	Thorax (%)	Distal (%)
Pairolero	T1 N0	170	6	15
	T2 N0	158	6	23
	T1 N1	18	28	39
Mountain	T3 N0/1	69	12	25
	T1/3 N2	92	1	32
Martini	T1 N1	17	0	47
	T2 N1	58	14	36
Iascone	T1 N0	16	19	6
	T2 N0	20	25	5

- Local recurrence rate was three times greater for the patients receiving limited resection, although no statistically significant difference was detected in survival.
- Various authors have reported on the rates of local and distal failure following surgical resection (see Table 2.8).
- Up to 28% and 47% of patients develop local and distal failure, respectively; therefore, trials of adjuvant chemotherapy and radiation therapy have attempted to address this issue. The major causes of mortality in these patients were distant disease and second primary cancers.
- Data obtained from the meta-analysis performed by the Non–Small Cell Lung Cancer Collaborative Group included 14 trials comparing surgical resection with or without chemotherapy that involved 4,357 patients with early stage disease. Five of the trials used long-term alkylating agents. Eight more recent trials were cisplatin based, using cyclophosphamide–adriamycin–cisplatin ($t = 3$), cisplatin–vindesine ($t = 3$), or cisplatin–adriamycin ($t = 2$). Alkylating agent–based therapy was associated with a 15% increase in the risk of death ($p = 0.005$). Cisplatin-based therapy was not associated with a statistically significant survival advantage.
- The Non–Small Cell Lung Cancer Collaborative Group also assessed data from seven trials comparing surgery with radiation therapy with or without chemotherapy involving 807 patients with early-stage disease. Six of the trials involved cisplatin-based regimens. The overall hazard ratio of 0.98 was not statistically significant.
- Although neither adjuvant chemotherapy nor radiation therapy can be recommended as the standard of care, patients should be encouraged to participate in clinical trials to evaluate new approaches.
- Because these patients are at increased risk for second primary tumors or recurrent disease, close follow-up is recommended (see Fig. 2.1).

Stage IIIA Disease

The management of patients with stage IIIA disease is difficult. The best treatment is unclear, and the therapeutic approach remains an area of active investigation. Randomized trials and institutional series have sought several different treatment strategies for potentially resectable stage IIIA (N2) disease, including preoperative chemotherapy and radiation therapy, or chemotherapy and radiation therapy without surgery.

- Surgical resection is the therapy of choice, but it requires an experienced and skilled thoracic surgeon.
- Patients with clinical (preoperative) N0 or N1 disease but microscopic pathologic (postresection) N2 disease survive longer than patients with clinical N2 disease, with 5-year survival rates of 34% and 9%, respectively.

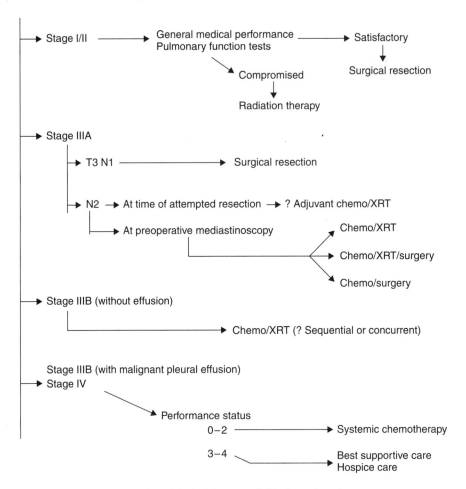

FIG. 2.1. An overview of current approaches in the treatment of patients with non–small cell lung cancer.

It is important to consider what clinical trials are available for each patient.
Patient should be encouraged to participate in clinical trials in order to improve the current therapeutics options.

- Neoadjuvant chemotherapy has the theoretical advantage of diminishing nodal involvement, thereby making surgical intervention less difficult, more likely to have an impact on survival, and provide immediate systemic therapy in patients at high risk for distal relapse. However, local treatment is delayed, and the tumor volume, if it does not respond adequately to the chemotherapy, may become unresectable.
- The continued presence of N2 nodal involvement following neoadjuvant chemotherapy is associated with a grave prognosis.
- Two prospective randomized phase III trials assessing the role of neoadjuvant chemotherapy showed a statistically significant survival advantage in favor of the chemotherapy arm (see Table 2.9). However, there were a number of potential flaws in these trials. Both trials were

TABLE 2.9. *Summary of selected phase III trials in patients with stage IIIA non–small cell lung cancer comparing surgical resection to neoadjuvant chemotherapy and resection showing a statistically significant difference in survival*

Author	No.	Chemotherapy	Schedule	Median survival	Actuarial survival (%)
Roth et al.	26	CEP	CEP–Surg.	64	56 at 3 yr
	32	—	Surg. alone	11	15 at 3 yr
Rosell et al.	30	MIC	MIC–Surg. Postop XRT (50 Gy)	26	25 at 2 yr
	30	—	Surg. alone Postop XRT (50 Gy)	8	0 at 2 yr

CEP, Cyclophosphamide, etoposide, and cisplatin; Surg., surgery; MIC, Mitomycin, ifosphamide, and cisplatin; Postop XRT, postoperative mediastinal radiation therapy.

terminated prematurely in view of the strong statistical significance at the interval evaluation, and so only a limited number of patients were treated per arm in each trial. In one of the trials (Rosell et al.), both arms received radiation therapy after the surgery. There was also stage heterogeneity within the Rosell study, as patients with stage T3 N0 M0 were included who would be considered as having stage II disease under the new staging classification (1). None of the patients in the control arm of this study was alive at 2 years, which was unexpected and did not reflect the usual survival rates of stage IIIA disease. In addition, there were a disproportionate number of patients with K-*ras* mutations within the control group, potentially biasing the results. This higher proportion of patients with K-*ras* mutations in the "surgery-alone" arm may have contributed to the poor outcome in this group.

Stage IIIB Disease (in Absence of Malignant Pleural Effusions)

- T4 lesions, bulky multilevel N2, or N3 involvement are not amenable to curative surgical resection. Traditionally, radiation therapy alone was the standard treatment in this setting. However, this was associated with 5-year failure rates of 90% and 50% to 70%, respectively, within the ipsilateral chest and systemically. Chemotherapy was added in an attempt to overcome the high relapse rates and poor outcomes with radiation therapy alone.
- The most appropriate scheduling of chemotherapy and radiation therapy is still under evaluation, as is the most efficacious fractionation of the radiation therapy.
- Various options are concurrent, sequential, or alternating schedules. Sequential scheduling aims to avoid the interactions between the two modalities, thereby limiting toxicity. Concurrent scheduling aims to maximize the therapeutic effect from chemosensitization but also results in potentiation of toxicity. Rapidly alternating schedules allow time for recovery from the acute toxicity of each modality.
- The various forms of radiation fractionation are standard, hyperfractionated, accelerated, continuous hyperfractionated accelerated radiation therapy (CHART), and hypofractionated split-course therapy.
- Data obtained from the Non–Small Cell Lung Cancer Collaborative Group's meta-analysis included 22 trials with 3,033 patients, in which radical radiation therapy with or without chemotherapy was assessed. Five trials included long-term alkylating agents. Eleven trials (1,780 patients) included cisplatin-based therapy. Chemotherapy showed a significant overall benefit, with a hazard ratio of 0.90 ($p = 0.006$) and a 10% reduction in the risk of death, which translates into an absolute benefit of 3% at 2 years and 2% at 5 years. Trials using cisplatin-based therapy yielded the strongest evidence for a positive chemotherapy effect, with a hazard ratio of 0.87 ($p = 0.005$).

TABLE 2.10. *Summary of selected phase III trials showing a statistically significant difference in survival in patients with locally advanced Non–small Cell Lung Cancer*[a]

					Survival %		
	No. of patients	Chemotherapy	XRT (Gy)	MST (mo)	1 yr	3 yr	p value
Sequential therapy							
Dillman et al.	78	PV	60	13.8	55	23	0.007
	77		60	9.7	40	11	
Le Chevalier et al.	176	VCPC	65	12.0	50	11	0.02
	177		65	10.0	41	5	
Concurrent therapy							
Schaake-Koning et al.	107	P daily	55	NR	54	16	0.009
	110	P weekly	55	NR	44	13	
	114		55	NR	46	2	
Concurrent versus sequential therapy Furuse et al.							
Concurrent	156	MVC	56	16.5	NR	22	0.04
Sequential	158	MVC	56	13.3	NR	15	

XRT, mediastinal radiation therapy; MST, median survival time; PV, cisplatin vinorelbine; VCPC, vindesine lomustine cisplatin cyclophosphamide; P, paclitaxel; NR, not reported; MVC, methotrexate vinblastine cisplatin.

[a]The trials compared sequential or concurrent chemoradiation therapy to radiation alone, and sequential chemoradiation to concurrent therapy.

- Two phase III trials comparing sequential chemoradiation and one phase III trial evaluating concurrent chemoradiation therapy showed statistically significant increases in patient survival compared to radiation therapy alone (see Table 2.10). The chemotherapy regimens tested to date in these settings have been predominantly cisplatin based.
- The sequential schedule was associated with similar local control in both groups but with lower rates of distal metastases, which may be responsible for the prolonged survival of patients in the combined modality arm of the trials. The concurrent schedule was associated with improved local control with no influence on systemic metastases.
- A recent phase III study in patients with unresectable stage III NSCLC comparing concurrent and sequential radiation therapy, in association with mitomycin, vindesine, and cisplatin chemotherapy, reported a significantly increased response rate and enhanced median survival duration in favor of the concurrent approach.
- The role of triple therapy (chemotherapy, radiation therapy, and surgical resection) over combination chemoradiation is under investigation.

Pancoast Tumor/Superior Sulcus Tumor

The Pancoast tumor described by Pancoast in 1924 comprises the characteristic and constant clinical phenomenon of pain in the distribution of the 8th cervical and 1st and 2nd thoracic spinal nerves, Horner syndrome, radiologic evidence of a small homogenous density at the apex of the lung, and minor or major destruction of the ribs and vertebral infiltration.

- Superior sulcus tumors are at least T3 and may be T4.
- Nodal involvement is a prognostic indicator of poor outcome as are positive resection margins and metastatic disease.

- Sixty percent of patients have adenocarcinoma.
- Untreated patients have an average survival of 10 to 14 months.
- Several early reports suggest that external beam radiation therapy could produce long-term survival. Combination radiation therapy and surgical resection appear most advantageous, when possible, and represents the standard of care. Five-year survival rates of up to 15% to 50% have been reported with this approach. No direct randomized clinical trial has been performed to compare the sequencing of radiation therapy and surgery in these patients. Indirect evidence from Ginsberg et al. suggests similar results with either pre- or postsurgical radiation therapy.
- T4 lesions (invasion of vertebral bodies, subclavian vessel) pertain to a poorer prognosis with 5-year survival rates of 9% to 11%. In those patients with suspected subclavian vessel involvement, an anterior approach is critical to facilitate resection. Rib involvement may have no impact on survival rates in resectable cases (5-year survival is 45% to 56%); although one study with 23 such patients revealed a statistically significant disadvantage on progression-free survival (PFS) (2-year PFS 37% versus 25%). Of 75 patients, from six studies, with resected N2 N3 disease, the 4-year survival was 8%.
- Ipsilateral supraclavicular nodal involvement (N3) seems to have a better prognosis than ipsilateral mediastinal nodes (N2).
- In a nonrandomized review of 100 patients with resected superior sulcus tumors, the 5-year survival of patients treated with lobectomy was twice that of patients treated with wedge resections (65% versus 30%, respectively; $p = 0.06$). All patients had chest wall resection in addition to the pulmonary resection. The local recurrence rates were similar (23% versus 38%, respectively).
- Most common sites of residual disease are the brachial plexus, the neural foramina, the vertebral bodies, and the subclavian veins. The most common sites of metastases are brain and bone.
- Patients with incomplete resections have overall survival rates similar to those who did not undergo resection.
- It appears that there is no survival benefit to postoperative irradiation in patients with incompletely resected disease.
- There are insufficient data on the use of combination chemotherapy and radiation therapy and surgery in patients with superior sulcus tumors.

Advanced Disease (Stage IIIB with Malignant Pleural Effusions and Stage IV)

- The survival of patients with advanced-stage (stage IIIB with malignant effusions and stage IV) NSCLC is extremely poor.
- The therapeutic approach includes consideration of systemic chemotherapy, or supportive therapy alone if the patient's general condition is not suitable for systemic chemotherapy.
- Best supportive care (BSC) produces median survival rates of 16 to 17 weeks and 1-year survival rates of 10% to 15%.
- Data obtained from the meta-analysis performed by Non–Small Cell Lung Cancer Collaborative Group included 1,190 patients with NSCLC from 11 trials and a comparison of supportive care to supportive care plus chemotherapy was evaluated. Eight of the trials included cisplatin-based regimens. Most of the trials, however, included patients with both unresectable locally advanced and systemically advanced disease. Therapy with alkylating agents had a negative impact on survival (hazard ratio 1.26), but the result was based on only two trials.
- The cisplatin-based trials showed a benefit of chemotherapy with a hazard ratio of 0.73 ($p<0.0001$), equivalent to an absolute improvement in survival of 10% (5% to 15%) at 1 year or an increase in median survival of 1.5 months (1 to 2.5 months).
- Completed prospective randomized trials including quality-of-life analyses show that cisplatin-based therapeutic regimens also improve quality of life in these patients.

- On the basis of this collective data, the guidelines of the American Society of Clinical Oncology on advanced NSCLC recognize the survival and quality-of-life advantage that chemotherapy can impart to patients with advanced-stage NSCLC. However, the greatest benefit is associated with patients with good PS [Eastern Cooperative Oncology Group (ECOG) PS 0-1]. Treatment-related toxicity is increased in patients with lower PS (ECOG PS 3,4).
- Agents in phase III trials in patients with advanced NSCLC include the taxanes (paclitaxel and docetaxel), vinca alkaloid (vinorelbine), antimetabolite (gemcitabine), and camptothecin (irinotecan). These agents have all shown promise in both phase I and II trials, both as single agents or in combination with a platinum agent. One-year survival rates of up to 40% have been commonly reported.
- Because of the modest results from chemotherapy, predictable toxicity, and high costs of new chemotherapy agents, there has been concern about the clinical benefits and economic value of chemotherapy in these patients. However, data from Canada, which compared patients with advanced-stage NSCLC treated either with BSC or with platinum-based chemotherapy, confirmed that systemic chemotherapy is more cost effective than BSC. More recent economic comparisons have focused on newer agents versus older regimens and have reported favorable findings.
- The optimal duration of therapy remains an important issue. Three recent randomized trials have addressed this issue in stage IIIB/IV NSCLC. No benefit in response rate, symptom relief, quality of life, or survival was noted for the longer duration of therapy; however, cumulative toxicities occurred more frequently in those patients randomized to longer treatment durations. These trials suggest that the duration of first-line therapy in advanced, metastatic NSCLC should be brief (three to four cycles).
- Second-line therapy has a survival and quality-of-life impact in advanced NSCLC; therefore, patients with a PS of 0–2 should be offered further treatment following progression.

Best Supportive Care

At all stages of disease, it is important to attend to the symptoms experienced by patients.

- These symptoms include therapy-related factors such as nausea, vomiting, anemia, and disease-related issues such as pain, dyspnea (from either parenchymal involvement or effusions), ataxia (cerebral involvement or peripheral neuropathy), and confusion (metabolic effects).
- Adequate antiemetic coverage pre- and postchemotherapy is essential and should be based on the emetogenic potential of the chemotherapeutic agent(s) prescribed.
- Anxiety is a common problem in patients with cancer and can be debilitating.
- Patients who stop smoking when their lung cancer is diagnosed are prone to develop depression.
- When chemotherapy no longer has a role, extra support for the patient and family is available through hospice services.

NOVEL THERAPEUTIC APPROACHES

In view of modest results with current therapeutic approaches, it is important to maintain interest in developing new approaches to therapy. New agents are being designed to more specifically target tumor pathways in an effort to reduce treatment-related side effects while preserving or enhancing efficacy. Listed below are several of the current directions in new treatment approaches:

- Photodynamic therapy
- Endobronchial implants
- Hypoxic cytotoxins (e.g., tirapazamine)
- Monoclonal antibodies to tumor factor receptors (e.g., trastuzumab)
- Signal transduction modulators (e.g., bryostatin, UCN-01, and farnesyl transferase inhibitors)

- Matrix metalloproteinase inhibitors or antiangiogenesis agents (e.g., marimastat, anti-VEGF, and endostatin)
- Gene replacement therapy (e.g., Ad-p53)
- Vaccine-based therapy
- Immunotherapy

Targeted Therapies

Epidermal Growth Factor Receptor (EGFR) is overexpressed in lung cancer, with the reported frequency of EGFR expression in NSCLC being 40% to 80%. The more promising new agents include gefitinib and erlotinib, both capable of inhibiting EGFR tyrosine kinase *in vitro*. Recent evidence from clinical trials suggests that these agents may have their greatest value in patients whose cancers possess particular mutations in the EGFK tyrosine kinase.

- Two phase II trials (IDEAL-1 and IDEAL-2) showed gefitinib monotherapy–induced tumor regression in 10% to 20% of NSCLC patients with recurrent, previously treated disease.
- Tumor-related symptoms improved in approximately 35% to 40% of patients.
- The median duration of response was 7 months.
- Two further large, randomized controlled phase III trials (INTACT I and II) showed no benefit from adding gefitinib to standard, platinum-based chemotherapy in chemotherapy-naïve patients with advanced NSCLC. However, no clinical trials of other triplets of chemotherapy have shown an advantage over doublets in terms of survival.
- A large phase III randomized trial compared single agent erlotinib with placebo in patients with NSCLC who failed at least one prior chemotherapeutic regimen and found a statistically significant survival advantage for those patients treated with erlotinib.

Screening

Screening for lung cancer remains an issue of great debate, both in terms of the most appropriate approach and the expected impact. Four prospective randomized trials evaluating early detection of NSCLC by chest x-ray failed to demonstrate a significant reduction in lung cancer mortality resulting from screening. They included 37,724 male cigarette smokers. No women were included. Two of the studies, the Memorial Sloan–Kettering Lung Project (MSKLP) and the Johns Hopkins Lung Project (JHLP), were designed to assess the impact of the addition of four monthly sputum cytology to annual chest x-ray evaluations. The studies concluded that sputum cytology added no benefit to chest x-ray alone. The long-term survival rates in the experimental and control groups in the MSKLP and JHLP were superior to the surveillance, epidemiology, and end results (SEER) data during the same period.

The other two studies, the Mayo Lung Project (MLP) and the Czechoslovakia study (CS), compared regular screening with chest x-rays in the experimental group and infrequent or no rescreening in the control group. Both studies found advantages favoring the experimental population in stage distribution, resectability, and survival.

In view of the lack of significant reduction in mortality, screening for the detection of early stage lung cancer is not recommended by any major public-policy advisory organization.

Retrospective data shows an increased risk of a second lung cancer following a diagnosis of prior lung cancer. Each year, 1% to 2% of patients with NSCLC will develop a second primary cancer. New techniques such as low-dose spiral CT scan, autofluorescent bronchoscopy, and molecular markers in sputum cytology need to be evaluated. The National Lung Screening Trial, opened for enrollment in September 2002, will compare spiral CT scan and standard chest x-ray, and aims to show whether either test is better at reducing deaths from lung cancer; it will also examine the risks and benefits of spiral CT scans compared to chest x-rays.

Chemoprevention

No strategy has been proven effective for preventing NSCLC in at-risk individuals.

Two large trials using development of lung cancer as a primary endpoint have now been completed. Both trials demonstrated an adverse risk of lung cancer with ß-carotene. The first study involved 29,133 men aged 50 to 69 from Finland, who were heavy cigarette smokers at entry (average one pack per day for 36 years). The study randomized participants to receive supplemental ß-carotene, α-tocopherol, the combination, or placebo for 5 to 8 years. Unexpectedly, participants receiving ß-carotene (alone or in combination with α-tocopherol) had a statistically significant 18% increase in lung cancer incidence [relative risk (RR), 1.18; 95% confidence interval (CI), 1.03 to 1.36] and an 8% increase in total mortality (RR, 1.08; 95% CI, 1.01 to 1.16) relative to participants receiving placebo. Supplemental ß-carotene did not appear to affect the incidence of other major cancers occurring in this population.

The finding of an increased incidence of lung cancer in ß-carotene–supplemented smokers has been replicated in the CARET (Carotene and Retinol Efficacy Trial). CARET was a multicenter lung cancer prevention trial of supplemental ß-carotene and retinol versus placebo in asbestos workers and smokers. This trial was terminated prematurely because interim analyses of the data indicated that the supplemented group was developing more lung cancer, not less, consistent with the results of the Finnish trial. Overall, lung cancer incidence was increased by 28% in the supplemented subjects (RR, 1.28; 95% CI, 1.04 to 1.57) and total mortality was also increased (RR, 1.17; 95% CI, 1.03 to 1.33). The increase in lung cancer following supplementation with ß-carotene and retinol was observed for current but not former smokers.

cis-Retinoic acid has been shown to be beneficial in patients with leukoplakia and head and neck cancer. The chemopreventive potential of 13-*cis*-retinoic acid in patients with stage I NSCLC following resection has been assessed. The trial closed in April 1997, and the mature data is awaited. Continued research and patient participation is required to define the best approach toward chemoprevention.

SUGGESTED READING

Incidence

Jemal A, Murray T, Samuels A, et al. Cancer statistics, 2003. *CA Cancer J Clin* 2003;53:5–26.

Smoking

Garfinkel L, Silverberg E. Lung cancer and smoking trends in the United States over the past 25 years. *CA Cancer J Clin* 1991;41:137–145.

Villeneuve PJ, Mao Y. Lifetime probability of developing lung cancer, by smoking status, Canada. *Can J Public Health* 1994;85:385–388.

Wiencke JK, Thurston SW, Kelsey KT, et al. Early age at smoking initiation and tobacco carcinogen DNA damage in the lung. *J Natl Cancer Inst* 1999;91:614–619.

Wingo PA, Ries LA, Giovino GA, et al. Annual report to the nation on the status of cancer, 1973-1996, with a special section on lung cancer and tobacco smoking. *J Natl Cancer Inst* 1999;91:675–690.

Pathology and Molecular Features

Salgia R, Skarin A. Molecular abnormalities in lung cancer. *J Clin Oncol* 1998;16:1207–1217.

The World Health Organization. Histological typing of lung tumors. *Am J Clin Pathol* 1982;77:123–1136.

Therapeutic Approaches

Albain KS, Rusch VW, Crowley JJ, et al. Concurrent cisplatin/etoposide plus chest radiotherapy followed by surgery for stages IIIA(N2) and IIIB non-small-cell lung cancer: mature results of Southwest Oncology Group phase II study 8805. *J Clin Oncol* 1995;13(8):1880–1892.

Bunn PA, Kelly K. New chemotherapeutic agents prolong survival and improve quality of life in non-small cell lung cancer: a review of the literature and future directions. *Clin Cancer Res* 1998;5:1087–1100.

Dillman RO, Seagren SL, Propert KJ, et al. A randomized trial of induction chemotherapy plus high-dose radiation versus radiation alone in stage III non-small-cell lung cancer. *N Engl J Med* 1990; 323:940–945.

Furuse K, Fukuoka M, Kawahara M, et al. Phase III study of concurrent versus sequential thoracic radio-therapy in combination with mitomycin, vindesine, and cisplatin in unresectable stage III non-small cell lung cancer. *J Clin Oncol* 1999;17:2692–2699.

Ginsberg RJ, Rubenstein LV. Randomized trial of lobectomy versus limited resection for T1 N0 non-small cell lung cancer. *Ann Thorac Surg* 1995;60:615–623.

Le Chevalier T, Arriagada R, Quoix E, et al. Radiotherapy alone versus combined chemotherapy and radiotherapy in nonresectable non-small-cell lung cancer: first analysis of a randomized trial in 353 patients. *J Natl Cancer Inst* 1991;83(6):417–423.

Non-Small Cell Lung Cancer Collaborative Group. Chemotherapy in non-small cell lung cancer: a meta-analysis using updated data on individual patients from 52 randomized clinical trials. *Br Med J* 1995;311:899–909.

PORT Meta-analysis Trialists Group. Postoperative radiotherapy in non-small-cell lung cancer: systematic review and meta-analysis of individual patient data from nine randomised controlled trials. *Lancet* 1998;352(9124): 257–263.

Rosell R, Gomez-Codina J, Camps C, et al. A randomized trial comparing preoperative chemotherapy plus surgery with surgery alone in patients with non-small-cell lung cancer. *N Engl J Med* 1994;330:153–158.

Roth JA, Fossella F, Komaki R, et al. A randomized trial comparing perioperative chemotherapy and surgery with surgery alone in resectable stage IIIA non-small-cell lung cancer. *J Natl Cancer Inst* 1994;86:673–680.

Schaake-Koning C, Van dan Bogaert W, Dalesio O, et al. Effects of concomitant cisplatin and radiotherapy on inoperable non-small-cell lung cancer. *N Engl J Med* 1992;326(8):524–530.

Souquet PJ, Chauvin F, Boissel JP, et al. Polychemotherapy in advanced non small cell lung cancer: a meta-analysis. *Lancet* 1993;342(8862):19–21.

Clinical Guidelines

American Society of Clinical Oncology. Clinical practice guidelines for the treatment of unresectable non-small-cell lung cancer. *J Clin Oncol* 1997;15:2996–3018.

Ettinger DS, Cox JD, Ginsberg RJ, et al. NCCN Non-Small-Cell Lung Cancer Practice Guidelines. The National Comprehensive Cancer Network. *Oncology (Huntingt)* 1996;10:81–111.

Second Cancers and Screening

Henschke CI, McCauley DI, Yankelevitz DF, et al. Early lung cancer action project: overall design and findings from baseline screening. *Lancet* 1999;354:99–105.

Johnson BE. Second lung cancers in patients after treatment for an initial lung cancer. *J Natl Cancer Inst* 1998;90(18):1335–1345.

Strauss GM, Gleason RE, Sugarbaker DJ. Chest X-ray screening improves outcome in lung cancer. A reappraisal of randomized trials on lung cancer screening. *Chest* 1995;107:270S–279S.

3

Small Cell Lung Cancer

Neelima Denduluri and Martin E. Gutierrez

*Medical Oncology Clinical Research Unit, National Cancer Institute,
National Institutes of Health, Bethesda, Maryland*

Small cell lung cancer (SCLC) constitutes approximately 15% to 25% of all lung cancers. SCLC has an aggressive natural history with a rapid doubling time, and a much greater propensity for regional and distant metastases than the other major types of lung cancers. In addition, SCLC differs from non–small cell lung cancer (NSCLC) in being highly sensitive to initial chemotherapy and radiation therapy. Therefore, the principles of management for this class of tumors differ significantly from those pertaining to NSCLC.

EPIDEMIOLOGY AND ETIOLOGY

Approximately 35,000 to 40,000 new cases of SCLC are diagnosed in the United States every year, comprising 18% of all lung cancers as assessed by the National Cancer Institute's Surveillance, Epidemiology, and End Results data. Epidemiologic data suggest that SCLC is increasing in incidence, particularly in women.

Risk factors implicated in the development of SCLC include cigarette smoking and exposure to uranium and radon gas.

MOLECULAR ABNORMALITIES

- SCLC is distinguished from all other human cancers by its high incidence of tumor-suppressor gene inactivation. More than 90% of patients with SCLC exhibit loss of the short arm on chromosome 3. Approximately 80% of SCLC inactivates p53 function (which is an important sensor of DNA damage and regulates progression through cell-cycle checkpoints) and more than 90% of SCLC inactivates Rb function, a major determinant of the G_1/S cell-cycle checkpoint.
- Other important molecular abnormalities seen in SCLC include *c-myc* amplification found in 44% of the cell lines after progression from cytotoxic chemotherapy and *BCL-2* gene overexpression in approximately 72% of SCLC cases.
- There are also abnormalities in the receptor tyrosine kinase/ligand; insulinlike growth factor-1 (IGF-1), and associated receptor in more than 95% of SCLC. The IGF-1/IGF-1R (insulin-like growth factor-1 receptor) autocrine loop plays a prominent role in the growth of SCLC. Phosphatidyl inositol 3-kinase (PI3K)-Akt signaling initiated by IGF-1 protects cells from apoptosis.
- c-Kit is co-expressed in 70% of SCLC, and the HGF/c-Met pathway has been involved in angiogenesis, cell motility, growth, invasion, and differentiation.
- Telomerase, which is believed to block senescence by preventing telomeric shortening, is overexpressed in SCLC.

PATHOLOGY

An accurate pathologic diagnosis is essential for treatment planning. This is aided by obtaining tissue blocks wherever possible because crush artifacts in needle aspirations or bronchoscopy can lead to mistaken diagnoses of SCLC. The older term, "oat-cell," is believed to reflect the morphology of crush artifact.

The cell from which SCLC originates is undefined, but it is believed to be the peptide hormone–secreting basal neuroendocrine or Kulchitsky cell. These cells often stain with silver and have demonstable neurosecretory granules.

The current pathologic classification of SCLC recognizes three classes:

- Small cell carcinoma (comprising more than 90% of all SCLCs).
- Mixed small and large cell variant.
- Combined small and non–small cell carcinoma.

No consistent clinical or prognostic differences have been identified among these groups. Atypical neuroendocrine carcinoid tumors and NSCLCs with neuroendocrine differentiation exhibit a genetic pattern and a clinical course distinct from those of SCLC.

CLINICAL FEATURES

Most SCLCs have an identifiable pulmonary lesion. Most frequently, SCLCs begin in a central, endobronchial location; local symptoms may include cough, dyspnea, wheezing, hemoptysis, chest pain, postobstructive pneumonia, superior vena cava (SVC) syndrome, hoarseness, and dysphagia. Approximately 4% of SCLCs may only be in extrapulmonary sites (i.e., cervix, head and neck, esophagus, colon, prostate, and others). Approximately two-thirds of patients have distant metastases at diagnosis. Common sites of extranodal metastases include bone, liver, central nervous system (CNS), and bone marrow. A significant number of metastases to endocrine organs are also seen.

Symptoms related to distant metastases include headaches, seizures, visual disturbances, jaundice, transaminitis, bone marrow involvement with resultant pancytopenia, bone pain, neurologic weakness secondary to cord compression, and anorexia. Because of the neuroendocrine nature of SCLC, several paraneoplastic syndromes are associated with SCLC. These include hyponatremia [syndrome of inappropriate secretion of antidiuretic hormone (SIADH), secretion of excess atrial natriuretic peptide], Cushing syndrome secondary to ectopic adrenocorticotropic hormone (ACTH) production, Eaton-Lambert syndrome, cerebellar ataxia, and subacute sensory neuropathy.

STAGING

The intensity of treatment regimens that are currently recommended (treatment-related mortality of up to 5%) dictates the need for accurate staging. The main goal of staging is to identify those patients who may benefit from combined-modality treatment (combining chemotherapy with concurrent thoracic radiation) (see Table 3.1).

The most frequently used staging system is the Veterans Administration Lung Group (Table 3.1). The TNM classification suggested by the American Joint Commission for Cancer (AJCC) is rarely used; it is applied primarily to select the exceedingly small population of patients (stage I) who may benefit from surgical resection in addition to combination chemotherapy.

Necessary components of an adequate staging evaluation include a complete history and physical examination, chest x-ray (CXR), computerized tomography (CT) scan, bronchoscopy if chest CT scan/CXR are nonrevealing, complete blood count (CBC), comprehensive metabolic panel including lactate dehydrogenase (LDH) and alkaline phosphatase levels, CT scan of the liver and adrenal glands, and a bone scan. Magnetic resonance imaging (MRI) of the

TABLE 3.1. *Veterans Affairs Lung Cancer Study Group staging of small cell lung cancer and prognosis*

		Survival	
Stage	%	Untreated	Combination chemotherapy
Limited-stage disease Tumor confined to one hemithorax and regional lymph nodes that can be encompassed within a radiotherapy por[a]	30–40	12 wk	12–20 mo
Extensive-stage disease Disease extending beyond the limits described for limited-stage disease[b]	60–70	5 wk	7–11 mo

[a]Contralateral hilar, mediastinal, or supraclavicular nodes usually included in limited-stage disease.
[b]Ipsilateral malignant pleural effusion is considered extensive disease.

head, if possible, is indicated; if there is a contraindication to MRI, a CT scan of the head with contrast is recommended at miniminum, and a positron emission tomography (PET) scan is also indicated. One must consider a bone marrow biopsy if pancytopenia may be an issue to dictate treatment.

TREATMENT

Although several single agents show activity against SCLC, significantly superior response rates and survival with use of multiagent therapy have made combination chemotherapy the standard approach in initial treatment. Optimal regimens yield 80% to 90% response rates, 50% to 60% complete response rates, and 2-year survival rates of 15% to 40%. Five-year survival is 15% to 25% (see Table 3.2).

The most important factors that predict a favorable outcome are extent of disease, good performance status, biology of the small cell tumor, and smoking cessation. Several combinations have been used successfully (see Table 3.3). The most commonly used regimen currently is etoposide and cisplatin (EP) because of its favorable toxicity profile. Schiller et al. (1) considered adding topotecan after four cycles of etoposide/cisplatin to ascertain whether this therapy would improve survival in patients with platinum-sensitive disease (not recurring within 60 days or progressing within 60 days after receiving cisplatin-based therapy). Adding topotecan versus observation only did not translate to increased survival.

TABLE 3.2. *Stage-dependent treatment of SCLC*

Stage	Treatment
Limited-stage disease	• Combination chemotherapy • Hyperfractionated thoracic radiation • Prophylactic cranial irradiation may be considered in complete responders
Extensive-stage disease	• Combination chemotherapy • Referrals to clinical trials or single-agent chemotherapy are acceptable alternatives in selected patients

TABLE 3.3. *Summary of commonly used chemotherapeutic regimens*

Regimen	Dose	Duration
EP		
Etoposide	120 mg/m^2 i.v. d 1–3	
Cisplatin	60 mg/m^2 i.v. d 1	Cycles repeated every 4 wk, for four cycles
Etoposide	100 mg/m^2 i.v. d 1–3	
Carboplatin	AUC 6 i.v. d 1	
Etoposide	100 mg/m^2 i.v. d 1–3	
Cisplatin	25 mg/m^2 i.v. d 1–3	
Etoposide	80 mg/m^2 i.v. d 1–3	Cycles repeated every 3 wk, for four cycles
Cisplatin	80 mg/m^2 i.v. d 1	
CI		
Cisplatin	60 mg/m^2 i.v. on d 1	Every 4 wk, for four cycles
Irinotecan	60 mg/m^2 i.v. on d 1, 8, and 15	
CAV		
Cyclophosphamide	1,000 mg/m^2 i.v. d 1	Cycles repeated every 3 wk, continued for four to six cycles
Doxorubicin	45 mg/m^2 i.v. d 1	
Vincristine	1 mg/m^2 i.v. d 1	
CAE		
Cyclophosphamide	1,000 mg/m^2 i.v. d 1	Cycles repeated every 3 wk, continued for four to six cycles
Doxorubicin	45 mg/m^2 i.v. d 1	
Etoposide	50 mg/m^2 i.v. d 1–3	
CAVE		
Cyclophosphamide	1,000 mg/m^2 IV d 1	Cycles repeated every 3 wk, continued for four to six cycles
Doxorubicin	50 mg/m^2 i.v. d 1	
Vincristine	1.5 mg/m^2 i.v. d 1	
Etoposide	60 mg/m^2 i.v. d 1–5	

AUC, area under the curve; EP, etoposide/cisplatin; CI, cisplatin/irinotecan; CAV, cyclophosphamide/doxorubicin/vincristine; CAE, cyclophosphamide/doxoruicin/etoposide; CDVE, cyclophosphamide/doxorubicin/vincristine/etoposide.

The optimal duration of chemotherapy is four to six cycles (or two cycles beyond best response). Longer duration of treatment has not been shown to be of any benefit. High-dose chemotherapy with autologous stem-cell reinfusion has not been demonstrated to be superior to conventional therapy in phase III trials and is currently used only in clinical trials.

Thoracic radiation provides a marginal survival advantage and reduced local recurrence rates when added to chemotherapy in limited-stage disease. Most regimens incorporating radiation therapy use a total dose of 45 to 50 Gy. The optimal timing of radiotherapy is concurrent with chemotherapy. Takada et al. (2) demonstrated an increase in response rate (35% versus 54%) and in 5-year survival rate with concurrent radiation therapy and chemotherapy. In a study of 231 patients, the median survival was 19.7 months in the sequential arm and 27.2 months in the concurrent arm. Turrisi et al. (3) demonstrated that chemotherapy (cisplatin and etoposide) and concurrent twice-daily radiation therapy are better than daily radiation alone, with a median survival of 19 months versus 23 months.

Use of prophylactic cranial irradiation (PCI) has received considerable attention because the risk of developing CNS metastases in 2-year survivors otherwise approaches 50% to 60%.

Auperin et al. (4) conducted a meta-analysis of 987 patients; the relative risk of death was 0.84 in the patients who received PCI. PCI improved both overall survival rate at 3 years (by 5.4%) and disease-free survival rate among patients with SCLC in complete remission. Therefore, PCI is recommended in patients with complete remission. PCI has not been shown to result in clinically significant neuropsychological sequelae.

Extensive-Stage Disease

Combination chemotherapy without thoracic irradiation is the cornerstone of therapy. Combination chemotherapies identical to those used in limited-stage disease are used with overall response rates of 60% to 80%, complete response rates of 15% to 20%, and median survival of 7 to 11 months. Five-year survival is less than 5%. Radiation therapy is used in local control of distant disease (CNS and other isolated metastatic sites not responding to systemic chemotherapy).

In this setting, cisplatin and carboplatin are thought to be equivalent in efficacy. The most efficacious regimens seem to be irinotecan/cisplatin or cisplatin/etoposideg–based regimens. Noda et al. (5) reported increases in survival rate with irinotecan/cisplatin compared with etoposide/cisplatin (12.8 versus 9.4 months 5-year survival and 19.5% versus 5.2% 2–year), survival with greater diarrhea toxicity but better hematologic toxicity. Currently there are two randomized clinical trials in the United States comparing irinotecan/cisplatin combination versus the standard-of-care regimen of cisplatin/etoposide.

Recurrent Disease or Disease Progressing with Initial Therapy

Recurrent disease or disease progressing with initial therapy has an extremely poor prognosis, with a median survival of 2 to 3 months. Treatment options in this group are limited. Thoracic irradiation should be considered in those patients whose recurrence is confined to the thorax and who have not previously received irradiation but need symptomatic relief. Patients who have not received a platinum-containing regimen or who have not relapsed for 6 months after receiving cisplatin or carboplatin may benefit from combinations containing cisplatin.

Platinum-refractory SCLC is defined as progression during first-line therapy or progression in a period less than or equal to 3 months after completing first-line therapy. In this setting, response rates are poor. However, multiple single-agent regimens have been shown to have some activity in patients who have recurrence of disease after 3 months, including taxol with a 34% response rate, docetaxel with a 26% response rate, and topotecan/irinotecan with a 40% to 60% response rate. Three-drug combinations have been studied with no improvement in disease response or survival. Patients may be referred to clinical trials that are testing new pharmacologic agents currently under development that target oncogenes and signaling pathways.

Long-Time Survivors of SCLC Are at High Risk for Developing Second Primary Tumors of NSCLC in Addition to Recurrent SCLC

Patients who are able to quit smoking seem to do better than patients who continue to smoke. These patients should be considered for chemoprevention strategies.

REFERENCES

1. Schiller JH, Adak S, Cella D. Topotecan versus observation after cisplatin plus etoposide in extensive-stage small-cell lung cancer: E7593—a phase III trial of the eastern cooperative oncology group. *J Clin Oncol* 2001;19(8):2114–2122.
2. Takada M, Fukuoka M, Kawahara M, et al. Phase III study of concurrent versus sequential thoracic radiotherapy in combination with cisplatin and etoposide for limited-stage small-cell lung cancer: results of the japan clinical oncology group study 9104. *J Clin Oncol* 2002;20(14):3054–3060.

3. Turrisi AT III, Kim K, Blum R, et al. Twice-daily compared with once-daily thoracic radiotherapy in limited small-cell lung cancer treated concurrently with cisplatin and etoposide. *N Engl J Med* 1999;340(4):265–271.
4. Auperin A, Arriagada R, Pignon JP, et al. Prophylactic Cranial Irradiation Overview Collaborative Group. Prophylactic cranial irradiation for patients with small-cell lung cancer in complete remission. *N Engl J Med* 1999;341(7):476–484.
5. Noda K, Nishiwaki Y, Kawahara M. Irinotecan plus cisplatin compared with etoposide plus cisplatin for extensive small-cell lung cancer. *N Engl J Med* 2002;346(2):85–91.

SELECTED READINGS

Adjei AA, Marks RS, Bonner JA. Current guidelines for the management of small cell lung cancer. *Mayo Clin Proc* 1999;74:809–816.
Demetri G, Elias A, Gershenson D, et al. NCCN small-cell lung cancer practice guidelines. *Oncology* 1996;10(Suppl. 11):179–194.
Ihde DC, Pass HI, Glatstein E. Small cell lung cancer. In: De Vita VT, Hellman S, Rosenberg SA, eds. *Cancer: principles and practice of oncology*, 5th ed. Philadelphia, PA: Lippincott-Raven Publishers, 1997:911–949.
Kelly K, Mikhaeel-Kamel N. Medical treatment of lung cancer. *J Thorac Imaging* 1999;14:257–265.
Sandler AB. Current management of small cell lung cancer. *Semin Oncol* 1997;244:463–476.
Teng M, Choy H, Ettinger D. Combined chemoradiation therapy for limited-stage small-cell lung cancer. *Oncology* 1999;13(10 Suppl. 5):107–115.

SECTION 3

Digestive System

4

Esophageal Cancer

Gregory D. Leonard*, David P. Kelsen†, and Carmen J. Allegra‡

*The Royal College of Physicians, Dublin, Ireland; †Gastrointestinal Oncology Service, Memorial Sloan-Kettering Cancer Center, New York, New York; and ‡Network for Medical Communication and Research, Atlanta, Georgia

Esophageal cancer is the ninth most commonly occurring cancer worldwide and the sixth most common cause of cancer mortality (1). It is highly curable in its earliest stages; however, it usually presents in the advanced disease. Despite the last two decades of progress in clinical research, the median survival time for a patient with symptoms of a primary esophageal cancer is less than 18 months. Most research and controversy in the treatment of esophageal cancer currently focuses on the role of chemoradiotherapy as either adjuvant or as primary therapy for esophageal cancer.

EPIDEMIOLOGY

United States:

- Esophageal cancer was estimated to account for 1% of all malignancies and 6% of all gastrointestinal malignancies in 2003 (2). The age-adjusted incidence from 1996 to 2000 is 4.5 cases per 100,000 population (http://seer.cancer.gov/csr/1975_2000/).
- Approximately 13,900 new cases and 13,000 deaths were estimated for 2003.
- The median age at diagnosis is 67 years. This cancer rarely occurs in patients younger than 25 years.
- Esophageal cancer is two to four times more frequent in men than in women. Siewert type 1 tumors [adenocarcinoma (ADC)] are eight to nine times more common in men than in women.
- Rates of occurrence of esophageal cancer are approximately threefold higher among blacks than among whites.
- Squamous cell carcinoma (SCC) is more common in black men; ADC is more common in white men.
- Five-year relative survival rates were 5% from 1974 to 1976 and 13% from 1992 to 1998.

Rest of the world:

- There are approximately 500,000 cases of esophageal cancer in the world, but there is marked geographic variation. Regions with clusters of high rates include China (e.g., Linxian), Iran, France, and South Africa.
- In the 1970s, approximately 90% of esophageal cancers were SCCs. The incidence of ADCs has increased dramatically and currently accounts for approximately 60% to 70% of new cases—a rate of acceleration greater than that of any other cancer in the United States.

ETIOLOGY

Adenocarcinoma

• Barrett esophagus
• Obesity
• Gastroesophageal reflux disease (GERD), which can be caused by obesity and might result in Barrett esophagus.

Squamous Cell Carcinoma

• Tobacco
• Alcohol
• Predisposing conditions:
  – Tylosis (SCC)
  – Achalasia
  – Esophageal diverticula and webs (SCC)
  – Plummer–Vinson syndrome
  – Human papillomavirus (HPV)
  – Celiac disease
• Less significant causes include environmental exposure and dietary factor.

BARRETT ESOPHAGUS

Barrett esophagus, perhaps as a result of GERD, is the most important risk factor (100 times risk increase over other factors) for ADC.

Screening recommendations (no randomized trial data for surveillance practices) are as follows:

• For no dysplasia, endoscopy every 2 to 3 years
• For low-grade dysplasia, endoscopy every 6 months for 12 months and then yearly
• For high-grade dysplasia, esophagectomy or three monthly endoscopies or photodynamic therapy (PDT).

CLINICAL PRESENTATION

The most common clinical presentations of esophageal cancer are listed in Table 4.1 and are usually related to local compression or infiltration symptoms or generalized malaise and anorexia.

The classic triad for presentation of esophageal cancer is as follows:

• Asthenia
• Anorexia
• Analgesia (for dysphagia).

TABLE 4.1. *Clinical presentation of esophageal cancer*

Symptoms	Patients with symptoms (%)
Dysphagia (solids usually before liquids)	80–96
Weight loss	42–46
Odynophagia	≤50
Epigastric or retrosternal pain	≤20
Cough or hoarseness	≤5
Tracheoesophageal fistula	1–13

DIAGNOSIS

- Symptoms
  - Dysphagia or odynophagia
  - Hematemesis
  - Dyspepsia
  - Hoarseness
  - Dyspnea
  - Anorexia.
- Signs (usually late presentation)
  - Horner syndrome
  - Left supraclavicular lymphadenopathy (Virchow node)
  - Cachexia
  - Hepatomegaly
  - Bone metastases (rare but paraneoplastic hypercalcemia can occur).
- Upper gastrointestinal endoscopy
- This diagnostic procedure is the gold standard. The combination of endoscopic biopsies and brush cytology has an accuracy of greater than 90% in making a tissue diagnosis of esophageal cancer.
- Barium contrast radiography
- This diagnostic procedure can document contour and motility abnormalities and unexpected airway fistula and may be useful when the entire esophagus has not been visualized endoscopically. However, a tissue diagnosis is needed for definitive diagnosis.

PATHOLOGY

- Most newly diagnosed patients have ADC, but there are contrasting reports on their relative prognosis. Less than 1% of esophageal tumors are lymphoma, melanoma, carcinosarcoma, or small cell carcinoma.
- Fifty percent of tumors arise in the lower one-third of the esophagus, 25% arise in the upper esophagus, and 25% of tumors occur in the middle one-third of the esophagus (2).

STAGING

The American Joint Commission for Cancer (AJCC) has designated staging of cancer by TNM classification, which defines the anatomic extent of disease (3) (see Table 4.2). Of note, cervical adenopathy in tumors in the lower one-third of esophagus is M1 as opposed to N1.

The Siewert classification subclassifies gastroesophageal junction tumors into three types according to their anatomic location: Type 1 are distal esophagus tumors, type II are cardia tumors, and type III are subcardia gastric tumors (4).

Staging work-up can include the following:

- **Computerized tomography scan (CT) scan:** CT scan of the chest and abdomen can demonstrate evidence of spread of tumor to lymph nodes or distant metastases to the liver (35%), lungs (20%), bone (9%), and adrenals (5%). CT scan may underestimate the depth of tumor invasion and peri-esophageal lymph node involvement in up to 50% of cases. Magnetic resonance imaging (MRI) provides similar results to CT.
- **Endoscopic ultrasound (EUS):** EUS may be helpful when metastases are not detected by CT or other imaging modalities. EUS is the optimal technique for locoregional staging. A meta-analysis demonstrated greater than 71% sensitivity in staging preoperative depth of invasion (T) and greater than 60% sensitivity for locoregional lymph nodes (N); specificity was greater than 67% and greater than 40%, respectively (5).

TABLE 4.2. *Definition of TNM and stage grouping*

TNM stage:

Primary tumor (T)

TX: Primary tumor cannot be assessed
T0: No evidence of primary tumor
Tis: Carcinoma *in situ*
T1: Tumor invades lamina propria or submucosa
T2: Tumor invades muscularis propria
T3: Tumor invades adventitia
T4: Tumor invades adjacent structures

Regional lymph nodes (N)

N1: Regional lymph node metastasis
NX: Regional lymph nodes cannot be assessed
N0: No regional lymph node metastasis

Distant metastasis (M)

MX: Distant metastasis cannot be assessed
M0: No distant metastasis
M1: Distant metastasis
Tumors of the lower thoracic esophagus
M1a: Metastasis in celiac lymph nodes
M1b: Other distant metastasis
Tumors of the midthoracic esophagus
M1a: Not applicable
M1b: Other distant metastasis
Tumors of the upper thoracic esophagus
M1a: Metastasis in cervical nodes
M1b: Other distant metastasis

Stage Grouping

Stage 0	Tis	N0	M0
Stage I	T1	N0	M0
Stage IIA	T2	N0	M0
	T3	N0	M0
Stage IIB	T1	N1	M0
	T2	N1	M0
Stage III	T3	N1	M0
	T4	Any N	M0
Stage IV	Any T	Any N	M1
Stage IVA	Any T	Any N	M1a
Stage IVB	Any T	Any N	M1b

- **Positron emission tomography (PET):** PET is useful when CT is negative for metastatic disease, and the diagnosis can change management of cancer in 20% to 25% of patients (6). Bronchoscopy is required in tumors less than 25 to 26 mm from the incisors, to exclude invasion of the posterior membranous trachea or tracheoesophageal fistula.

TREATMENT

Surgery

- Surgery alone remains a standard treatment for esophageal cancer with resectable local or locoregional disease. In 1993, surgery was used as a component of treatment in 34% of patients. Surgery alone was used in 18% of patients (7).
- Recent improvements in staging techniques and patient selection have improved surgical morbidity and mortality. Operative mortality rates are now less than 5%. Surgical expertise is a major contributor to survival, with better outcomes in high-volume centers. Resection is possible in approximately 50% of patients (8). Five-year survival in patients with surgical resection is 5% to 25%.
- Surgical principles include a wide resection of the primary tumor by aiming for an R0 resection (no residual tumor), including more than 5-cm resection margins plus regional lymphadenectomy. Intraoperative frozen section can assess for residual disease, which, if present, is considered an R1 (microscopic tumor) or R2 (macroscopic tumor) resection.
- In general, patients with cervical carcinoma of the esophagus are not considered candidates for surgical resection; chemoradiation is favored in these patients.

- Surgical approaches include the following:

  - **Transthoracic resection:** En bloc esophagectomy requires laparotomy and thoracotomy, for example, total thoracic or transthoracic (Lewis) procedures. A three-field lymph node dissection (extended lymphadenectomy) includes superior mediastinum and cervical lymphadenectomy. It is the treatment of choice in Japan but is associated with increased toxicity and has a questionable survival advantage.
  - **Transhiatal esophagectomy:** This includes laparotomy and cervical anastomosis. This technique avoids thoracotomy.

Chemoradiotherapy (Combined-modality Approach)

Although no large prospective randomized trials have directly compared primary chemoradiation with surgery, definitive chemoradiation for locoregional carcinoma of the esophagus is considered to be an alternative to surgery.

- Interest in chemoradiotherapy is based on the Radiation Therapy Oncology Group (RTOG) 85-01 trial (9) that demonstrated a survival advantage (14 versus 9 months median survival and 27% versus 0% 5-year survival) in favor of chemoradiotherapy over radiotherapy alone in inoperable patients (see Table 4.3). A number of randomized trials of chemoradiotherapy versus radiotherapy alone have failed to duplicate the results of RTOG 85-01; however, a recent Cochrane review has confirmed the superiority of chemoradiotherapy versus radiotherapy in fit, motivated patients (10).
- Chemoradiotherapy is now the standard of care for patients with unresectable esophageal cancer or an alternative to surgery for patients with resectable cancers.

Chemoradiotherapy as Definitive Therapy in Resectable Cancer

Upper thoracic esophageal (above the aortic arch) tumors and T4 or N1 tumors are usually considered unresectable.

- The outcomes of chemoradiotherapy in RTOG 85-01 were comparable to those found in surgical therapy (11). Results from the randomized trials of preoperative chemoradiotherapy have demonstrated pathological complete response rates of greater than 25% and are associated with an improved survival.
- Trials that used surgery after chemoradiotherapy in patients who responded and higher doses of radiation for patients who did not respond failed to show a benefit for the group receiving surgery.

TABLE 4.3. *Radiation Therapy Oncology Group (RTOG) 85-01 trial of chemoradiotherapy versus radiotherapy alone in esophageal cancer*

Number of patients	Histology	Treatment	Median survival	5-Year survival	p-value
121	SCC = 88% ADC = 12%	Cisplatin 75 mg/m^2 d 1 5-FU 1,000 mg/m^2/d d 1–4 50 Gy of radiation wk 1, 5 Cisplatin/5-FU wk 8, 11 versus 64 Gy of radiation 2Gy/fx	14.1 mo vs. 9.3 mo	27% vs. 0%	0.0001

SCC, squamous cell carcinoma; ADC, adenocarcinoma; 5-FU, 5-fluorouracil; Gy, Gray of radiation; fx, fraction of radiation.
From Cooper JS, Guo MD, Herskovic A, et al. Chemoradiotherapy of locally advanced esophageal cancer long-term follow-up of a prospective randomized trial (RTOG 85-01). *JAMA* 1999;281:1623–1627, with permission.

- A better determinant of the role of surgery after chemoradiotherapy is evident from two recent trials:
  - In the first trial, patients with locally advanced but resectable tumors were treated with chemoradiotherapy, and patients with at least a partial response were randomized to continued chemoradiotherapy or surgery (12). There was no difference in overall survival (19.3 versus 17.7 months, respectively), but early mortality and duration of hospital stay were less in the chemoradiotherapy-only arm.
  - The second trial randomized patients with locally advanced tumors to either definitive chemoradiotherapy or chemoradiotherapy (lower doses of radiation) and surgery (13). There was no significant difference in survival outcomes (15 versus 16 months, respectively) between the two groups of patients. There was improved survival in a subgroup of patients receiving surgery because they did not respond to chemoradiotherapy.
- No prospective randomized trial has compared chemoradiation to surgery alone in resectable tumors.
- Local recurrence rates, however, remain greater than 45%.
- Radiation dose escalation has not proved to be beneficial. A recent trial examining this approach was closed after an interim analysis indicated that there would be no advantage with higher doses of radiation.

Preoperative Chemoradiotherapy (Trimodality Approach)

- The rationale for preoperative chemoradiotherapy was first studied by Leichman et al. in 21 patients with SCC. Patients were treated with 3,000 cGy of radiation and with two cycles of concurrent 5-fluorouracil (5-FU) and cisplatin (14). An additional 2,000 cGy of radiation was given postoperatively when residual tumor was seen at surgery. The pathologically complete response was 37% with a median survival of 18 months.
- Eight prospective randomized phase III trials (two reported in abstract form) have addressed the issue of whether preoperative chemoradiotherapy offers any benefit over surgery alone (11). Much debate exists about the interpretation of these trials (see Table 4.4). Only Walsh et al. have demonstrated significant benefits in median survival (16 versus 11 months; $p = 0.01$) and 3-year survival (32% versus 6%; $p = 0.01$) of patients receiving preoperative chemoradiotherapy (15). However, limitations of this trial include poor surgical outcome, small numbers of patients studied, and the fact that all patients had ADC.

TABLE 4.4. *Randomized phase III trials of trimodality therapy compared to surgery*

Study	Number of evaluable patients	Histology	3-Year survival trimodality therapy vs. surgery
Nygaard (16)	88	SCC	17% vs. 9%[a]
Apintop (17)	69	SCC	24% vs. 10%[b]
Le Prise (18)	86	SCC	19% vs. 14%
Walsh (15)	113	ADC	32% vs. 6%
Bosset (19)	282	SCC	30% vs. 31%[c]
Urba (20)	100	SCC 25% ADC 75%	30% vs. 16%
Burmeister (21)	505	SCC 29% ADC 61%	21.7 mo vs. 18.5 mo[d]
Lee (22)	102	NA	28.2 mo vs. 27.3 mo[d]

SCC, squamous cell carcinoma; ADC, adenocarcinoma; NA, not available.
[a]2×2 factorial design; [b]5-year survival; [c]median follow-up of 55 mo; [d]median survival.

- Other trials failed to duplicate these results, although many showed nonsignificant median survival benefits, disease-free survival benefits, and, overall, showed a trend toward an improvement in outcome when preoperative chemoradiotherapy was added.
- Use of new chemotherapeutic agents such as paclitaxel and irinotecan have shown promise.

Postoperative Chemoradiotherapy

- There are fewdata on the use of postoperative chemoradiotherapy in esophageal cancer.
- A recent trial found a statistically significant survival advantage for postoperative chemora- diotherapy compared to surgery alone in gastroesophageal and gastric cancers (see Table 4.5) (23). On the basis of these data, adjuvant chemoradiotherapy has been recommended for ADC tumors of the lower esophagus. It is possible that the survival benefit associated with the use of chemoradiotherapy results from reductions in local recurrences and thus compen- sates for inadequate surgery (only 10% of patients had the recommended D2 resection).

Radiation Therapy

- Radiation therapy alone is generally considered palliative and is used in patients who are unable to tolerate chemoradiotherapy.

Preoperative Radiotherapy:

- No randomized trials of preoperative single-modality radiotherapy have demonstrated a sur- vival benefit in patients.

Postoperative Radiotherapy:

- Similarly, there is no benefit of single-modality postoperative radiotherapy in patients.

Chemotherapy

- Single-agent chemotherapy demonstrates response rates of 15% to 25%. Combination chemotherapy response rates are 25% to 45%, but this has not definitively improved survival in advanced disease states.
- Cisplatin with 5-FU is the most frequently used regimen for both combined-modality therapy in locoregional disease and systemic therapy for palliation.
- SCC may be more sensitive to chemotherapy, but there is no difference in long-term outcome between SCC and ADC.
- New chemotherapeutic agents have demonstrated encouraging response rates (see Table 4.6).

TABLE 4.5. *Intergroup-116 trial of adjuvant chemoradiotherapy versus surgery alone in gastric or gastroesophageal adenocarcinomas*

Number of patients	Surgery	Treatment	Median survival	3-Year survival	*p*-value
556	D0 54% D1 36% D2 10%	Surgery followed by 5-FU 425 mg/m^2/d d 1–5 LV 20 mg/m^2/d d 1–5[a] 4,500 cGy radiation d28,180 cGy/d 5 d/wk for 5 wk vs. surgery alone	36 mo vs. 27 mths	50% vs. 41%	0.005

5-FU, 5-fluorouracil; LV, leucovorin.

[a]Two further courses of chemotherapy were given 1 mo apart after radiation. Additional 5-FU 400 mg/m^2 and LV 20 mg/m^2 were given on the first 4 d and the last 3 d of radiotherapy.

TABLE 4.6. *New chemotherapeutic agents in esophageal cancer*

Chemotherapy	Dose ranges	Combination chemotherapy	Response rates (%)
Paclitaxel	50–200 mg/m^2	Cisplatin Carboplatin Etoposide	26–100[a]
Docetaxel	60–100 mg/m^2	Cisplatin 5-FU	18–24
Irinotecan	65–125 mg/m^2	Cisplatin 5-FU	22–58
Oxaliplatin	85–130 mg/m^2	5-FU Epirubicin Capecitabine	48–81
Capecitabine	1,000–1,250 mg/m^2	Epirubicin 5-FU Cisplatin Oxaliplatin	54

5-FU, 5-fluorouracil.
[a]Some trials included radiation therapy.

Preoperative (Neoadjuvant) Chemotherapy

- The poor survival, even for patients with clinically localized carcinoma of the esophagus, suggests that occult metastases are present at diagnosis, thereby providing the impetus to add systemic therapy early during patient management.
- In the two largest trials examining preoperative chemotherapy, the Intergroup (INT 0113) trial (24) showed no survival benefit, whereas the Medical Research Council (MRC) trial (25) demonstrated a 3-month median survival advantage for chemotherapy over surgery alone (see Table 4.7).The following differences in the two studies may have contributed to their different outcomes:
  - Chemotherapy was of longer duration and was with higher doses in INT 0113. This therapy may have been detrimental by delaying access to surgery and causing more toxicity.
  - Surgery was performed in only 80% of the patients in the chemotherapy arm in INT 0113 compared to 92% in the MRC trial. Outcome for surgery alone was poor in the MRC trial, thereby possibly exaggerating the benefits of chemotherapy.
  - Radiation therapy off protocol (equally distributed between treatment arms) was available in the MRC trial.
  - A larger sample size in the MRC trial may have facilitated detection of a statistically significant result.

Postoperative Chemotherapy

- Most trials of postoperative chemotherapy also involved preoperative chemotherapy.
- As with preoperative chemotherapy, there is renewed interest in this approach on the basis of the MRC data, although it has yet to be adopted as a standard approach
- A recent trial assessed the use of perioperative epirubicin, cisplatin, and 5-FU (ECF) chemotherapy or surgery alone in esophagogastric cancer. In 503 patients, 15% had esophagogastric cancer and 11% had esophageal cancer. Adjuvant chemotherapy increased progression-free survival and resectability rates and showed a trend toward improved survival ($p = 0.06$) (26).

TABLE 4.7. *Comparison of the two largest preoperative chemotherapy trials*

	Intergroup 0113	Medical Research Council (MRC)
Patient number	467	802
Histology	ADC = 54%, SCC = 46%	ADC = 66%, SCC = 31%
Treatment	Cisplatin 100 mg/m^2 D1	Cisplatin 80 mg/m^2 D1
	5-FU 1,000 mg/m^2/d d 1–5	5-FU 1,000 mg/m^2/d d 1–4
	for q4wk × 3 followed by surgery	For q3wk × 2 followed by surgery
	vs. surgery alone	vs. surgery alone
	Postoperative CT to patients with stable disease or response to preoperative CT	
	Three further cycles but with cisplatin 75 mg/m^2	
Resectability	80% CT + surgery	92% CT +surgery
	96% surgery alone	97% surgery alone
Median survival	14.9 mo CT + surgery	16.8 mo CT + surgery
	16.1 mo surgery alone	13.3 mo surgery alone

ADC, adenocarcinoma; SCC, squamous cell carcinoma; CT, chemotherapy; 5-FU, 5-fluorouracil.

Palliation

- Palliative options can be split into local or systemic options.
- Local therapies include external beam and brachytherapy radiation. This approach can palliate dysphagia in approximately 80% of patients. PDT has also been approved by the U. S. Food and Drug Administration (FDA) for this indication. For rapid palliation, laser or balloon dilatation and stenting is recommended. The placement of a gastrostomy or jejunostomy tube may improve the patient's nutritional status.
- The systemic chemotherapy options in esophageal cancer are improving (Table 4.6). However, no trial has identified a reference regimen specific to esophageal cancer.
- Cisplatin combined with 5-FU is the most commonly used regimen, but this did not demonstrate a statistically significant benefit over cisplatin alone when tested in a randomized trial of patients with advanced SCC of the esophagus (27).
- Most data on chemotherapy in advanced esophageal cancer are extrapolated from trials in gastric cancer that often include gastroesophageal tumors. In Europe, ECF is frequently used because of its superior survival compared to 5-FU, doxorubicin, and methotrexate (FAMTX) in advanced esophagogastric cancer (28).
- A recent trial in metastatic or unresectable gastric and gastroesophageal cancer evaluated docetaxel, cisplatin, and 5-FU (DCF) and cisplatin and 5-fluorouracil (CF). Time to disease progression improved from 3.7 months to 5.2 months (hazard ratio 1.704), and median overall survival improved from 8.5 months to 10.2 months ($p = 0.0053$) in patients receiving DCF compared to those receiving CF (29).

DISTRIBUTION, TREATMENT, AND SURVIVAL FOR ESOPHAGEAL CANCER BY STAGE IN THE UNITED STATES

The distribution, treatment, and survival in patients with esophageal cancer according to stage in the United States are given in Table 4.8.

TABLE 4.8. *Stage, distribution, treatment and survival of esophageal cancers in the United States*

Stage	Distribution (%)	Treatment	5-Year relative survival rates (%)
Localized (I + II)	25	Surgery Chemoradiotherapy if surgery not possible Adjuvant chemoradiotherapy indicated for GE or lower esophageal ADC tumors	27
Regional (III)	28	Surgery if possible (e.g., T3 N0 lesions) Definitive chemoradiotherapy Neoadjuvant chemoradiotherapy followed by surgery Adjuvant chemoradiotherapy indicated for GE or lower esophageal ADC tumors	13
Distant (IV)	25	Best supportive care/palliation *Local:* Radiation therapy or brachytherapy Intraluminal intubation or dilatation Laser or endocoagulation Photodynamic therapy *Chemotherapy:* Cisplatin 100 mg/m^2 i.v. d 1 q21d 5-FU 1,000 mg/m^2 i.v. d 1–5 continuous q21d treatment until progression or intolerable toxicity Or Epirubicin 50 mg/m^2 i.v. d 1 q21d Cisplatin 60 mg/m^2 i.v. d 1 q21d 5-FU 200 mg/m^2/d i.v. continuous infusion treatment for maximum of 6 mo	2

ADC, adenocarcinoma; GE, gastroesophageal; 5-FU, 5-fluorouracil.

FOLLOW-UP FOR PATIENTS WITH LOCOREGIONAL DISEASE

There is no standard surveillance scheme.

- History and physical examination, complete blood count (CBC), urea, electrolytes, and liver function tests are recommended every 4 months for 1 year, every 6 months for 2 years, and then annually (www.nccn.org).
- Chest radiograph should be obtained as indicated.
- CT scans of the chest/abdomen should be obtained as clinically indicated.
- Upper gastrointestinal endoscopy should be performed as clinically indicated.

REFERENCES

1. Day NE, Varghese C. Oesophageal cancer. *Cancer Surv* 1994;19220:43–54.
2. Jemal A, Murray T, Samuels A, et al. Cancer Statistics, 2003. *CA Cancer J Clin* 2003;53:5–26.
3. American Joint Committee on Cancer. *Cancer staging manual*, 6th ed. New York: Springer-Verlag, 2002:91–98.
4. Stein HJ, Feith M, Siewert JR. Cancer of the esophagogastric junction. *Surg Oncol* 2000;9:35–41.
5. Kelly S, Harris KM, Berry E, et al. A systematic review of the staging performance of endoscopic ultrasound in gastro-oesophageal carcinoma. *Gut* 2001;49:534–539.

6. Flamen P, Lerut A, Cutsem Van, et al. Utility of positron emission tomography for the staging of patients with potentially operable esophageal carcinoma. *J Clin Oncol* 2000;18:3202–3210.
7. Daly JM, Karnell LH, Menck HR. National cancer database report on esophageal carcinoma. *Cancer* 1996;78:1820–1828.
8. Sagar PM, Gauperaa T, Sue-Ling H, et al. An audit of the treatment of cancer of the esophagus. *Gut* 1994;35:941–945.
9. Cooper JS, Guo MD, Herskovic A, et al. Chemoradiotherapy of locally advanced esophageal cancer long-term follow-up of a prospective randomized trial (RTOG 85-01). *JAMA* 1999;281:1623–1627.
10. Rebecca WO, Richard MA, Combined chemotherapy and radiotherapy (without surgery) compared with radiotherapy alone in localized carcinoma of the esophagus. *Cochrane Database Syst Rev* 2003;(1):CD002092.
11. Leonard GD, McCaffrey JA, Maher M. Optimal therapy for esophageal cancer. *Cancer Treat Rev* 2003;29:275–282.
12. Stahl M, Wilke MK, Walz S, et al. Randomized phase III trial in locally advanced squamous cell carcinoma (SCC) of the esophagus: chemoradiation with and without surgery. *Proc Am Soc Clin Oncol* 2003;22:250 (abstract 1001).
13. Bedenne L, Michel P, Bouche O, et al. Randomized phase III trial in locally advanced esophageal cancer: radiochemotherapy alone (FFCD 9102). *Proc Am Soc Clin Oncol* 2002;21:130a (abstract 519).
14. Leichman L, Steiger Z, Seydel HG, et al. Preoperative chemotherapy and radiation therapy for patients with cancer of the esophagus: a potentially curative approach. *J Clin Oncol.* 1984;2:15–79.
15. Walsh TN, Nooman N, Hollywood D, et al. A comparison of multimodal therapy and surgery for esophageal adenocarcinoma. *N Engl J Med.* 1996;335:462–467.
16. Nygaard K, Hagen S, Hansen HS, et al. Pre-operative radiotherapy prolongs survival in operable esophageal carcinoma: a randomised multicenter study of pre-operative radiotherapy and chemotherapy: the second Scandinavian trial in esophageal cancer. *World J Sun* 1992;16:1104–1110.
17. Apinop C, Puttisak P, Precha N. A prospective study of combined therapy in esophageal cancer. *Hepatogastroenterology* 1994;41:391–393.
18. Leprise E, Etienne PL, Meunier B, et al. A randomised study of chemotherapy, radiation therapy, anti-surgery vs surgery for localised squamous cell carcinoma of the esophagus. *Cancer* 1994;73:1779–1784.
19. Bosset JF, Gignoux M, Triboulet JP, et al. Chemoradiotherapy followed by surgery compared with surgery alone in squamous cell cancer of the esophagus. *N Engl J Med* 1997;337:161–167.
20. Urba S, Orringer M, Turrisi JP, et al. Randomised trial of peroperative chemoradiation versus surgery alone in patients with locoregional esophageal carcinom. *J Clin Oncol* 2001;19:305–313.
21. Burmeister BH, Smithers B, Fitzgerald L, et al. A randomized phases III trial of preoperative chemoradiation followed by surgery (CR-S) versus surgery alone(S) for localized resectable cancer of the esophagus. *Proc Am Soc Clin Oncol* 2002;21:130a (abstract 518).
22. Lee JL, Kim SB, Jung HY. A single institutional phase III trial of preoperative chemotherapy with hyperfractionation radiotherapy plus surgery (CRT-S) versus surgery(S) alone for stage II, III resectable esophageal squamous cell carcinoma (SCC): An interim analysis. *Proc Am Soc Clin Oncol* 2003;23:260 (abstr 1043).
23. MacDonald JS, Smalley SR, Benedetti J, et al. Chemoradiotherapy after surgery compared with surgery alone for adenocarcinoma of the stomach or gastroesophageal junction. *N Engl J Med* 2001;345:725–730.
24. Kelsen D, Ginsberg R, Pajak TF, et al. Chemotherapy followed by surgery compared with surgery alone for localized esophageal cancer. *N Engl J Med* 1998;339:1979–1984.
25. Medical Research Council Oesophageal Cancer Working Party. Surgical resection with or without preoperative chemotherapy in oesophageal cancer: a randomised controlled trial. *Lancet* 2002; 359:1727–1733.
26. Bleiberg H, Conroy T, Paillot B, et al. Randomized phase II study of cisplatin and 5-fluororuacil (5-FU) versus cisplatin alone in advanced squamous cell oesophageal cancer. *Eur J Cancer* 1997;33:1216–1220.
27. Webb A, Cunningham D, Scarffe JH, et al. A randomised trial comparing ECF with FAMTX in advanced esophagogastric cancer. *J Clin Oncol* 1997;15:261–267.
28. Ajani JA, Van Cutsem E, Moiseyenko S, et al. Docetaxel (D), cisplatin, 5-fluorouracil compare to cis-platin (C) and 5-fluorouracil (F) for chemotherapy-naïve patients with metastatic or locally recurrent, unresectable gastric carcinoma (MGC): interim results of a randomized phase III trial (V325). *Proc Am Soc Clin Oncol* 2003;22:249 (abstract 999).
29. Allum W, Cunningham D, Weeden S. Perioperative chemotherapy in operable gastric and lower oesophageal cancer: a randomised, controlled trial (the MAGIC trial, ISRCTN 93793971). *Proc Am Soc Clin Oncol* 2003;22:249 (abstract 998).

5

Gastric Cancer

M. Wasif Saif

University of Alabama at Birmingham, Birmingham, Alabama

EPIDEMIOLOGY

Worldwide, gastric carcinoma represents the second or third most common malignancy. The frequency of occurrence of gastric carcinoma at different sites within the stomach has changed in the United States over recent decades. Cancer of the distal half of the stomach has been decreasing in the United States since the 1930s. However, over the last two decades, the incidence of cancer of the cardia and gastroesophageal junction has been rapidly rising. The incidence of this cancer has increased dramatically, especially in patients younger than 40 years. An estimated 22,400 new cases and 12,100 deaths from gastric carcinoma were expected in the United States in 2003.

RISK FACTORS

- Age at onset: fifth decade
- Male-to-female ratio is 1.67:1.0
- African American–to–white ratio is 1.5:1
- Precursor conditions include chronic atrophic gastritis and intestinal metaplasia, pernicious anemia (10% to 20% incidence), partial gastrectomy for benign disease, *Helicobacter pylori* infection (especially childhood exposure—three- to fivefold increase), Ménétrier disease, and gastric adenomatous polyps. These precursor lesions are largely linked to distal (intestinal type) gastric carcinoma.
- Family history: first degree (two- to threefold); the family of Napoleon Bonaparte is an example; familial clustering; patients with hereditary nonpolyposis colorectal cancer (Lynch syndrome II) are at increased risk; recently, germline mutations of E-cadherin have been linked to the rare entity of familial diffuse gastric cancer.
- Tobacco use results in a 1.5 to threefold increased risk for cancer.
- Fermenting and smoking of food results in high salt and nitrosamines content.
- Deficiencies of vitamins A, C, and E; β-carotene; selenium; and fiber are risk factors for cancer.
- Blood type A
- Alcohol
- The marked rise in the incidence of gastroesophageal and proximal gastric adenocarcinoma appears to be strongly correlated to the rising incidence of Barrett esophagus.

PATHOPHYSIOLOGY

Most gastric cancers are adenocarcinomas (more than 90%) of two distinct histologic types: intestinal and diffuse. The other gastric cancers are predominantly non-Hodgkin lymphomas or leiomyosarcomas. Differentiating between adenocarcinoma and lymphoma is critical because the prognosis and treatment for these two entities differ considerably.

Intestinal Type

The "epidemic" form of cancer is further differentiated by gland formation and is associated with precancerous lesions, gastric atrophy, and intestinal metaplasia. The intestinal form accounts for most distal cancers and is stable or its incidence is declining. These cancers in particular are associated with *H. pylori* infection, as proposed by Correa. In this carcinogenesis model, the interplay of environmental factors leads to glandular atrophy, relative achlorhydria, and increased gastric pH. This results in bacterial overgrowth, and *H. pylori* and bacteria produce nitrites and nitroso compounds causing further development of gastric atrophy and intestinal metaplasia, thereby increasing the risk of cancer.

This form is more common in areas of the world where gastric carcinoma is endemic. The recent decline in gastric carcinoma in the United States is likely the result of a decline in the incidence of intestinal type lesions.

Intestinal type lesions are associated with an increased frequency of overexpression of epidermal growth-factor receptor, *erbB-2* and *erbB-3*.

Diffuse Type

The "endemic" form of carcinoma is more common in younger patients and exhibits an undifferentiated signet-ring histology. There is a predilection for submucosal spread because of lack of cell cohesion, leading to linitis plastica. Contiguous spread of the carcinoma to the peritoneum is common. Precancerous lesions have not been identified, and a carcinogenesis model has not been proposed although it is also associated with *H. pylori* infection. Genetic predispositions to endemic forms of carcinoma have been reported, as have associations between carcinoma and individuals with type A blood. These cancers occur in the proximal stomach where increased incidence has been observed worldwide; stage for stage, these cancers have a worse prognosis than do distal cancers.

Diffuse lesions have been linked to abnormalities of fibroblast growth-factor systems, including the *K-sam* oncogene (see Fig. 5.1).

Molecular Analysis

- loss of heterozygosity of chromosomes 5q or APC gene (deleted in 34% of gastric cancers), 17p, and 18q (DCC gene)
- microsatellite instability, particularly, of transforming growth factor-ß (TGF ß) type II receptor, with subsequent growth-inhibition deregulation
- p53 is mutated in approximately 40% to 60% cases by allelic loss and base transition mutations
- reduced E-cadherin expression, a cell adhesion mediator, is observed in diffuse-type undifferentiated cancers
- *Her2/neu* and *erbB-2/erbB-3* (epidermal growth factors) are overexpressed, especially in intestinal forms
- Epstein–Barr viral genomes are detected
- *ras* mutations are rarely reported, in contrast to other gastrointestinal cancers.

DIAGNOSIS

Gastric carcinoma, when superficial and surgically curable, typically produces no symptoms. Among 18,365 patients analyzed by the American College of Surgeons, patients presented with the following symptoms:

- weight loss (62%)
- abdominal pain (52%)

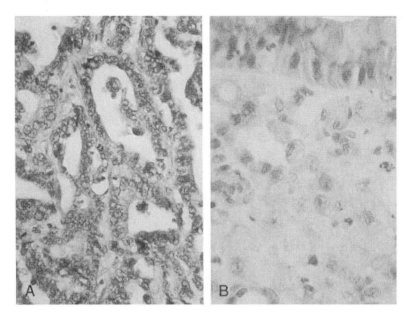

FIG. 5.1. Two histological types of gastric adenocarcinoma. **A:** Intestinal **B:** Diffuse.

- nausea (34%)
- anorexia (32%)
- dysphagia (26%)
- melena (20%)
- early satiety (18%)
- ulcer-type pain (17%) and
- lower extremity edema (6%).

Clinical findings at presentation may demonstrate the following symptoms:

- anemia (42%)
- hypoproteinemia (26%)
- abnormal liver functions (26%)
- fecal occult blood (40%).

Gastric carcinomas spread by direct extension, invading into adjacent structures. The disease may also spread by lymphatic vessels:

- to intra-abdominal nodes and left supraclavicular nodes (Virchow node)
- along peritoneal surfaces, resulting in a periumbilical nodule (Sister Mary Joseph node, named after the nurse in the operating room of Mayo Clinic, or "periumbilical lymph nodes," which form as tumor spreads along the falciform ligament to subcutaneous sites)
- to Irish node, a left anterior axillary lymph node resulting from the spread of proximal primary cancer to lower esophageal and intrathoracic lymphatics
- to enlarged ovary (Krukenberg tumor; ovarian metastases)
- to a mass in the cul-de-sac (Blumer shelf), which is palpable on rectal examination or
- to frank peritoneal carcinomatosis and malignant ascites.

The liver is the most common site of hematogenous dissemination, although pulmonary metastases are also seen.

Paraneoplastic Syndromes

Skin syndromes:

- Acanthosis nigricans
- Dermatomyositis
- Circinate erythemas
- Pemphigoid
- Seborrheic keratoses: Leser–Trélat sign, acute onset.

Central nervous system (CNS) syndromes:

- Dementia
- Cerebellar ataxia.

Miscellaneous syndromes:

- Thrombophlebitis
- Microangiopathic hemolytic anemia
- Membranous nephropathy.

Tumor Markers

- Carcinoembryonic antigen (CEA) is elevated in 40% to 50% of cases, useful in follow-up but not for screening
- α-Fetoprotein and CA 19-9 are elevated in 30% of patients with gastric cancer
- Medically refractory persistent peptic ulcer may prompt barium or endoscopic evaluation.

Endoscopic Findings

- Initial upper gastrointestinal endoscopy and double-contrast barium swallow identify suggestive lesions and have diagnostic accuracy of 95% and 75%, respectively.
- Computerized tomographic scanning is then useful for assessing local extension, lymph node involvement, and presence of metastasis, although understaging occurs in most cases.
- Endoscopic ultrasonography assesses the depth of tumor invasion and lymph node status with 80% accuracy, supplementing preoperative evaluations.

STAGING

The American Joint Committee on Cancer (AJCC) has designated staging by TNM classification (see Table 5.1).

PROGNOSIS

a. Pathological staging remains the most important determinant of prognosis.
b. Other prognostic variables that have been reported to be associated with an unfavorable outcome include:
   - older age
   - location of tumor (see Table 5.2)
   - weight loss greater than 10%
   - diffuse versus intestinal histology (5-year survival after resection, 16% versus 26%, respectively)

TABLE 5.1. *TNM classification of cancer staging designated by the American Joint Committee on Cancer (AJCC)*

Primary Tumor
Tis: Carcinoma *in situ*
T1: Invasion of lamina propria or submucosa
T2: Invasion of muscularis propria
T3: Invasion of serosa
T4: Invasion of adjacent structures

Lymph Node Status
N0: No regional lymph node involvement
N1: Metastases to 1 to 6 regional lymph nodes
N2: Metastases to 7 to 15 regional lymph nodes
N3: Metastases to more than 15 regional lymph nodes

Metastatic Disease
M0: No distant metastases
M1: Distant metastases present

Stage

0	Tis	N0	M0
IA	T1	N0	M0
IB	T1	N1	M0
	T2	N0	M0
II	T1	N2	M0
	T2	N1	M0
	T3	N0	M0
IIIA	T2	N2	M0
	T3	N1	M0
	T4	N0	M0
IIIB	T3	N2	M0
IV	T4	N1–3	M0
	T1–3	N3	M0
	T1–4	N0–2	M1

Two-thirds of patients are first seen with stage III or IV disease. Lymphadenectomy should contain at least 15 lymph nodes for proper staging.

- high-grade or undifferentiated tumors
- four or more lymph nodes involved
- aneuploid tumors
- elevations in epidermal growth factor or P-glycoprotein level
- overexpression of thymidylate synthase
- overexpression of ERCC1, p53, and Her-2
- loss of p21 and p27.

TABLE 5.2. *Five-year survival with respect to location of tumor*

Site	5-yr survival after surgical resection (%)
Proximal stomach	10
Distal stomach	25
Entire stomach	5

MANAGEMENT OF GASTRIC CANCER

Standard of Care

Although surgical resection remains the cornerstone of gastric cancer treatment, the optimal extent of nodal resection remains controversial, with randomized studies failing to show that the D2 procedure improves survival when compared with D1 dissection. The high rate of recurrence and poor survival of patients following surgery provides a rationale for the early use of adjuvant treatment. Adjuvant chemotherapy or adjuvant radiotherapy, when used alone, does not improve survival following resection. However, the results of the Intergroup 0116 study are promising in showing that the combination of 5-fluorouracil (5-FU)–based chemotherapy with radiotherapy significantly prolongs disease-free and overall survival when compared to no adjuvant treatment. In advanced gastric cancer, chemotherapy enhances quality of life and prolongs survival when compared with the best supportive care. There is no agreed standard of treatment in this setting. Of the commonly used regimens, epirubicin plus cisplatin and 5-FU (ECF) probably has the strongest claim to this role. However, there is a pressing need for assessing new agents, both cytotoxic and molecularly targeted, in both the advanced and adjuvant settings.

Surgery

Although complete surgical resection of the tumor and adjacent lymph nodes remains the only chance for cure, up to 80% of gastric cancer in patients in the United States is advanced at diagnosis. Surgical extirpation of gastric cancer is indicated in patients with stages I, II, and III disease, with minimal lymph node involvement. Tumor size and location dictate the type of surgical procedure to be used (Table 5.2).

Current issues are:

a. subtotal versus total gastrectomy
b. extended lymphadenectomy
c. prophylactic splenectomy.

Subtotal versus Total Gastrectomy

- Subtotal gastrectomy (SG) may be performed in case of proximal cardia or distal lesions, provided that the fundus or cardioesophageal junction is not involved.
- Proximal gastrectomy is associated with increased postoperative complications, mortality, and quality-of-life decrement, necessitating thorough consideration of complete gastric resection.
- Total gastrectomy (TG) is more appropriate if tumor involvement is diffuse and arises in the body of the stomach, with extension to within 6 cm of the cardia (see Figs. 5.2 and 5.3).

Extended Lymph Node Dissection

The regional lymph nodes include N1 and N2 lymph node groups (lesser and greater curvature of perigastric, left gastric, common hepatic, splenic, and celiac axis nodes). D2 lymphadenectomy involves more extensive N2 lymph-node–group resection and is reported to improve survival in patients with T1, T2, and some serosa-involved T3 lesions. Factors such as operative time, hospitalization length, and transfusion requirements, and thus morbidity, are all increased. The greatest benefit of extended lymph node dissection (ELD) may occur in early gastric cancer lesions with small tumors and superficial mucosal involvement because up to 20% of such lesions have occult lymph node involvement. The routine use of D2 lymphadenectomy continues to be studied.

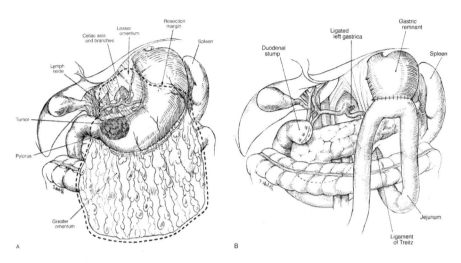

FIG. 5.2. (A and B) Subtotal gastrectomy (SG).

Prophylactic Splenectomy

Routine splenectomy for tumors that do not adhere to or invade the spleen is not beneficial. *Palliative surgery* is considered in patients with obstruction, bleeding, or pain, and despite operative mortalities of 25% to 50%, the results from the gastrojejunostomy bypass surgery alone indicate a twofold increase in mean survival. The selection of patients most likely to benefit from this palliative effort requires further evaluation.

Radiation Therapy

- Gastric carcinoma is relatively resistant to radiotherapy; consequently, for patients with locally recurrent or metastatic disease, moderate doses of external-beam irradiation are used only to palliate symptoms and not to improve survival.
- Local or regional recurrence in the gastric or tumor bed, the anastomosis, or regional lymph nodes occur in 40% to 65% of patients after gastric resection with curative intent (see Table 5.3). The frequency of such relapses makes regional radiation an attractive possibility for adjuvant therapy. This modality is limited by the technical challenges inherent in abdominal irradiation, optimal definition of fields, and the generally diminished performance status, in particular, nutritional state, of potential candidates.

TABLE 5.3. *Failure areas following surgery*

Failure area	MGH clinical (130) no. (%)	MINN reoperation (105) no. (%)	MCNEER autopsy (92) no. (%)
Gastric bed	27 (21%)	58 (55%)	48 (52%)
Anastomosis or stump	33 (25%)	28 (27%)	55 (60%)
Lymph nodes	11 (8%)	45 (43%)	48 (52%)

no., total number of patients; MGH, Mass achusetts general hospital; MINN, Minnesota; MCNEER, Massey Cancer Center.

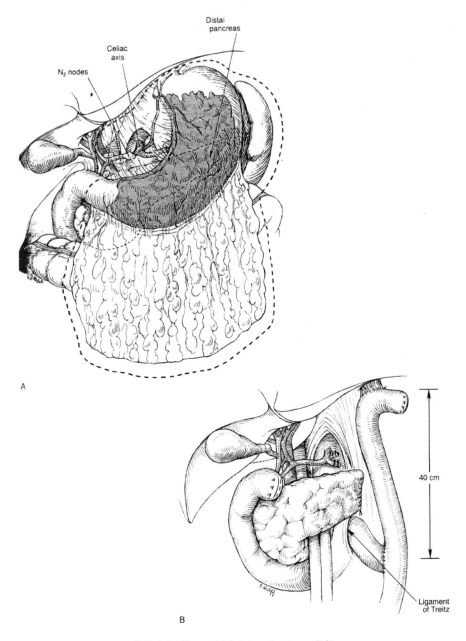

Distal
pancreas

Celiac
axis

N₂ nodes

A

40 cm

Ligament
of Treitz

B

FIG. 5.3. (A and B) Total gastrectomy (TG).

- Serial studies of the Gastrointestinal Tumor Study Group (GITSG) of patients with locally unresectable pancreatic and gastric adenocarcinoma have shown that combined-modality therapy is superior to either optimal radiotherapy or chemotherapy alone. On the basis of this concept, combined chemoradiation typically in combination with 5-FU chemotherapy has been evaluated both in the neoadjuvant and the adjuvant settings.
- Palliative radiation is important in managing pain, obstructions, and bleeding.
- Investigators at the National Cancer Institute randomized 60 patients who underwent curative resection to either receive intraoperative radiotherapy (IORT) or not receive IORT. IORT failed to afford a benefit over conventional therapy in overall survival.

Adjuvant Chemoradiotherapy

- In 1993, a meta-analysis of 11 randomized, controlled trials concluded that postoperative chemotherapy offered no significant survival benefit beyond that associated with curative resection. However, this meta-analysis was later criticized for lacking sufficient power to detect a difference and for its choice of trials. There have been several randomized trials published since the meta-analysis of Hermans et al. Earle and Maroun recently conducted another meta-analysis of all studies through 1999. A small survival benefit was noted for patients randomized to adjuvant therapy [relative risk = 0.94; 95% confidence interval (CI), 0.89 to 1.00].
- A prospective randomized trial from the British Stomach Cancer Group failed to demonstrate a survival benefit for postoperative adjuvant radiation alone, although locoregional failures had decreased from 27% to 10.6%.
- Adjuvant external-beam radiation therapy with combined chemotherapy has been evaluated in the United States. In a phase III intergroup trial (INT-0166), 556 patients with completely resected stage IB to stage IV M0 adenocarcinoma of the stomach and gastroesophageal junction were randomized to receive surgery alone or surgery plus postoperative chemotherapy (5-FU and leucovorin) and concurrent radiation therapy (45 Gy). A significant survival benefit has been reported for adjuvant combined-modality therapy with 5-year median follow-up. Median survival was 36 months for the adjuvant chemoradiation group as compared to 27 months for the surgery alone arm ($P = 0.005$). Three-year overall survival and relapse-free survival were 50% and 48%, respectively, for adjuvant chemoradiation and 41% and 31%, respectively, for surgery alone ($P = 0.005$).

Neoadjuvant Chemoradiotherapy

The available data on the role of neoadjuvant preoperative therapy are not yet conclusive. Although neoadjuvant therapy may reduce the tumor mass in many patients, several randomized, controlled trials have shown that, compared with primary resection, a multimodal approach does not result in a survival benefit in patients with locoregional, that is, potentially resectable, tumors. In contrast, in patients with locally advanced tumors (i.e., patients in whom complete tumor removal with primary surgery seems unlikely), neoadjuvant therapy increases the likelihood of complete tumor resection on subsequent surgery. However, only those patients with objective histopathologic response to preoperative therapy seem to benefit from this approach.

Chemotherapy

The most commonly administered chemotherapeutic agents with objective response rates in gastric cancer include 5-FU, doxorubicin, cisplatin, methotrexate, mitomycin, etoposide, and doxorubicin.

TABLE 5.4. *Chemotherapy versus best supportive care (BSC)*

Regimen	Patients	Survival BSC (mo)	Survival chemo (mo)
FAMTX	36	3	12
FAMTX	40	3	10
ELF	37	3	7.5+
ELF	18	4	10

BSC, best supportive care; FAMTX, fluorouracil, doxorubicin, and methotrexate; ELF, etoposide, fluorouracil, and leucovorin.

Chemotherapy versus Best Supportive Care

Four studies have randomized patients with metastatic gastric cancer to either combination chemotherapy or best supportive care (BSC). Two studies used fluorouracil, doxorubicin, and methotrexate (FAMTX) and two studies used etoposide, fluorouracil, and leucovorin (ELF) as the primary chemotherapeutic agents. In all four studies, a significant survival benefit was noted for patients randomized to chemotherapy (see Table 5.4).

Single Agents versus Combination Regimens

Single Agents

Monotherapy with single agents results in 15% to 20% response rates. 5-FU is the most extensively studied, producing a 20% response rate. In addition, mitomycin-C (MMC), adriamycin, and carmustine (BCNU) have shown similar results. More recent studies using well-defined response criteria, have, however, failed to produce such results, showing response rates of less than 10% for 5-FU and adriamycin. Cisplatin has been used recently and has shown promising results in more than one study. Complete responses with single agents are, however, rare, and partial regressions are relatively brief. Newer agents being investigated include taxotere, taxol, oxaliplatin, irinotecan, and oral forms of 5-FU (see Table 5.5).

Combination Chemotherapy

Better understanding of the pharmacology of many chemotherapeutic agents, including 5-FU, the main drug used in advanced gastric cancer, has led to the development of combination regimens. Various combinations of active agents have been reported to improve the response rate among patients with advanced gastric carcinoma, approaching 30% to 60%. However, the

TABLE 5.5. *Single-agent chemotherapy in advanced gastric cancer*

Drug	n patients	RR (%)
5-FU	392	21
MMC	211	30
Cisplatin	36	22
CCNU	37	8
MTX	28	11
Adriamycin	68	25
BCNU	23	17

RR, response rate; 5-FU, 5-fluorouracil; MMC, mitomycin-C; CCNU, 1-(2-chloroethyl)-3-cyclohexyl-1-nitrosourea; MTX, methotrexate; BCNU, adriamycin, and carmustine.

TABLE 5.6. *Combination regimens*

Drugs	No. of patients	RR (%)	MS	Comment
FAM	656	30	12.5 mo	Until recently, was the most widely prescribed regimen
FAMe	141	28	—	—
FAP	234	34	30 wk	Significant toxicity
EAP	197	46	10–17 mo	Benefits patients with *more locally advanced disease* but is less beneficial in patients with peritoneal carcinomatosis and other M1 disease Treatment-related deaths in 10% of patients
FAMTX	364	41	7–10 mo	12% complete responders
ELF	>100	9–48	10 mo	Useful in *elderly and renally impaired patients*
Taxotere/CDDP	47	53	9 mo	Despite hematologic toxicity, overall well-tolerated
CDDP/CPT-11	44	48	9 mo	Active against both gastric and GEJX
	25	51		—
ECF	135	45	8.7 m	1-yr survival: 36%
MLP-F		82	16 m	33% complete responders The percentage of complete responders was influenced by supplemental local therapies (i.e., radiation to 50%)

RR, response rate; MS, median survival; FAM, fluorouracil, doxorubicin, mitomycin-C; FAMe, 5-FU, doxorubicin, and semustine; FAP, 5-FU, doxorubicin, and cisplatin; EAP, Etoposide, doxorubicin, cisplatin; FAMTX, fluorouracil, doxorubicin, and methotrexate; ELF, etoposide, fluorouracil, and leucovorin; CDDP, cisplatin; CPT-11, irinotecan; ECF, epirubicin plus cisplatin and 5-FU; MLP-F, Methotrexate, Leucovorin, 5-Fu and cisplatin.

North Central Cancer Treatment Group (NCCTG) observed *no difference in overall survival* among 252 patients randomized to receive 5-FU, doxorubicin, and semustine (methyl-CCNU) (FAMe); 5-FU, doxorubicin, and cisplatin (FAP); or 5-FU alone.

Most commonly used combination regimens include FAM (fluorouracil, doxorubicin, mitomycin-C), FAP, ECF, ELF, FLAP (fluorouracil, leucovorin, doxorubicin, cisplatin), PELF (cisplatin, epidoxorubicin, leucovorin, fluorouracil with glutathione and filgrastim), FAMTX, and FUP (fluorouracil, cisplatin) (Tables 5.6, 5.7, and 5.8).

TABLE 5.7. *Randomized studies in advanced gastric cancer using second-generation regimens*

	n patients	RR (%)	MS
FAMTX vs. FAM	213	41 vs. [a]	42 wk vs. 29 wk[a]
PELF vs. FAM	147	43 vs. 15[a]	35 wk vs. 23 wk
FAMTX vs. EAP	60	33 vs. 20	7.3 mo vs. 6.1 mo
ECF vs. FAMTX	274	45 vs. 21[a]	8.9 mo vs. 5.7 mo[a]

RR, response rate; MS, median survival; FAMTX, fluorouracil, doxorubicin, and methotrexate; FAM, fluorouracil, doxorubicin, mitomycin-C; PELF, cisplatin, epidoxorubicin, leucovorin, fluorouracil with glutathione and filgrastim; ECF, epirubicin plus cisplatin and 5-FU.
[a]Difference is statistically significant.

TABLE 5.8. *Regimens and doses of agents*

Drug combinations	Doses in mg/m^2/schedule	RR/CR
FAMTX		
Methotrexate	1,500 d1, h0	30%–70%/12%
Leucovorin	15 PO q6 × 8, starting h0	
5-FU	1,500 d1, h1	
Doxorubicin	30 d15	
ELF		
Leucovorin	300 d1–3	48%/12%
Etoposide	120 d1–3	
5-FU	500 d1–3	
CPT-11/CDDP		
CPT-11	60 d1, 8, 15, 22	30%–40%
CDDP	25–30 d1, 8, 15, 22	
ECF		
Epirubicin	50 d1	37%–45%/17%
CDDP	60 d1	
5-FU	200 qd by continuous i.v. × 21 wk	

RR, response rate; CR, complete remission.

Newer Agents

Newer chemotherapeutic agents, including irinotecan, gemcitabine, oxaliplatin, and taxanes, show promising activity and are currently being tested in phase III trials.

Taxotere has already been investigated in two phase II clinical trials. In the European trial, a 24% response rate was reported in a series of 33 patients with advanced gastric cancer. It is interesting that patients who had their primary tumor removed responded better than those patients who did not. In a Japanese study, 20% of patients who showed no response to previous chemotherapy had a partial response to 60 mg per m^2 of 3- or 4-weekly doses of taxotere. Docetaxel has also been shown to lack cross-resistance with other drugs in the treatment of gastric cancer and is likely to be at least additive to cisplatin and 5-FU. Phase II results of docetaxel–cisplatin has yielded response rates similar to those achieved by ECF and PELF. Adding 5-FU to docetaxel–cisplatin has achieved an objective response rate (ORR) of 52% versus 45% for docetaxel–cisplatin alone in a randomized phase II trial. Docetaxel-based regimens demonstrate acceptable tolerability despite predictable hematotoxicity. Neutropenia, the major toxicity, is manageable by dose modification or by using prophylactic granulocyte colony stimulating factor. Several phase III trials are now ongoing, including a large-scale trial of docetaxel–cisplatin–5-FU versus cisplatin–5-FU.

Irinotecan (CPT-11) has also been used alone or in combination with cisplatin in phase I–II clinical studies. Response rates of 23% and 41%, respectively, with acceptable toxicity were reported. In the first study, objective responses were observed in 20% of pretreated patients (mostly with 5-FU).

Using *Capecitabine (Xeloda)* instead of 5-FU in combination regimen is also under evaluation in randomized trials.

S-1 is a novel oral fluoropyrimidine derivative composed of tegafur (5-FU prodrug), 5-chloro-2,4-dihydroxypyridine (inhibitor of 5-FU degradation), and potassium oxonate (inhibitor of gastrointestinal toxicities). A phase II trial has revealed a response rate of 53.6%, whereas a retrospective study showed an overall response rate of 32% (44% of patients were chemo naïve).

Use of Stents

The *use of plastic and expansile metal stents* has been associated with successful palliation of obstructive symptoms in more than 85% of patients with tumors in the gastroesophagus and in the cardia.

TREATMENT OF GASTRIC CANCER ACCORDING TO STAGE

Stage 0 Gastric Cancer

Stage 0 indicates gastric cancer confined to the mucosa. On the basis of experience in Japan, where stage 0 is diagnosed frequently, it has been found that more than 90% of patients treated by gastrectomy with lymphadenectomy will survive beyond 5 years. An American series has confirmed these findings.

Stage I Gastric Cancer

a. One of the following surgical procedures is recommended for stage I gastric cancer:
  - distal SG (if the lesion is not in the fundus or at the cardioesophageal junction)
  - proximal SG or TG, with distal esophagectomy (if the lesion involves the cardia), of the tumors that often involve the submucosal lymphatics of the esophagus
  - TG (if the tumor involves the stomach diffusely or arises in the body of the stomach and extends to within 6 cm of the cardia or distal antrum)
  - regional lymphadenectomy, which is recommended with all of the previously noted procedures
  - splenectomy, which is not routinely performed.
b. Postoperative chemoradiotherapy is recommended for patients with node-positive (T1 N1) and muscle-invasive (T2 N0) disease.
c. Neoadjuvant chemoradiotherapy is under clinical evaluation.

Stage II Gastric Cancer

a. One of the following surgical procedures is recommended for stage II gastric cancer:
  - distal SG (if the lesion is not in the fundus or at the cardioesophageal junction)
  - proximal SG or TG (if the lesion involves the cardia)
  - TG (if the tumor involves the stomach diffusely or arises in the body of the stomach and extends to within 6 cm of the cardia)
  - regional lymphadenectomy is recommended with all of the above procedures
  - splenectomy is not routinely performed.
b. Postoperative chemoradiotherapy is also recommended.
c. Neoadjuvant chemoradiotherapy is under clinical evaluation.

Stage III Gastric Cancer

a. Radical surgery: Curative resection procedures are confined to patients who do not have extensive nodal involvement at the time of surgical exploration.
b. Postoperative chemoradiotherapy is also recommended.
c. Neoadjuvant chemoradiotherapy is under clinical evaluation.

Stage IV Gastric Cancer

Patients with No Distant Metastases (M0)

- Radical surgery is performed if possible, followed by postoperative chemoradiation.
- Neoadjuvant chemoradiation therapy is under clinical evaluation.

Patients with Distant Metastases (M1)

All newly diagnosed patients with hematogenous or peritoneal metastases should be considered as candidates for clinical trials if possible. In some patients, chemotherapy may provide substantial palliative benefit and occasional durable remission, although it does not prolong life or provide a cure.

INTRAPERITONEAL SPREAD

In approximately 50% of patients with advanced gastric cancer, the disease recurs locally or at an intraperitoneal site, and this recurrence has a negative effect on survival. Investigators have reported their experience with systemic and intraperitoneal (IP) 5-FU and cisplatin in conjunction with R0 resection of high-risk gastric cancer. Thirty-four patients (17 male and 17 female; median age 59 years, range 26 to 77 years) received an R0 resection (18 patients received SG, 2 patients received proximal gastrectomy, and 14 received TG) and adjuvant IV or IP 5-FU or cisplatin for histologically confirmed T2–4 N0–3 gastric adenocarcinoma at Memorial Sloan-Kettering Cancer Center. Patients who received radiation therapy or preoperative chemotherapy were excluded. A case-matched analysis of these 32 patients and 170 randomly selected matched controls was performed. The control group was chosen from a pool of 614 patients who underwent resection alone between 1985 and 1997, excluding those patients who had M1 disease or preoperative chemotherapy. A 5:1 match ratio was used to select patients by sex, T staging, and N staging. At a median follow-up of 131 months for survivors, the median survival was found to be 25 months in the IP group versus 26 months for the matched-control group. five- and 10-year actuarial survival was 37% and 37% for the IP group versus 30% and 18% for the matched controls. None of these findings were statistically significant. The recurrence rate was 61% in the IP chemotherapy group, with 66% occurring locally or at an intraperitoneal site, which was not better than the matched controls. All patients were evaluated for toxicity, and there was one death from cardiac arrest during IP chemotherapy treatment. Acute grade III or IV toxicity was observed in 14 (44%) patients, consisting of nausea or vomiting, diarrhea, and hematologic toxicity, but all the toxic responses resolved. It was concluded that adjuvant IP 5-FU and cisplatin can be delivered with low mortality and significant morbidity. This regimen did not alter survival or alter the pattern of recurrence. Better agents are needed to improve the efficacy of this mode of therapy. Patients at higher risk, with serosal involvement or contiguous structure invasion, can also receive prophylaxis with continuous hyperthermic peritoneal perfusion (CHPP) perioperatively.

POSTSURGICAL FOLLOW-UP

- Follow-up in patients following complete surgical resection should include clinic visits, with liver function tests and CEA measurements being performed.
- A chest radiograph is also warranted.
- Intervals of every 3 months for the first 2 years, then every 6 months for 3 years, and then every year have been suggested.
- If TG is not performed, yearly upper endoscopy is dictated by a 1% to 2% incidence of second primary tumors.
- Vitamin B_{12} deficiency develops in most TG patients and 20% of SG patients, typically within 4 to 10 years. Vitamin B_{12} supplementation is administered at 1,000 µg intramuscularly every month.

SCREENING

In most countries, screening of the general populations is not practical because of low incidence of gastric cancer. However, screening is worthwhile in Japan where the incidence of gastric cancer is high. Japanese screening guidelines include initial upper endoscopy at age 50, with follow-up endoscopy for abnormalities. No such guidelines are available in the United States.

PRIMARY GASTRIC LYMPHOMA

Epidemiology and Pathology

Primary gastric lymphoma (PGL) is an uncommon malignancy that is increasing in incidence and represents approximately 2% to 7% of primary gastric malignancies. In the United States, there will be an estimated 22,400 cases of gastric malignancy per year, which indicates that an estimated 448 to 1,568 new cases of gastric lymphoma would have occurred in 1997. The incidence of PGL has been increasing over the last 20 years without any clear explanation. Incidence of PGL increases with age, with a peak in the sixth to seventh decades. A slight male predominance has been reported in several series. There are three types of gastric lymphomas:

  a. PGL is defined as an extranodal lymphoma arising in the stomach, which is the most common site of extranodal lymphoma. PGL can spread to regional lymph nodes and can become disseminated. Most PGLs are of B cell origin, although occasional cases of T-cell and Hodgkin lymphoma are seen.
  b. Secondary gastric lymphoma indicates involvement of the stomach as a part of a diffuse lymphoma arising elsewhere. In an autopsy series, patients who died from disseminated non-Hodgkin lymphoma (NHL) showed involvement of the gastrointestinal tract in 50% to 60% of cases.
  c. Tertiary gastric lymphoma is recurrent lymphoma involving the stomach after treatment of a nodal lymphoma and is uncommon.

Pathology

Most gastric lymphomas are B-cell lymphoma, most commonly having diffuse, large cell features. Most gastric lymphomas appear to arise in the lamina propria from which they infiltrate into the submucosa, eventually spreading to regional lymph nodes.

Up to 40% of gastric lymphomas are low-grade mucosa-associated lymphoid tissue (MALT) lymphomas. These indolent, low-grade lymphomas are characterized by aggregates of lymphoid tissue in mucosal sites with the following features: large reactive follicles, prominent marginal zones containing cells with angular nuclei reminiscent of centrocytes, infiltration of the gastric epithelium by lymphoid cells, and plasma cells underlying the superficial epithelium. Heavy- and light-chain gene rearrangements of monoclonal immunoglobin are identified in the lymphomas.

Clinical Presentation

Symptoms of PGL that are most common at presentation are abdominal pain and weight loss. Bleeding is less common, and patients rarely present with perforation.

Stage IE and stage IIE PGL present in patients with an equal prevalence. Stage IE disease is seen in 36% to 72% of patients at presentation and stage IIE disease is seen in 28% to 64% of patients.

Presentation with high-grade and low-grade disease is also equal, with 34% to 65% of disease presenting as high-grade lymphoma, 12% to 17% presenting as intermediate-grade lymphoma, and 35% to 65% presenting as low-grade lymphoma.

Diagnosis

Diagnosis of PGL by endoscopic evaluation has markedly improved over the last decade. In recent series, successful endoscopic diagnosis of lymphoma was made in 92% to 100% of the patients. A large review of 3,157 patients with PGL reported data on the sensitivity of endoscopic diagnosis for 848 patients. A diagnosis of cancer was made in 79% of patients, with a diagnosis of lymphoma made in only 54%. This indicates that 25% of the patients were diagnosed with cancer that was not thought to be lymphoma. The review also stated that the success of endoscopic evaluation and biopsy in diagnosing gastric lymphoma has improved markedly in recent decades. In a review of patients treated from 1980 to 1990, the correct pre-operative diagnosis was made in only 57% of patients, but an improvement was noted over time. A diagnosis rate of 44% was seen between 1980 and 1984 compared with 64% from 1985 to 1990. Other series report a correct diagnosis by endoscopy in 38% to 92% of patients. Techniques that have led to a higher rate of success include the use of larger biopsy forceps, multiple biopsies, and the use of brushings. If an ulcer is present, the biopsy should be at the edge of the ulcer crater at multiple sites.

Staging

Staging of gastric lymphoma based upon the Ann Arbor system includes stage IE, which indicates a disease limited to the stomach, without nodal spread. Stage IIE_1 is a tumor in the stomach that spreads to adjacent contiguous lymph nodes. Stage IIE_2 is a tumor in the stomach that spreads to lymph nodes that are noncontiguous with the primary tumor.

Treatment

Treatment of PGL is highly variable, with no consensus established on the most effective therapy. To date, only one randomized clinical trial comparing treatments has been published. Treatment decisions must, therefore, be based on retrospective studies that address the treat-ment of this uncommon malignancy. These retrospective studies are difficult to compare and mostly represent nonrandomized data with significant stage and grade variation. Selection bias is evident in some series; patients with more advanced disease and more aggressive histology receive more aggressive therapy. There is a need for prospective randomized trials to evaluate the different treatments of this malignancy.

Impact of Association with H. Pylori on Treatment of PGL

Evidence for a strong association between gastric lymphoma and gastric infection by *Helicobacter pylori* has been shown. A simplified treatment algorithm that outlines the treat-ment of low-grade lymphoma is shown in Fig. 5.4.

Treatment of Low-grade and High-grade Primary Gastric Lymphoma

The initial therapy is based upon the type of PGL. Low-grade MALT lymphoma is treated initially by eradicating *H. pylori*. Complete regression after proven eradication is followed with serial endoscopies. For patients with stages IE and IIE_1 non-MALT lymphoma and low-grade MALT lymphoma not responding to treatment of *H. pylori* infection, surgical resection is indicated. Surgical resection has the advantage of allowing accurate staging, grading, and cure with surgery alone. This allows chemotherapy to be given only to those patients with high-grade lymphoma and avoids chemotherapy in those patients with favorable histology. Chemotherapy after surgical resection is indicated in those patients with positive lymph nodes, residual disease, and high-grade lymphoma found in the pathologic specimen. We feel that all high-grade lym-phomas, both MALT and non-MALT in origin, should be treated initially with chemotherapy. This is shown in Fig. 5.5.

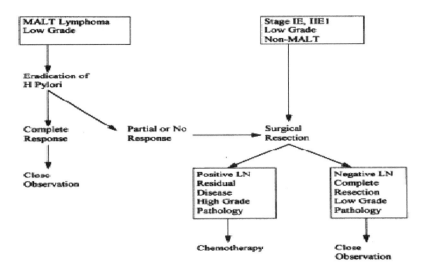

FIG. 5.4. Simplified algorithm outlining the treatment of low-grade lymphoma.

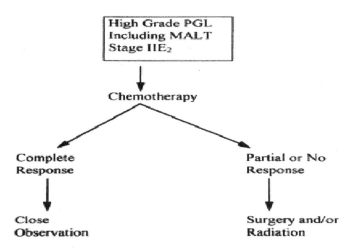

FIG. 5.5. Mucosa-associated lymphoid tissue (MALT) and non-MALT should be initially treated with chemotherapy.

SELECTED READINGS

Adachi Y, Yasuda K, Inomata M, et al. Pathology and prognosis of gastric carcinoma: well versus poorly differentiated type. *Cancer* 2000;89(7):1418–1424.
Bonenkamp JJ, Hermans J, et al. Extended lymph-node dissection for gastric cancer: Dutch Gastric Cancer Group. *N Engl J Med* 1999;340:908–914.

Chang HM, Jung KH, Kim TY, et al. A phase III randomized trial of 5-fluorouracil, doxorubicin, and mito-mycin C versus 5-fluorouracil and mitomycin C versus 5-fluorouracil alone in curatively resected gastric cancer. *Ann Oncol* 2002;13(11):1779–1785.

Cullinan SA, Moertel CG, Wieard HS, et al. Controlled evaluation of three drug combination regimens versus fluorouracil alone for the therapy of advanced gastric cancer: North Central Cancer Treatment Group. *J Clin Oncol* 1994;12:412–416.

Earle CC, Maroun JA, Adjuvant chemotherapy after curative resection for gastric cancer non-Asian patients: revisiting a meta-analyses of randomised trials. *Eur J Cancer* 1999;35(7):1059–1064.

Gastrointestinal Tumor Study Group. A comparison of combination chemotherapy and combined modality therapy for locally advanced gastric carcinoma. *Cancer* 1982;49:1771–1777.

Gunderson LL, Sosin H. Adenocarcinoma of the stomach: areas of failure in a re-operation series (second or symptomatic look) clinicopathologic correlation and implications for adjuvant therapy. *Int J Radiat Oncol Biol Phys* 1982;8(1):1–11.

Hermans J, Bonenkamp JJ, Boon MC. et al. Adjuvant therapy after curative resection for gastric cancer: meta-analysis of randomized trials. *J Clin Oncol* 1993;11:1441–1447.

Macdonald JS, Smalley SR, Benedetti J, et al. Chemoradiotherapy after surgery compared with surgery alone for adenocarcinoma of the stomach or gastroesophageal junction. *N Engl J Med* 2001;345(10):725–730.

Stephens J, Smith J. Treatment of primary gastric lymphoma and gastric mucosa-associated lymphoid tissue lymphoma. *J Am Coll Surg* 1998;187(3):312–320.

Waters JS, Norman A, Cunningham D, et al. Long-term survival after epirubicin, cisplatin and fluorouracil for gastric cancer: results of a randomized trial. *Br J Cancer* 1999;80(1-2):269–272.

6

Biliary Tract Cancer

Gregory D. Leonard*, Eileen M. O'Reilly†, and Carmen J. Allegra‡

*The Royal College of Physicians, Dublin, Ireland; †Department of Medicine,
Memorial Sloan-Kettering Cancer Center, New York, New York; and
‡Network for Medical Communication and Research, Atlanta, Georgia

Carcinomas of the biliary tract include those cancers arising either in the gallbladder or the bile duct. There were estimated to be 6,800 new cases of gallbladder and biliary tract cancers (excluding intrahepatic biliary tract cancer) and 3,500 deaths from these cancers in 2003 (1). Gallbladder cancer is twice as common as cholangiocarcinoma. The term cholangiocarcinoma was initially used to designate tumors of the intrahepatic bile ducts, but, more recently, it refers to the entire spectrum of tumors arising in the intrahepatic, perihilar, and distal bile ducts. The epidemiology, clinical features, staging, and surgical treatment are distinct for carcinomas arising in the gallbladder and bile duct, and these are described separately. The palliative treatment options are similar and are discussed together at the end of the chapter.

CARCINOMA OF THE GALLBLADDER

Epidemiology

- The age-adjusted incidence of carcinoma of gallbladder is 1.2 per 100,000 population in the United States from 1996 to 2000 (http://seer.cancer.gov/csr/1975_2000/).
- It affects women two to six times more commonly than men and has a 50% greater incidence in whites as compared to black individuals (2). The highest incidence is among Native Americans and in South America (particularly Chile), Japan, and Eastern Europe, and the lowest incidence is in Singapore, Nigeria, and the United States.
- The mean age at diagnosis of the carcinoma is 65 years.

Etiology

- **Cholelithiasis (gallstones):** Of patients with gallbladder carcinoma, 65% to 90% have gallstones, whereas only 1% to 3% of patients with gallstones develop gallbladder cancer. The risk increases with increase in size of the stones.
- **Infection:** *Salmonella typhi*, *Escherichia coli*, and *Helicobacter pylori* infections also cause gallbladder carcinomas.
- **Gallbladder polyps or porcelain gallbladder:** Polyps >1 cm diameter have the greatest malignancy potential. Porcelain gallbladder due to extensive calcium deposition in the wall is a pathological finding and can be associated with carcinoma in less than 20% of patients.
- **Miscellaneous:** Anomalous pancreaticobiliary duct junction resulting in backflow of pancreatic juice and biliary stasis may cause gallbladder cancer. Obesity, estrogens, and chemicals from the rubber industry have also been associated with this disease.

Clinical Features

- Pain (82%)
- Weight loss (72%)
- Anorexia (74%)
- Nausea or vomiting (68%)
- Mass in the right upper quadrant (65%)
- Jaundice (44%)
- Abdominal distension (30%)
- Pruritus (20%)
- Incidental (15% to 20%)
- Courvoisier law states that if the gallbladder is enlarged and if the patient has painless jaundice, the cause is unlikely to be gallstones.
- In elderly patients, gallbladder cancer may present as cholecystitis.

Diagnosis

- Abnormal serology can occur with elevations in levels of alkaline phosphatase, γ-glutamyl transpeptidase, bilirubin, carcinoembryonic antigen (CEA), or CA 19-9, but these factors are more commonly elevated in cholangiocarcinoma.
- Plain radiograph of the abdomen may detect calcifications from porcelain gallbladder.
- Ultrasound is usually abnormal (thickened wall, mass, and loss of gallbladder or liver interface) but may not be specific for gallbladder cancer.
- Computerized tomography (CT) scan gives better visualization of the extent of tumor growth and nodal status and is useful in gallbladder cancer where distant metastases are common.
- Magnetic resonance cholangiopancreatography (MRCP) and cholangiography by endoscopic retrograde cholangiopancreatography (ERCP) are the optimal imaging modalities to outline local anatomy for preoperative planning (2).
- Biopsies prior to surgery may result in tumor seeding; therefore, the diagnosis is usually made at the time of surgery.

Pathology

- Adenocarcinoma accounts for more than 85% of cases. It is subcharacterized into papillary, tubular, mucinous, or signet cell type. Other histologies include anaplastic, squamous cell, small cell, and carcinoid carcinoma.

Staging

- Gallbladder cancers have been classified by Nevin et al. (3) or by using the TNM staging system (4) (see Table 6.1).
- A staging laparoscopy is a useful adjunct to imaging modalities because it may detect intra-abdominal metastases, thereby sparing radical and potentially morbid surgery in patients.

Treatment

Surgery

- Only 10% to 30% of patients can be considered for potentially curative surgery (2).
- Surgery can be a simple cholecystectomy or a radical (extended) cholecystectomy.
- A radical procedure involves wedge resection of the gallbladder bed, excision of the supraduodenal extrahepatic bile duct, en bloc dissection of regional lymph nodes, and

TABLE 6.1. *Staging systems for gallbladder cancer AJCC 6th edition TNM stage*

Stage IA	T1 N0 M0	T1a: invades lamina propria
		T1b: invades the muscle layer
Stage IB	T2 N0 M0	T2: invades perimuscular connective tissue
Stage IIA	T3 N0 M0	T3: perforates the serosa and/or directly invades the liver or one other adjacent organ
Stage IIB	T1–3 N1 M0	N1: metastases in cystic duct, choledochal, and/or hilar lymph nodes
Stage III	T4 N0–1 M0	T4: tumor invades portal vein or hepatic artery or multiple extrahepatic organs or structures
Stage IV	Any T any N M1	M1: distant metastases
Nevin stage		
Stage I	Intramucosal only	
Stage II	Extends to muscularis	
Stage III	Extends through serosa	
Stage IV	Transmural involvement and cystic lymph nodes are involved	
Stage V	Direct extension to liver or distant metastases	

resection of segments V and IVB of the liver (some physicians advocate pancreaticoduodenectomy) (5).

- Stage I disease can be treated successfully with a simple cholecystectomy, with survival rate being greater than 85%, but some physicians advocate radical surgery (Table 6.2).
- Up to 40% of stage IIA (formerly stage II) cancers are found to have lymph node involvement at surgery, upstaging them to pathological stage IIB (formerly stage III). Because of this upstaging, most surgeons advocate radical surgery for stage II and above. Many studies have demonstrated improvements in survival in patients reoperated with a radical procedure compared to those receiving only a simple cholecystectomy (6).
- Some authors have reported extended survivals with radical surgery even in stage IV patients studied by Nevin et al. (7).

Radiation

- In patients with unresectable tumors, radiation alone is rarely a successful palliative procedure (8).
- A number of reports have documented improvements in survival rates in cases of intraoperative or postoperative adjuvant radiotherapy. No prospective randomized controlled trials have been performed to address this issue.

TABLE 6.2. *Treatment and 5-year survival of gallbladder cancers according to stage*

TNM stage	Treatment	Median survival	5-yr survival (%)
I	Simple cholecystectomy	19 mo	60–100
	Radical cholecystectomy		
II	Radical cholecystectomy	7 mo	10–20
	+/– Radiation therapy (not standard)		
III	Radical cholecystectomy	4 mo	5
	+/– Radiation therapy (not standard)		
IV	Palliation with stent placement	2 mo	0
	Surgery or radiation or chemotherapy or combination of these		

Chemotherapy and Palliation

The benefits and options available for chemotherapy and palliation of carcinoma of the gallbladder are the same as those for cholangiocarcinoma and are discussed in the sections Chemotherapy and Palliation.

Survival

The various aspects of survival following treatment of gallbladder cancers according to stage are given in Table 6.2.

CARCINOMA OF THE BILE DUCTS (CHOLANGIOCARCINOMA)
Epidemiology

- Cholangiocarcinoma is subdivided into proximal extrahepatic (perihilar or Klatskin tumor; 50% to 60%), distal extrahepatic (20% to 25%), intrahepatic (peripheral tumor; 20% to 25%), and multifocal (5%) tumors (9).
- The incidence of intrahepatic bile duct tumors was 0.9 cases per 100,000 population between 1996 and 2000 and for other biliary tumors was 1.5 cases per 100,000 population. The incidence has increased, partly because of increased recognition of the intrahepatic form of the disease.
- Cholangiocarcinoma is more common in men (10).

Etiology

- **Inflammatory conditions:** Primary sclerosing cholangitis is associated with a 5% to 15% lifetime risk. Ulcerative colitis and chronic intraductal gallstone disease also increase risk.
- **Bile duct abnormalities:** Caroli disease (cystic dilatation of intrahepatic ducts), bile duct adenoma, biliary papillomatosis, and choledochal cysts increase risk.
- **Infection:** In Southeast Asia, risk can be increased 25- to 50-fold by parasitic infestation from *Opisthorchis viverrini* and *Clonorchis sinensis*. Hepatitis C cirrhosis is also a risk factor.
- **Miscellaneous:** Smoking, thorotrast (a radiologic contrast agent), asbestos, radon, and nitrosamines are also known to increase risk (5).

Clinical Features

- Intrahepatic cholangiocarcinoma may present as a mass, be asymptomatic, or produce vague symptoms such as pain, anorexia, weight loss, night sweats, and malaise.
- Extrahepatic cholangiocarcinoma usually presents with symptoms and signs of cholestasis (icterus, pale stools, dark urine, and pruritus or cholangitis, which includes pain, icterus, and fever).

Diagnosis

- A cholestatic serologic picture (as discussed in gallbladder cancer) may be seen. A value of CA 19-9 >100 U per mL is highly suggestive of malignancy and is elevated in up to 85% of patients with cholangiocarcinoma (9).
- Ultrasonography is the first-line investigation for suspected cholangiocarcinoma. Biliary dilatation is usually seen. This technique can often overlook masses and is poor at delineating anatomy.
- CT scan is better at defining anatomy and can be used to direct CT scan–guided biopsies.
- MRCP is the optimal imaging modality.

- ERCP provides anatomical information (cholangiography) that is useful for planning surgery, but, more importantly, it may provide a tissue diagnosis. However, because these tumors are desmoplastic, cytology brushings have a low yield (30%) in making the diagnosis. When brushings and biopsy are combined, the yield improves to 40% to 70%. Endoscopic ultrasound and positron emission tomography (PET) may provide further information on local and distant disease, respectively.
- The diagnosis of cholangiocarcinoma is frequently made on the basis of the clinical scenario, serology, and radiology but without histologic confirmation, but such a diagnosis in the absence of tissue should be made only after efforts are taken to prove the diagnosis by use of cytologic or pathologic evaluation preoperatively.

Pathology

- Adenocarcinomas account for 95% of tumors.

Staging

- Up to 50% of patients have lymph node involvement at presentation and 10% to 20% have peritoneal involvement. In one series, laparoscopy prevented unnecessary surgery in one third of patients (11).
- Staging is based on the TNM classification (4). Other classifications such as the classification by Bismuth et al. (12) define the extent of ductal involvement (Table 6.3).

Treatment

Surgery

- Surgery is the only curative option and may be possible in 30% to 60% of patients (10). The goals of surgery are (a) tumor removal and (b) establishing or restoring biliary drainage.
- Surgery for extrahepatic hilar cholangiocarcinomas is based on the stage of disease, and the goal of surgical intervention is to obtain a tumor-free margin >5 cm (see Table 6.4).
- Long-term survival has been reported after liver transplantation in three studies, but transplantation is not a standard approach (5).

TABLE 6.3. *Staging systems for extrahepatic bile duct cancers AJCC 6th edition TNM classification*

Stage IA	T1 N0 M0	T1: tumor confined to the bile duct
Stage IB	T2 N0 M0	T2: tumor invades beyond the bile duct wall
Stage IIA	T3 N0 M0	T3: Tumor invades liver, gallbladder, pancreas, unilateral branches of portal vein, or hepatic artery
Stage IIB	T1–3 N1 M0	N1: Regional lymph node
Stage III	T4 any N M0	T4: tumor invades main portal vein or bilateral branches, common hepatic artery or other adjacent structures
Stage IV	Any T any N M1	M1: distant metastases

Intrahepatic cancers are classified as per liver tumors
Ampulla of Vater cancers have a separate staging classification (4)

Bismuth classification

Type I	Tumors below the confluence of left and right hepatic ducts
Type II	Tumors reaching the confluence but not involving the left or right hepatic ducts
Type III	Tumors occluding the common hepatic duct and either the right or left hepatic duct
Type IV	Tumors that are multicentric or that involve the confluence of the right and left hepatic ducts

TABLE 6.4. *Treatment and survival of cholangiocarcinomas according to location*

Location	Treatment	Median survival	5-yr survival (%)
Extrahepatic (hilar)	Type I + II En bloc resection of extrahepatic bile ducts, gallbladder, regional lymphadenectomy, and Roux-en-Y hepaticojejunostomy Type III As above plus right/left hepatectomy Type IV As above plus extended right/left hepatectomy	12–24 mo	9–18
Extrahepatic (distal)	Pancreaticoduodenectomy	12–24 mo	20–30
Intrahepatic	Resect involved segments or lobe of liver	18–30 mo	10–45

Radiation

- In patients with unresectable disease, there have been reports of long-term survival with combined-modality chemoradiotherapy. One report documented a median survival of 21 months in patients with unresectable cancer or those with residual disease after surgery (13).
- Adjuvant radiation is not recommended because there is limited and conflicting data on this subject. One retrospective series reported a significant improvement in 5-year survival for those treated with radiation therapy and surgery compared to surgery alone (39% versus 13%) (14). However, the mortality with surgery in the surgery alone group was 10%.

Chemotherapy

- Chemotherapy appears to provide palliative benefit to patients with biliary tract cancer, although definitive proof of a survival benefit is lacking (15).
- There are now many chemotherapy options for cholangiocarcinoma and gallbladder cancer (5,16). Many of these trials are reported in abstract form or sample sizes are small, so the treatment of choice has not been established. Usual response rates are between 10% and 20%, and high response rates found in single-institution studies have not been reproducible in larger multi-institution trials.
- Historically, fluoropyrimidines have been the cytotoxic therapy of choice, but the likelihood of response is less than 10%. Increasingly, gemcitabine is considered as the standard of care.
- Gemcitabine combinations, for example, cisplatin and gemcitabine, have demonstrated high response rates of 20% to 60% and median survival up to 20 months, but as yet there have been no randomized comparisons showing clear-cut superiority over single-agent therapy.
- Mitomycin, as a single-agent or as combination therapy, has demonstrated response rates of up to 47% and median survivals of 9.5 months.
- Other single agents with activity include docetaxel, irinotecan, raltitrexed, anthracyclines, carboplatin, and oxaliplatin.

Palliation

- Patients with unresectable or metastatic disease may benefit from palliative surgery, radiation, or chemotherapy, or a combination of these.
- Biliary drainage can be achieved by Roux-en-Y choledochojejunostomy, bypass of the site of obstruction to left or right hepatic duct, or endoscopic or percutaneously placed stents

(metal-wall stents have a larger diameter and are less prone to occlusion or migration and are preferably used in patients with a life expectancy of greater than 6 months and/or in those who have unresectable disease).
• Celiac plexus block or photodynamic therapy are other options (17).

REFERENCES

1. Jemal A, Murray T, Samuels A, et al. Cancer Statistics, 2003. *CA Cancer J Clin* 2003;53:5–26.
2. Misra S, Chaturvedi A, Misra NC, et al. Carcinoma of the gallbladder. *Lancet Oncol* 2003;4:167–176.
3. Nevin JE, Moran TJ, Kay S, et al. Carcinoma of the gallbladder, staging, treatment and prognosis. *Cancer* 1976;37:141–148.
4. American Joint Committee on Cancer. *Cancer staging manual*, 6th ed. New York: Springer-Verlag, 2002:139–156.
5. Yee K, Sheppard BC, Domreis J, et al. Cancers of the gallbladder and biliary ducts. *Oncology* 2002;16:939–957.
6. Todoroki T, Kawamoto T, Takahashi H, et al. Treatment of gallbladder cancer by radical resection. *Br J Surg* 1999;86:622–627.
7. Fong Y, Jarnagin W, Blumgart LH. Gallbladder cancer: comparison of patients presenting initially for definitive operation with those presenting after prior noncurative intervention. *Ann Surg* 2000;232:557–569.
8. Houry S, Haccart V, Huguier M, et al. Gallbladder cancer: role of radiation therapy. *Hepatogastroenterology* 1999;46:1578–1584.
9. Khan SA, Davidson BR, Goldin R, et al. Guidelines for the diagnosis and treatment of cholangiocarcinoma: consensus document. *Gut* 2002;51(Suppl. VI):vi1–vi9.
10. de Groen PC, Gores GJ, LaRusso NF, et al. Biliary tract cancers. *N Engl J Med* 1999;341:1368–1378.
11. Corvera CU, Weber SM, Jarnagin WR. Role of laparoscopy in the evaluation of biliary tract cancer. *Surg Oncol Clin North Am* 2002;11:877–891.
12. Bismuth H, Castaing D, Traynor O, et al. Resection or palliation: priority of surgery in the treatment of hilar cancer. *World J Surg* 1988;12:39–47.
13. Morganti AG, Trodella L, Valentini V, et al. Combined modality treatment in unresectable extrahepatic biliary carcinoma. *Int J Radiat Biol Phys* 2000;46:913–999.
14. Todoroki T, Ohara K, Kawamoto T, et al. Benefits of adjuvant radiotherapy after radical resection of locally advanced main hepatic duct carcinoma. *Int J Radiat Biol Phys* 2000;46:581–587.
15. Glimelius B, Hoffman K, Sjoden PO, et al. Chemotherapy improves survival and quality of life in advanced biliary and pancreatic cancer. *Ann Oncol* 1996;7(6):793–600.
16. Henja M, Pruckmayer M, Raderer M. The role of chemotherapy and radiation in the management of biliary cancer: a review of the literature. *Eur J Cancer* 1998;34:977–986.
17. Berr F, Wiedmann M, Tannapfel A, et al. Photodynamic therapy for advanced bile duct cancer: evidence for improved palliation and extended survival. *Hepatology* 2000;31:291–298.

7

Primary Cancers of the Liver

Gregory D. Leonard*, William R. Jarnagin†, and Carmen J. Allegra‡

*The Royal College of Physicians, Dublin, Ireland; †Department of Surgery Weill Medical College of Cornell University, New York, New York; and ‡Network for Medical Communication and Research, Atlanta, Georgia

Primary liver cancers arise predominantly from the parenchymal liver cells or hepatocytes (90%) and are called *hepatocellular carcinoma* (HCC). Tumors arising from the intrahepatic bile ducts (10%) are called *cholangiocarcinomas* and are discussed primarily in Chapter 6. HCC is the fifth leading cause of cancer in the world, with an annual incidence of one million cases (1). The incidence in the United States has increased by approximately 75% in the last decade, likely because of increases in incidence of chronic hepatitis infection (2). Research on vaccinations for hepatitis B and its consequences have prevented the development of HCC in many regions of the world. Further progress in the treatment of HCC is necessary to significantly reduce mortality from this common global disease.

EPIDEMIOLOGY

- In the United States, the incidence of clinically significant metastatic carcinoma to the liver is 20 times more common than primary liver cancer.
- The age-adjusted incidence of HCC from 1996 to 2000 is 5 per 100,000 population (http://seer.cancer.gov/csr/1975_2000/). In 2003, 17,300 (includes intrahepatic bile duct cancers) new cases of primary liver cancer and 14,400 deaths from this disease were estimated in the United States (3).
- There is marked geographic variation in the incidence of HCC, with the highest incidences of up to 30 per 100,000 population occurring in sub-Saharan Africa and Asia.
- Men are affected twice as often as women. The mean age at diagnosis is between 50 and 60 years.

ETIOLOGY

- Cirrhosis is present in 80% of patients with HCC. Therefore, risk factors for cirrhosis are also risk factors for HCC.
- Hepatitis B virus (HBV) infection increases the risk of developing HCC by 100-fold. HBV causes 80% of HCC in the world. HCC develops from chronic hepatitis due to HBV at a rate of 0.5% per year.
- Hepatitis C virus (HCV) infection accounts for 30% to 50% of HCC in the United States. HCC develops from HCV at a rate of 5% per year.
- Alcoholic cirrhosis accounts for 15% of of HCC.
- Hemochromatosis, hereditary tyrosinemia, and autoimmune chronic active hepatitis are other causes of cirrhosis and are associated with a significant risk for developing HCC (6).

99

- There is less convincing evidence for the risk of developing HCC from:
  - Aflatoxin B_1 (chemical product of Aspergillus)
  - Androgenic steroids
  - Thorotrast (radiology contrast agent) and
  - Oral contraceptives.

CLINICAL FEATURES

- The most common symptoms or signs of HCC are (7):
  - Pain (91%)
  - Weight loss (35%)
  - Vomiting (8%)
  - Hepatomegaly (89%)
  - Abdominal swelling (43%) and
  - Jaundice (7% to 41%).
- Paraneoplastic manifestations can also occur. They include hypoglycemia, hypercalcemia, carcinoid, erythrocytosis, hypercholesterolemia, hyperthyroidism, and osteoporosis.

DIAGNOSIS

- Serologic tests may reveal abnormalities in the liver profile. α-Fetoprotein (AFP) is elevated in 50% to 90% of patients with HCC but can also be elevated in other liver abnormalities. AFP values >400 µg per dL in patients without hepatitis or >4,000 µg per mL in patients positive for hepatitis B surface antigen and with radiographic abnormalities suggest the diagnosis of HCC (www.nccn.org). If surgery is planned in these patients, an open biopsy at laparotomy is usually preferred to decrease the risk of tumor seeding, bleeding, or rupture. Des-γ-carboxy prothrombin protein, induced by the absence of vitamin K, is increased in about 91% of patients with HCC, but is also elevated in other causes of hepatitis. Carcinoembryonic antigen (CEA) is less useful in HCC and is more likely to be elevated in cholangiocarcinoma.
- Ultrasonography is considered the best screening tool in conjunction with AFP for high-risk populations. Triphasic computerized tomography (not contrast enhanced, arterial phase, and portal phase) provides better definition, can assess for metastatic disease, and is used to guide percutaneous biopsies. Gadolinium-enhanced magnetic resonance (MR) imaging may improve characterization of small lesions. MR angiography is used to plan for surgery.
- Laparoscopy is recommended to improve staging and to prevent unnecessary laparotomy (10).

PATHOLOGY

- There are many histologic types of HCC including trabecular, pseudoglandular or acinar, compact, scirrhous, clear cell, and fibrolamellar.
- Fibrolamellar carcinoma is a histologic variant accounting for 1% of HCC. It occurs more commonly in women, is not associated with cirrhosis, and has a better prognosis than HCC.

STAGING

- The TNM staging system (see Table 7.1) has been criticized because it does not evaluate the underlying liver disease, which is clearly a major prognostic factor in patients regardless of tumor stage (11).
- The Child-Pugh grading system has been incorporated into the management of HCC because it evaluates the status of the underlying liver function and influences treatment (12) (see Table 7.2).

TABLE 7.1. *The American Joint Committee on Cancer (AJCC) 6th edition TNM stage groupings*

Stage I	T1 N0 M0	T1: solitary tumor with no vascular invasion
Stage II	T2 N0 M0	T2: solitary tumor with vascular invasion or multiple tumors none >5 cm
Stage IIIA	T3 N0 M0	T3: multiple tumors >5 cm or involving a major branch of the portal or hepatic vein
Stage IIIB	T4 N0 M0	T4: tumor directly invading adjacent organs other than gallbladder or perforating visceral peritoneum
Stage IIIC	Any T N1 M0	N1: regional lymph node metastases
Stage IV	Any T any N M1	M1: distant metastases

TREATMENT

Surgery

- Surgery remains the only possiblity for cure in HCC. The treatment algorithm for HCC is determined by two factors: Tumor extent and the severity of the underlying hepatic parenchymal disease (Fig. 7.1).
- **Partial hepatectomy:** Hepatic resection remains the mainstay of surgical therapy for this disease. Only 13 to 35% are surgical candidates. The majority have either disease that is beyond surgical correction or have poor hepatic reserve or both. Small tumors have the best outcomes. Recurrence is most commonly seen in the remnant liver. Repeat hepatectomy is possible in 10 to 29% of patients.

  Operative mortality is <5% but is higher in the presence of cirrhosis.

  Five-year survival is 30 to 40%, but is lower (12 to 37%) in patients with large tumors, tumors with vascular invasion and more advanced cirrhosis (2).
- **Total hepatectomy and liver transplantaion:** Transplantation is indicated in patients with severe cirrhosis or where extensive resection leaving minimal liver reserve is required.

  Criteria for transplantation are: a solitary tumor ≤5cm, 2 or 3 tumors ≤3cm in size, and the absence of vascular invasion. Based on these criteria four-year survival was reported as 75%, however, 12 of the 14 non-operative deaths were due to transplant complications as opposed to tumor recurrence (13). Patients with intrahepatic cholangiocarcinoma are not considered transplant candidates as results with transplantation in this disease have been poor.

  Survival outcomes often appear more favorable compared to resection but may be due to patient selection, inclusion of incidental tumors, and lack of intention to treat analyses where survival outcomes are poorer due to disease progression while waiting for transplant (10). Survival outcomes may be further improved by living donor transplantation, although this remains controversial.

TABLE 7.2. *Child-Pugh scoring system*

Chemical and biochemical parameters	Score attributed to each parameter		
	1	2	3
Encephalopathy	None	1–2	3–4
Ascites	None	Slight	Moderate
Albumin (g/dL)	>3.5	2.8–3.5	<2.8
Prothrombin time prolonged (s)	1–4	4–6	>6
Bilirubin (mg/dL)	1–2	2–3	>3

Class A = 5–6 points, Class B = 7–9 points, Class C = 10–15 points.

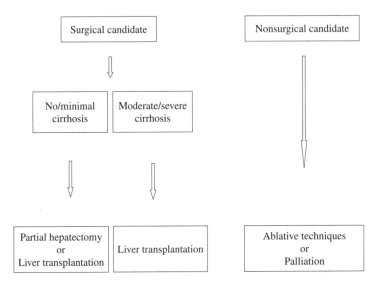

FIG. 7.1. Treatment algorithm for the management of hepatocellular carcinoma (HCC).

Disadvantages of transplantation are the expense, the lack of specialty centers perform-ing operations and the lack of donor livers (currently 18,505 patients on the waiting list, 40% have been waiting for over 2 years).

Preoperative chemoembolization is often used as a temporizing modality while waiting for a liver, but the value of this approach is not yet proven.

Ablative Techniques

Ablative techniques have a role in patients who are not candidates for resection (12). Abla-tion of solitary, small lesions may be as effective as resection but a prospective comparison between surgery and one of these methods has yet to be performed. Ablation of large tumors (>5cm) has been shown to be associated with very high local recurrence rates.

- Percutaneous ethanol injection into tumors causes cellular dehydration, coagulative necro-sis and localized tissue ischemia. It is frequently used for up to three localized tumors of <5cm that are not surgical candidates usually due to cirrhosis. It is relatively inexpensive and well tolerated.
- Radiofrequency ablation is performed percutaneously using ultrasound guidance and causes focal coagulative necrosis of tumors via thermal energy. It is most efficacious for tumors <3cm where complete necrosis can occur in up to 90% of tumors.
- Cryotherapy is also safe and more effective than RFA for larger tumors but is less suited to a percutaneous approach.
- Hepatic artery chemoebolization is based on the principal that 80% of the blood supply to tumors is from the hepatic artery which supplies only 20–30% of normal liver parenchyma. Ligation or embolization of the hepatic artery can induce temporary tumor responses but when combined with chemotherapy can be more efficacious. Further discussion on this topic is in the chemotherapy section.

Radiation

- External beam radiotherapy has a limited role in HCC owing to the poor tolerance of radiation by the liver. However, safe and effective doses can be given to palliate the pain.
- Radioactive isotopes have demonstrated efficacy in the adjuvant treatment of HCC.

    Iodine-131 combined with lipiodol (a dye used for lymphangiography that is known to concentrate in tumors when given by hepatic arterial infusion) given by the hepatic artery has been compared to the observation in 43 patients in Hong Kong who had curative resections for HCC (12). At interim analysis, the study was closed owing to an improved disease-free survival from 13.6 months to 57.2 months with the radioactive isotope. This provocative study has yet to be validated in a multicenter trial.

Chemotherapy

- Single-agent chemotherapy has demonstrated response rates of approximately 15% to 30%, which increases to 20% to 35% with combination therapy. Cisplatin and anthracycline combinations have been studied most extensively, but there is no reference regimen for this disease (14).
- Although most chemotherapy trials are in phase II, some trials have demonstrated a statistically significant survival advantage compared to resection alone (15) (see Table 7.3). Chemotherapy is usually used for palliation in patients with unresectable disease and should only be used for adjuvant therapy as part of a clinical trial.
- The PIAF regimen (intravenous cisplatin, recombinant interferon alfa 2b, doxorubicin, and 5-fluorouracil) demonstrated a 50% objective response rate in 50 patients with unresectable disease from Hong Kong (16). Nine of the 13 responding patients were operated on and four were found to have complete pathological remission. In addition to highlighting a potentially active regimen, this trial also demonstrates that radiologic assessment may underestimate tumor cell kill.

TABLE 7.3. *Selection of trials demonstrating a survival advantage with the use of chemotherapy*

Author	n	Stage	Treatment	1-, 2-, and 3-yr survival	p-value
Lai et al. (17)	106	unresectable	Doxorubicin vs. observation	11 wk vs. 7 wk[a]	0.036
Nakashima et al. (18)	74	Adjuvant	HAI cisplatin or HAI 5-FU, doxorubicin and mitomycin C vs. observation	63%, 50%, 7% vs. 39%, 22%, 12%	<0.05
Lai et al. (19)	66	Adjuvant	Epirubicin, HAI iodized oil with cisplatin	69%, 53%, 48% vs. 50%, 36%, 18%	0.03

HAI, hepatic arterial infusion; 5-FU, 5-fluorouracil.
[a]Median overall survival.

Regional Chemotherapy

- Hepatic arterial infusion chemotherapy acts on the premise that tumor blood supply is by the hepatic artery. Response rates are often higher with this therapy. Trials comparing efficacy of various systemic chemotherapies are contradictory. At the University of California, less than 10% of patients with HCC were candidates for surgical placement of infusion pumps. Pump insertion requires a laparotomy, is expensive, and is performed only in certain specialized centers.
- Chemoembolization involves regional administration of chemotherapy followed by embolization of specific arteries using gelatin sponges, collagen, alcohol, or microspheres. Embolization can cause tumor ischemia and increases the potential for improved chemotherapeutic exposure to the tumor. Patients with portal vein thrombosis or poor liver reserve are usually excluded because normal liver parenchyma relies on the hepatic arterial blood supply. Lipiodol is commonly used for embolization because it can transport lipophilic chemotherapeutic agents and can be radiolabeled. No trials have compared the outcomes for different chemotherapeutic administration techniques in HCC.

Prevention and Novel Therapies

- Tamoxifen, antiandrogen therapy, and octreotide have been extensively investigated and do not have a beneficial effect on patients with HCC. HMG-CoA reductase inhibitors such as pravastatin have had more encouraging results (20).
- Interferon-α reduces the onset of liver damage and its progression to cirrhosis in 10% to 30% of patients with chronic hepatitis B.
- Refrigerated storage of food grains and transportation of grains in refrigerated vehicles should help reduce the risk of ingesting aflatoxin.
- Acyclic retinoid, polyprenoic acid, reduces the incidence of second primary of HCC after initial resection and requires further investigation.
- Screening of high-risk populations with α-fetoprotein at 4-month intervals and with ultrasound at yearly intervals has been shown to identify patients with earlier stages of HCC and may improve survival in high-risk groups (21).

REFERENCES

1. Jemal A, Murray T, Samuels A, et al. Cancer Statistics, 2003. *CA Cancer J Clin* 2003;53:5–26.
2. Cha CH, Ruo L, Fong Y, et al. Resection of hepatocellular carcinoma in patients otherwise eligible for transplantation. *Ann Surg* 2003;238:315–323.
3. Schafer DF, Sorrell MF. Hepatocellular carcinoma. *Lancet* 1999;353:1253–1257.
4. Valea FA. Liver and hepatic duct cancer. *Clin Obstet Gynecol* 2002;45:939–951.
5. El S, Mason AC. Rising incidence of hepatocellular carcinoma in the United States. *N Engl J Med* 1999;340:745–750.
6. Okuda K, Obata H, Nakajima Y, et al. Prognosis of primary hepatocellular carcinoma. *Hepatology* 1984;4S:3S.
7. American Joint Committee on Cancer. *Cancer staging manual*, 6th ed. New York: Springer-Verlag, 2002:131–138.
8. Pugh RN, Murray L, Dawson JL, et al. Transection of the esophagus for bleeding esophageal varices. *Br J Surg* 1973;60:646–649.
9. Bismuth H, Chiche L, Adam R, et al. Liver resection versus transplantation for hepatocellular carcinoma in cirrhotic patients. *Ann Surg* 1993;218:145–151.
10. Llovet JM, Fuster J, Bruix J. Intention-to-treat analysis of surgical treatment of early hepatocellular carcinoma: resection versus transplantation. *Hepatology* 1999;30:1434–1440.
11. Lau W, Leung W, Ho S, et al. Adjuvant intraarterial iodine-131-labelled lipiodol for respectable hepatocellular carcinoma. A prospective randomized trial. *Lancet* 1999;353:797–801.
12. Venook AP. Regional strategies for managing hepatocellular carcinoma. *Oncology* 2000;14:347–354.

13. Mazzaferro V, Regalia E, Doci R, et al. Liver transplantation for the treatment of small hepatocellular carcinomas in patients with cirrhosis. *N Engl J Med* 1996;334:693–699.
14. Johnson PJ. Are there indications for chemotherapy in hepatocellular carcinoma. *Surg Oncol Clin North Am* 2003;12:127–134.
15. Haskell CM. Liver: chemotherapy. In: Haskell CM, ed. *Cancer treatment*, 5th ed. Philadelphia, PH: W. B. Saunders, 2001:778–785.
16. Leung TWT, Patt YZ, Lau WY, et al. Complete pathological remission is possible with systemic combination chemotherapy for inoperable hepatocellular carcinoma. *Clin Cancer Res* 1999;5:1676–1681.
17. Lai CL, Wu PC, Chan GC, et al. Doxorubicin versus no antitumor therapy in inoperable hepatocellular carcinoma. A prospective randomized trial. *Cancer* 1988;62:479–483.
18. Nakashima K, Kitano S, Kim YI, et al. Postoperative adjuvant arterial infusion chemotherapy for patients with hepatocellular carcinoma. *Hepatogastroenterology* 1996;43:1410–1414.
19. Lai EC, Lo CM, Fan ST, et al. Postoperative adjuvant chemotherapy after curative resection of hepatocellular carcinoma: a randomized controlled trial. *Arch Surg* 1998;133:183–188.
20. Kawata S, Yamasaki E, Nagase T, et al. Effect of pravastatin on survival in patients with advanced hepatocellular carcinoma. A randomized controlled trial. *Br J Cancer* 2001;84:886–891.
21. Yang B, Zhang B, Xu Y, et al. Prospective study of early detection for primary liver cancer. *J Cancer Res Clin Oncol* 1997;123:357–360.

8

Colorectal Cancer

George P. Kim[*], Chris H. Takimoto[†], and Carmen J. Allegra[‡]

[*]Gastrointestinal Cancer Section, Mayo Clinic Cancer Center, Jacksonville, Florida;
[†]Institute for Drug Development, Cancer, Therapy & Research Center, San Antonio, Texas;
and [‡]Network for Medical Communication and Research, Atlanta, Georgia

EPIDEMIOLOGY

- Colorectal cancer (CRC) is the second overall, that is, men and women combined, leading cause of cancer death in the United States and is the third most common cause of cancer, separately, in men and in women.
- It was estimated that approximately 146,940 new cases of CRC would have been diagnosed in 2004 in the United States, and one-third of patients would have died as a result of the disease (1).
- The lifetime risk of developing CRC is 1:18.
- Surgery will cure almost 50% of all diagnosed patients, although almost 80,000 people develop metastatic CRC each year.
- The incidence of colon cancer is higher in the more economically developed regions, such as the United States or Western Europe, than in Asia, Africa, or South America.
- Between 1973 and 1998, the U.S. incidence of CRC continued to decline, and so did mortality, which declined by 23.5% during this interval.

RISK FACTORS

Although certain conditions predispose patients to develop colon cancer, up to 70% of patients have no identifiable risk factors:

- **Age:** More than 90% of colon cancer occur in patients older than 50 years.
- **Gender:** The incidence of colon cancer is higher in women, whereas rectal cancer is more common in men.
- **Ethnicity:** The occurrence of cancer is more common in African Americans than in whites, and mortality increases by 32% in African Americans.
- **History of colorectal cancer or adenomas:**
  - tubular adenomas (lowest risk)
  - tubulovillous adenomas (intermediate risk)
  - villous adenomas (highest risk).
- **Tobacco use:** About 2.5-fold increased risk of adenomas is observed in smokers.
- **Obesity**
- **Dietary factors:** high-fiber, low caloric intake, and low animal-fat diets may reduce the risk of cancer.
- **Calcium deficiency:** Daily intake of 1.25 to 2.0 g of calcium was associated with a reduced risk of recurrent adenomas in a randomized placebo-controlled trial.

- **Micronutrient deficiency:** Folate and vitamin E and D deficiency may increase the risk of cancer.
- **Inflammatory bowel disease:** Ulcerative colitis increases risk by 7-fold to 11-fold, especially with the duration of colitis (8 to 12 years) and with the detection of dysplasia. Crohn disease is associated with a twofold increased risk of CRC.
- **Nonsteroidal antiinflammatory drugs:** An American Cancer Society study reported 40% lower mortality in regular aspirin users, and similar reductions in mortality were seen in prolonged nonsteroidal antiinflammatory drug (NSAID) use in patients with rheumatologic disorders. The cyclooxygenase-2 (COX-2) inhibitor celecoxib is approved by the U.S. Food and Drug Administration (FDA) for adjunctive treatment of patients with familial adenomatous polyposis (FAP). Its role in the prevention of cancer development in nonheretidary cohorts is under investigation.
- **Family history:** In the general population, if one first-degree relative develops cancer, it increases the relative risk for other family members to 1.72, and if two relatives are affected, the relative risk increases to 2.75; increased risk is also observed when a first-degree relative develops an adenomatous polyp before age 60. True hereditary forms of cancer account for only 6% of CRCs.

Familial Adenomatous Polyposis Syndrome

FAP is an autosomal-dominant inherited syndrome with more than 90% penetrance, manifested by hundreds of polyps developing by late adolescence. The risk of developing invasive cancer over time is virtually 100%. Germline mutations in the adenomatous polyposis coli (APC) gene on chromosome 5q21 have been identified. The loss of the APC gene results in altered signal transduction with increased transcriptional activity of ß-catenin.

Attenuated FAP: These FAPs are flat adenomas that arise at an older age than FAPs do; mutations tend to occur in the proximal and distal portions of the APC gene.

Gardner syndrome: This syndrome is associated with desmoid tumors, lipomas, and fibromas of the mesentery or abdominal wall.

Turcot syndrome: This syndrome involves tumors of the central nervous system (CNS).

Peutz–Jeghers syndrome: This syndrome shows nonneoplastic hamartomatous polyps throughout the gastrointestinal tract and perioral melanin pigmentation.

Juvenile polyposis: These are hamartomas in colon, small bowel, and stomach.

Hereditary Nonpolyposis Colorectal Cancer

The Lynch syndromes, named after Henry T. Lynch, include Lynch I or the colonic syndrome, which is an autosomal-dominant trait characterized by distinct clinical features including proximal colon involvement, mucinous or poorly differentiated histology, pseudodiploidy, and the presence of synchronous or metachronous tumors. Increased survival has been observed in patients despite colon cancer developing before 50 years, with a lifetime risk of cancer approximating 75%. The Lynch II or extracolonic individuals are susceptible to malignancies in the endometrium, ovary, stomach, hepatobiliary tract, small intestine, and genitourinary tract.

The "Amsterdam Criteria" were established to identify potential kindreds and include:

- Histologically verified CRC in at least three family members, one being a first-degree relative of the other two members
- CRC involving at least two successive generations and
- At least one family member being diagnosed by 50 years.

Inclusion of extracolonic tumors and clinicopathological and age modifications were introduced by the "Bethesda Criteria" in 1997. Germline defects in DNA mismatch-repair genes (*hMSH2*, *hMLH1*, *hPMS1*, and *hPMS2*) have been detected, and resultant microsatellite instability (MSI) can be identified in virtually all hereditary nonpolyposis colorectal cancer (HNPCC) kindreds and in 15% to 20% of sporadic colon cancers.

SCREENING

The American Cancer Society has developed screening guidelines for the early detection of colon cancer. There are a variety of available early detection tests for colon cancer. Starting at age 50, both men and women should discuss the full range of testing options with their physicians and choose one of the following:

- Yearly fecal occult blood test (FOBT)
- Flexible sigmoidoscopy every 5 years
- Yearly FOBT and flexible sigmoidoscopy every 5 years (preferred over either FOBT alone or flexible sigmoidoscopy alone)
- Double-contrast barium enema every 5 years
- Colonoscopy every 10 years.

It should be noted that all positive tests should be followed up with colonoscopy. Individuals with a family or personal history of colon cancer or polyps or a history of chronic inflammatory bowel disease should be tested earlier and may need to undergo testing more often.

Virtual Colonoscopy

A virtual colonoscopy or computerized tomographic colonography is an emerging technology in which a spiral computerized tomography (CT) scan of the colon is obtained and three-dimensional images are created and reviewed by a radiologist. A recent study demonstrated comparable sensitivity to conventional colonoscopy (88.7% versus 92.3% for polyps at least 6 mm in dimension). Earlier studies using two-dimensional technology and inexperienced radiologists observed equivocal results. Patients still require bowel preparation and colonic distension as well as ingestion of oral contrast. Additional studies are required before this technique can be used routinely.

Carcinoembryonic Antigen

Carcinoembryonic antigen (CEA) is not useful for general CRC screening purposes. CEA has a low positive predictive value whereby approximately 60% of cancers are missed.

K-*ras* Detection

The K-*ras* gene is mutated in 50% of CRCs, and its detection in stool represents a potential powerful screening strategy. This is currently an active area of clinical investigation.

PATHOPHYSIOLOGY

Colon carcinogenesis involves progression from hyperproliferative mucosa to polyp formation, with dysplasia, and transformation to noninvasive lesions and subsequent tumor cells with invasive and metastatic capabilities. CRC is a unique model of multistep carcinogenesis resulting from the accumulation of multiple genetic alterations. Stage-by-stage molecular analysis has revealed that this progression involves several types of genetic instability, including loss of heterozygosity, with chromosomes 8p, 17p, and 18q representing the most common chromosomal losses. The 17p deletion accounts for loss of p53 function, and 18q contains the tumor-suppressor genes deleted in colon cancer (i.e., DCC) and the gene deleted in pancreatic 4 (i.e., DPC4). The loss of heterozygosity of chromosome 18q has prognostic significance.

Colon carcinogenesis also occurs as a consequence of defects in the DNA mismatch repair system. The loss of *hMLH1* and *hMSH2*, predominantly, in sporadic cancers leads to accelerated accumulation of additions or deletions in repeating DNA nucleotide units. This MSI contributes to the loss of growth inhibition mediated by transforming growth factor-ß (TGF-ß) due to a mutation in the type II receptor. Mutations in the APC gene on chromosome 5q21 are responsible for FAP and are involved in cell signaling and in cellular adhesion, with binding of ß-catenin. Alterations in the APC gene occur early in tumor progression. Mutations in the protooncogene *ras* family, including K-*ras* and N-*ras*, are important for transformation and also are common in early tumor development.

More than 90% of CRCs are adenocarcinomas, with proximal tumors becoming increasingly more common. Left-sided cancers tend to be annular, leading to obstruction, whereas right-sided cancers are more commonly polypoid and clinically silent. One-third of patients will initially be seen with metastatic disease, whereas 50% will eventually develop metastases.

DIAGNOSIS

Signs and Symptoms

- Abdominal pain, typically intermittent and vague
- Weight loss
- Bowel changes, such as pencil stools
- Early satiety
- Gastrointestinal bleeding
- Fatigue
- Obstruction, perforation, acute or chronic bleeding, or liver metastasis, all of which contribute to symptom development
- Unusual presentations including patients with deep venous thrombosis, *Streptococcus bovis* bacteremia, and nephrotic-range proteinuria
- Clinical findings including anemia, weight loss, electrolyte abnormalities, and liver enzyme elevations.

Diagnostic Evaluation

- A double-contrast barium enema may be more cost effective as an initial evaluation, but endoscopic studies provide histologic information, potential therapeutic intervention, and overall greater sensitivity and specificity.
- Basic laboratory studies including complete blood count, electrolytes, and liver and renal function tests, chest radiograph, and CT scan of the abdomen and pelvis are useful in initial cancer diagnosis, although the relative contributions of these various modalities are undefined.
- CEA elevations occur in non–cancer-related conditions, reducing the specificity of CEA measurements in the initial detection of colon cancer.

STAGING

The American Joint Committee on Cancer (AJCC) (1) staging of colon cancer using the TNM classification was updated in 2003 (see Fig. 8.1). Patients with stage II and III disease have been further stratified, and vascular or lymphatic invasion has been included (see Table 8.1). The tumor designation, or T stage, defines the extent of bowel wall penetration, as opposed to tumor size. The AJCC staging system accounts for the number of lymph nodes involved as a significant predictor of survival. Four or more positive lymph nodes or gross versus microscopic bowel wall penetration lead to diminished survival. Some patients with stage

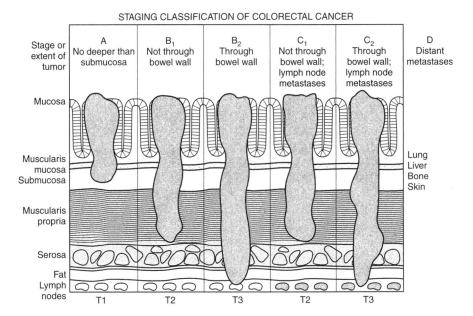

FIG. 8.1. Staging classification of colorectal cancer. Classification is based on modifications of Dukes' system. Stages B3 and C3 (not shown) signify invasion of contiguous organs or structures (T4). Prognosis is also determined by the number of positive lymph nodes: more than four (N2) lymph nodes predicts a worse outcome than one to three (N1) lymph nodes, and a poor histopathological differentiation, vascular or lymphatic invasion, and a positive preoperative CEA value of >5 ng per mL implies a worse outcome. According to the revised TNM classification system, stage I equals T1 or T2 N0 (Dukes' stage A and B$_1$); stage II equals T3 or T4 N0 (Dukes' stage B$_2$ and B$_3$); stage III equals any T plus N1, N2, or N3 (Dukes' stage C$_1$, C$_2$ and C$_3$); and stage IV equals any T any N plus M1 (Dukes' stage D).

II disease exhibit a heterogeneous outcome and are at high risk for relapse, with outcomes similar to those of node-positive patients (see Table 8.2).

PROGNOSIS

Adverse Prognostic Factors

The adverse prognostic factors include:

- Advanced stage
- Serosal penetration
- Advanced age of patient
- High tumor grade
- More than four lymph nodes being involved
- Bowel obstruction or perforation at presentation
- MSI caused by a defective DNA mismatch-repair system (altered *MLH1*, *MSH2*), which is associated with an improved outcome
- Biochemical and molecular markers such as elevated thymidylate synthase, p53 mutations, or loss of heterozygosity of chromosome 18q, which are associated with a poor prognosis (2,3).

TABLE 8.1. *American Joint Committee on Cancer (AJCC) staging classification (2003)*

Primary tumor: T
  TX: Primary tumor cannot be assessed
  T0: No evidence of primary tumor
  Tis: Carcinoma *in situ*—intraepithelial or invasion of the lamina propria[a]
  T1: Tumor invades submucosa
  T2: Tumor invades muscularis propria
  T3: Tumor invades through the muscularis propria into the subserosa or into nonperitonealized pericolic or perirectal tissues
  T4: Tumor directly invades other organs or structures, and/or perforates visceral peritoneum[b,c]

Regional lymph nodes: N[d]
  NX: Regional nodes cannot be assessed
  N0: No regional lymph node metastasis
  N1: Metastasis in 1 to 3 regional lymph nodes
  N2: Metastasis in 4 or more regional lymph nodes

Distant metastases: M
  MX: Presence of distant metastases cannot be assessed
  M0: No distant metastases
  M1: Distant metastases are present. Metastasis in the external iliac or common iliac lymph node is classified as M1

Stage grouping	Dukes'/MAC
Stage 0:	Tis N0 M0
Stage I	T1 N0 M0—A A
	T2 N0 M0—A B1
Stage IIA	T3 N0 M0—B B2
Stage IIB	T4 N0 M0—B B3
Stage IIIA	T1—T2 N1 M0—C C1
Stage IIIB	T3–T4 N1 M0—C C2/C3
Stage IIIC	Any T N2 M0—C C1/C2/C3
Stage IV	Any T Any N M1—D

- Stage group II is subdivided into IIA and IIB on the basis of whether the primary tumor is T3 or T4, respectively
- Stage III is subdivided into IIIA (T1–2 N1 M0), IIIB (T3–4 N1 M0), or IIIC (any T N2 M0)

Stage at initial diagnosis:	
Stage I	14%
Stage II/III	65%
Stage IV	21%

[a]Tis includes cancer cells confined within the glandular basement membrane (intraepithelial) or lamina propria (intramucosal) with no extension through the muscularis mucosae into the submucosa.

[b]Direct invasion in T4 includes invasion of other segments of the colorectum through the serosa, for example, invasion of the sigmoid colon by a carcinoma of the cecum.

[c]Tumor that is macroscopically adherent to other organs or structures is classified T4. However, if no tumor is present in the adhesion microscopically, the classification should be pT3. The V and L substaging should be used to identify the presence or absence of vascular or lymphatic invasion.

[d]Smooth metastatic nodules in the pericolic or perirectal fat are considered lymph node metastases and will be counted in the N staging. In contrast, irregularly contoured metastatic nodules in the peritumoral fat are considered as a vascular invasion and will be coded as an extension of the T category as either V1 (microscopic vascular invasion) if it is only microscopically visible or as V2 (macroscopic vascular invasion) if it is grossly visible.

TABLE 8.2. *Five-year survival prognosis by stage*

Stage 0–I	>90%
Stage II	70–85%
Stage III	55–70%
Stage IV	<10%

MANAGEMENT ALGORITHM

Surgery

- The primary curative intervention requires en bloc extirpation of the involved bowel segment along with mesentery by laparotomy, with pericolic and intermediate lymphadenectomy for both staging and therapeutic intent. Negative proximal, distal, and lateral surgical margins are of paramount importance.
- Surgical intervention is indicated if polypectomy pathology reveals muscularis mucosal involvement or penetration.
- Surgical palliation may include colostomy or even resection of metastatic disease for symptoms of acute obstruction or persistent bleeding.
- The number of lymph nodes resected and pathologically examined is critical to accurate staging. The probability of true node negativity in T1 or T2 tumors is less than 25% when at least 18 nodes are examined, whereas in T3 and T4 tumors, fewer than 10 nodes need to be evaluated to achieve the same probability. On average, at least 12 to 14 lymph nodes should be examined.

Radiation Therapy

- Administration of radiotherapy is limited by bowel-segment mobility. Small bowel toxicity, in particular, limits abdominal radiation, and patients with comorbidities such as diabetes, previous surgery with adhesion formation, and previous 5-fluorouracil (5-FU) exposure are at higher risk than patients without comorbidities. Bowel toxicity ranging from 4% to 8% is expected.
- Local control and improved disease-free survival (DFS) have been reported in retrospective series of patients with T4 lesions or perforations, nodal disease, and subtotal resections who have been treated with 5,000 to 5,400 cGy directed at the primary tumor bed and draining lymph nodes. However, there are no randomized data to support the use of radiation in the management of colon cancer.

Adjuvant Chemotherapy for Colon Cancer

Intergroup 035

This large Intergroup trial of 5-FU and levamisole (Lev) is of historic importance because it reported a 41% reduction in the relapse rate and a 33% decrease in overall cancer mortality (4). This study resulted in the National Institutes of Health consensus panel recommending that 5-FU–based adjuvant therapy be administered to all patients with resected stage III colon cancer.

Intergroup 0089

Intergroup 0089 is a landmark study that randomized 3,759 patients with stage II or III disease to one of four arms (5). The results demonstrated that the 5-FU and leucovorin (LV)–containing schedules (Mayo Clinic and Roswell Park) were equivalent and that the three-drug combination only increased toxicity. The 5-FU and Lev arm was effective but required 12 months of treatment versus the 6-month schedules of the 5-FU and LV arm.

The 5-year DFS and overall survival (OS) for each of the four arms in the study were as follows:

- 5-FU + Lev for 12 months; DFS = 56%, OS = 63%
- 5-FU + high-dose LV; DFS = 60%, OS = 66%
- 5-FU + low-dose LV; DFS = 60%, OS = 66%
- 5-FU + LV + Lev; DFS = 60%, OS = 67%.

MOSAIC

A European study of 2,219 patients with stage II (40%) and III (60%) disease who were treated with infusional 5-FU with LV modulation versus the same combination with oxaliplatin (FOLFOX4) every 2 weeks for 6 months (6) demonstrated a 3-year DFS benefit favoring the FOLFOX4 combination [78.2% for 5-FU and LV versus 72.9% for FOLFOX4, hazard ratio (HR) 0.77; 95% CI, 0.65 to 0.92, $p = 0.002$], although the OS between the two arms was not statistically different when the study was reported. A 3-year disease-free endpoint was chosen because a recent retrospective analysis of more than 17,400 patients demonstrated that the 3-year disease-free endpoint is equivalent to the conventional 5-year OS benchmark. Treatment with FOLFOX4 was well tolerated, with 41% patients having grade 3 and 4 neutropenia, with only 0.7% being associated with fever. Anticipated peripheral neuropathy or paresthesias were observed (grade 2–32% and grade 3–12%) but was almost entirely resolved 1 year later (grade 2–5% and grade 3–1%).

X-ACT

A 1987 study of patients with stage III disease compared capecitabine (1,250 mg per m^2 b.i.d. for 14 days, every 3 weeks) with the Mayo Clinic bolus of 5-FU and LV (7). The study was designed to demonstrate equivalency, with a primary endpoint of 3-year DFS. The capecitabine arm demonstrated a trend toward superiority in this endpoint (64.2% versus 60.6%, HR 0.87; 95% CI, 0.75 to 1.00, Log-rank $p = 0.0526$).

CALGB 89803

CALGB 89803 was a study of irinotecan with bolus 5-FU and LV (IFL) versus weekly 5-FU in patients with stage III disease (8). Increased grade 3 and 4 neutropenia and early deaths were observed in the experimental arm, and a higher number of patients withdrew from the study. Overall, IFL was not better than the 5-FU and LV arm. The use of the IFL regimen in the adjuvant setting cannot be recommended at present. An important study of irinotecan in combination with infusional 5-FU or FOLFIRI (continuous infusion 5-FU with biweekly irinotecan) has completed accrual of 1,800 patients, and preliminary analyses report no significant increases in treatment-related toxicity.

Adjuvant Chemotherapy Regimens for Colon Cancer

On the basis of these adjuvant chemotherapy studies, the use of one of the following regimens is recommended for patients with stage III colon cancer. The results with capecitabine are promising in the adjuvant setting.

5-Fluorouracil and Calcium Leucovorin:

- **Mayo Clinic (bolus) regimen:** 5-FU, 425 mg per m^2 daily for 5 days; preceded by LV, 20 mg per m^2 daily every 4 weeks for six cycles *OR*
- **Roswell Park (weekly) regimen:** 5-FU, 500 mg per m^2 with LV, 500 mg per m^2 weekly for 6 weeks, repeated every 8 weeks for 8 months.

The toxicity profile of these two regimens differs. Myelosuppression and oral mucositis are more common with the daily Mayo Clinic regimen, whereas diarrhea may be more severe with the weekly schedule. Cryotherapy with ice held in the mouth during the 5-FU infusion may help lessen the mucositis associated with the therapy.

Oxaliplatin, 5-Fluorouracil (Infusional and Bolus), and Leucovorin (FOLFOX4):

- Oxaliplatin 85 mg per m^2 on day 1 only, followed by bolus 5-FU 400 mg per m^2 on days 1 and 2, with LV 200 mg per m^2 on days 1 and 2. Infusional 5-FU 600 mg per m^2 is then given for 22 hours on days 1 and 2.

FOLFOX6, which omits the day 2 bolus 5-FU and LV, uses 2,400 mg per m^2 of continuous 5-FU over 46 hours and appears to have activity equivalent to that of FOLFOX4 in the advanced disease setting. The oxaliplatin dose is increased to 100 mg per m^2, but ongoing studies are evaluating the 85 mg per m^2 dose.

Adjuvant Chemotherapy for Stage II Colon Cancer

Despite the 75% 5-year survival with surgery alone, some patients with stage II disease have a higher risk of relapse, with outcomes being similar to those of node-positive patients. Adjuvant chemotherapy provides up to 33% OS advantage, resulting in an absolute treatment benefit of approximately 5%.

Several analyses have reported varying outcomes in patients with stage II disease who received adjuvant treatment:

- The National Surgical Adjuvant Breast and Bowel Project (NSABP) summary of protocols (C-01 to C-04) of 1,565 patients with stage II disease reported a 32% relative reduction in mortality (cumulative odds, 0.68; 95% CI, 0.50 to 0.92; $p = 0.01$). This reduction in mortality translated into an absolute survival advantage of 5% (9).
- A meta-analysis by Erlichman et al. (10) detected a nonsignificant 2% benefit (82% versus 80%, $p = 0.217$) in 1,020 patients with high-risk T3 and T4 cancer treated with 5-FU and LV for 5 consecutive days.
- Schrag reviewed Medicare claims for chemotherapy within the Surveillance, Epidemiology and End Results (SEER) Database and identified 3,700 patients with resected stage II disease among whom 31% received adjuvant treatment (11). No survival benefit was detected with 5-FU compared to surgery alone (74% versus 72%) even with patients considered to be at high risk because of obstruction, perforation, or T4 lesions.
- In the recent MOSAIC study, FOLFOX4 chemotherapy showed benefits in patients with stage II disease (40%), although this was not statistically significant [86.6% versus 83.9% 5-FU and LV, HR 0.82 (0.57–1.17), relative risk reduction, 18%].
- The Quasar Collaborative Group study reported an OS benefit of 1% to 5% in 3,238 patients (91% Dukes B colon cancer) randomized to chemotherapy versus surgery alone. With a median follow-up of 4.2 years, the risk of death (HR 0.88; 95 % CI, 0.75 to 1.05; $p = 0.15$) and recurrence rate (HR 0.82; 95% CI, 0.70 to 0.97; $p = 0.02$) favored 5-FU and LV chemotherapy.
- The American Society of Clinical Oncology Panel recently concluded that the routine use of adjuvant chemotherapy for patients with stage II disease could not be recommended (12). A review of 37 randomized controlled trials and 11 meta-analyses found no evidence of a statistically significant survival benefit with postoperative treatment. Treatment needed to be considered for specific subsets of patients (e.g., T4 lesions, perforation, poorly differentiated histology, or inadequately sampled nodes), and patient input was critical.

Immunotherapy (Edrecolomab, 17-1A)

Riethmuller et al. (13) treated 189 patients postoperatively with the monoclonal antibody edrecolomab, resulting in a 27% decrease in recurrence rate and a 30% reduction in mortality rate. In a comparison of patients with stage III disease treated with 5-FU–based chemotherapy without or with edrecolomab, a survival advantage was suggested for the latter (HR 0.785; 95% CI, 0.638 to 0.967). The results from a study of edrecolomab in patients with stage II disease are pending.

Adjuvant Treatment for Rectal Cancer

In contrast to colon cancer, treatment failures after potentially curative resections tend to occur more locally in 10% to 18% of patients. Combined-modality adjuvant chemotherapy and radiation therapy is now the standard therapy for patients with stages II and III rectal cancer (T3, T4, and nodal disease N+).

Intergroup 0114

A four-arm study of 1,695 patients compared 5-FU alone, 5-FU and LV combination, 5-FU and Lev combination, and 5-FU and LV and Lev combination (14). Two cycles of·chemotherapy was administered before and after chemotherapy in combination with external beam radiation (50.4 Gy to 45 Gy with 5.4 Gy boost). The chemotherapy during the radiation was given as a bolus with or without LV. The DFS and OS was similar in all treatment arms, leading to the conclusion that 5-FU alone was as effective as other combinations.

NCCTG 86-47-51

Both DFS and OS advantages were observed in patients receiving continuous infusion of 5-FU during radiation when compared with those receiving bolus 5-FU (15). This survival benefit has led to continuous infusion 5-FU during radiation being considered as the standard.

Adjuvant Combined-modality Regimens for Rectal Cancer

- 5-FU by intravenous bolus injection at 500 mg/m^2/day on days 1 to 5 and on days 36 to 40, followed by
  - radiation therapy given in 180-cGy fractions over 5 weeks, starting day 64, to a total dose of 4,500 to 5,400 cGy along with 5-FU, 225 mg/m^2/day, by ambulatory infusion pump during the entire 5-week period of radiation therapy, followed by
  - intravenous bolus of 5-FU, 450 mg/m^2/day, given daily for 5 days on days 134 to 138 and on days 169 to 173 for a total treatment period of 6 months.
- On the basis of the improvements in these earlier studies and in the adjuvant chemotherapy for colon cancer, one can consider the administration of either Mayo Clinic or Roswell Park regimen 2 months before 5-FU chemotherapy–radiation, followed by an additional two cycles.
- Studies have shown that preoperative chemoradiation (preop chemoRT) is better than postoperative chemoradiation (postop chemoRT) for survival and preservation of anal function. Many physicians in the United States now use preop chemoRT followed by surgery and by additional chemoRT to complete a 6-month course of chemotherapy, that is, approximately 4 months of treatment after surgery.
- Capecitabine, which mimics infusional 5-FU, is being investigated in conjunction with radiation, and no increased toxicity has been observed. Additionally, oxaliplatin is being evaluated as a radiation sensitizer for patients with rectal disease.

FOLLOW-UP AFTER ADJUVANT TREATMENT

Eighty percent of recurrences are seen within 2 years of initial therapy. The American Cancer Society recommends total colonic evaluation with either colonoscopy or double-contrast barium enema within 1 year of resection, followed every 3 to 5 years if findings remain normal. Synchronous cancers must be excluded during initial surgical extirpation, and metachronous malignancies in the form of polyps must be detected and excised before more malignant behavior develops.

TREATMENT FOR ADVANCED DISEASE

5-Fluorouracil–Based Chemotherapy

Single-arm phase II studies of 5-FU and LV chemotherapy regimens in advanced CRC have reported response rates ranging from 0% to 70%, but most larger studies have observed objective response rates of 15% to 20%, with median survival of 8 to 12 months.

Continuous Infusion of 5-Fluorouracil

The efficiency of continuous infusion of 5-FU may be equivalent to or slightly better than that of bolus 5-FU and LV and is generally well tolerated despite the inconvenience of a prolonged intravenous infusion apparatus (16,17). 5-FU at 300 mg/m^2/day is infused continuously by an ambulatory infusion pump. Toxicities include mucositis; however, myelosuppression is less common. Palmar–plantar erythrodysesthesia (hand–foot syndrome) is common and may respond to pyridoxine, 50 to 150 mg/m^2/day. Continuous infusions of 5-FU may have modest activity in patients who have progressed on a bolus 5-FU regimen.

Oxaliplatin

Oxaliplatin is an agent that differs structurally from other platinums in its 1,2-diaminocyclohexane (DACH) moiety. At doses resulting in equivalent cytotoxicity, oxaliplatin forms fewer DNA adducts than does cisplatin, suggesting that oxaliplatin lesions are more lethal than *cis*-platinum adducts. Oxaliplatin exhibits synergy with 5-FU because increased response rates as high as 66% have been observed even in patients who are refractory to 5-FU. Despite its unique toxicities (i.e., reversible peripheral neuropathy, laryngopharyngeal dysesthesias, and cold hypersensitivities), oxaliplatin lacks the emetogenic and nephrogenic toxicities of cisplatin.

Oxaliplatin was approved for second-line therapy in metastatic patients on the basis of a study comparing FOLFOX4 with oxaliplatin alone and with infusional or bolus 5-FU and LV. In this study, response rate, time to progression, and relief of tumor-related symptoms were improved with FOLFOX4 when compared to the other treatment arms. Despite the improved time to progression, the OS difference was not statistically significant (9.8 versus 8.7 and 8.1 months, respectively).

The North Central Cancer Treatment Group (N9741) conducted a trial comparing first-line FOLFOX4 versus IFL versus IROX (irinotecan in combination with oxaliplatin). The study, designed by Richard Goldberg et al. (18), originally consisted of six arms, but three were eliminated on the basis of changes in the standard of care or toxicity. In addition, a higher 60-day mortality was detected in the IFL arm, resulting in a dose reduction to 100 mg per m^2. The response rate, time to progression, and OS were significantly better in the FOLFOX4 arm than in the IFL arm. Interestingly, survival in the patients on IROX regimen was better than in the IFL-treated patients and was not significantly different from those on the FOLFOX combination. Imbalances in the second-line chemotherapy administered to patients in this study may confound the survival differences. Approximately 60% of the oxaliplatin failures were treated with irinotecan, whereas only 24% of patients who are refractory to irinotecan received oxaliplatin. In addition, the study was not designed to address the effect of infusional 5-FU. The observed toxicities in the study were reflective of the specific drug combinations and included grade 3 or higher paresthesias (18%) in the FOLFOX arm and a 28% incidence of diarrhea in the IFL arm. Despite a higher degree of neutropenia (50% in FOLFOX versus 40% in IFL) with FOLFOX, febrile neutropenia was significantly greater in the IFL arm (15% with FOLFOX versus 4% with IFL). IROX also exhibited significant toxicities. Oxaliplatin has been approved by the FDA for use in the first-line treatment of patients with metastatic CRC largely on the basis of this study.

Although FOLFOX is clearly a superior regimen compared to IFL, the use of infusional 5-FU with irinotecan may produce results similar to those seen using FOLFOX. Tournigand et al. reported an equivalent median survival of 21.5 months with FOLFIRI followed by FOLFOX and a median survival of 20.6 months with the opposite sequence ($p = 0.99$) (19). The conclusion is that similar survival is observed in patients receiving either sequence. Other investigators have suggested that the use of all active agents results in the best survival in patients with advanced CRC.

Irinotecan/CPT-11

Irinotecan is a topoisomerase I–targeting agent, with activity in patients with advanced CRC and in patients deemed refractory to 5-FU. Response rates as high as 20% are observed, and an additional 45% of patients achieve disease stabilization. Significant survival advantages have been shown for irinotecan as second-line therapy after 5-FU compared with supportive care or with continuous-infusion 5-FU regimens. Several schedules are typically administered with and without 5-FU:

- The first schedule followed the IFL regimen (20)—irinotecan is infused at a dose of 125 mg per m^2 over 90 minutes weekly for 4 weeks followed by a 2-week rest. In a phase III study comparing this regimen to the 5-FU bolus Mayo Clinic regimen, a higher response rate (39% versus 21%, $p = 0.0001$) and OS (14.8 versus 12.6 months, $p = 0.042$) were observed for this regimen.

  Delayed-onset diarrhea is common and requires close monitoring and aggressive management (high-dose loperamide, 4 mg initially and then 2 mg every 2 hours until diarrhea stops for at least 12 hours). Neutropenia and mild nausea and vomiting also are common. This combination of toxicities can be severe and life threatening, which was evident in a large phase III study, NCCTG 9741, comparing irinotecan and oxaliplatin combination regimens (see subsequent text). A higher 60-day mortality was observed (4.5% versus 1.8%), and the dose of the irinotecan weekly regimen reduced to 100 mg per m^2.

- A second schedule administered 350 mg per m^2 of irinotecan over a 90-minute period once every 3 weeks and produced responses in 13.7% of patients and stable disease in another 44% of patients (21). In patients who are refractory to 5-FU, a median survival of 10.5 months was reported.

- A third schedule combined infusional 5-FU with biweekly irinotecan, as reported by Douillard et al. (22). Improvements in response (35% versus 22%, $p<0.005$), median survival (17.4 versus 14.1 months, $p = 0.031$), and quality of life were observed in the irinotecan-treated arm. Neutropenia was equivalent to that found in the weekly irinotecan regimen, although febrile neutropenia and diarrhea were markedly reduced in this third regimen.

- Finally, the administration of weekly irinotecan alone has been reported by Pitot et al. (23) In patients receiving 5-FU earlier, a 13% response rate and an 7.7 median response duration were observed.

Capecitabine

Capecitabine, the oral fluoropyrimidine prodrug, undergoes a series of three enzymatic steps in its conversion to 5-FU. The final enzymatic step is catalyzed by thymidine phosphorylase, which is overexpressed in tumor than in normal tissues. Subsequently, the tumor tissue achieves higher concentrations of 5-FU, with thymidine phosphorylase preferentially activating the tumor tissue. Two phase III studies have compared single-agent capecitabine to the Mayo Clinic 5-FU and LV regimen and demonstrated higher response rates for the former but equivalent time to progression and median survival (24). The toxicity profile favored the capecitabine arm because decreased gastrointestinal and hematologic toxicities and fewer hospitalizations were observed in this arm. An increased frequency of hand–foot syndrome and hyperbilirubinemia were noted with capecitabine. Early phase II studies with capecitabine in combination with either oxaliplatin or irinotecan demonstrated promising response rates as high as 50% to 65%, and several large phase III studies are ongoing.

Bevacizumab

Bevacizumab (BV) is a recombinant humanized anti–vascular endothelial cell growth factor (anti-VEGF) monoclonal antibody with amino acid sequence similarity of 97% to that of human IgG1. BV blocks VEGF-induced angiogenesis with an exceptionally high affinity for VEGF. One of the initial trials with BV in untreated CRC patients combined BV (doses of either 5 or 10 mg per kg every 2 weeks) with weekly 500–mg per m^2 dose of 5-FU and LV. Interestingly, a 40% response rate and 21.5-month median survival was observed in the 5–mg per kg cohort. The major toxicities included thrombosis (13 patients with three treatment discontinuations and one patient death), proteinuria, and hypertension. Updated toxicity data reveals that full-dose anticoagulation can be administered with BV and that there is no increased risk of deep venous thrombus formation. The intriguing results presented by Hurwitz et al. (25) also reports a higher response rate (45% versus 35%, $p<0.0029$) and a longer median survival (20.3 versus 15.6 months) when BV is combined with IFL. A large phase III trial combining BV with FOLFOX as second-line treatment is awaited. BV has been approved by the FDA, largely on the basis of the results of these trials, for the treatment of patients with advanced CRC in combination with any intravenous 5-FU–based regimen.

Cetuximab

Cetuximab is a chimerized IgG1 antibody that prevents ligand binding to the epidermal growth factor receptor (EGFR) and its heterodimers. Cetuximab exhibits higher affinity (subnanomolar) or approximately 1-log greater binding than the natural ligands for EGFR. The agent blocks receptor dimerization, tyrosine kinase phosphorylation, and subsequent downstream signal transduction. Cetuximab is administered at a dose of 400 mg per m^2 in the first week and then at a 250 mg per m^2 dose each week thereafter.

In a study with patients refractory to irinotecan who were treated with the combination of cetuximab and irinotecan versus cetuximab alone, improvements in the response rate (22.9% versus 10.8%, 0.0074) and time to progression (4.1 versus 1.5 months, <0.0001) were reported (26). Despite manageable toxicity, no improvements in survival outcomes were observed. A correlation between the intensity of the skin rash and median survival was noted. Cetuximab has been approved by the FDA for the treatment of patients with EGFR-positive advanced CRC that is refractory to or intolerant of irinotecan.

CHEMOTHERAPY REGIMENS FOR METASTATIC COLORECTAL CANCER

First Line

- Oxaliplatin based: FOLFOX4 or 6 or CAPOX
- Irinotecan based: FOLFIRI
- BV in combination with intravenous 5-FU regimen: 5-FU and LV, IFL, FOLFIRI, or FOLFOX.

Other Regiments

- Capecitabine alone
- Irinotecan alone (350 mg/m^2) or IFL
- XELOX (Oxaliplatin and capecitabine)

- XELIRI (Irinotecan and capacitabine)
- 5-FU alone as continuous infusion.

Second Line

- Any alternative, non–cross resistant regimen to first-line treatment (i.e., FOLFOX followed by FOLFIRI)
- Cetuximab either alone or in combination with irinotecan.

CONTROVERSIES

Carcinoembryonic Antigen

CEA is an acid glycoprotein localized to the cell membrane, facilitating release into blood and surrounding body fluids. CEA is elevated in nonneoplastic processes such as smoking and inflammatory bowel disease and in cancers involving the breast, lungs, or pancreas. The degree of tumor differentiation correlates with CEA expression; up to 30% of colon cancers, in particular poorly differentiated tumors, exhibit no CEA elevation. Elevation is typically defined as a concentration >5 ng per mL and is associated with increased recurrence rate and decreased survival. A measurement of concentration >25 ng per mL is highly suggestive of metastatic disease. In patients preoperatively evaluated with CEA measurements, a sensitivity of 43% and a specificity of 90% were reported.

Persistent elevation of CEA postoperatively may suggest residual tumor or early metastasis. The routine use of CEA alone for evaluating treatment response is not recommended because up to 20% of patients exhibit conflicting declines in CEA levels despite disease progression. Patients with initially negative levels of CEA can subsequently exhibit positive levels. Serial CEA measurements after completion of postoperative chemotherapy may identify patients who are eligible for a curative resection, in particular, patients with a solitary liver or lung metastasis, but this is rare. Data from studies such as the Ohio State study report a 31% 5-year survival in select populations with aggressive CEA surveillance and second-look laparotomy to detect early recurrences. A joint National Institutes of Health (NIH) and U.K. trial failed to demonstrate survival differences with serial CEA measurements. The American Society of Clinical Oncology recommends CEA testing in patients with previous CRC diagnoses who would be eligible or be considered for surgical resection.

Hepatic-only Metastasis

The liver is the most common site for metastasis, with one third of instances involving only the liver; liver is involved in two-thirds of patients dying from colon cancer. Approximately 25% of liver metastases are resectable, with certain patient subsets showing 30% to 40% 5-year survival after resection and 3% to 5% operative morbidity and mortality. Intraoperative ultrasound is the most sensitive test for initial detection, followed by CT scan or magnetic resonance imaging (MRI).

Nonresectable patients with disease limited to the liver can be treated with locoregional [by hepatic artery infusion (HAI)] or systemic chemotherapy. Postoperative chemotherapy trials have exhibited some benefit. Kemeny et al. (27) reported a 4-year DFS and hepatic disease-free benefit in patients with resected liver metastases who had received intraarterial floxuridine with systemic 5-FU compared to those who did not receive any postoperative therapy, although there was no statistically significant difference in OS (62% versus 53%, $p = 0.06$).

The feasibility of converting an initially unresectable disease to a potentially curative disease has been investigated by Bismuth and colleagues (28). Metastectomy was possible in 99 patients with either down-staged or stable disease, and the 3-year survival was encouraging (58% for responders, 45% for patients with stable disease). Similar observations have been reported by

Alberts using preoperative FOLFOX4 on 41% of patients undergoing resection with an observed median survival of 31.4 months (95% CI, 20.4 to 34.8) for the entire cohort (29).

REFERENCES

1. American Joint Committee on Cancer. *AJCC cancer staging manual*, 5th ed. Philadelphia, PA: Lippincott–Raven Publishers; 1997.
2. Johnston PG, Fisher ER, et al. The role of thymidylate synthase expression in prognosis and outcome of adjuvant chemotherapy in patients with rectal cancer. *J Clin Oncol* 1994;12:2640–2647.
3. Popat S, Matakidou A, Houlston RS. Thymidylate synthase expression and prognosis in colorectal cancer: a systematic review and meta-analysis. *J Clin Oncol* 2004;22:529–536.
4. Moertel CG, Fleming TR, Macdonald JS, et al. Levamisole and fluorouracil for adjuvant therapy of resected colon carcinoma [see comments]. *N Engl J Med* 1990;322:352–358.
5. Haller DG, Catalano PJ, MacDonald JS, et al. Fluorouracil (FU), leucovorin (LV) and levamisole (LEV) adjuvant therapy for colon cancer: five-year final report of INT-0089. *Proc Am Soc Clin Oncol* 1998;16:256a.
6. Andre T, Boni C, Mounedji-Boudiaf L, et al. Multicenter international study of oxaliplatin/5-fluorouracil/leucovorin in the adjuvant treatment of colon cancer (MOSAIC) investigators. Oxaliplatin, fluorouracil, and leucovorin as adjuvant treatment for colon cancer. *N Engl J Med* 2004;350:2343–2351.
7. Cassidy J, Scheithauer W, McKendrick H, et al. Capecitabine (X) vs bolus 5-FU/leucovorin (LV) as adjuvant therapy for colon cancer (the X-ACT study): efficacy results of a phase III trial. *Proc Am Soc Clin Oncol* 2004;23:3509.
8. Saltz LB, Niedzwiecki D, Hollis D, et al. Irinotecan plus fluorouracil/leucovorin (IFL) versus fluorouracil/leucovorin alone (FL) in stage III colon cancer (CALGB C89803). *Proc Am Soc Clin Oncol* 2004;23:3500.
9. Mamounas E, Wieand S, Wolmark N, et al. Comparative efficacy of adjuvant chemotherapy in patients with Dukes' B versus Dukes' C colon cancer: results from four National Surgical Adjuvant Breast and Bowel Project adjuvant studies (C01, C02, C03, and C04). *J Clin Oncol* 1999;17:1349–1355.
10. Erlichman. Efficacy of adjuvant fluorouracil and folinic acid in B2 colon cancer. International multicenter pooled analysis of B2 colon cancer trials (IMPACT B2) investigators. *J Clin Oncol* 1999;17(5):1356–1363.
11. Schrag D, Rifas-Shiman S, Saltz L, et al. Adjuvant chemotherapy use for medicare beneficiaries with stage II colon cancer. *J Clin Oncol* 2002;20:3999–4005.
12. Benson AB, Schrag D, Somerfield MR, et al. American Society of Clinical Oncology recommendations on adjuvant chemotherapy for stage II colon cancer. *J Clin Oncol* 2004;22:3408–3419.
13. Riethmuller G, Schneider-Gadicke E, Schlimok G, et al. Randomised trial of monoclonal antibody for adjuvant therapy of resected Dukes' C colorectal carcinoma: German Cancer Aid 171A Study Group. *Lancet* 1994;343:1177–1183.
14. Krook JE, Moertel CG, Gunderson LL, et al. Effective surgical adjuvant therapy for high-risk rectal carcinoma [see comments]. *N Engl J Med* 1991;324:709–715.
15. O'Connell MJ, Martenson JA, Wieand HS, et al. Improving adjuvant therapy for rectal cancer by combining protracted infusion fluorouracil with radiation therapy after curative surgery. *N Engl J Med* 1994;331:502–507.
16. Leichman CG, Fleming TR, Mussia FM, et al. Phase II study of fluorouracil and its modulation in advanced colorectal cancer: a Southwest Oncology Group study. *J Clin Oncol* 1995;13:1303–1311.
17. Falcone A, Allegrini G, Lenconi M, et al. Protracted continuous infusion of 5-fluorouracil and low-dose leucovorin in patients with metastatic colorectal cancer resistant to 5-fluorouracil bolus-based chemotherapy: a Phase II study. *Cancer Chemother Pharmacol* 1999;44:159–163.
18. Goldberg RM, Sargent DJ, Morton RF, et al. A randomized controlled trial of fluorouracil plus leucovorin, irinotecan, and oxaliplatin combinations in patients with previously untreated metastatic colorectal cancer. *J Clin Oncol* 2004;22:23–30.
19. Tournigand C, Andre T, Achille E, et al. FOLFIRI followed by FOLFOX6 or the reverse sequence in advanced colorectal cancer: a randomized GERCOR study. *J Clin Oncol* 2004;22(2):229–237.
20. Saltz LB, Cox JV, Blanke C et al, Irinotecan Study Group. Irinotecan plus fluorouracil and leucovorin for metastatic colorectal cancer. *N Engl J Med* 2000;343:905–914.
21. Cunningham D, Pyrhonen S, James RD, et al. Randomised trial of irinotecan plus supportive care versus supportive care alone after fluorouracil failure for patients with metastatic colorectal cancer. *Lancet* 1998;352:1413–1418.

22. Douillard JY, Cunningham D, Roth AD, et al. Irinotecan combined with fluorouracil compared with fluorouracil alone as first-line treatment for metastatic colorectal cancer: a multicentre randomised trial. *Lancet* 2000;355:1041–1047.
23. Pitot HC, Wender DB, O'Connell MJ, et al. Phase II trial of irinotecan in patients with metastatic colorectal carcinoma. *J Clin Oncol* 1997;15(8):2910–2919.
24. Van Cutsem E, Hoff PM, Harper P, et al. Oral capecitabine vs intravenous 5-fluorouracil and leucovorin: integrated efficacy data and novel analyses from two large, randomised, phase III trials. *Br J Cancer* 2004;90:1190–1197.
25. Hurwitz H, Fehrenbacher L, Novotny W, et al. Bevacizumab plus irinotecan, fluorouracil, and leucovorin for metastatic colorectal cancer. *N Engl J Med* 2004;350:2335–2342.
26. Cunningham D, Humblet Y, Siena S, et al. Cetuximab monotherapy and cetuximab plus irinotecan in irinotecan-refractory metastatic colorectal cancer. *N Engl J Med* 2004;351:337–345.
27. Kemeny MM, Adak S, Gray B, et al. Combined-modality treatment for resectable metastatic colorectal carcinoma to the liver: surgical resection of hepatic metastases in combination with continuous infusion of chemotherapy—an intergroup study. J Clin Oncol 2002;20:1499–1505.
28. Bismuth H, Adam R, Levi F, et al. Resection of nonresectable liver metastases from colorectal cancer after neoadjuvant chemotherapy. *Ann Surg* 1996;224:509–520.
29. Alberts SR, Donohue JH, Mahoney MR, et al. Liver resection after 5-fluorouracil, leucovorin and oxaliplatin for patients with metastatic colorectal cancer (MCRC) limited to the liver *A North Central Cancer Treatment Group (NCCTG) Phase II Study Meeting:2003 Asco Annual Meeting* Abstract No:1053.

9

Pancreatic Cancer

George P. Kim[*], James L. Gulley[†], and Chris H. Takimoto[‡]

[*]Gastrointestinal Cancer Section, Mayo Clinic Cancer Center, Jacksonville, Florida;
[†]Laboratory of Tumor Immunology and Biology, Center for Cancer Research, National
Cancer Institute, National Institutes of Health, Bethesda, Maryland; and [‡]Institute for
Drug Development, Cancer Therapy & Research Center, San Antonio, Texas

EPIDEMIOLOGY

- In 2004, it was estimated that 31,860 new cases of pancreatic cancer would have been diagnosed and 31,270 patients would have died from this malignancy.
- It is the fourth leading cause of death from cancer in the United States.
- The 5-year survival of patients with pancreatic cancer remains less than 5%.
- Men and African Americans are at a higher risk for developing pancreatic cancer and thus exhibit higher mortality rates.
- Incidence of pancreatic cancer increases at the age of 50 and peaks in the seventh decade (Table 9.1).

Pathophysiology

The pancreas performs both endocrine and exocrine functions; however, approximately 80% of the cells in the pancreas are acinar cells and 10% to 15% are ductal cells. Approximately 95% of malignant pancreatic cancer arises in the exocrine pancreas, with two-thirds arising in the head of the pancreas. The sites where the cancer arises determine the symptoms: lesions arising in the head of the pancreas causing duct obstruction, jaundice, and pain, whereas tumors arising in the body or tail of the pancreas are less likely to cause symptoms before metastasis.

- Pain caused by localized disease is usually described as mid to upper back pain resulting from tumor invasion of the celiac and mesenteric plexi.
- Most patients develop glucose intolerance and some degree of pancreatic insufficiency.
- K-ras mutations are associated with most cases of pancreatic cancer (see Fig. 9.1).
- Mucinous cystic neoplasm and intraductal papillary mucinous neoplasm are relatively benign lesions, but the presence of severe dysplasia or invasion warrant further investigation and probable resection. Despite the evolution of malignant clones within these lesions, the overall survival is better than with ductal adenocarcinoma.

STAGING

The American Joint Committee for Cancer/International Union Against Cancer (AJCC/UICC) staging classification of pancreatic cancer is done using the TNM classification, as shown in Table 9.2 (1).

TABLE 9.1. *Risk factors*

Environmental	
Cigarette smoking	N-nitrosoamines may increase risk by twofold to threefold. Accounts for roughly 30% of pancreatic cancers.
Dietary factors	Decreased with fruits and vegetables, increased risk with fat and meat. No caffeine association, and alcohol link is controversial.
Disease states	
Diabetes mellitus	Maximal risk at time of diagnosis of diabetes and for the subsequent 5 y.
Chronic pancreatitis	Relative risk as high as 16-fold.
Genetic	
FAMM	p16 mutation, 13- to 22-fold increased risk
Hereditary pancreatitis	PRSS1 or cationic trypsinogen gene, 20-fold increased risk
HNPCC	Lynch syndrome II
BRCA2	10-fold risk
Peutz-Jeghers syndrome	Manifested by hamartomatous gastrointestinal polyps and perioral pigmented spots, mutation of serine–threonine kinase (STK)11
Occupational	
Chemicals	Petrochemical products, benzidine, and β-naphthylamine.

PROGNOSIS

Tumor size, presence of lymph node metastasis, and histologic differentiation each have independent prognostic values, with larger tumors, lymph node metastasis, and poor differentiation having worse prognoses. The 36-month survival for node-negative patients is between 25% and 30%, whereas there is only a 6- to 8-month median survival for node-positive patients. Long-term survival is seen in about 20% of patients who successfully undergo a potentially curative surgical resection (Fig. 9.2).

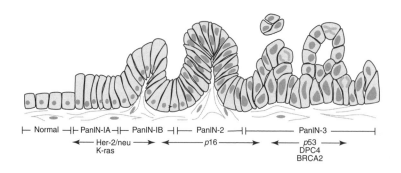

FIG. 9.1. Neoplastic progression model—pancreatic intraepithelial neoplasia (PanIN-1 through PanIN-3). (From Hruban RH, Goggins M, Parsons J, et al. Progression model for pancreatic cancer. *Clin Can Res* 2000;6:2969–2972, with permission.)

TABLE 9.2. *American Joint Committee for Cancer/International Union Against Cancer (AJCC/UICC) staging classification (2002)*

Primary tumor
  TX Primary tumor cannot be assessed
  T0 No evidence of primary tumor
  Tis Carcinoma *in situ*
  T1 Tumor limited to the pancreas ≤2 cm
  T2 Tumor limited to the pancreas >2 cm
  T3 Tumor extends beyond the pancreas but without involvement of the celiac axis or the superior mesenteric artery
  T4 Tumor involves the celiac axis or the superior mesenteric artery (unresectable primary tumor)

Regional lymph nodes
  NX Regional lymph nodes cannot be assessed
  N0 No regional lymph node metastasis
  N1 Regional lymph node metastasis

Distant metastasis
  MX Distant metastasis cannot be assessed
  M0 No distant metastasis
  M1 Distant metastasis

Stage grouping

Stage			
Stage 0	Tis	N0	M0
Stage IA	T1	N0	M0
Stage IB	T2	N0	M0
Stage IIA	T3	N0	M0
Stage IIB	T1–3	N1	M0
Stage III	T4	Any N	M0
Stage IV	Any T	Any N	M1

From Exocrine Pancreas. In: American Joint Committee on Cancer. AJCC Cancer Staging Manual. 6th edition New York, NY: Springer, 2002, 157–164.

DIAGNOSIS

- **Screening tests:** There are no good screening tests for pancreatic cancer. CA 19-9, a sialated Lewis antigen, is elevated in 70% to 90% of patients with pancreatic cancer; however, it is not useful as a screening test because of low specificity. The CA 19-9 may have greater utility in monitoring recurrent or advanced disease.
- **Imaging techniques:** Imaging techniques include chest radiographs, abdominal computerized tomography (CT), ultrasound, endoscopic retrograde cholepancreatography (ERCP), and endoscopic ultrasound (EUS):
  - Dual-phase contrast, helical CT—its sensitivity is 67% for lesions <1.5 cm and almost 100% for tumors >1.5 cm; it has a 95% positive predictive value in defining resectability if major vessel tumor encasement is present.
  - Endoscopic ultrasound—it is excellent for tumor and nodal staging, and also for detecting the presence of portal vein invasion; fine needle aspiration (FNA) is used for diagnosing tumor with minimal risk; it is also used for visualizing and sampling hepatic lesions; limitations include assessment of blood vessel encasement or superior mesenteric artery (SMA) invasion.
  - Pathologic diagnosis may be achieved with ERCP, laparoscopy, peritoneal cytology, or CT-guided biopsy.
- Most common metastasis to pancreas is from renal cell cancers.

Resectable disease   5-year Survival
                                                                         17.5%

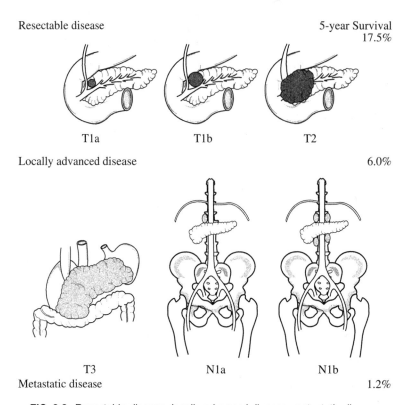

Locally advanced disease   6.0%

Metastatic disease   1.2%

FIG. 9.2. Resectable disease, locally advanced disease, metastatic disease.

MANAGEMENT

For management considerations, pancreatic cancer can be divided into resectable disease (potentially curable), locally advanced disease, and metastatic disease (see Fig. 9.3).

Resectable Disease

Less than 10% of patients with pancreatic cancer have resectable disease at diagnosis. Resectable disease is confined to the pancreas without encasement of the celiac axis or superior mesenteric artery and with a patent superior mesenteric–portal vein confluence. However, patients may have isolated involvement of the superior mesenteric vein, portal vein, or hepatic artery. A Whipple or modified, pylorus-sparing procedure is the surgical procedure of choice. The stomach (distal third), gallbladder, cystic and common bile ducts, duodenum, and proximal jejunum are resected, with resultant pancreatico-, choledocho-, and gastrojejunostomy. The peripancreatic, superior mesenteric, and hepatoduodenal lymph nodes are also staged. Even after complete resection, the risk of locoregional recurrence is greater than 70%. This risk has led to numerous studies of adjuvant chemotherapy and radiation therapy after surgical resection. The original Gastrointestinal Study Group (GITSG) trial (2) randomized 21 patients to chemoradiation versus 22 patients to surgery alone. The chemoradiation arm consisted of split-course administration of 4,000 cGy radiation in 200-cGy fractions concomitantly with bolus 5-fluorouracil

Management algorithm

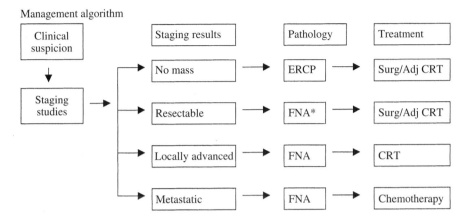

FIG. 9.3. Staging studies should include computerized tomography (CT) (spiral with contrast preferred) or magnetic resonance imaging (MRI), endoscopic ultrasound (EUS), as well as laparoscopy for potentially resectable cancers. (*) indicates that for CT-guided FNA, there is a controversy about tumor seeding in potentially curable (i.e., resectable) disease, and in some centers, patients undergo a planned Whipple procedure to obtain tissue at the time of surgery. Adj CRT, adjuvant chemoradiation; FNA, fine needle aspiration; ERCP, endoscopic retrograde cholangiopancreatography.

(5-FU; 500 mg/m^2/day for the first 3 days of each 2,000-cGy segment of radiotherapy). 5-FU alone (500 mg/m^2/week) was administered for up to two additional years. A significantly prolonged median survival of 20 months for the patients on chemoradiation versus 11 months for controls was observed. In addition, 43% 2-year actuarial survival (versus 18% for the control arm) and 25% 5-year overall survival were observed.

This relatively small trial established the benefit from postoperative combined-modality therapy. More recent approaches include: (a) administration of up to 5,040 cGy radiation as a continuous-course schedule instead of the split-course schedule; (b) combination with 5-FU at a dose of 500 mg/m^2/day daily for the first 3 days and the last 3 days of radiation therapy or administration of continuous infusion 5-FU at a dose of 225 to 250 mg/m^2/day during the entire radiation portion (3); and (c) the postradiation treatment of weekly 5-FU has also been shortened from 2 years to 4–6 months, and weekly gemcitabine at a dose of 1,000 mg per m^2 for 3 of every 4 weeks has been used instead of 5-FU.

Several randomized trials have also provided additional information about the effectiveness of conventional adjuvant therapy. A European Organization for Research and Treatment of Cancer trial (4) treated 114 patients with a combined-modality approach similar to that of the GITSG trial except for the maintenance 5-FU versus no adjuvant treatment. The median survival was 17.1 months in the experimental arm versus 12.6 months in surgery-alone patients ($p = 0.099$), and 2-year survival (37% versus 23%) also suggested benefit. The study was considered negative but may more accurately be described as being underpowered. A recent trial from the European Study Group for Pancreatic Cancer (ESPAC-1) used a 2 × 2 factorial randomization design and suggested that chemotherapy alone in the adjuvant setting was more effective than chemotherapy–radiation (5). Unfortunately, the conclusion from this study is limited by selection bias and considerable treatment variability. The results, nonetheless, are intriguing. Finally, the recently completed Radiation Therapy Oncology Group trial 97-04 compared gemcitabine to 5-FU alone prior to combined-modality therapy (5,040 cGy external beam radiation and continuous infusion 5-FU at a dose of 225 mg per m^2) followed by three additional months of gemcitabine or 5-FU. The study represents the first pancreatic adjuvant trial in several decades and serves as the foundation for further studies with contemporary radiation and chemotherapeutic approaches.

Locally Advanced Disease

Approximately 25% of patients have regional involvement at diagnosis, and treatment with combined chemotherapy and radiation has been shown to improve survival more significantly than treatment with either modality alone. In locally advanced, unresectable patients with good performance status, one commonly administered regimen is 4,500 to 5,400 cGy radiation with 5-FU at a dose of 500 mg/m^2/day daily on the first and last 3 days of radiation (6). The treatment schema is identical to that used for adjuvant treatment of resectable disease. Median survival is approximately 10 months with treatment. Administration of non–split-course radiation and continuous infusion of 5-FU (maximum tolerated dose is 250 g/m^2/day) are acceptable approaches.

Use of gemcitabine as a radiation-sensitizing agent is undergoing evaluation in patients with locally advanced disease. Initial studies of gemcitabine at a dose of 400 to 600 mg/m^2/week and 5,040 cGy irradiation reported tolerability (mainly gastrointestinal toxicity and myelosuppression) and objective responses in patients. Alternatively, in an effort to maximize the systemic effects of gemcitabine, a full dose of 1,000 mg per m^2 every week has been combined with a maximally tolerated 4,200 cGy radiation (administered as 280-cGy fractions over 3 weeks). The 8- to 11-month median survival with gemcitabine radiosensitization is similar to that observed with 5-FU.

Several studies have evaluated the use of preoperative chemotherapy–radiation in an effort to convert unresectable to resectable disease. Despite reports of improvements, this approach is of limited benefit, and only 8% to 13% of patients will achieve a complete resection.

Metastatic Disease

Approximately 50% of newly diagnosed pancreatic cancer patients have metastasis, and palliative treatment with systemic chemotherapy should be offered to patients with a good performance status [Eastern Cooperative Oncology Group (ECOG) 0–2]. Gemcitabine is the first-line standard treatment in patients with metastatic pancreatic cancer (7). This is based on a study in which 126 untreated patients were randomized to receive gemcitabine, 1,000 mg per m^2 intravenously weekly for 3 of 4 weeks, or single-agent 5-FU, 600 mg per m^2 intravenous bolus weekly. Despite an objective response rate of less than 10%, a benefit in quality-of-life scores (clinical benefit response 23.8% versus 4.8%, [$p = 0.0022$) and median survival (5.7 versus 4.4 months, $p = 0.0025$) was observed with the gemcitabine therapy. The 1-year survival also favored the gemcitabine arm (18% versus 2%).

Several clinical trials studies attempting to surpass survival outcomes with gemcitabine alone have been performed. These two- and three-drug combination studies report median survival of 6 to 10 months and 1-year survival of approximately 20% to 35%. To overcome saturation of intracellular drug accumulation, prolonged infusion of gemcitabine at a fixed-dose rate of 10 mg/m^2/minute has also been evaluated in a phase II study by Tempero et al. (8). Gemcitabine at a dose of 1,500 mg per m^2 given over 150 minutes resulted in a response rate of 11.6%, median survival of 8.0 months, and 1-year survival of 23.8%.

The combination of gemcitabine and oxaliplatin (GEMOX) is promising, as reported by Louvet et al. (9,10). In the initial study, 64 patients with pancreatic cancer (45% locally advanced, 55% metastatic) were treated with gemcitabine (1,000 mg per m^2 at a fixed dose rate of 10 mg/m^2/minute on day 1) followed by oxaliplatin (100 mg per m^2 on day 2) on an every 2-week schedule. The objective response rate was 30.6% and the clinical benefit response was 40%. The median survival was 9.2 months and the 1-year survival was reported as 36%. Louvet recently reported results from a larger phase III study comparing 30-minute infusion of gemcitabine to the GEMOX regimen. Although response rate and progression-free survival favored GEMOX, no statistically significant improvement in 6-month and 1-year survival was observed. Possible explanations for the lack of survival benefit include the better-than-expected survival observed in the control arm and the use of second-line, platinum-containing regimens. Nonetheless, an ongoing Eastern Cooperative Group Study comparing standard 30-minute gemcitabine to fixed–dose-rate gemcitabine and to GEMOX will determine the impact of the fixed–dose-rate approach and the contribution of oxaliplatin.

Novel agents such as bevacizumab (Avastin) and cetuximab (Erbitux) are also being evaluated.

- Abbruzzese (11) evaluated gemcitabine and cetuximab (initial dose of 400 mg per m^2 followed by 250 mg per m^2 weekly) in a trial with 41 patients and observed a partial response rate of 12.5%, median survival of 6.7 months, and 1-year survival of 33%.
- Kindler et al. (12) evaluated gemcitabine and Avastin (10 mg per kg every 2 weeks) in a trial with 19% partial response rate and with 48% of patients exhibiting stabilized disease symptoms; median survival was 8.7 months, time to progression was 5.8 months, and 1-year survival was 29%.

Palliation

Pain remains a significant problem with pancreatic cancer and can be palliated with narcotics, external beam radiation, and, if indicated, a nerve block to an involved plexus. Biliary and intestinal obstruction is also a common local issue and can be relieved with stents or surgical bypass.

TREATMENT OPTIONS

Localized Disease

Whipple procedure followed by adjuvant chemoradiation with a continuous course of 45- to 50.4-Gy external beam radiation in 1.8-Gy fractions split course can be considered in older patients (allowing greater dosage adjustment secondary to toxicity) with

- 5-FU, 500 mg/m^2/day by intravenous bolus for the first 3 days of each 20-Gy segment of radiotherapy (total dose per 3-day course of fluorouracil, 1,500 mg per m^2), or alternatively, 5-FU, 225 to 250 mg/m^2/day continuous infusion concomitantly with radiation followed by
- gemcitabine, 1,000 mg/m^2/week intravenously weekly for 3 weeks (days 1, 8, and 15) followed by 1 week without gemcitabine for 4 to 6 months.

Locally Advanced Disease

For those patients with good performance status (PS 0–2), clinical trials are the preferred mode of treatment, with chemoradiation or gemcitabine available as standard treatments. The chemoradiation is given as described earlier, and chemotherapy after chemoradiation consists of

- gemcitabine, 1,000 mg/m^2/week intravenously weekly for 3 weeks (days 1, 8, and 15) followed by 1 week without gemcitabine. Treatment cycles are repeated every 28 days for 4 to 6 months.

For those patients with poor performance status, supportive care is recommended. The goal of treatment for locally advanced disease is to prolong survival.

Metastatic Disease

For patients with good performance status, clinical trials are the preferred mode of treatment, with gemcitabine or supportive care available as standard approaches.

- Gemcitabine, 1,000 mg/m^2/week intravenous weekly for 3 weeks (days 1, 8, and 15), followed by 1 week without gemcitabine (total dose per cycle: 3,000 mg per m^2). Treatment cycles are repeated every 28 days.

The goal of treatment for metastatic disease is to decrease symptoms.

REFERENCES

1. American Joint Committee on Cancer. *AJCC cancer staging manual*, 6th ed. New York: Springer, 2002:157–164.
2. Gastrointestinal Study Group. Further evidence of effective adjuvant combined radiation and chemotherapy following curative resection of pancreatic cancer. *Cancer* 1987;59:2006–2010.
3. Yeo CJ, Abrams RA, Grochow LB, et al. Pancreaticoduodenectomy for pancreatic adenocarcinoma: postoperative adjuvant chemoradiation improves survival. *Ann Surg* 1997;225:621–636.
4. Klinkenbijl JH, Jeekel J, Sahmoud T, et al. Adjuvant radiotherapy and 5-fluorouracil after curative resection of cancer of the pancreas and periampullary region: phase III trial of the EORTC gastrointestinal tract cancer cooperative group. *Ann Surg* 1999;230:776–784.
5. Neoptolemos JP, Stocken DD, Friess H, et al. European Study Group for Pancreatic Cancer. A randomized trial of chemoradiotherapy and chemotherapy after resection of pancreatic cancer. *N Engl J Med* 2004;350:1200–1210.
6. Moertel CG, Frytak S, Hahn RG, et al. Therapy of locally unresectable pancreatic carcinoma: a randomised comparison of high dose (6000 rads) radiation alone, moderate dose radiation (4000 rads) + 5-fluorouracil, and high dose radiation + 5-fluorouracil. *Cancer* 1981;48:1705–1710.
7. Burris HA III, Moore MJ, Andersen J, et al. Improvements in clinical survival and clinical benefit with gemcitabine as first line therapy for patients with advanced pancreas cancer: a randomized trial. *J Clin Oncol* 1997;15:2403–2413.
8. Tempero M, Plunkett W, Ruiz Van Haperen V, et al. Randomized phase II comparison of dose-intense gemcitabine: thirty-minute infusion and fixed dose rate infusion in patients with pancreatic adenocarcinoma. *J Clin Oncol* 2003;21:3402–3408.
9. Louvet C, Andre T, et al. Gemcitabine combined with oxaliplatin in advanced pancreatic adenocarcinoma: final results of a GERCOR multicenter phase II study. *J Clin Oncol* 2002;20:1512–1518.
10. Louvet C. GemOx (gemcitabine + oxaliplatin) versus Gem (gemcitabine) in non resectable pancreatic adenocarcinoma: final results of the GERCOR /GISCAD intergroup phase III. *Proc Am Soc Clin Oncol* 2004;Abstract 4008.
11. Xiong HQ, Rosenberg A, LoBuglio A, et al. Cetuximab, a monoclonal antibody targeting the epidermal growth factor receptor, in combination with gemcitabine for advanced pancreatic cancer: a multicenter phase II trial. *J Clin Oncol* 2004;22:2610–2616.
12. Kindler HL, Friberg G, Stadler WM, et al. Bevacizumab plus gemcitabine in patients with advanced pancreatic cancer: updated results of a multi-center phase II trial. *Proc Am Soc Clin Oncol* 2004;23:314, Abstract 4009.

10

Anal Cancer

M. Wasif Saif

University of Alabama at Birmingham, Birmingham, Alabama

Anal cancer is an uncommon malignancy, accounting for only a small percentage (4%) of all cancers of the lower alimentary tract. Overall, the risk of anal cancer is rising, with data suggesting that individuals with human papillomavirus (HPV) and male homosexuals, in particular, are at increased risk for developing anal cancer. The three major prognostic factors are site (anal canal versus perianal skin), size (primary tumors <2 cm have a better prognosis), and differentiation (well-differentiated tumors are more favorable than poorly differentiated tumors). Concomitant radiotherapy [5-fluorouracil (5-FU) and mitomycin C] has proved to be useful in locally advanced anal canal carcinoma. Nevertheless, this conservative treatment has a failure rate of 30%. The tolerance and efficiency of a neoadjuvant chemotherapy [5-FU and cisplatin (CDDP)] have been validated by a phase II trial using 80 patients, which observed 73% colostomy-free survival and 70% relapse-free survival at 3-year follow-up in patients. Its usefulness is being studied in an ongoing phase III trial, as well as the dose escalation of the radiation boost, from 15 Gy to 25–25 Gy.

EPIDEMIOLOGY

In the United States, the annual incidence of anal cancer is 6 per 1,000,000 population in whites and is more frequent in female than in male subjects, showing an incidence of 9 of 1,000,000 in nonwhite women versus 5 per 1,000,000 in white and Hispanic men (F/M ratio is 2:1). However, cancer of the anal margin is more frequent in men. More than 80% of anal cancer develops in patients 50 to 60 years of age. Epidemiologic studies during the last decade suggest that the incidence of anal cancer has increased in men younger than 35 years, reversing the gender ratio in this age group; it also is related to receptive anal intercourse.

ETIOLOGY AND RISK FACTORS

No etiologic factor has been recognized in most cases of anal cancer. Environmental factors are predominantly implicated in the carcinogenesis of anal cancer. The most common risk factors can be classified as follows:

Risk Factors with Strong Evidence:

1. HPV infection (anogenital warts)
2. History of receptive anal intercourse
3. History of sexually transmitted disease
4. More than 10 sexual partners
5. History of cervical, vulvar, or vaginal cancer
6. Immunosuppression after solid-organ transplantation.

Risk Factors with Moderately Strong Evidence:

1. Human immunodeficiency virus (HIV) infection
2. Long-term use of corticosteroids
3. Cigarette smoking.

PATHOLOGY

Anatomy

1. The *anal canal* extends from the anorectal ring to a zone approximately halfway between the pectinate (or dentate) line and the anal verge.
2. The *anal margin* consists of the anal area distal to the anal canal, including perianal skin.

The World Health Organization (WHO) defines carcinoma of the anal canal as lesions arising from the anorectal ring proximally up to the dentate line distally, whereas carcinoma of the anal margin is defined as lesions arising distal to the dentate line to the junction between perineal skin and the hair-bearing skin of the buttocks (see Fig. 10.1).

HISTOLOGY

The histologic types of carcinomas and the features of each type of carcinoma are given in Table 10.1.

Frequency

The frequency of occurrence of each histologic type of carcinoma is given in Table 10.2. The table indicates that squamous cell carcinoma is the commonest form of anal cancer.

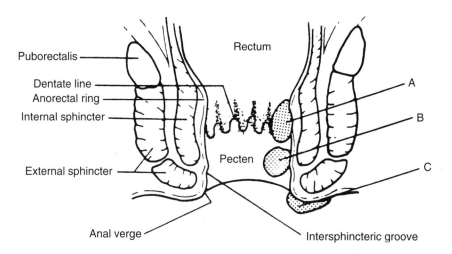

FIG. 10.1. Anatomy of the anal canal. A tumor in location *A* is always considered anal canal cancer; in location *C*, it is anal margin cancer. A tumor in location *B* was called *canal* or *margin cancer*, depending on institutional preference, but now should be called *anal canal cancer* by the American Joint Committee on Cancer/Union Internationale Contre le Cance (AJCC/UICC) definition.

TABLE 10.1. *Features of different types of anal cancer*

Histologic types	Features
• Squamous cell (epidermal) carcinoma	Occurs in the lower anus, often ulcerating
• Cloacogenic (also called basaloid, cuboidal, or transitional) carcinoma	Develops high in the anal canal in the transitional zone between glandular mucosa of the rectum and the squamous epithelium of the distal anus
• Intraepithelial squamous cell carcinoma (Bowen disease)	Premalignant lesion of the perirectal skin
• Intraepithelial mucous adenocarcinoma (Paget disease)	Develops in apocrine or mucous glands

TABLE 10.2. *Frequency of occurrence of different types of anal cancer*

Squamous cell carcinoma	113	(55%)
Cloacogenic (basaloid) carcinoma	64	(31%)
Intraepithelial adenocarcinoma (Paget disease)	8	(4%)
Melanoma	7	(2%)
Basal cell carcinoma	6	
Adenocarcinoma	6	
Total	204	

Presentation

Symptoms

The incidence of different presenting symptoms in three types of anal carcinoma is shown in Table 10.3. Bleeding seems to be the common symptom in squamous cell carcinoma and in basaloid squamous carcinoma, whereas pruritus is the most common presenting symptom in perianal carcinoma.

Signs

Physical examination should include digital anorectal examination, anoscopy, proctoscopy, and palpation of inguinal lymph nodes.

TABLE 10.3. *Frequency of occurrence of symptoms in different types of anal cancer*

Presenting symptoms	Squamous cell carcinoma	Perianal	Basaloid squamous carcinoma
Bleeding	50	9	32
Pain	41	5	17
Mass	27	5	16
Constipation	11	1	10
Diarrhea	5	0	7
Pruritus[a]	22	17	1
Other	16	6	12
Asymptomatic	25	6	14

[a]$p < 0.001$. Differences not statistically significant for other lesions.
From Beahrs OH, Wilson SM. Carcinoma of the anus. *Ann Surg* 1976;184(4):422–428, with permission.

BIOPSY

An incisional biopsy is preferred for confirming diagnosis. Suggestive inguinal lymph nodes should be examined to rule out metastatic disease.

STAGING AND PROGNOSTIC FACTORS

Staging work-up should include physical examination, with special attention to digital rectal and pelvic examination and inguinal nodes, chest radiograph, and liver function tests. Pelvic computerized tomography (CT) scan and endoscopic ultrasound (EUS) of the anal canal may be beneficial.

The UICC (Union Internationale Centre le Cancer) and AJCC (American Joint Committee on Cancer) have proposed a practical staging system for anal cancer. Cancer of the anal margin is staged identically to squamous cell cancer of skin. The staging system for both types of tumors is outlined in Tables 10.4 and 10.5.

TABLE 10.4. *American Joint Committee on Cancer (AJCC) classification of anal canal tumors*

Primary tumor (T)
- TX Primary tumor cannot be assessed
- T0 No evidence of primary tumor
- Tis Carcinoma *in situ*
- T1 Tumor ≤2 cm in greatest dimension
- T2 Tumor >2 cm but <5 cm in greatest dimension
- T3 Tumor >5 cm in greatest dimension
- T4 Tumor of any size that invades adjacent organs (e.g., vagina, bladder, and urethra; involvement of sphincter muscle(s) alone is not classified as T4)

Regional lymph nodes (N)
- NX Regional lymph nodes cannot be assessed
- N0 No regional lymph node metastasis
- N1 Metastasis in perirectal lymph node(s)
- N2 Metastasis in unilateral internal iliac and/or inguinal lymph node(s)
- N3 Metastasis in perirectal and inguinal lymph node(s) and/or bilateral internal iliac and/or inguinal lymph nodes

Distant metastasis (M)
- MX Distant metastasis cannot be assessed
- M0 No distant metastasis
- M1 Distant metastasis

Grade (G)
- GX Grade of differentiation cannot be assessed
- G1 Well differentiated
- G2 Moderately differentiated
- G3 Poorly differentiated
- G4 Undifferentiated

Stage groupings

Stage	T	N	M
Stage 0	Tis	N0	M0
Stage I	T1	N0	M0
Stage II	T2	N0	M0
	T3	N0	M0
Stage IIIA	T1–3	N1	M0
	T4	N0	M0
Stage IIIB	T4	N1	M0
	Any T	N2–3	M0
Stage IV	Any T	Any N	M1

TABLE 10.5. *TNM classification of anal margin tumors*

Primary tumor (T)[a]			
T4	Tumor invades deep extradermal structures		
Regional lymph nodes (N)			
N1	Ipsilateral inguinal nodes		
Metastases (M)			
M1	Distant metastases		
Stage groupings[b]			
Stage III	T4	N0	M0
	Any T	N1	M0

[a]Designation as for anal canal tumors, except T4.
[b]Stage groupings as for anal canal tumors, except stage III (no stage IIA or IIIB).
From Sobin LH, Wittekind C (eds). *UICC International Union Against Cancer: TNM classification of malignant tumors.* 5th ed. New York: John Wiley & Sons, 1997, with permission.

MAJOR PROGNOSTIC FACTORS

There are four major prognostic factors:

- **Site:** anal canal versus perianal skin
- **Size:** <5 cm versus >5 cm
- **Differentiation:** well-differentiated tumors have more favorable outcomes than poorly differentiated tumors
- **Lymph Node Involvement:** absence of nodal involvement or local extension.

When balanced with other factors, the prognosis for patients with squamous cell carcinoma of the anus and for those with cloacogenic carcinoma is similar.

TREATMENT

Surgery

Anal Canal Lesions

Because anal cancer is a rare tumor, most studies have involved a small number of patients who have been included over several years. The absence of data from randomized trials makes treatment difficult in certain circumstances. The location of the primary tumor is a major determinant of appropriate treatment.

Traditionally, the standard (and sole) form of therapy for anal canal lesions has been surgical resection, often involving an anteroposterior (AP) resection with inguinal node dissection. Despite such radical procedures, the most common site of failure is the pelvis, with local recurrences occurring in 30% of patients (see Table 10.6). Although postoperative (adjuvant) radiation therapy has been used to reduce the local recurrence rate, the potential benefit of such a practice has not been documented through a controlled trial.

Tumors that (a) involve the dentate line, (b) are larger than 2 cm, or (c) involve more than 50% of the bowel circumference are probably best managed with combined-modality treatment. This integrated approach improves overall survival and may allow avoidance of radical surgery. In the last several years, several studies have used combined-modality treatments with radiation and chemotherapy after local resection. Therefore, the primary therapeutic modalities for anal cancer are a combination of chemotherapy and radiation therapy. Combined chemoradiation is aimed at cure and preservation of anal function. AP resection is used as salvage therapy in patients with chemoradiation-resistant disease. Table 10.6 shows the results of a few of these trials.

TABLE 10.6. *Anal canal lesions*

Surgical results	5-Yr survival (%)
Nodes negative	54–70
Metachronous nodal spread	51
Synchronous nodal spread	16

Anal Margin Lesions

For anal margin lesions, a wide local excision without the need for a colostomy seems to be adequate (see Table 10.7).

Radiation Therapy

a. **Potential advantages compared to radical surgery:**

   i. no operative mortality
   ii. no colostomy
   iii. no sexual impotence.

b. **Disadvantages in comparison with surgery:**

   i. Although the abdominal–perineal resection (APR) has remained a standard procedure for the last 25 years, radiotherapeutic techniques and equipment have changed markedly, permitting, in recent years, the delivery of a far higher, precisely defined dose (approximately 6,000 cGy) with less toxicity; *that is, as such, the substandard dosages of the past (3,500 to 4,000 cGy), which were occasionally accompanied by significant toxicity, do not reflect the present clinical situation.*
   ii. The extent of local and nodal involvement among patients receiving primary irradiation is usually not determined.
   iii. The two techniques cannot be compared prospectively because the issue of a permanent colostomy is an unacceptable variable in a clinical trial.

Radiation therapy has been given using

- external beam treatment
- interstitial treatment
- external and interstitial treatment.

TABLE 10.7. *Results: 5-year survival after local excision in anal margin cancer (31 patients)*

	Tumor size (cm)				
	0–2	2–5	>5	NC	Total
Alive without recurrence	7	9	3	1	20
Alive with recurrence	0	1	0	0	1
Lost to follow-up	0	1	0	0	1
Died from recurrence	2	0	0	1	3
Died from unrelated causes	2	4	0	0	6
Total	11	15	3	2	31

NC, not classified.
From Greenall MJ, Quan SH, Stearns MW, et al. Epidermoid cancer of the anal margin. Pathologic features, treatment, and clinical results. *Am J Surg* 1985;149(1):95–101, with permission.

The overall 45% to 50% rate of "cure" reported in the series of select patients who were treated primarily with radiation therapy is quite similar to that reported in surgically treated patients. Recent series utilizing external beam and interstitial treatment or very high dose external beam irradiation have shown encouraging responses, suggesting a local control rate of 70% to 80%, but will require further confirmation before receiving full acceptance.

Combined Radiation Therapy and Chemotherapy

In an attempt to enhance the efficacy of radical surgery in patients with anal cancer, in 1972, Nigro et al. (1) from Wayne State University began giving patients preoperative concomitant radiation (3,000 cGy external beam irradiation) and chemotherapy (by 5-FU continuous infusion and mitomycin C). When this attempt was last updated, 45 patients had been followed for a median period of 50 months; 38 of 45 patients (84%) achieved a complete biopsy-proven response after only radiation and chemotherapy, including all patients whose initial lesion was <5 cm; none of these 30 patients developed local or distant tumor recurrence, whereas all 7 of the patients who had recurrent disease after preoperative treatment developed distant spread of the tumor and subsequently died despite an APR.

Although the original treatment plan called for an APR following the radiation and chemotherapy, this program was altered after five of the first six patients who underwent the radical operation were found to have no tumor in the operative specimen; subsequently, surgery has been performed only on those patients who have been found to have residual tumor in the anal canal during the posttreatment biopsy. Most patients have been cured of their anal cancers without the need for a colostomy and with relatively mild toxicity. These highly encouraging results from the group from Wayne State University have now been confirmed and extended by others in randomized trials.

Radiation Therapy Alone versus Chemoradiation Therapy

European Organization for Research and Treatment of Cancer (EORTC) randomized 110 patients with bulky tumors to receive 4,500 to 6,500 cGy of pelvic radiotherapy (RT) alone or in combination with 5-FU and mitomycin C. Statistically significant benefits for complete response rate, local regional control, and colostomy-free survival favored the combined-modality approach.

United Kingdom Coordinating Committee on Cancer Research (UKCCCR) randomized 585 patients to receive 4,500 cGy of pelvic RT alone or in combination with 5-FU and mitomycin C. Local-failure rate was reduced by 46% in patients given the combined-modality approach.

Value of Mitomycin C in the Combined-modality Regimen

Radiation Therapy Oncology Group (RTOG) randomized 310 patients to receive 4,500 to 5,040 cGy of pelvic RT with 5-FU or the same and 5-FU with mitomycin C. A statistically significant benefit for disease-free survival was observed in the patient cohort who received mitomycin C. The substitution of cisplatin for mitomycin C (when combined with 5-FU and radiation therapy) has been explored in phase II trials (Doci et al.); the initial results are promising. Induction therapy with 5-FU and cisplatin followed by RT and 5-FU and cisplatin is presently being compared with "standard" RT and 5-FU and mitomycin C combination in an ongoing Intergroup protocol (see Tables 10.8, 10.9, and 10.10).

Treatment options according to the stage are shown in Table 10.11. The overall management of anal cancer has been shown in Fig. 10.2.

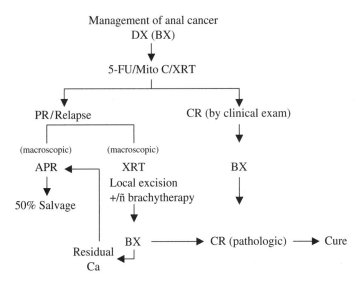

Management of anal cancer
DX (BX)

5-FU/Mito C/XRT

PR/Relapse
CR (by clinical exam)

(macroscopic) (macroscopic)

APR ◄   XRT   BX
Local excision
+/ñ brachytherapy

50% Salvage

BX ───► CR (pathologic) ───► Cure

Residual
Ca

FIG. 10.2. Management of anal cancer.

Stage 0

Surgical resection is the treatment of choice for the lesions of the perianal area that do not involve the anal sphincter.

Stage I

Stage I involves

- Tumors of the perianal skin or anal margin not involving the anal sphincter: wide local excision (for small tumors)
- Anal canal cancer.

Stage I involving tumors of the anal sphincter and those that are too large for complete local resection are treated with external beam radiation therapy with or without chemotherapy. Results from the UKCCCR randomized trial of RT alone versus RT, 5-FU, and mitomycin C revealed that combined chemoradiation is more effective than radiation therapy alone (Table 10.11).

TABLE 10.8. *Multimodality studies*

Group	No. of patients	Regimen	XRT	APR	5-Yr survival
Wayne State	104	5-FU 1 g/m^2/24 h × 4 d Mito C 10–15 mg/m^2 d 1	30 Gy	31	83%
Memorial Sloan-Kettering	42	5-FU 750 mg/m^2/24 h × 5 d Mito C 15 mg/m^2 d 1	30 Gy	23	82%
RTOG/ ECOG	79	5-FU 1g/m^2/24 h × 4 d Mito C 10 mg/m^2 d	40 Gy	8	73%
Fresno Community Hospital	30	5-FU 1 g/m^2/ 24 h × 4 d Mito C 10–15 mg/m^2 d	41–50 Gy	1	90%
	255			63 (25%)	82%

XRT, radiation therapy; APR, abdominal–perineal resection; 5-FU, 5-fluorouracil; Mito C, mitomycin C; RTOG/ECOG, Radiation Therapy Oncology Group/Eastern Cooperative Oncology Group.

TABLE 10.9. *Selected results of concurrent radiation and fluorouracil and mitomycin C*

Chemotherapy regimens	Radiation (dose/fractions/time)	Primary tumor control	Regional node control	5-yr survival	Reference
Fluorouracil, 1,000 mg/m²/d, CIVI for 8 d, days 1–4, 29–32 (total dose/course, 8,000 mg/m²) Mitomycin C, 15 mg/m² i.v. bolus d 1 (total dose/course, 15 mg/m²)	30 Gy/15/d 1–21	31/34 (91%) (≤5 cm)	NS	80% crude	Leichman et al. (1985) (2)
Fluorouracil, 1,000 mg/m²/d, CIVI for 8 d, days 2–5, on days 28–31 (total dose/course, 8,000 mg/m²) Mitomycin C, 10 mg/m² i.v. bolus d 1 (total dose/course, 10 mg/m²)	40.8 Gy/24/ d 1–35	22/26 (85%) (≥3 cm)	32/50 (64%) (≤3 cm)	NA	73%, 3 yr actuarial	Sischy et al. (1989) (3)
Fluorouracil, 1,000 mg/m²/d, CIVI for 8 d, d 1–4, 43–46 (total dose/course, 8,000 mg/m²) Mitomycin C, 10 mg/m²/dose i.v. bolus for 2 doses, d 1 and 43 (total dose/course, 20 mg/m²)	48–50 Gy/20–24/d 1–58 (split course)	25/27 (93%) (≤5 cm)	16/20 (80%) (≥5 cm or T)	4/5	65%, actuarial	Cummings et al. (1982) (4)
Fluorouracil, 1,000 mg/m²/d, CIVI for 8 d, d 1–4, 29–32 (total dose/course, 8,000 mg/m²) Mitomycin C, 10 mg/m²/dose IV bolus for 2 doses, d 1 and 29 (total dose/course, 20 mg/m²)	50 Gy/25–28/d 1–35 ± boost	21/22 (95%) (≤X cm)	14/19 (74%) (<5 cm or T4)	3/4	77%, actuarial	Schneider et al. (1992) (5)
Fluorouracil, 600 mg/m²/d, CIVI for 5 d, d 1–5 (total dose/course, 3,000 mg/m²) Mitomycin, 12 mg/m² i.v. bolus day 1 (total dose/course, 12 mg/m²)	42 Gy/10/d 1–19 plus interstitial boost	57/70 (81%) (≥4 cm)	No data in original publication	NS	NS	Papillon and Montbarbon, (1987) (6)
Fluorouracil, 1,000 mg/m²/d, CIVI for 4 d, d 1–4 (total dose/course, 4,000 mg/m²) Mitomycin, 10–15 mg/m² i.v. bolus d 1 (total dose/course, 10–15 mg/m²)	50–54 Gy/25–27/ d 1–35 (≤5 cm)	28/30 (93%) (≥5 cm or T4)	42/56 (75%)	NS	72%, actuarial	Tanum et al., (1991) (7)
Fluorouracil, 1,000 mg/m²/d, CIVI for 4 d, d 1–4 (total dose/course, 4,000 mg/m²) Mitomycin C, 10 mg/m² i.v. bolus d 1 (total dose/course, 10 mg/m²)	50 Gy/20/d 1–28 (≤5 cm)	3/3 (≥5 cm or T4)	11/13 (85%)	3/3	75%, actuarial	Cummings et al., (1984) (8)
Fluorouracil, 750 mg/m²/d, CIVI for 8 d, d 1–5, 43–47 (total dose/course, 8,000 mg/m²) Mitomycin C, 15 mg/m²/dose i.v. bolus for 3 doses, d 1, 43, and 85 (total dose/course, 45 mg/m²)	54–60 Gy/30–33/ d 1–53 (split course)	28/38 (74%) (≤5 cm)	9/17 (53%) (≥5 cm)	8/8	81%, actuarial	Doci et al., (1992) (9)

CIVI, continuous intravenous infusion; NS, not stated; NA, not applicable; T, tumor invading adjacent organs; T4, tumor invading deep extradermal structures. From Cohen AM, Winawer SJ, eds. *Cancer of the colon, rectum and anus.* New York: McGraw Hill, 1995, with permission.

TABLE 10.10. *Dosage of chemoradiation in anal cancer*

Treatment modality	Dose
External beam radiation	4,500–5,000 cGy
RTOG	170 cGy/d for 27 d, d 2–28 (total dose, 4,500–5,000 cGy)
Milan	180 cGy/d for 4 wk followed by a 2-wk rest (total dose, 5,400 cGy)
Chemotherapy	
Mitomycin C	
RTOG	Mitomycin C, 10 mg/m^2 i.v. bolus on d 2
Milan	Mitomycin C, 15 mg/m^2 i.v. bolus on d 1
Fluorouracil	
RTOG	Fluorouracil, 1,000 mg/m^2/d CIVI for d 2–4 and 28–32 (total dose/course, 8,000 mg/m^2)
Milan	Fluorouracil, 750 mg/m^2/d CIVI for 5 d, d 1–5 (total dose/course, 3,750 mg/m^2)

RTOG, Radiation Therapy Oncology Group; i.v., intravenous.

Radical resection is reserved for residual cancer in the anal canal after chemoradiation therapy. Interstitial iridium-192 implantation after external beam RT may aid some patients with residual disease to have complete response.

The optimal dose of external beam radiation with concurrent chemotherapy still must be determined.

Stage II

Stage II involves

- Tumors of the perianal skin or anal margin not i nvolving the anal sphincter: wide local resection (of small tumors)
- Cancers of the anal canal (involving the anal sphincter and those that are too large to be completely excised locally)
- **Chemoradiation therapy:** (Table 10.8, 10.9, and 10.10). Salvage chemotherapy with fluorouracil and cisplatin, combined with a radiation boost may avoid a permanent colostomy in patients with residual tumor after initial nonoperative therapy, as suggested by a phase III randomized intergroup study (Flam et al.)
- **Resection:** Radical resection for residual disease in the anal canal after the initial nonoperative treatment is also an option.

TABLE 10.11. *Treatment options for anal cancer*

Stage	Treatment options
0	Surgery
I	Radiation
	Chemoradiation
	Surgery
	Interstitial iridium-192 after external beam radiation
II	Chemoradiation
	Surgery
IIIa	Treatment as for I and II
IIIb	Chemoradiation with surgical resection of residual disease
IV	Palliative surgery
	Palliative irradiation
	Palliative chemoradiation
	Clinical trials

Stage IIIA

Stage IIIA anal cancer presents clinically as stage II anal cancer in most patients but is upstaged to IIIA by the presence of perirectal nodal disease or adjacent organ involvement. EUS (endoanal or endorectal) may help in staging.

- Treatment is similar to that for stage I and II disease involving chemoradiation.
- Salvage chemotherapy combined with a radiation boost is an option, as shown by Flam et al.
- Postoperative radiation therapy is also used.

Stage IIIB

Although curing stage IIIB disease is possible, the presence of metastatic disease secondary to the involvement of inguinal lymph nodes (unilateral or bilateral) constitutes a poor prognostic sign.

- Chemoradiation (as described for stage II) with surgical resection of residual disease at the primary site plus unilateral or bilateral superficial and deep inguinal lymph node dissection is a mode of treatment.
- Because of the poor prognosis of these patients, they should be recruited for clinical trials whenever possible.

Stage IV

There is no standard chemotherapy for stage IV disease. Palliation of symptoms constitutes the backbone of management. Patients with stage IV anal cancer should be included in clinical trials. Various treatment modalities for stage IV disease are as follows:

- Palliative surgery
- Palliative radiation therapy
- Palliative combined chemotherapy and radiation therapy
- Clinical trials.

RECURRENT ANAL CANCER

Local recurrences after initial treatment with either chemoradiation or surgical resection can be effectively controlled by alternate treatment options (Table 10.8) including

- surgical resection after radiation (salvage APR)
- postoperative radiation.

FOLLOW-UP

Patients with anal cancer should be monitored

- every 3 months for the first 3 years
- every 6 months for an additional 2 years
- and then annually.

The following specific recommendations should be undertaken:

- Medical history
- Physical examination
- Complete blood counts
- Liver function tests
- Chest radiograph
- CT scan every 6 to 12 months for the first 3 years.

TABLE 10.12. *5-year disease-free survival rates*

Stage	%
Primary disease	65–80
Persistent or recurrent disease	40–50

Prognosis: 5-year disease-free survival for primary and persistent disease is given in Table 10.12. (See Fig.10.2).

Prevention

The physician can create an awareness and a high-risk group (homosexual men, patients with cervical or vulvar cancer) can be recognised to aid patients by early detection of the disease. Yearly anoscopy may be indicated in such a group. Role of the Papanicolaou smear still must be studied.

ANAL CARCINOMA IN HUMAN IMMUNODEFICIENCY VIRUS–INFECTED PATIENTS

The incidence of anal cancer is increasing in patients with HIV infection, especially with the advent of new antiretroviral medications.

Epidemiology

The San Francisco Study revealed that the incidence of anal carcinoma in homosexual men was between 25 and 87 cases per 100,000 population, as compared with 0.7 cases per 100,000 in the entire male population (10).

Etiology

• HPV, especially oncogenetic serotypes 16 and 18, which are found to be associated with anal intraepithelial neoplasia (AIN), which designates a precursor lesion. The same subtypes of HPV that are implicated in malignant transformation in cervical cancer are implicated in malignant transformation in anal cancer.
• Perianal herpes simplex
• Anal condylomas
• Anal-receptive behavior in homosexual or bisexual men, especially with multiple sexual partners.

Clinical Presentation

The clinical presentation of anal carcinoma in HIV-infected patients include:

• Rectal pain
• Rectal bleeding
• Rectal discharge
• Symptoms secondary to obstruction.

Diagnosis

Diagnostic work-up is similar to the determination of the extent of local disease and staging for dissemination in immunocompetent patients.

Pathology

- Squamous cell carcinoma
- Grading for AIN is similar to that for cervical intraepithelial neoplasia (CIN).

Staging

The staging of anal cancer in HIV-infected patients is similar to that in HIV-negative patients.

Prognosis

HIV-infected patients with severe immunosuppression, as evidenced by CD4 counts of <50 per mm^3, may experience more aggressive and advanced disease.

Treatment

- The treatment of choice for squamous cell carcinoma of the anus is combined-modality therapy with
  - mitomycin C, 10 mg per m^2, day 1 (total dose per course, 10 mg per m^2) intravenous bolus
  - 5-FU, 1,000 mg/m^2/day continuous intravenous infusion (CIVI) for 4 days, days 1 to 4 (total dose/course, 4,000 mg per m^2) *PLUS*
  - external beam radiation therapy.
- Appropriate radiation dosage still must be investigated in HIV infection. Anecdotal experience indicates that HIV-infected patients have a decreased tolerance to full pelvic RT, resulting in myelotoxicity and mucositis, thereby limiting the size of treatment fields. Surgical excision with or without local RT may be considered for small localized cancer with minimal depth of invasion.
- **Treatment of AIN:** Treatment of AIN in HIV-infected patients is similar to the treatment of CIN in women and may include electrocautery, cryoablation, or laser ablation.

Screening

Anal Papanicolaou smears have a reported sensitivity of approximately 70% (equal to that associated with uterine cervix Papanicolaou testing). There are currently no standard recommendations for screening of anal cancer in this population. Anoscopy with anal cytologic evaluation should be undertaken in patients with abnormal discharge, bleeding, pruritus, bowel irregularity, rectal, or pelvic pain, and in those with a history of previous preinvasive lesions or abnormal Papanicolaou smears. Other patients who should be screened include HIV-negative men with a history of anal-receptive intercourse, HIV-positive men and women with CD4 cell counts <500 per mm^3, and HIV-positive and HIV-negative women with a history of high-grade CIN.

REFERENCES

1. Nigro ND, Seydel HG, Considine B, et al. Combined preoperative radiation and chemotherapy for squarnous cell carcnoma of the anal canal cancer. *Cancer* 1983;51:1826–1829.
2. Leichman L, Nigro N, Vatikevicius VK, et al. Cancer of the anal canal. Model for preoperative adjuvant combined modality therapy. *Am J Med* 1985;72(2):211–5.
3. Sischy B, Doggett RL, Krall JM, et al. Definitive irradiation and chemotherapy for radiosensitization in management of anal carcinoma: interim report on radiation therapy oncology group study no. 8314. *J Natl Cancer Inst* 1989;81(11):850–6.
4. Cummings BJ, Rider WD, Harwood AR, et al. Combined radical radiation therapy and chemotherapy for primary squamous cell carcinoma of the anal canal. *Cancer Treat Rep* 1982;66(3):489–92.
5. Schneider IH, Grabenbauer GG, Reck T, et al. Combined radiation and chemotherapy for epidermiod carcinoma of the anal canal. *Int J Colorectal Dis* 1992;7(4):192–6.

6. Papillon J, Montbarbon JF. Epidermoid carcinoma of the anal canal. A series of 276 cases. *Dis Colon Rectum* 1987;30(5):324–33.
7. Tanum G, Tveit K, Karlsen KO, et al. Chemotherapy and radiation therapy for anal carcinoma. Survival and late morbidity. *Cancer* 1991;67(10):2462–6.
8. Cummings B, Keane T, Thomas G, et al. Results and toxicity of the treatment of anal canal carcinoma by radiation therapy or radiation therapy and chemotherapy. *Cancer* 1984;54(10):2062–8.
9. Doci R, Zucali R, Bombelli L, et al. Combined chemoradiation therapy for anal cancer. A report of 56 cases. *Ann Surg* 1992;215(2):150–6.
10. Palefsky JM, Holly EA, Ralston ML, et al. High incidence of anal high grade squamous intraepithelial lesions among HIV- positive and HIV- negative homosexual and bisexual men. *AIDS* 1998;12:495–503.

SUGGESTED READINGS

Allal AS, Laurencet FM, Raymond MA, et al. Effectiveness of surgical salvage therapy for patients with locally uncontrolled anal carcinoma after sphincter conserving treatment. *Cancer* 1999;86:405–409.
Bartelink H, Roelofson F, Eschwege F, et al. Concomitant radiotherapy and chemotherapy is superior to radiotherapy alone in the treatment of locally advanced anal cancer: results of a phase III randomized trial of the European Organization for Research and Treatment of Cancer radiotherapy and gastrointestinal cooperative groups. *J Clin Oncol* 1997;15:2040–2049.
Doci R, Zucali R, LaMonica G, et al. Primary chemoradiation therapy with fluorouracil and cisplatin for cancer of the anus: results in 35 consecutive patients. *J Clin Oncol* 1996;14:3121–3125.
Flam M, John M, Pajak TF, et al. Role of mitomycin in combination with fluorouracil and radiotherapy, and of salvage chemoradiation in the definitive nonsurgical treatment of epidermoid carcinoma of the anal canal: results of a phase III randomized intergroup study. *J Clin Oncol* 1996;14:2527–2539.
Martenson JA Jr, Gunderson LL. External radiation therapy without chemotherapy in the management of anal cancer. *Cancer* 1993;71:1736–1740.
Melbye M, Cote TR, Kessler L, et al. High incidence of anal cancer among AIDS patients. *Lancet* 1994;343:636–639.
Palefsky JM, Holly EA, Hogoboom CJ, et al. Anal cytology as a screening tool for anal squamous intraepithelial lesion. *J Acquir Immun Defic Syndr Hum Retrovirol* 1997;14:415–422.
Peddada AV, Smith DE, Rao AR, et al. Chemotherapy and low-dose radiotherapy in the treatment of HIV-infected patients with carcinoma of the anal canal. *Int J Radiat Oncol Biol Phys* 1997;37:1101–1105.
Ryan DP, Compton CC, Mayer RJ. Carcinoma of the anal canal. *N Engl J Med* 2000;342:792–800.
Schraut F, Wang CH, Dawson PI, et al. Depth of invasion, location, and size of cancer of the anus dictate operative treatment. *Cancer* 1983;51:1291–1296.
Sischy B, Scotte Doggett RL, Krall JM, et al. Definitive irradiation and chemotherapy for radio sensitization in management of anal carcinoma: interim report on Radiation Therapy Oncology Group Study No. 8314. *J Natl Cancer Inst* 1989;81:850–856.
UKCCCR Anal Cancer Trial Working Party. Epidermoid anal cancer: results from the UKCCCR randomized trial of radiotherapy alone versus radiotherapy, 5-fluorouracil, and mitomycin. *Lancet* 1996;348:1049–1054.

11

Other Gastrointestinal Tumors

M. Wasif Saif

University of Alabama at Birmingham, Birmingham, Alabama

GASTROINTESTINAL STROMAL TUMOR

Introduction

Gastrointestinal stromal tumors (GISTs), a type of sarcoma, are the most common non-epithelial tumors of the digestive tract that arise from precursors of connective tissue cells located in the gastrointestinal (GI) tract. Most GI soft tissue neoplasms, previously classified as leiomyomas, schwannomas, leiomyoblastomas, or leiomyosarcomas, are presently classified as GIST on the basis of molecular and immunohistologic features. GISTs are strongly and uniformly positive for CD117 (c-kit), a type III receptor tyrosine kinase. c-kit mutations, mostly in exon 11, leading to ligand-independent constitutive activation, are supposed to play a major role in the pathogenesis of GIST.

Epidemiology

The incidence of GIST is estimated to be approximately 10 to 20 cases per 1,000,000 population; the median age at diagnosis has been reported to be 55 to 65 years. GISTs most commonly occur in the stomach (70%) or duodenum, followed by the small intestine (20% to 30%), and 10% are found elsewhere in the GI tract. Early stage GIST typically manifests as a localized tumor (i.e., in the stomach). Approximately 50% of patients present with metastatic disease at first diagnosis, predominantly in the liver or peritoneum.

Diagnosis

GIST cells express c-kit, a growth factor receptor with tyrosine kinase activity derived from the protooncogene c-*kit*. In fact, the most specific criterion for the diagnosis of GIST is immunohistochemical staining of CD117, which allows the expression of c-*kit* to be detected. Mutations in the protooncogene that activate the tyrosine kinase function of c-*kit* are observed in most GISTs and are considered to be a central part of pathogenesis of the disease.

The positron emission tomography (PET) and computerized tomography (CT) scans are sensitive and reliable indicators of tumor response to therapy, particularly with imatinib. 2-fluoro-2-deoxy-d-glucose (FDG). PET improves staging, accurately separates responders from nonresponders in an early phase, and is helpful during follow-up of patients.

Prognostic Factors

Prognostic factors have recently been identified for GIST and include tumor size, mitotic rate, and other minor factors (Table 11.1).

TABLE 11.1. *The prognostic factors that define different risk groups for gastrointestinal stromal tumors (GISTs)*

Risk group	Definition
Intermediate risk	Tumor size <5 cm and 6–10 mitoses/50 HPFs OR
	Tumor size 5–10 cm and ≤5 mitoses/50 HPFs
High risk	Tumor size >5 cm and >5 mitoses/50 HPFs OR
	Tumor size >10 cm and any mitotic rate OR
	Any tumor size and >10 mitoses/50 HPFs
Overly malignant risk	Metastatic spread at primary diagnosis

HPFs, high-power fields.

Treatment

Surgery

At present, surgery is the standard treatment for primary resectable GIST. However, often, surgical removal of GISTs either is not feasible or is palliative in nature. Overall 5-year survival after surgical resection of GIST is approximately 60%.

Chemotherapy

Recurrent or malignant GIST does not respond to conventional cytotoxic agents; the response rate of this fatal disease to doxorubicin has been reported to be less than 5%. Other commonly used chemotherapeutic agents yield similarly poor responses in GIST.

Radiotherapy

The effectiveness of radiation therapy, another typical component of cancer treatment, in treating GIST also has not been proven.

Targeted Therapy

The development of a tyrosine kinase inhibitor has changed the management of unresectable GIST. Imatinib mesylate (STI571, Glivec), a tyrosine kinase inhibitor, which inhibits the c-kit receptor, has been proven to be highly effective against GIST and has improved survival in metastatic GIST.

Early results from clinical trials confirm the high activity of this novel treatment, with response rates of approximately 60% and arrest of tumor progression seen in more than 80% of patients, resulting in fast relief of symptoms (see Table 11.2).

Imatinib is approved at a dose of 400 to 600 mg daily for GIST. Some investigators have attempted to determine the most effective dose of imatinib in GIST patients. A large international randomized phase III trial compared the efficacy of two different doses of imatinib in GIST patients. The study randomized 946 patients to receive either 400 mg of imatinib once daily (with crossover to 800 mg per day with disease progression) or 400 mg twice daily (for a daily dose of 800 mg). The interim analysis presented at American Society of Clinical Oncology (ASCO) meeting showed that patients responded well to both doses of imatinib, with an objective response of 43% observed in each arm of the trial. Complete response was similar between the two arms—5.6% and 3.9%, respectively, for the 400-mg and 800-mg groups. Most patients, however, showed either partial response (44.7% and 47.2%, respectively) or stable disease (32.7% and 33.3%, respectively). Data also showed that progression-free survival (PFS), the primary end point of the study, was significantly higher in patients who received the 800-mg dose of imatinib ($p = 0.0216$; see Fig. 11.1).

TABLE 11.2. *Responses to imatinib mesylate in a phase II trial of patients with advanced gastrointestinal stromal tumors (GISTs)*

Confirmed overall responses[a]	400-mg dose of imatinib (n = 73) (%)	600-mg dose of imatinib (n = 74) (%)	Either dose (n = 147) (%)
Partial response	62	65	63
Stable disease	15	20	20
Progressive disease	16	18	12
Clinical benefit	77	85	83

[a]15-month follow-up.

Treatment with imatinib is generally well tolerated, although most common toxicities include grade 1 or 2 adverse events—most commonly nausea, diarrhea, periorbital edema, muscle cramps, fatigue, headache, and dermatitis.

Future Treatments

The role of adjuvant treatment after potentially curative resection of GIST is being evaluated in ongoing clinical trials. An investigational agent, SU11248, has also shown promising results against imatinib-resistant GIST in early trials. Other novel agents that are being tested include RAD001 and PKC412.

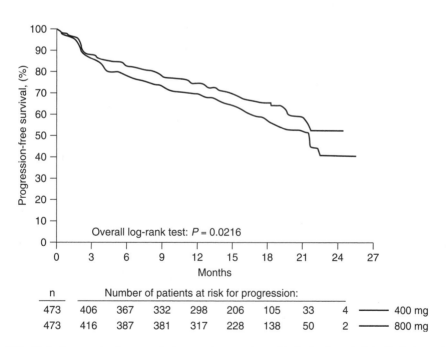

FIG. 11.1. Progression-free survival curve from a phase III study of gastrointestinal stromal tumors (GISTs); patients treated with 400 or 800 mg of imatinib mesylate. [From Verweij J, Casali PG, Zalcberg J, et al. Progression-free survival in gastrointestinal stromal tumors with high-dose Imatinib: randomized trial. *Lancet* 2004; 364(9440):1127–1134, with permission.]

SMALL BOWEL ADENOCARCINOMA
Epidemiology

Cancer of the small bowel is a relatively rare malignancy, accounting for approximately 2% of GI tumors. Approximately 5,300 new cases of small bowel adenocarcinoma and 1,100 deaths from the disease are reported annually in the United States. An estimated 40% of small bowel cancers are adenocarcinomas, 40% are carcinoids, 15% are sarcomas (GIST), and less than 5% are lymphomas. Limited information is available on the incidence, prognosis, and role of chemotherapy in the treatment of this disease.

Etiology

An increased risk of developing small bowel adenocarcinoma has been described in patients with:

- Crohn disease (40-fold to 100-fold increase in relative risk)
- Familial adenomatous polyposis [(FAP), 50-fold to 300-fold increase in relative risk]
- Hereditary nonpolyposis colorectal cancer [(HNPCC), greater than 100-fold increase in relative risk]
- K-*ras* mutations at codon 12 in duodenal tumors (1)
- Expression of p53 in carcinoma arising from the ampulla of Vater (2)
- Expression of c-erbB-2, Ki-67, and tenascin (3).

Familial clustering of small bowel adenocarcinomas with multicentric colorectal cancer and gastric cancer has been identified (4).

Pathology

An estimated 40% of small bowel cancers are adenocarcinomas, 40% are carcinoids, 15% are sarcomas (GISTs), and less than 5% are lymphomas.

Small bowel adenocarcinoma includes adenocarcinomas arising in the duodenum, jejunum, and ileum. Whereas adenocarcinomas arising from the ampulla of Vater and the periampullary region are typically included in the category of small bowel adenocarcinomas, those arising from the ileocecal valve, appendix, and Meckel diverticulum are excluded.

Small bowel adenocarcinomas are similar to their colonic counterparts in the adenoma–carcinoma sequence and demonstrate similar pathologic features, with slight differences in frequency of histologic types and immunohistochemical markers.

Most small bowel adenocarcinomas are solitary, sessile lesions, often appearing in association with adenomas. They are usually moderately well differentiated and are almost always positive for acid mucin.

Small bowel adenocarcinomas can be positive for carcinoembryonic antigen (CEA), carbohydrate antigen 19-9 (CA 19-9), and p53. Expression of c-erbB-2, Ki-67, and tenascin has also been described. Small bowel adenocarcinomas arising from the ileum may show staining with neuroendocrine markers.

Clinical Presentation

The clinical presentation of small bowel adenocarcinoma depends on the location of the primary tumor, its growth pattern, and the extent of metastatic spread. In general, symptoms are initially nonspecific and include anemia, bleeding, abdominal pain, nausea and vomiting, or obstruction and/or perforation in cases of locally advanced tumor. Because of a vague presentation of small bowel adenocarcinoma, the time between initial development of symptoms and diagnosis is often relatively long, approximately 6 to 8 months, and contributes to the higher percentage of advanced cases at the time of diagnosis (in contrast to colorectal cancer). Common sites of metastases include locoregional lymph nodes, liver, lung, and the peritoneum.

Diagnosis

The staging workup of small bowel adenocarcinoma includes the following:

- Upper GI series with small bowel follow-through (SBFT) is abnormal in 53% to 83% of patients and delineates the tumor in 30% to 44% of patients.
- CT scanning of the abdomen and pelvis detects abnormalities in 97% of cases and predicts the presence of cancer in 80% of cases. The characteristic CT finding may include a partially obstructing, concentric narrowing in the proximal small bowel (especially with primary tumors >3 cm).
- Upper GI barium series and endoscopies have varying rates of success, but remain the mainstay in identifying proximal small bowel adenocarcinoma. Although cases with elevation of CEA, CA 19-9, or CA 125 levels have been reported, no clear role for such tumor markers has been established for diagnosis.

Staging

Small bowel adenocarcinomas are staged according to the tumor–node–metastasis (TNM) criteria, as used for colon cancer. Staging is based on the extent to which the tumor is present in the bowel wall, the regional nodal status, and the presence or absence of distant metastasis.

Prognosis

Resectability is the key prognostic factor. Other factors include age older than 75 years, performance status, well-differentiated and moderately differentiated versus undifferentiated small bowel adenocarcinomas, tumor location (arising in the duodenum), and presence of distant metastasis. The prognostic significance of lymph node status for survival is controversial.

Survival

The median survival of patients with localized, locally advanced, and metastatic disease is 50.1, 22.2, and 8.6 months, respectively.

Treatment of Localized Disease

Surgery

Surgical resection is the mainstay of treatment for small bowel adenocarcinomas because it offers a potential cure. A large review of the Department of Defense database from 1970 to 1996 found that 47% of 144 small bowel malignancies were small bowel adenocarcinomas; 91% of these patients underwent surgical resection, 45% with curative surgery. During a median follow-up of 38.9 months (range 1 to 405 months), the median survival was 182 months versus 33 months and the 5-year survival rate was 81% versus 42% after curative surgery and incomplete resection, respectively. In patients not amenable to surgery, the median survival was 10 months with a 5-year survival of 39%. Rose et al. found that among 79 patients with primary duodenal small bowel adenocarcinomas, the patients with completely resected disease (node-negative) had a median survival of 86 months and a 5-year survival of 60%, whereas patients with completely resected disease (node-positive) had a median survival of 41 months and a 5-year survival of 43% (5). Patients who either had palliative surgery or who did not undergo surgery had a median survival of 9 months, and no patient was alive at 5 years. This study, although small, suggested that resection of the primary tumor, even with known locoregional involvement, may provide survival benefit.

Adjuvant Therapy

Adjuvant Chemotherapy

Data for adjuvant therapy involving agents such as 5-fluorouracil (5-FU), obtained from the experience gained in the treatment of colorectal cancer and the information obtained from patients with metastatic small bowel disease are scarce. No prospective phase II or randomized phase III data are currently available. A review of the National Cancer Data Base from 1985 to 1995 was published by Howe et al. in *Cancer* in 1999, which revealed an increasing use of adjuvant chemotherapy for regionally advanced disease—from 28% from 1985 to 1990 to more than 40% from 1990 to 1995—a practice based on the current treatment standards for colorectal cancer. It is estimated that 14% of patients in the United States with only localized small bowel adenocarcinoma receive some form of adjuvant chemotherapy. An intensified adjuvant therapy—protracted intravenous infusion of 5-FU modulated with leucovorin with an intense-dose external-beam radiotherapy to liver, regional lymph nodes, and tumor bed—was evaluated in patients with pancreatic or periampullary adenocarcinoma. The regimen was found to be very toxic, with no survival benefit when compared to the historical data from patients who were receiving more conventional doses of chemotherapy or radiation. Median disease-free survival was approximately 8 months, with earlier recurrences suggesting that the disease may promptly develop resistance to chemotherapy and radiation.

Chemoradiation

Coia L et al. treated four patients with resectable duodenal cancer at Fox Chase Cancer Center as part of a clinical study for pancreatic cancer with neoadjuvant or preoperative chemoradiation (6). The regimen consisted of two cycles of 5-FU at a dosage of 1 g/m^2/day for 4 days on days 2 to 5 and days 29 to 32 and mitomycin C at a dosage of 10 mg per m^2 on day 2 given with concurrent radiation administered at a dose of 1.8 Gy per day to a total dose of 50.4 Gy. Surgical resection was performed 4 to 6 weeks after completion of chemoradiation. All four patients underwent surgical resection and achieved complete pathologic response. At a median follow-up of 4.5 years, all patients were alive without recurrence, with actual survival durations of 12, 23, 35, and 90 months, respectively.

Treatment of Metastatic Disease

Surgery

The role of surgical resection is limited to either palliative measures or prevention of bowel obstruction or bleeding in patients with metastatic small bowel adenocarcinoma.

Chemotherapy

The choice of chemotherapeutic agents and the actual efficacy of such treatment in metastatic disease are less defined. This is partly because of the lack of well-controlled clinical trials and partly because this disease is not very common. The National Cancer Data Base indicates that 37% of all patients with advanced disease received some form of chemotherapy, 12% received external-beam radiation with or without surgery, and 25% received no cancer-related therapy. Historically, the most commonly used chemotherapy includes 5-FU alone or 5-FU–based regimens. Other chemotherapy regimens include tegafur, thiotepa, mitomycin C, and cisplatin, anthracyclines, or alkylating agents. Regimens such as ECF (epirubicin, cisplatin, and 5-FU) have been tested in a small group of patients with advanced small bowel cancer at the Royal Marsden Hospital (7). Patients received epirubicin at 50 mg per m^2, cisplatin at 60 mg per m^2, each given every 3 weeks, and protracted venous infusion (PVI) of 5-FU at a dose of 200 mg per m^2. The overall response rate was 37%. The median progression-free survival was 7.8 months, with a median overall survival of 13 months. The authors concluded that small bowel adenocarcinoma is sensitive to infusional 5-FU and that chemotherapy appears to have clinical benefit over palliative surgery alone. In summary, lack of prospective, randomized trials; the minimal benefit, if any, reported in clinical series; and the associated toxicity should be taken into account. The decision to treat should be individualized, and the risks and benefits should be carefully explained to the patient.

REFERENCES

1. Younes N, Fulton N, Tanaka R, et al. The presence of K-12 ras mutations in duodenal adenocarcinomas and the absence of ras mutations in other small bowell adenocarcinomas and carcinoid tumors. *Cancer* 79:1804–1808, 1997.
2. Park SH, Kim YI, Park YH, et al. Clinicopathologic correlation of p53 protein overexpression in adenoma and carcinoma of the ampulla of Vater. *World J Surg* 24(1):54–59, 2000.
3. Vaidya P, Yosida T, Skakura T, et al. Combined analysis of expression of c-erb B-2, Ki-67 antigen and tenascin provides a better prognostic indicator of carcinoma of the papilla of Vater. *Pancreas* 12:196–201, 1996.
4. Stemmermann GN, Goodman MT, Nomura AMY. Adenocarcinoma of the proximal small intestine: A marker for familial and multicentric cancer? *Cancer* 70:2766–2771, 1992.
5. Rose DM, Hochwald SN, Klimstra DS, et al. Primary duodenal adenocarcinoma: A ten-year experience with 79 patients. *J Am Coll Surg* 183:89–96, 1996.
6. Coia L, Hoffman J, Scher R, et al. Preoperative chemoradiation for adenocarcinoma of the pancreas and duodenum. *Int J Radiat Oncol Biol Phys* 30:161–167, 1994.
7. Crawley C, Ross P, Norman A, et al. The Royal Marsden Experience of small bowel adenocarcinoma treated with protracted venous infusion 5-fluorouracil. *Br J Cancer* 78:508–510, 1998.

SUGGESTED READINGS

Abrams RA, Grochow LB, Chakravarthy A, et al. Intensified adjuvant therapy for pancreatic and periampullary adenocarcinoma: survival results and observations regarding patterns of failure, radiotherapy dose and CA 19-9 levels. *Int J Radiat Oncol Biol Phys* 1999;44:1039–1046.

Buemming P, Meis-Kindblom JM, Kindblom LG, et al. Is there an indication for adjuvant treatment with imatinib mesylate in patients with aggressive gastrointestinal stromal tumors (GISTs)?. Presented at: 39th Annual Meeting of the American Society of Clinical Oncology, Chicago, IL, May 31, June 3, 2003, Abstract 3289.

Casali G, Verweij J, Zalcberg J, et al. Imatinib (Gleevec) 400 and 800 mg daily in patients with gastrointestinal stromal tumors (GIST): a randomized phase III trial from EORTC Soft Tissue and Bone Sarcomas Group, the Italian Sarcoma Group (ISG), and the Australasian Gastro-intestinal Trials Group (AGITG). A toxicity report. Presented at: 38th Annual Meeting of the American Society of Clinical Oncology, Orlando, FL, May 1824, 2002, Abstract 1650.

Choi H, Charnsangavej C, Macapinlac HA, et al. Correlation of computerized tomography (CT) and proton emission tomography (PET) in patients with metastatic GIST treated at a single institution with imatinib mesylate. Presented at: 39th Annual Meeting of the American Society of Clinical Oncology, Chicago, IL, May 31, June 3, 2003, Abstract 3290.

Crawley C, Ross P, Norman A, et al. The Royal Marsden Experience of small bowel adenocarcinoma treated with protracted venous infusion 5-fluorouracil. *Br J Cancer* 1998;78:508–510.

Demetri GD, von Mehren M, Blanke CD, et al. Efficacy and safety of imatinib mesylate in advanced gastrointestinal stromal tumors. *N Engl J Med* 2002;347:472–480.

Howe JR, Karnell LH, Menck HR, et al. Adenocarcinoma of the small bowel, review of the National Cancer Data Base, 1985–1995. *Cancer* 1999;86:2693–2696.

Joensuu H, Roberts PJ, Sarlomo-Rikala M, et al. Effect of the tyrosine kinase inhibitor STI571 in a patient with a metastatic gastrointestinal stromal tumor. *N Engl J Med* 2001;344:1052–1056.

Veyrieres M, Baillet P, Hay JM, et al. Factors influencing long-term survival in 100 cases of small intestine primary adenocarcinoma. *Am J Surg* 1997;173:237–239.

SECTION 4

Breast

12

Breast Cancer

Hamid R. Mirshahidi and Jame Abraham

*Section of Hematology/Oncology, Mary Babb Randolph Cancer Center,
West Virginia University, Morgantown, West Virginia*

Breast cancer is the most common cancer diagnosed in women in North America, and it is second only to lung cancer as a cause of death from cancer in women. When diagnosed early, breast cancer can be treated primarily using surgery, radiation, and systemic therapy (chemotherapy or hormonal therapy). At the time of diagnosis, more than 90% of patients will have only localized disease.

EPIDEMIOLOGY

- In the United States, an estimated 211,240 new cases of invasive breast cancer were diagnosed in women in 2005.
- It had been estimated that in 2005 approximately 40,410 new cases of noninvasive breast cancer [ductal carcinoma *in situ* (DCIS)] would be diagnosed in the United States.
- In 2004, 40,110 women were expected to die from breast cancer in the United States.
- Approximately 1,450 cases of breast cancer had been estimated to be diagnosed in men in 2004.
- Lifetime risk of developing breast cancer in North American women (who live up to the age of 85) is one in eight.
- The incidence of breast cancer increases with age, but the rate of increase in incidence slows after menopause.
- The 5-year survival rate of all patients with breast cancer is 87.5%.

RISK FACTORS

The risk factors for developing breast cancer in women are listed in Table 12.1.

GENETICS

- Approximately 5% to 10% of all women with breast cancer may have a germ-line mutation of the genes *BRCA1* or *BRCA2*.
- Mutations of *BRCA1* (chromosome 17q21) and *BRCA2* (chromosome 13q12–13q13) are responsible for 90% of hereditary breast cancer.
- Specific mutations of *BRCA1* and *BRCA2* are more common in women of Ashkenazi Jewish ancestry.
- The estimated lifetime risk for developing breast cancer in women with a *BRCA1* or *BRCA2* mutation is 40% to 85%, and the risk for developing bilateral breast cancer is 20% to 40%.
- Mutations in either gene also confer a 20% to 40% increased lifetime risk for developing ovarian cancer.

TABLE 12.1. *Risk factors for breast cancer in women*

History of breast cancer
BRCA1 or *BRCA2* mutations
Increasing age
Early menarche
Late menopause
Nulliparity
First birth after the age of 30
Atypical lobular hyperplasia or atypical
   ductal hyperplasia
Prior breast biopsies
Long-term postmenopausal estrogen replacement
Early exposure to ionizing radiation

Indications for Genetic Testing

The indications for genetic testing for breast cancer and ovarian cancer are as follows:

- Two or more family members with breast and/or ovarian cancer at age less than 50 years
- Breast cancer and or ovarian cancer at a very young age
- Known *BRCA1* or *BRCA2* mutations in a family member
- Same patient being diagnosed with both breast cancer and ovarian cancer
- One or more family members younger than 50 years with breast cancer and having Ashkenazi Jewish ancestry
- Patients with ovarian cancer having an Ashkenazi Jewish ancestry.

Genetic testing is available commercially (Myriad Genetics). All patients should undergo genetic counseling before the test.
If the test is positive patients have many options including:

- Intense screening using mammogram or magnetic resonance imaging (MRI)
- Chemoprevention using tamoxifen may be considered
- Bilateral prophylactic mastectomy, which could prevent breast cancer in 90% to 100%
- Prophylactic oophorectomy alone reduces breast cancer by 50%.

PATHOLOGY

Eighty percent of breast cancers are invasive ductal carcinoma. Pathologic classification of breast cancer includes:

- Carcinoma, NOS (not otherwise specified)
- Ductal
  - Intraductal (DCIS)
  - Invasive with predominant intraductal component
  - Invasive, NOS
  - Comedo
  - Inflammatory
  - Medullary with lymphocytic infiltrate
  - Mucinous (colloid)
  - Papillary
  - Scirrhous
  - Tubular
  - Other

- Lobular
  - *In situ*
  - Invasive with predominant *in situ* component
  - Invasive
- Nipple
  - Paget disease, NOS
  - Paget disease with intraductal carcinoma
  - Paget disease with invasive ductal carcinoma
- Others
  - Undifferentiated carcinoma.

The following tumor subtypes occur in the breast but are not considered to be typical breast cancers:

- Cystosarcoma phyllodes
- Angiosarcoma
- Primary lymphoma.

The following high-risk lesions are known to occur in breast cancer:

- Atypical ductal hyperplasia (ADH)
- Lobular carcinoma *in situ* (LCIS) or lobular neoplasia.

CHEMOPREVENTION

Tamoxifen

- National Surgical Adjuvant Breast and Bowel Project (NSABP) P-1 study showed a 49% reduction in the incidence of invasive breast cancer in high-risk subjects who took tamoxifen at a dose of 20 mg daily for 5 years.
- Women eligible for this trial were at least 35 years old and were assessed to have an absolute risk of at least 1.67% over the period of 5 years using Gail Model or a pathologic diagnosis of LCIS.
- Gail model is a statistical model that calculates a woman's absolute risk of developing breast cancer by using the following criteria: age, age at menarche, age at first live birth, number of previous biopsies, history of ADH, and number of first-degree relatives with breast cancer. For a free computer disk of this model, call 1-800-4-CANCER or visit the National Cancer Institute (NCI) website (http://www.nci.nih.gov).
- The reduction in the incidence of breast cancer following treatment with tamoxifen is associated with an increase in endometrial cancer (risk ratio of 2.53) and thrombotic events (e.g., pulmonary embolism, with a risk ratio of 3.01) in patients who are older than 50 years.
- Use of tamoxifen for breast cancer should be individualized, and must be considered after weighing the risk–benefit ratio for each patient.

Raloxifene

The NSABP P-2 Study of Tamoxifen and Raloxifene (STAR), in which tamoxifen is being compared with raloxifene in postmenopausal women for prevention of breast cancer, has recently completed accrual of patients.

Aromatase Inhibitors

Aromatase inhibitors are being investigated for breast cancer prevention.

SCREENING

Mammogram

- Regular mammographic screening results in early diagnosis of breast cancer and a 25% to 30% decrease in mortality in women older than 50 years.
- A 17% reduction in mortality is seen in women between 40 and 49 years.
- The NCI recommends annual mammography for women aged 40 years and older.

Magnetic Resonance Imaging of the Breast

- MRI is found to be superior to mammogram and ultrasound in young women at high risk for breast cancer and/or in women with *BRCA1* or *BRCA2* mutations.

SCREENING FOR HIGH-RISK FAMILY

Women with families at high risk for breast cancer, especially with *BRCA1* and *BRCA2* mutations, are often advised to undergo mammographic screening from the age of 25, or 5 years earlier than the earliest age at which another family member was diagnosed with breast cancer.

CLINICAL FEATURES

Clinical features could include a breast lump, skin thickening or alteration, peau d'orange, dimpling of the skin, nipple inversion or crusting (Paget disease), unilateral nipple discharge, and so on. Patients could instead present with signs and symptoms of metastatic disease.

DIAGNOSIS

The diagnosis of breast cancer includes the following:

1. History and physical examination.
2. Bilateral mammogram (80% to 90% accuracy).
3. Biopsy: Any distinct mass should be considered for a biopsy, even if the mammograms are negative.
   The standard methods of diagnosis are:
   - Fine-needle aspiration
   - Core-needle biopsy
   - Incisional or excisional biopsy.
   The options in nonpalpable breast lesions are:
   - Ultrasound-guided core-needle biopsy
   - Stereotactic core-needle biopsy under mammographic localization
   - Needle localization under mammography, followed by surgical excision
   - MRI-guided biopsy.
4. Laboratory studies:
   - Complete blood count, liver function tests, and alkaline phosphatase level
   - Routine use of breast cancer markers such as CA 27:29 or 15:3 are not recommended but are used widely.
5. Pathology review to determine:
   - Histology and diagnosis (invasive versus *in situ*)
   - Pathologic grade of the tumor
   - Tumor involvement of the margin
   - Special studies—estrogen receptor/progesterone receptor (ER/PR) status, HER2/neu status, and indices of proliferation (e.g., mitotic index, Ki-67, or S phase)

- HER2/neu status is studied by immunohistochemistry (IHC) and a result of 3+ is considered positive
- If the IHC result is 2+ (indeterminate), fluorescent *in situ* hybridization (FISH) should be performed for gene amplification.

6. Radiographic studies are performed on the basis of the findings of the history and physical examination and screening blood tests:
   - Computerized tomography (CT) scan of the chest and abdomen
   - Imaging of the brain with CT or MRI
   - Bone scan
   - Chest radiograph.

STAGING OF BREAST CANCER

The American Joint Committee on Cancer (AJCC) staging of breast cancer and the pathologic classification are listed in Tables 12.2, 12.3, and 12.4.

TABLE 12.2. *Staging of breast cancer (American Joint Committee on Cancer)*

Primary tumor (T)

TX:	Primary tumor cannot be assessed
T0:	No evidence of primary tumor
Tis:	Carcinoma *in situ*; intraductal carcinoma, lobular carcinoma *in situ*, or Paget disease of the nipple with no associated tumor. Note: Paget disease associated with a tumor is classified according to the size of the tumor.
T1:	Tumor ≤2.0 cm in greatest dimension
T1mic:	Microinvasion ≤0.1 cm in greatest dimension
T1a:	Tumor >0.1 but ≤0.5 cm in greatest dimension
T1b:	Tumor >0.5 cm but ≤1.0 cm in greatest dimension
T1c:	Tumor >1.0 cm but ≤2.0 cm in greatest dimension
T2:	Tumor >2.0 cm but ≤5.0 cm in greatest dimension
T3:	Tumor >5.0 cm in greatest dimension
T4:	Tumor of any size with direct extension to (a) chest wall or (b) skin
T4a:	Extension to chest wall
T4b:	Edema (including peau d'orange) or ulceration of the skin of the breast or satellite skin nodules confined to the same breast
T4c:	Both of the above (T4a and T4b)
T4d:	Inflammatory carcinoma

Regional lymph nodes (N)

NX:	Regional lymph nodes cannot be assessed (e.g., previously removed)
N0:	No regional lymph node metastasis
N1:	Metastasis to movable ipsilateral axillary lymph node(s)
N2a:	Metastasis to ipsilateral axillary lymph node(s) fixed or matted
N2b:	Metastasis in clinically apparent[a] ipsilateral internal mammary nodes in the absence of clinical evident axillary lymph node metastasis
N3a:	Metastasis in ipsilateral infraclavicular lymph node(s)
N3b:	Metastasis to ipsilateral internal mammary lymph node(s) and axillary node(s)
N3c:	Metastasis in ipsilateral supraclavicular lymph node(s)

[a]Clinically apparent is defined as being detected by imaging studies (excluding lymphoscintigraphy) or by clinical examination or being grossly visible on histopathologic evaluation.

TABLE 12.3. *Pathologic classification (pN)*

pNX:	Regional lymph nodes cannot be assessed (not removed for pathologic study or previously removed)
pN0:	No regional lymph node metastasis histologically, no additional examination for isolated tumor cells (ITC)
pN0(i–):	No regional lymph node metastasis histologically, negative IHC
pN0(i+):	No regional lymph node metastasis histologically, positive IHC, no IHC cluster >0.2 mm
pN0(mol–):	No regional lymph node metastasis histologically, negative molecular finding (RT-PCR)
pN0(mol+):	No regional lymph node metastasis histologically, positive molecular finding (RT-PCR)
pN1:	Metastasis in 1–3 axillary lymph node(s) and/or in internal mammary node(s), with microscopic disease detected by sentinel lymph node dissection but not clinically apparent[a]
pN1mi:	Only micrometastasis (>0.2 mm, <2.0 mm)
pN1a:	Metastasis in 1–3 axillary lymph node(s)
pN1b:	Metastasis in internal mammary node(s), with microscopic disease detected by sentinel lymph node dissection but not clinically apparent[a]
pN1c:	Metastasis in 1–3 axillary lymph node(s) and in internal mammary node(s), with microscopic disease detected by sentinel lymph node dissection but not clinically apparent[a]
pN2:	Metastasis in 4–9 axillary lymph nodes or in clinically apparent[b] internal mammary lymph nodes in the absence of axillary lymph node metastasis
pN2a:	Metastasis in 4–9 axillary lymph nodes (at least one tumor deposit >2.0 mm)
pN2b:	Metastasis in clinically apparent[b] internal mammary lymph nodes in the absence of axillary lymph node metastasis
pN3:	Metastasis in ten or more axillary lymph nodes, or in infraclavicular lymph nodes, or clinically apparent[b] ipsilateral internal mammary lymph nodes in the presence of one or more positive axillary lymph nodes; or in more than three axillary lymph nodes, with clinically microscopic metastasis in internal mammary lymph nodes or in ipsilateral supraclavicular lymph nodes
pN3a:	Metastasis in ten or more axillary lymph nodes (at least one tumor deposit >2.0 mm), or metastasis to the infraclavicular lymph nodes
pN3b:	Metastasis in clinically apparent[b] ipsilateral internal mammary lymph nodes in the presence of one or more positive axillary lymph nodes; or in more than three axillary lymph nodes and in internal mammary lymph nodes, with microscopic disease detected by sentinel lymph node dissection but not clinically apparent[a]
pN3c:	Metastasis in ipsilateral supraclavicular lymph nodes

Distant metastasis (M)

MX:	Presence of distant metastasis cannot be assessed
M0:	No distant metastasis
M1:	Distant metastasis present

IHC, immunohistochemistry; RT-PCR, reverse-transcription polymerase chain reaction.

[a]Not clinically apparent is defined as not being detected by imaging studies (excluding lymphoscintigraphy) or clinical examination, or by not being grossly visible on histopathologic evaluation.

[b]Clinically apparent is defined as being detected by imaging studies (excluding lymphoscintigraphy) or clinical examination, or by being grossly visible pathologically.

From AJCC Cancer Staging Manual. Sixth Edition 2002. Springer Publication, with permission.

TABLE 12.4. *American Joint Committee on Cancer stage groupings*

Stage 0	Tis	N0	M0
Stage I	T1	N0	M0
Stage IIA	T0	N1	M0
	T1	N1	M0
	T2	N0	M0
Stage IIB	T2	N1	M0
	T3	N0	M0
Stage IIIA	T0	N2	M0
	T1	N2	M0
	T2	N2	M0
	T3	N1	M0
	T3	N2	M0
Stage IIIB	T4	N0—N2	M0
Stage IIIC	Any T	N3	M0
Stage IV	Any T	Any N	M1

From AJCC Cancer Staging Manual. Sixth Edition 2002, Springer Publication, with permission.

Prognostic Factors

1. Number of positive axillary lymph nodes
   - This is one of the most powerful prognostic indicators.
2. Tumor size
   - Tumors smaller than 1 cm have a good prognosis in patients without lymph node involvement.
3. Histologic or nuclear grade
   - Patients with poorly differentiated histology and high nuclear grade have a worse prognosis than others.
   - Scarff–Bloom–Richardson (SBR) grading system and Fisher nuclear grade are commonly used systems.
4. ER/PR status
   - ER- and or PR-positive tumor has better prognosis.
5. Histologic tumor type
   - Prognoses of infiltrating ductal and lobular carcinoma are similar.
   - Mucinous (colloid) and typical medullary and tubular histologies have good prognosis if the size is <3 cm.
   - Inflammatory breast cancer has poor prognosis.
6. HER2/neu overexpression is clearly associated with poor prognosis.
   - Median survival of patients with tumors exhibiting HER2/neu overexpression is 3 years compared to HER2/neu–negative patients who have a median survival of 6 to 7 years.
7. Gene Expression Profiles
   - Oncotype DX is a new diagnostic genomic assay based on an NSABP study. This assay can accurately and precisely quantify the likelihood of cancer recurrence in women with newly diagnosed, stage I or II, node-negative, ER-positive breast cancer. Patients are divided into low-risk, intermediate-risk, and high-risk groups on the basis of the expression of a panel of 21 genes. The recurrence score determined by this assay is found to be a better predictor of outcome than standard measures such as age, tumor size, and tumor grade.

MANAGEMENT OF BREAST CANCER
High-risk Lesions

Patients with high-risk lesions may be eligible for breast cancer prevention studies.

Atypical Ductal Hyperplasia

- There is a fourfold to fivefold increase in the risk of developing breast cancer in patients with ADH.
- There is wide variation in the criteria used in the diagnosis of ADH.
- ADH is managed by close follow-up of patients.
- Clinical breast examination and mammogram are the preferred screening methods.
- Tamoxifen 20 mg PO for 5 years: NSABP P-1 study showed 86% reduction in the risk for developing invasive breast cancer in patients who received tamoxifen.

Lobular Carcinoma In Situ

- LCIS is not considered a form of cancer but a marker of increased risk for developing invasive breast cancer.
- It is usually multicentric and bilateral.
- There is a 21% chance of developing breast cancer in patients within 15 years of developing LCIS.
- It is managed by close follow-up of patients.
- Clinical breast examination every 4 to 12 months and annual mammogram is essential.
- Tamoxifen may be used for prevention of breast cancer (56% reduction in risk as per the NSABP P-1 study).

Noninvasive Breast Cancer
Ductal Carcinoma In Situ

- With the extensive use of mammograms, the diagnosis of DCIS has increased over the last few years.
- Microcalcification or soft-tissue abnormality is seen in the mammogram in cases of DCIS.

Different Histologic Types of Ductal Carcinoma In Situ

- Comedocarcinoma has a poor prognosis.
- Non–comedocarcinoma includes micropapillary, papillary, solid, and cribriform carcinoma.

Treatment

- Lumpectomy followed by radiation treatment plus tamoxifen is the standard treatment option.
- Other treatment options are:
  - Total mastectomy with or without tamoxifen
  - Breast-conserving surgery without radiation therapy, which could be considered in select patients with low Van Nuys Prognostic Index (VNPI), which combines four predictors of local recurrence (tumor size, margin width, pathologic classification, and age).
- In patients who previously had lumpectomy and radiation, tamoxifen reduced the risk of breast cancer recurrence (ipsilateral and contralateral; NSABP B-24). Recent subset analysis of B-24 showed that the benefit was more obvious in patients with ER/PR-positive DCIS.
- The role of aromatase inhibitors such as anastrozole is being investigated for receptor-positive DCIS in a large NSABP (B-35) study.

Invasive Breast Cancer

Early stage Breast Cancer

Surgery

No survival difference is seen in patients who are treated with modified radical mastectomy versus those treated with lumpectomy plus radiation. Breast preservation with lumpectomy plus radiation therapy is the preferred treatment for breast cancer.

Contraindications for lumpectomy:

- Two or more tumors in separate quadrants of the breast
- Diffuse, indeterminate, or malignant-appearing microcalcifications
- Central location of the tumor mass.

Contraindications for radiation:

- History of therapeutic irradiation to the breast
- Connective tissue disorders (scleroderma)
- Pregnancy.

Axillary lymph node dissection:

- Axillary lymph node dissection (ALND) primarily provides prognostic information. It has minimal therapeutic benefit, especially in clinically negative axillae.
- Histologically positive axillary lymph nodes are the most important prognostic factor.
- Among patients with clinically negative axillary lymph nodes, 30% will have positive histology after dissection.
- It is associated with approximately 10% to 25% risk of lymphedema, which can be mild to severe. This varies with the level of axillary node dissection.

Sentinel node biopsy:

- Sentinel node biopsy (SNB) is a minimally invasive procedure for axillary staging.
- A radioactive substance or blue dye is injected into the area around the tumor.
- The ipsilateral axilla is explored and the node that has taken up the dye or radioactive material is excised and examined pathologically.
- In expert hands, this procedure identifies a node in more than 92% to 98% of patients.

Reconstruction:

Reconstructive surgery may be used for patients who opt for a total mastectomy. It may be done at the time of the mastectomy (immediate reconstruction) or it can be delayed.

Radiotherapy

- Radiotherapy (RT) is an integral part of breast-conserving treatment (lumpectomy).
- Radiation boost up to 4,500 to 5,000 cGy ± 1,000 to 1,500 cGy to the tumor bed of the breast is effective.
- In patients who need chemotherapy, RT is usually done after chemotherapy.
- Postmastectomy radiation treatment to the chest wall and supraclavicular lymph nodes decreases the risk of locoregional recurrence in patients with four or more positive lymph nodes and in patients with tumor size >5 cm.
- Two randomized trials showed improvement in overall survival (OS) for postmastectomy radiation in patients with one to three positive lymph nodes, and it is being evaluated in more clinical trials.

Newer radiation techniques under investigation:

1. **Partial breast irradiation (PBI)** is under investigation and may be used in clinical trial at this point.

2. **Partial breast brachytherapy (PBB)** or interstitial brachytherapy is also undergoing clinical trials in stage I and II patients with free resected margins and zero to three positive lymph nodes. In the PBB method, patients receive ten fractions of radiations of 3.4 Gy within 5 days.
3. **Mammosite Radiation Therapy System (RTS)** was approved by the U.S. Food and Drug Administration (FDA) on May 6, 2002, for patients with T2 N0 M0 breast cancer. Radiation of 34-Gy is delivered in ten fractions within 5 days through a balloon inserted at the lumpectomy site during surgery.

Systemic Treatment for Early Breast Cancer

Chemotherapy is recommended for most of the patients with node-positive disease. For node-negative patients, the treatment is based on many factors, such as the tumor size, ER/PR status, nuclear or histologic grade (Table 12.5).

Adjuvant Chemotherapy:
Multiple systemic chemotherapy regimens are used including AC (doxorubicin and cyclophosphamide), CMF [cyclophosphamide, methotrexate, and 5-fluorouracil (5-FU)], AC followed by a taxane, EC, CAF (cyclophosphamide, doxorubicin, 5-FU), CEF (cyclophosphamide, epirubicin, 5-FU), FAC (5-FU, doxorubicin, and cytoxan), TAC (taxotere, adriamycin, and cytoxan).

- CALGB 9344 and NSABP B-28 trials showed that adding four cycles of paclitaxel to four cycles of AC improves the disease-free survival (DFS) and OS in node-positive patients.
- CALGB 9741 trial showed that dose-dense chemotherapy in which node-positive patients received the same total doses of AC followed by paclitaxel on a 2-week regimen rather than a 3-week schedule with growth factor support had a superior DFS and OS.
- BCIRG 001 trial showed improvement in DFS and OS in node-positive early stage breast cancer patients who were treated with TAC versus the standard FAC regimen (see Table 12.6 and Fig. 12.1).

Antiestrogen therapy in the adjuvant setting:
Antiestrogen therapy is recommended only for ER-positive and/or PR-positive patients.

Tamoxifen:

- Tamoxifen is a selective estrogen-receptor modulator (SERM).
- In early stage breast cancer, tamoxifen decreases the risk of recurrence by 42% and the absolute risk of death by 22% in both pre- and postmenopausal women with ER-positive tumors.

TABLE 12.5. *Risk categories for patients with node-negative breast cancer*

Factors	Min/low risk (all factors)	Intermediate risk (between the two categories)	High risk (at least one factor)
Tumor size	≤1 cm	1–2 cm	>2 cm
ER and/or PR status	Positive	Positive	Negative
Grade	Grade 1 (uncertain relevance for tumors ≤1 cm)	Grade 1–2	Grade 2–3
Age	>35		<35

ER, estrogen receptor; PR, progesterone receptor.
From Baum M, Bianco AR, Buzdar A, et al. Anastrozole alone or in combination with tamoxifen versus tamoxifen alone for adjuvant treatment of postmenopausal women with early stage breast cancer. *Cancer* 2003;98:1802–1810, with permission.

TABLE 12.6. *Commonly used combination chemotherapy regimens*

Regimen	Drugs	Route	Cycles	Source
AC	Doxorubicin 60 mg/m^2	i.v. on d 1	q21d/4 cycles	1
	Cyclophosphamide			
	600 mg/m^2	i.v. on d 1		
CMF	Cyclophosphamide			2–3
	100 mg/m^2	PO on 1–14 d	q28d/6 cycles	
	Methotrexate 40 mg/m^2	i.v. on d 1 and 8		
	Fluorouracil 600 mg/m^2	i.v. on d 1 and 8		
	Or			
	Cyclophosphamide			
	600 mg/m^2	i.v. on d 1	q21d/4 cycles	
	Methotrexate 40 mg/m^2	i.v. on d 1		
	Fluorouracil 600 mg/m^2	i.v. on d 1		
AC + P	Doxorubicin 60 mg/m^2	i.v. on d 1	q21d/4 cycles	4
	Cyclophosphamide			
	600 mg/m^2	i.v. on d 1		
	Followed by			
	Paclitaxel 175 mg/m^2	i.v. on d 1	q21d/4 cycles	
Dose-Dense Chemotherapy				5
AC + P	Doxorubicin 60 mg/m^2	i.v. on d 1	q14d/4 cycles	
	Cyclophosphamide			
	600 mg/m^2	i.v. on d 1	q14d/4 cycles	
	Followed by			
	Paclitaxel 175 mg/m	i.v. on d 1	q14d/4 cycles	
	Filgrastim with each cycle			
CAF	Cyclophosphamide			6
	500 mg/m^2	i.v. on d 1	q21d/4 cycles	
	Doxorubicin 50 mg/m^2	i.v. on d 1		
	Fluorouracil 500 mg/m^2	i.v. on d 1		
CEF	Cyclophosphamide			7–8
	75 mg/m^2	PO on 1–14 d	q28d/6 cycles	
	Epirubicin 60 mg/m^2	i.v. on d 1 and 8		
	Fluorouracil 500 mg/m^2	i.v. on d 1 and 8		
	Or			
	Cyclophosphamide			
	500 mg/m^2	i.v. on d 1	q21d/4 cycles	
	Epirubicin 100 mg/m^2	i.v. on d 1		
	Fluorouracil 500 mg/m^2	i.v. on d 1		
TAC	Doxorubicin 50 mg/m^2	i.v. on d 1	q21d/4 cycles	9
	Cyclophosphamide			
	500 mg/m^2	i.v. on d 1		
	Docetaxel 75 mg/m^2	i.v. on d 1		

Source:

1. Modified from Fisher B, Brown AM, Dimitrov NV, et al. Two months of doxorubicin-cyclophosphamide with and without interval reinduction therapy compared with 6 months of cyclophosphamide, methotrexate, and fluorouracil in positive-node breast cancer patients with tamoxifen nonresponsive tumors: results from the National Surgical Adjuvant Breast and Bowel Project B-15. *J Clin Oncol* 1990;8(9):1483–1496, with permission.

2. From Bonadonna G, Valagussa P, Moliterni A, Zambetti M, Brambilla C. Adjuvant cyclophosphamide, methotrexate, and fluorouracil in node-positive breast cancer: the results of 20 years of follow-up. *N Engl J Med* 1995;332:901–906, with permission.

continued on next page

TABLE 12.6. *Continued*

3. From Bonadonna G, Zambetti M, Valagussa P. sequential or alternating doxorubicin and CMF regimens in breast cancer with more than three positive nodes: ten-year result. *JAMA* 1995;273:542–547, with permission.

4. From Henderson IC, Berry D, Demetri G, et al. Improved disease free (DFS) and overall survival (OS) from the addition of sequential paclitaxel but not from the escalation of doxorubicin dose in an adjuvant chemotherapy regimen for patients with node positive primary breast cancer. *J Clin Oncol* 2003;21:976–983, with permission.

5. From Citron ML, Berry DA, Cirrincione C, et al. Randomized trial of dose-dense versus conventionally Scheduled and sequential versus concurrent combination chemotherapy as postoperative adjuvant treatment of node-positive primary breast cancer: first report of inter-group trial C9741/Cancer and Leukemia Group B Trial 9741. *J Clin Oncol* 2003;21:1431–1439, with permission.

6. From Smalley RV, Lefante J, Bartolucci A, et al. A comparison of cyclophosphamide, adri-amycin, and 5-fluorouracil (CAF) and cyclophosphamide, methotrexate, and fluorouracil, vin-cristine, and prednisone (CMFVP) in patients with advanced breast cancer. *Breast Cancer Res Treat* 1983:3:209–220, with permission.

7. From Levine MN, Bramwell VH, Pritchard KI, et al. Randomized trial of intensive cyclophos-phamide, epirubicin, and fluorouracil chemotherapy compared with cyclophosphamide, methotrex-ate, and fluorouracil in premenopausal women with node-positive breast cancer. *J Clin Oncol* 1998;16:2651–2658, with permission.

8. From French Epirubicin Study Group. Epirubicin-based chemotherapy in metastatic breast cancer patients: role of dose intensity and duration of treatment. *J Clin Oncol* 2000;18: 3115–3124, with permission.

9. From Nabholtz JM, Pienkowski T, Mackey J, et al. Phase III trial comparing TAC with FAC in the adjuvant treatment of node-positive breast cancer patients: interim analysis of the BCIRG 001 study (abstract). *Proc Am Soc Clin Oncol* 2002;21:36a. Abstract 141, with permission.

- Tamoxifen decreases the incidence of breast cancer in the contralateral breast by approxi-mately 50%.
- Recommended treatment is tamoxifen, 20 mg per day PO for 5 years.

Anastrozole:
- Anastrozole is an aromatase enzyme inhibitor approved for adjuvant treatment of post-menopausal women.
- Arimidex, Tamoxifen, Alone or in Combination(ATAC) trial showed that anastrozole has a favorable side-effect profile (especially thromboembolic disease and endometrial cancer) and superiority over tamoxifen in contralateral breast cancer reduction, DFS, and OS.
- The dose of anastrozole is 1 mg PO everyday for 5 years.
- Major side effects include joint pain and osteopenia, osteoporosis, and fracture.

Letrozole:
A recent study showed approximately 43% reduction in recurrence in patients receiving 2.5 mg of letrozole after completing 5 years of tamoxifen (extended adjuvant therapy) (1).

Exemestane:
Exemestane therapy after 2 to 3 years of tamoxifen therapy significantly improved DFS and reduced the incidence of contralateral breast cancer as compared with the standard 5 years of tamoxifen therapy (2). A smaller but similar study from an Italian group showed an improve-ment in DFS by switching to anastrozole after 2 to 3 years of tamoxifen.

Locally Advanced Breast Cancer and Inflammatory Breast Cancer

Locally advanced breast cancer and inflammatory breast cancer have the following features:

- Tumor ≥5 cm
- Tumors of any size, with direct invasion of the skin of the breast or chest wall (T4)
- Any tumor with fixed or matted axillary lymphadenopathy (N2).

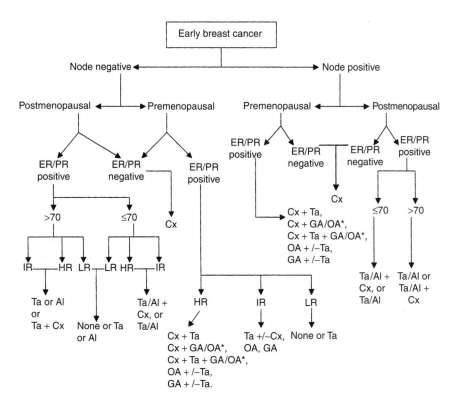

FIG. 12.1. Treatment algorithm for early breast cancer.
• LR = Low Risk, IR = Intermediate Risk, HR = High Risk, Chemotheraphy = Cx,
Tamoxifen = Ta, Aromatase inhibitor = Al, GnRH Analog = GA
Ovarian Ablation = OA
• Treatment in older women should be individualized.
*This treatment option is under clinical evaluation.
• Adapted from NCI PDQ.

Treatment

1. Initial surgery is limited to biopsy to confirm the diagnosis and to identify the receptor status.
2. Neoadjuvant (primary) chemotherapy: NSABP B-18 (AC for four cycles) and B-27 (AC followed by Taxotere for four cycles) showed a higher clinical and pathologic response rate in patients who received neoadjuvant chemotherapy.
3. Surgery is performed after the best response to preoperative chemotherapy.
4. Radiation therapy to the chest wall and supraclavicular area is performed after surgery.

Metastatic Breast Cancer

• The treatment goal is to palliate symptoms and to improve survival.
• All patients should be considered for ongoing clinical trials.

TABLE 12.7. *Hormonal agents used in metastatic breast cancer*

Selective Estrogen-Receptor Modifier (SERM) with combined estrogen agonist and estrogen antagonist activity
   Tamoxifen (Nolvadex, others), 20 mg/d PO
   Toremifene (Fareston), 60 mg/d PO

Estrogen Receptor-Down Regulator
Faslodex, 250 mg/mo i.m.

Aromatase inhibitors
   Anastrozole (Arimidex), 1 mg/d PO
   Letrozole (Femara), 2.5 mg/d PO
Exemestane (Aromasin), 25 mg/d PO

LHRH agonist analog in premenopausal women
   Leuprolide (Lupron Depot), 7.5 mg/dose i.m. monthly, or
   Leuprolide (Lupron Depot), 22.5 mg/dose i.m. every 3 mo, or
   Leuprolide (Lupron Depot), 30 mg/dose i.m. every 4 mo

GnRH agonist analog
   Goserelin (Zoladex), 3.6 mg/dose s.c. implant into the abdominal wall every 28 d or
   Goserelin (Zoladex), 10.8 mg/dose s.c. implant into the abdominal wall every 12 wk
   Used in patients who have tumors that express either ER or PR receptors or both receptors.

LHRH, luteinizing hormone releasing hormone; GnRH, gonadotropin-releasing hormone; ER, estrogen receptor; PR, progesterone receptor.

- In 5% to 15% of patients, durable complete remission can be achieved with systemic therapy.
- Local control may be achieved by surgery and/or radiation treatment.
- In hormone receptor–positive patients with soft-tissue, bone, or asymptomatic visceral disease, hormonal agents should be considered as the first-line therapy (see Table 12.7).
- Chemotherapy regimens can be used as the initial treatment in hormone receptor–negative disease or in patients with symptomatic visceral disease.
  - Quality of life should be an important consideration.
  - Most of the patients could be treated with sequential single agents, but in select patients, combination chemotherapy also could be used (see Fig. 12.2).

Bisphosphonates

- Bisphosphonates should be used in patients with bony metastatic disease because they prevent progression of lytic lesions, delay skeletal-related events, and decrease pain.
- Zoledronic acid (4 mg by 15-minute infusion) and pamidronate (90 mg by 2-hour infusion) are two available biphosphonates approved for bony metastatic disease.

Commonly used chemotherapy agents in metastatic breast cancer:

- Anthracyclines
  - Doxorubicin
  - Epirubicin
  - Liposomal doxorubicin
  - Mitoxantrone
- Taxanes
  - Paclitaxel
  - Docetaxel
- Alkylating agents
  - Cyclophosphamide
- Fluoropyrimidines
  - Capecitabine
  - 5-FU

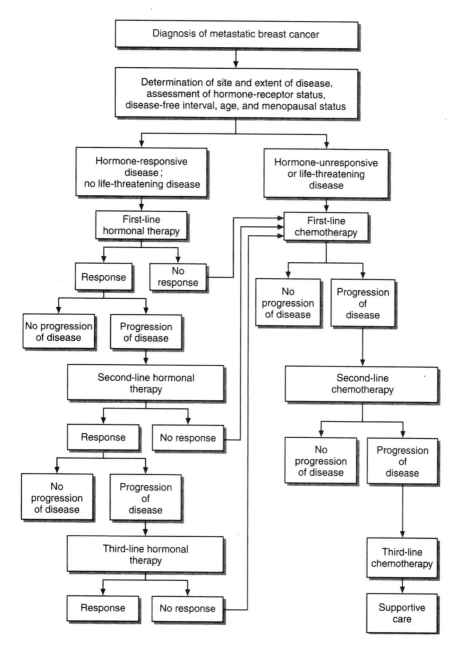

FIG. 12.2. Algorithm for the management of metastatic breast cancer (3).
(From Hortobagyi GN. Treatment of breast cancer. *N Engl J Med* 1998;339:974–984.)

- Antimetabolites
  - Methotrexate
- Vinca alkaloids
  - Vinorelbine
  - Vinblastine
  - Vincristine
- Platinum
  - Carboplatin
  - Cisplatin
- Other
  - Gemcitabine.

Trastuzumab (Herceptin)

- Trastuzumab (Herceptin) is a humanized monoclonal antibody that binds to the HER2/neu receptor.
  - It is indicated in patients with metastatic disease whose tumor overexpresses HER2/neu protein (3 + by IHC or FISH positive).
  - Approximately 25% of the patients overexpress HER2/neu.
- Herceptin is combined with many chemotherapy agents including docetaxel, paclitaxel, navelbine, gemcitabine, and carboplatin.
  - Initial dosage is trastuzumab, 4 mg per kg i.v. over 90 minutes, followed at weekly intervals by maintenance with trastuzumab, 2 mg per kg i.v. over 30 minutes if the initial infusion rate is well tolerated.
- Pharmacokinetic studies show that Herceptin could be given every 3 weeks (8 mg per kg loading dose and 6 mg per kg every 3 weeks), and many clinical trials are ongoing to test this regimen.
  - Preexisting cardiac disease and cardiomyopathies associated with prior treatments (e.g., anthracycline drugs and radiation to the chest) may be exacerbated by trastuzumab.
  - The probability of cardiac dysfunction is greatest in patients who receive the therapy concurrent with anthracycline drugs (e.g., doxorubicin).

Capecitabine (Xeloda)

It is an oral antimetabolite that is anabolized to 5-FU in tumors. It is the third-line therapy for metastatic breast cancer after anthracyclines and taxanes or second-line therapy if anthracyclines are not indicated. FDA-approved dosage is 1,250 mg per m^2 PO BID for weeks followed by 1 week rest and given every 3 weeks. Lower doses such as 900 to 1,000 mg per m^2 PO BID is widely used. Major side effect is hand–foot syndrome.

Abraxane

Abraxane is an albumin-stabilized nanoparticle formulation of paclitaxel. It eliminates the need for toxic solvents like cremophor and steroid pretreatment. FDA approved ABRAXANE.

Oophorectomy

- Oophorectomy can be considered in premenopausal patients.
- It can be done with surgical, radiation, or chemical methods.

Recurrent Breast Cancer
Local Recurrence

1. After mastectomy:
   - Eighty percent of local recurrences occur within 5 years.
   - The treatment of choice is surgical excision and RT.
   - Systemic therapy may be considered, although the survival advantage is not clear.
2. After lumpectomy:
   - Mastectomy is the treatment of choice for patients who have only isolated breast cancer recurrence.
   - The 5-year relapse-free survival is 60% to 75%, if treated only with mastectomy.

Breast Cancer in Pregnancy

- Breast cancer diagnosis may be delayed in pregnant women.
- Breast cancer during pregnancy was thought to be more aggressive, but the overall poor outcome is likely related to advanced stage at the time of diagnosis.
- Breast biopsy is safe in all stages of pregnancy and should be done for any suggestive mass.

Treatment

- Lumpectomy and axillary dissection can be performed in the third trimester, and RT can be safely delayed until after delivery.
- Modified radical mastectomy is the treatment of choice in the first and second trimesters because radiation treatment is contraindicated during pregnancy.

Chemotherapy

- Chemotherapy should not be administered during the first trimester.
- No chemotherapeutic agent has been found to be completely safe during pregnancy.
- An anthracycline combined with cyclophosphamide (e.g., AC given every 3 weeks for four cycles) has been used in the adjuvant setting during the second or third trimesters.
- Chemotherapy should be scheduled to avoid neutropenia and thrombocytopenia at the time of delivery.
- Paclitaxel is teratogenic and should not be used during pregnancy.
- Tamoxifen is teratogenic and should not be used in pregnant women.
- Therapeutic abortion does not change the survival rate.

Male Breast Cancer

- Male breast cancer is uncommon.
- Risk factors are family history, *BRCA2* germ-line mutation, Klinefelter syndrome, and radiation.
- Presence of gynecomastia is not a risk factor for breast cancer.
- It is first seen as a mass beneath the nipple or ulceration.
- The mean age of occurrence is 60 to 70 years.
- Eighty percent of male breast cancer is hormone-receptor positive.

Treatment

- Modified radical mastectomy.
- Lumpectomy is rarely done because it does not offer any cosmetic benefit.
- Systemic treatment with chemotherapy and antiestrogen should follow the general guidelines for female patients.
- None of the adjuvant treatment modalities has been tested in a randomized clinical trial setting in men.

FOLLOW-UP FOR PATIENTS WITH OPERABLE BREAST CANCER

1. History and physical examination every 3 to 6 months for the first 3 years, every 6 to 12 months for the next 2 years, and then annually.
2. Monthly breast self-examination.
3. Annual mammogram of the contralateral and ipsilateral (remaining breast after lumpectomy) breast.
4. Annual Papanicolaou smear and pelvic examinations in women who are taking, or who have taken, tamoxifen.
5. Complete blood count, liver function tests, and alkaline phosphatase levels obtained with physical examination.
   - Serum tumor markers (CA 27, 29, and CA 15-3) are not recommended.
   - Bone scan and imaging of the chest, abdomen, pelvis, and brain are not recommended routinely, but they are done if symptoms or laboratory abnormalities are present.
6. Rectal examination, occult blood testing, and skin examination must be performed annually or every 2 years.
7. (From recommendations by American Society of Clinical Oncology, with permission.)

REFERENCES

1. Gross PE, Ingle JN, Martino S, et al. A randomized trial of letrozole in postmenopausal women after five years of tamoxifen therapy for early-stage breast cancer. *NEJM* 2003;349:1793–1802
2. Charles Coombes R, HallE , Gibson LJ, et al. A randomized trial of exemestane after two to three years of tamoxifen therapy in postmenopausal women with primary breast cancer. *NEJM* 2004;350:1081–1092.
3. Hortobagyi GR. Treatment of breast cancer. *N Engl J Med* 1998;339:974–984.

SUGGESTED READINGS

Baum M, Bianco AR, Buzdar A, et al. Anastrozole alone or in combination with tamoxifen versus tamoxifen alone for adjuvant treatment of postmenopausal women with early-stage breast cancer. *Cancer* 2003;98:1802–1810.
Bear HD, Anderson S, Brown A, et al. The effect on tumor response of adding sequential preoperative docetaxel to preoperative doxorubicin and cyclophosphamide: preliminary results from National Surgical Adjuvant Breast and Bowel Project protocol B-27. *J Clin Oncol* 2003;21:4165–4174.
Coleman RE. Efficacy of zoledronic acid and pamidronate in breast cancer patients: a comparative analysis of randomized phase III trials. *Am J Clin Oncol* 2002;25:S25–S31.
Fisher B, Constatino JP, Wickerham DL, et al. Tamoxifen for prevention of breast cancer; report of NSABP P-1 study. *J Natl Cancer Inst* 1998;90:1371–1388.
Fisher B, Dignam J, Wolmark N, et al. Tamoxifen in the treatment of intraductal breast cancer: NSABP B-24 randomized controlled trial. *Lancet* 1999;353:1993–2000.
Goldhirsch A, Wood WC, Gelber RD, et al. Meeting highlights : International expert consensus on the primary therapy of early breast cancer. *J Natl Cancer Inst* 1998;90:1601–1608.
Gradishar WJ, Jordan VC. Hormonal therapy for breast cancer. *Hematol Oncol Clin North Am* 1999; 13:435–455.
Hartmann LC, Schaid DJ, Woods JE, et al. Efficacy of bilateral prophylactic mastectomy in women with a family history of breast cancer. *N Engl J Med* 1999;340:77–84.
Hortobagyi GN. Treatment of breast cancer. *N Engl J Med* 1998;339:974–984.
Jemal A, Murray T, Samuels A, et al. Cancer Statistics, 2004. *CA Cancer J Clin* 2004;53:5–26.
Struewing JP, Hartge P, Wacholder S, et al. The risk of cancer associated with specific mutations of BRCA1 and BRCA2 among Ashkenazi Jews. *N Engl J Med* 1997;336:1401–1408.

SECTION 5

Genitourinary

13

Renal Cell Cancer

Hung T. Khong*, Christopher Klebanoff†, and Susan Bates‡

*USA Cancer Research Institute, University of South Alabama, Mobile, Alabama;
†Emory School of Medicine, Atlanta, Georgia; ‡Cancer Therapeutics Branch, National
Cancer Institute, National Institutes of Health, Bethesda, Maryland.

EPIDEMIOLOGY

- In the year 2003, there was an estimated 3% of adult malignancies, with 31,900 new cases and 11,900 deaths from renal cancer.
- The male-to-female ratio for renal cancer is 2:1.
- In the United States, the incidence rates for renal cell carcinoma (RCC) are higher among blacks than among whites (Table 13.1).
- Age at diagnosis is usually greater than 40 years, with the median age in the mid-60s.
- Cancer of the renal tubular epithelium accounts for 90% of all malignancies arising in the kidney. Most of the remaining cases are transitional cell carcinoma of the renal pelvis.
- Surveillance, Epidemiology, and End Results (SEER) data indicate that the incidence and mortality rates for RCC have increased steadily in all race and sex groups from 1975 through 1995 (Figs. 13.1 and 13.2; Table 13.1).

ETIOLOGY AND RISK FACTORS

- Tobacco use contributes to one third of all cases of RCC in the United States—current smokers exhibit 40% higher risk than nonsmokers; the risk increases per pack-year history.
- High consumption of fried or sautéed meat is another risk factor.
- Obesity, particularly in women, contributes to the risk for developing RCC.
- Exposure to asbestos and petroleum products increases the chances of developing RCC.
- End-stage renal disease with development of acquired cystic disease of the kidney is a major risk factor; patients with cystic changes in the kidney who undergo dialysis exhibit a 30-times higher risk than the general population.

TABLE 13.1. *Age-adjusted incidence rates per 100,000 person-years*

Race/Sex	Incidence rate (%)	% increase/yr
White men	9.6	2.3
White women	4.4	3.1
Black men	11.1	3.9
Black women	4.9	4.3

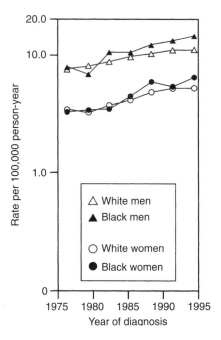

FIG. 13.1. Age-adjusted incidence rates for renal cell carcinoma.

- Hereditary disease:
  1. von Hippel-Lindau (VHL) disease is a familial syndrome with an autosomal dominant inheritance pattern, associated with retinal hemangiomas, central nervous system (CNS) hemangioblastomas, renal cysts and RCC, pheochromocytoma, and epididymal cysts. RCC is found to develop in 25% of VHL patients (data have been collected from literature reviews: total number of VHL patients is 706 and total number of RCC cases reported is 176). The mean age at onset is 44 years.
  2. Hereditary nonpapillary RCC develops because of translocation between the short arm of chromosome 3 (3p) and chromosome 6, 8, or 11, as is seen in some familial RCC kindreds.
  3. Hereditary papillary RCC (HPRCC) type I is associated with a mutation of the aMET protooncogene at 7q31.3. aMET encodes a transmembrane receptor tyrosine kinase.
  4. Hereditary leiomyomatosis and renal cell cancer (HLRCC) is an autosomal dominant disorder characterized by smooth-muscle tumors of the skin and uterus and/or renal cancer that was recently linked to mutations in the fumarate hydratase (FH) gene. The renal cancers may have either type II papillary or collecting duct morphology
  5. Renal chromophobe and oncocytoma is linked to the Birt–Hogg–Dubé syndrome, a dermatologic disorder characterized by cutaneous hair follicle tumors (fibrofolliculomas), pulmonary cysts, and renal tumors. The Birt–Hogg–Dubé syndrome gene has been found at 17p11.2 and is associated with chromophobe (34%), oncocytoma (5%), hybrid chromophobe–oncocytomas (50%), clear cell carcinoma (9%), and papillary renal cancer (2%).

PATHOLOGIC CLASSIFICATION

For pathologic classification, see Table 13.2.

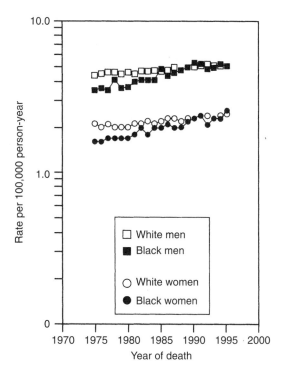

FIG. 13.2. Age-adjusted mortality rates for renal cell carcinoma.

TABLE 13.2. *Pathologic classification of renal cell carcinoma*

Type of carcinoma	Frequency (%)	Genetic changes	5-yr survival (%)
Clear cell	70–80	3p (81%–98%), von Hippel-Lindau (VHL) gene mutation (57%)[a]	55–60
Papillary	10–15	Trisomies (3q, 7, 12, 16, 17, and 20), Y, and c-met gene mutation	80–90
Chromophobe	5	Monosomy of multiple chromosomes (1, 2, 6, 10, 13, 17, and 21) and hypodiploidy	90
Collecting duct	<1	18 Y	<5
Unclassified	4–5		

Sarcomatoid variant is not a histologic type of renal cancer but a high-grade change that has been found to arise in all types.

[a]VHL gene, a tumor-suppressor gene, is located on chromosome 3p, which is deleted in 81%–98% of sporadic clear cell RCC. Therefore, 3p implies loss of one allele of the VHL gene. The remaining allele is mutated in 57% of cases.

CLINICAL PRESENTATION

The classic triad of hematuria, abdominal pain, and abdominal mass occurs in only 10% of patients (Tables 13.3 to 13.7).

DIAGNOSIS

For diagnosis of RCC in patients, see Table 13.8.

STAGING AND PROGNOSIS

Two commonly used staging systems for RCC are the modified Robson system and the tumor–node–metastases (TNM) system proposed by the American Joint Committee for Cancer

TABLE 13.3. *American Joint Committee for Cancer stage (1987 version: T1, ≤2.5 cm; T2, >2.5 cm) at diagnosis*

Stage	Frequency (%)
I	9.3
II	39.5
III	16
IV	24.6
Unknown	10.6

There is a shift from stage II to stage I under the 1997 version of the AJCC stage, which defines T1 as ≤7 cm and T2 as >7 cm. From one recent study, stage I is reported to be 45%, and stage II 13%, as per the 1997 version.

TABLE 13.4. *Common presenting symptoms or laboratory abnormality*

Symptom/lab finding	% of patients
Hematuria	56–59
Pain	38–41
Abdominal mass	36–45
Weight loss	28
Anemia	21
Fever	11
Nonmetastatic hepatic dysfunction (Stauffer syndrome)	7
Polycythemia	<5
Hypercalcemia	<5 (up to 25% in metastatic disease)
Acute varicocele	2

TABLE 13.5. *Common sites of metastatic involvement*

Site	%
Lung	75
Lymph node/soft tissue	36
Bone	20
Liver	18
Skin	8
CNS	8

CNS, central nervous system.

TABLE 13.6. *Adverse prognostic factors in patients with metastatic renal cell carcinoma*

Karnofsky performance status >80%
LDH <1.5 × upper limit of normal
Hemoglobin greater than lower limit of normal
Corrected serum calcium <10 mg/dL
Absence of prior nephrectomy

LDH, lactate dehydrogenase.

TABLE 13.7. *Risk groups based on the prognostic factors in Table 13.6*

Risk group	Number of risk factors listed in Table 13.6	Median survival time (mo)	Survival rate (%)		
			1-yr	2-yr	3-yr
Favorable	0	20	71	45	31
Intermediate	1 or 2	10	42	17	7
Poor	3 or more	4	12	3	0

(AJCC) (Table 13.9). The TNM system is preferred because it more accurately describes the extent of tumor involvement.

Prognosis: 5-year survival rates in patients with RCC based on gender and race is given in Table 13.10 (see Fig. 13.3).

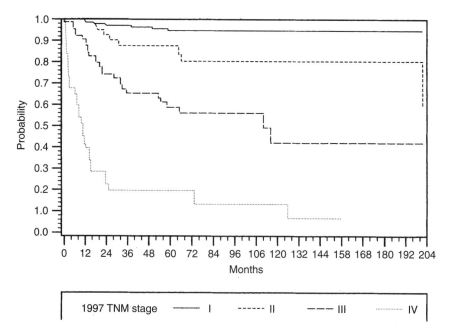

FIG. 13.3. Survival rates in renal cell carcinoma (RCC) given by American Joint Committee for Cancer/Union Internationale Contre le Cancer (AJCC/UICC) stage (1997 version) at diagnosis.

TABLE 13.8. *Initial evaluation*

H & P
CBC/Chemistry profiles (including PT/PTT)
Urinalysis
CT scan of the abdomen and pelvis with contrast
CXR
CT scan of the chest if
  1. Abnormal CXR or
  2. Large primary tumor or
  3. IVC involvement
Bone scan not done routinely unless
  1. bone pain is present or
  2. when serum alkaline phosphatase level is elevated

H&P, history and physical; CBC, complete blood count; PT/PTT, prothrombin time/partial thromboplastin time; CT, computerized tomography; CXR, chest x-ray; IVC, inferior vena cava; RCC, renal cell carcinoma.

A recent study found pelvic CT scan to have a negligible yield in the staging of 119 patients with RCC (no malignancy found).

TREATMENT

Surgery

- Nephrectomy is the only curative treatment for localized RCC.
- Radical nephrectomy is defined as resection of the kidney, ipsilateral adrenal gland, regional lymph nodes, and perirenal fat.
- Lymph node dissection is not therapeutic but allows more accurate staging.
- Ipsilateral adrenalectomy may be reserved for patients with large upper-pole disease and/or with tumor involvement of the adrenal gland, as suggested by computerized tomography (CT).
- Partial nephrectomy may be performed in patients for whom standard nephrectomy would significantly impair renal function. Recent studies have shown that in patients with localized tumors 4 cm or less in greatest dimension (including those patients with unilateral disease and a normal contralateral kidney), nephron-sparing surgery offers long-term disease survival comparable to that obtained after radical nephrectomy.
- In selected stage IV patients who present (or relapse) with a solitary metastasis, nephrectomy and resection of the metastasis may be the primary treatment of choice.
- Adjuvant therapies (radiation or systemic therapy) have not been shown to prevent or decrease relapse rates.
- Nephrectomy should be considered before systemic therapy in select patients with metastatic RCC. Studies have shown improved survival in patients who have undergone nephrectomy followed by immunotherapy for metastatic disease.

Systemic Treatment

Hormone Therapy and Chemotherapy

- Hormone therapy and chemotherapy appear to have little effect on the treatment of metastatic RCC.
- A review of 155 trials that studied 80 single chemotherapeutic agents showed a median overall response rate of 4%. The overall response rates for vinblastine and 5-fluorouracil (5-FU) and for vinblastine and 5-fluorodeoxyuridine (FUDR) were 6% to 9% and 5% to 8%, respectively. A recent trial combining gemcitabine with infusional 5-FU reported a 17% response rate. However, follow-up trials adding to that regimen yielded lower response rates.

TABLE 13.9. *TNM staging of renal cell carcinoma*

Primary tumor (T)

TX   Primary tumor cannot be assessed
T0   No evidence of primary tumor
T1   Tumor 7 cm or less in greatest dimension, limited to the kidney
T1a Tumor 4 cm or less in greatest dimension, limited to the kidney
T1b Tumor more than 4 cm but not more than 7 cm in greatest dimension, limited to the kidney
T2   Tumor more than 7 cm in greatest dimension, limited to the kidney
T3   Tumor extends into major veins or invades adrenal gland or perinephritic tissues but not beyond Gerota's fascia
T3a Tumor directly invades adrenal gland or perirenal and/or renal sinus fat but not beyond Gerota's fascia
T3b Tumor grossly extends into renal vein or its segmental (muscle-containing) branches, or vena cava below the diaphragm
T3c Tumor grossly extends into vena cava above diaphragm or invades the wall of the vena cava
T4   Tumor invades beyond Gerota's fascia

Regional lymph nodes (N)[a]

NX   Regional lymph nodes cannot be assessed
N0   No regional lymph node metastasis
N1   Metastasis in a single regional lymph node
N2   Metastasis in more than one regional lymph node

Distant metastasis (M)

MX   Distant metastasis cannot be assessed
M0   No distant metastasis
M1   Distant metastasis

Stage grouping

Stage	T	N	M
Stage I	T1	N0	M0
Stage II	T2	N0	M0
Stage III	T1	N1	M0
	T2	N1	M0
	T3	N0	M0
	T3	N1	M0
	T3a	N0	M0
	T3a	N1	M0
	T3b	N0	M0
	T3b	N1	M0
	T3c	N0	M0
	T3c	N1	M0
Stage IV	T4	N0	M0
	T4	N1	M0
	Any T	N2	M0
	Any T	Any N	M1

[a]Laterality does not affect the N classification.
Note: If a lymph node dissection is performed, then pathological evaluation would ordinarily include at least eight nodes.
Used with the permission of the American Joint Committee on Cancer (AJCC), Chicago, Illinois. The original source for this material is the *AJCC Cancer Staging Manual, Sixth Edition* (2002) published by Springer-Verlag New York, www.springer-ny.com.

TABLE 13.10. *Five-year survival rates (%) in renal cell carcinoma based on sex and race*[a]

Stage	White men (%)	White women (%)	Black men (%)	Black women (%)
Localized	89	86	75	84
Regional	62	59	52	44
Distant	9	7	7	8
Unstaged	31	21	21	35

[a]SEER, 1975–1995; Time period from 1986 to 1995.

- Patients should be encouraged to enroll in clinical trials.
  - A randomized placebo-controlled clinical trial testing the vascular endothelial growth factor (VEGF) antibody, bevacizumab (Avastin), demonstrated an improved time to progression in patients receiving the highest dose, that is, 10 mg per kg ($P<0.001$).
  - New therapeutic agents reported at the 2004 American Society of Clinical Oncology (ASCO) meeting indicated significant response rates in patients with metastatic disease. These agents include SU11248 and BAY 43-9006; both agents are tyrosine kinase inhibitors thought to inhibit the VEGF receptor. It has been reported in abstracts that 24% of patients treated with SU11428 have shown partial response.

Interleukin-2

- High-dose interleukin-2 (IL-2) is the only drug approved by the U.S. Food and Drug Administration (FDA) for the treatment of metastatic RCC (Table 13.11).
- Long-acting therapeutic response was seen in a small number of patients treated with high-dose IL-2. (8% of patients showed partial responses, with a median response duration of 54 months for all responses, and 7% of patients exhibited complete responses; median duration for all complete responses has not been reached.) These results have been confirmed in other clinical studies.
  - High dose of IL-2: 600,000 to 720,000 U per kg i.v. infused over 15 minutes once every 8 hours until toxicity or up to 14 doses for 5 days. The cycle is repeated once after a 7- to 10-day rest, with one or two additional courses repeated every 6 to 12 weeks if there is evidence of tumor stabilization or regression.
  - Low dose (i.v.): 72,000 U per kg i.v. bolus every 8 hours to a maximum of 15 doses every 7 to 10 days for two cycles (one course), with an additional course if there is evidence of tumor stabilization or regression. One or two additional courses may be given if further regression is observed.
- Low dose (s.c.): First 5-day cycle—18 million units per day s.c., for 5 days (week 1). Subsequent 5-day cycles—9 million units per day s.c., for 2 days, and then 18 million units per day s.c., 3 days per week (weeks 2 to 6).

Interferon-α

- Interferon-α (IFN-α) produces response rates of approximately 12% to 15%; 2% to 5% complete responses are generally seen in patients with pulmonary metastases.
- Usual regimens: 5 to 10 MU per m^2 s.c., three to five times a week or daily.
- A recent randomized study demonstrated a modest survival benefit for nephrectomy in patients with metastatic kidney cancer who were being treated with interferon; the survival in patients treated with interferon and nephrectomy was 11.1 months compared to 8.1 months for patients treated with interferon alone ($p = 0.05$). A survival advantage was also observed in a similar randomized trial from the European Organization for Research and Treatment of Cancer (EORTC) Genitourinary Group.

TABLE 13.11. *Treatment regimens with recombinant interleukin-2 (rIL-2)*
and/or recombinant interferon-α (rIFN-α)

Regimen	Treatment	Comment	Reference
High-dose rIL-2	600,000–720,000 U/kg i.v. over 15 min q8h until toxicity or 14 doses for 5 d	Repeat once after a 7- to 10-day rest	Fyfe G, Fisher RI, Rosenberg SA, et al., 1995
Low-dose rIL-2 (i.v.)	72,000 U/kg i.v. bolus q8h to a maximum of 15 doses q7–10d for 2 cycles (1 course)	One more course if tumor stabilization or regression occurs; one or two more courses if there is further tumor regression	Yang JC, Topalian SL, Parkinson D, et al., 2003
Low-dose rIL-2 (s.c.)	18 MU/d s.c. for 5 d, then 9 MU/d s.c. for 2 d, then 18 MU/d s.c. 3 d a wk, for 6 wk		Sleijfer DTh, Janssen RAJ, Buter J, et al., 1992
rIFN-α 2	5 to 10 MIU/m^2 s.c., 3 to 5 times a wk, or daily		Horoszewicz JS and Murphy GP, 1989
rIL-2 +	20 MU/m^2 s.c., d 3–5, wk1 and 4	Repeat cycle every 8 wk	Atzopodiem J, Kirchner H, Hannien EL, et al., 1993
	5 MU/m^2 s.c., d 1, 3, 5, wk 2, 3, 5, and 6		
rIFN-α 2	6 MU/m^2 s.c., d 1, wk 1 and 4		
	6 MU/m^2 s.c., d 1, 3, and 5, wk 2, 3, 5, and 6		

Combination of Interleukin-2 and Interferon-α

- Recombinant interleukin-2 (rIL-2): 20 million units per m^2 s.c., days 3 to 5, weeks 1 and 4; 5 million units per m^2 s.c., days 1, 3, and 5, weeks 2, 3, 5, and 6.
- Recombinant interferon-α 2 (rIFN-α 2): 6 million units per m^2 s.c., day 1, weeks 1 and 4; 6 million units per m^2 s.c., days 1, 3, and 5, weeks 2, 3, 5, and 6. Cycle is repeated every 8 weeks.

Notably, several trials reported response rates and overall survival of combination regimens (IL-2 and IFN-α, with or without 5-FU) similar to that of high-dose IL-2 alone.

Other Biologic Therapy

In a recent randomized, phase II trial, the anti-VEGF antibody, bevacizumab, was shown to significantly prolong the time to progression of disease in metastatic–renal cancer patients. There was no statistical difference in overall survival between the treatment and placebo groups in the last analysis.

SUGGESTED READINGS

Atzopodiem J, Kirchner H, Hannien EL, et al. European studies of interleukin-2 in metastatic renal cell carcinoma. *Semin Oncol* 1993;20:23.

Chow WH, Devesa SS, Warren JL, et al. Rising incidence of renal cell cancer in the United States *JAMA* 1999;281:1628–1631.

Flanigan RC, Salmon SE, Blumenstein BA, et al. Nephrectomy followed by interferon alfa-2b compared with interferon alfa-2b alone for metastatic renal-cell cancer. *N Engl J Med* 2001;345:1655–1659.

Fyfe G, Fisher RI, Rosenberg SA, et al. Results of treatment of 255 patients with metastatic renal cell carcinoma who received high-dose recombinant interleukin-2 therapy. *J Clin Oncol* 1995;13:688–696.

Horoszewicz JS, Murphy GP. An assessment of the current use of human interferons in therapy of urological cancers. *J Urol* 1989;142:1173–1180.

Javidan J, Stricker HJ, Tamboli P, et al. Prognostic significance of the 1997 TNM classification of renal cell carcinoma. *J Urol* 1999;162:1277–1281.

Minasian LM, Motzer RJ, Gluck L, et al. Interferon alfa-2a in advanced renal cell carcinoma: treatment results and survival in 159 patients with long-term follow-up. *J Clin Oncol* 1993;11:1368–1375.

Motzer RJ, Russo P. Systemic therapy for renal cell carcinoma. J Urol 2000;163:408–417.

Motzer RJ, Mazumdar M, Bacik J, et al. Survival and prognostic stratification of 670 patients with advanced renal cell carcinoma. *J Clin Oncol* 1999;17:2530–2540.

Motzer RJ, Mazumdar M, Bacik J, et al. Effect of cytokine therapy on survival for patients with advanced renal cell carcinoma. *J Clin Oncol* 2000;18:1928–1935.

NCI-PDQ Web-Page at http://www.nci.nih.gov/cancertopics/pdq/treatment/renalcell/Health Professional/. 2003.

Negrier S, Escudier B, Lasset C, et al. Recombinant human interleukin-2, recombinant human interferon alfa-2a, or both in metastatic renal-cell carcinoma. *N Engl J Med* 1998;338:1273–1278.

Parkinson DR, Sznol M. High-dose interleukin-2 in the therapy of metastatic renal cell carcinoma. *Semin Oncol* 2003;22:61–66.

Sleijfer DT, Janssen RAJ, Buter J, et al. Phase II study of subcutaneous interleukin-2 in unselected patients with advanced renal cell cancer on an outpatient basis. *J Clin Oncol* 1992;10:1119–1123.

Yang JC, Haworth L, Sherry RM, et al. A randomized trial of bevacizumab, an anti-vascular endothelial growth factor antibody, for metastatic renal cancer. *N Engl J Med* 2003;349:427–434.

Yang JC, Topalian SL, Parkinson D, et al. Randomized study of high-dose and low-dose interleukin-2 in patients with metastatic renal cancer. *J Clin Oncol* 2003;21:3127–3132.

14

Prostate Cancer

James L. Gulley* and William L. Dahut†

*Laboratory of Tumor Immunology and Biology, Center for Cancer Research, National Cancer Institute, National Institutes of Health, Bethesda, Maryland; †Medical Oncology Clinical Research Unit, Center for Cancer Research, National Cancer Institute, National Institutes of Health, Bethesda, Maryland

EPIDEMIOLOGY

Prostate cancer (CaP) is the most common noncutaneous malignancy occurring in American men and the second most frequent cause of cancer-related mortality in American men. The risk for developing CaP increases progressively with age, and although the median age at diagnosis is 72 years, there is no "peak" age. Black men have a lower median age at diagnosis than do white men. Incidence and mortality rates are higher in blacks than in whites.

Incidence and mortality rates were found to increase after the U.S. Food and Drug Administration (FDA) approved the use of prostate-specific antigen (PSA) screening in 1986. The age-adjusted mortality rates have now dropped below the rate in 1986, possibly because of decline in distant disease incidence (1).

Frequency of clinically aggressive disease varies geographically, although the frequency of occult tumors does not. This suggests a role of environmental factors in the etiology of CaP. Studies of Japanese immigrants to the United States show that the incidence of CaP increases after migration.

RISK FACTORS FOR PROSTATE CANCER

- Age (incidence increases with age)
- Family history (risk increases twofold with a first-degree relative)
- Race (in the United States, the incidence is highest among blacks followed by whites, and finally by Asians)
- Geographic location (lowest in Asia, high in Scandinavia and United States)
- Dietary fat (putative but not definitive).

SCREENING

Screening for CaP is performed with PSA and/or digital rectal examination (DRE). There is much debate about screening asymptomatic men for CaP. This debate centers on whether biologically and clinically significant cancers are actually being detected at an early enough stage to reduce mortality, or conversely, whether cancers detected by screening would never have caused clinically significant disease if these had not been detected or treated. Autopsy series have shown the rate of occult CaP in men in their 80s to be approximately 75%, and more men die with, rather than from, CaP. A recent study showed a decrease in CaP-specific mortality in men undergoing radical prostatectomy (RP) compared to those who underwent watchful waiting, but there was no difference in overall survival (OS). Thus, because local treatment is associated with significant morbidity, and no randomized controlled trial has convincingly shown a decrease in mortality from screening or early treatment, screening remains controversial.

Despite the controversy, there is widespread use of PSA for CaP screening in the United States. Advocates of screening recommend that annual screening should commence at the age of 50 for average-risk men and at the age of 40 for African American men and for men with a family history of CaP.

CHEMOPREVENTION

Chemoprevention trials examine the treatment of asymptomatic patients with therapeutic agents that may be capable of preventing cancer. The Prostate Cancer Prevention trial was a study that compared finasteride, a 5-α reductase inhibitor, to a placebo in the prevention of CaP in men older than 50 years who had a normal DRE and a PSA of 3.0 ng per mL or less (2). This trial had more than 9,000 men included in the final analysis. A surprisingly large number of patients in both arms developed CaP. There was a significant decrease in the incidence of CaP in the experimental arm, with 24.8% of placebo-treated men and 18.4% of finasteride-treated men being diagnosed with CaP ($p < 0.001$). There were several other differences seen between the two arms. Sexual dysfunction was more common in the finasteride-treated men, whereas urinary symptoms were more common in those receiving placebo. The finasteride group showed an increase in Gleason score (GS) of 7 to 10 tumors, with 6.4% of men being affected in comparison to 5.1% of men in the placebo group having this pathology. One possible explanation is that this is the effect of androgen-deprivation therapy (ADT) on the appearance of the pathologic specimen. Longer follow-up is needed to determine the clinical course of these patients.

A large-scale 2 × 2 factorial study compared dietary supplementation with vitamin E and/or β-carotene and/or placebo in male Finnish smokers (3). Although the Finnish trial showed an increase in lung cancer in the β-carotene arm, a secondary analysis showed that there were fewer CaPs and CaP-related deaths in those men who received vitamin E. Another separate, multi-institutional trial tested supplementation with selenium versus placebo in preventing skin cancer (4). In a secondary analysis, men who received selenium experienced only 37% as many CaPs as did men who received placebo, a statistically significant difference. A retrospective study of selenium levels in men with and without CaP also showed a protective effect in men who had the highest amount of selenium.

These interesting retrospective data have led to the development of a prospective placebo-controlled, 2 × 2 factorial study that is examining the effect of selenium and vitamin E in the prevention of CaP—the Selenium and Vitamin E Cancer Prevention Trial (SELECT) (5).

PATHOLOGY

Ninety-five percent of CaPs are adenocarcinomas; other histologies (sarcoma, lymphoma, small cell carcinoma, and transitional carcinoma) are rarely found. Although visceral metastases or osteolytic bone metastases are found in a few patients with metastatic adenocarcinoma of the prostate, a careful examination of pathology should be performed to determine whether a nonadenocarcinoma variant is present in this setting because treatment regimens differ for these variants.

Adenocarcinoma arises in the peripheral zone of the prostate in approximately 70% of cases.

The GS (see Table 14.1) is obtained by examining the histologic architecture of the biopsy. Primary and secondary Gleason grades are given to the biopsy of prostate gland tissue obtained at the time of surgery. The primary grade denotes the dominant histologic pattern, and the secondary grade is the pattern that represents the bulk of the nondominant pattern or a focal high-grade area. Both primary and secondary grades range from 1 (well differentiated) to 5 (poorly

TABLE 14.1. *Risk of metastatic disease*

Gleason score	Risk of developing metastatic disease (%)
2–4	20
5–7	40
8–10	75

differentiated). The two grades are added together, resulting in the GS (range 2 to 10). Total GS of 2 to 4, 5 to 6, 7, and 8 to 10 represent well-differentiated, moderately differentiated, moderately poorly differentiated, and poorly differentiated tumors, respectively. However, there is a growing belief that the highest score is most predictive of clinical outcome. There is often a change in GS at the time of RP, with 20% of cases being upgraded to a higher score.

CLINICAL MANIFESTATIONS AND DIAGNOSIS

Signs and Symptoms

Men with local or regional disease can be asymptomatic or can have lower–urinary tract symptoms similar to that of benign prostatic hypertrophy (BPH). Occasionally, men with regional disease have hematuria. The symptoms of the presence of metastatic disease include bone pain or weight loss, and, rarely, spinal cord compression. With the advent of widespread screening with PSA, most men are asymptomatic at the time of diagnosis.

Workup and Staging

CaP is usually detected by an abnormal PSA and/or DRE, followed by a transrectal ultrasound with core biopsy (generally 8 to 12 cores). Historically, a PSA level of >4 ng per mL was used as a threshold for biopsy, but recent data suggest that cancers can be seen with lower PSA levels. A negative biopsy should prompt reassessment in 6 months with PSA or DRE and repeat biopsy as needed.

Age enters into the decision-making process; men with low-volume tumors, with a GS of 5, or older men with major comorbid illnesses and limited life expectancy are less likely to benefit from definitive treatment than are younger and otherwise healthy men. In men with a life expectancy of less than 5 years with asymptomatic CaP, one option is deferral of further workup and treatment until presentation of symptoms; however, many patients prefer a more aggressive course.

If local treatment is planned, a bone scan is indicated for bone pain, T3 or T4, GS >7, or PSA >10 ng per mL. There is no clinical evidence that obtaining a "baseline" bone scan in other patients improves survival.

Computerized tomography (CT) scan or magnetic resonance imaging (MRI) is obtained for T3 and T4 lesions to detect the presence of enlarged lymph nodes in men for whom surgery is considered. If lymph nodes appear enlarged, a fine-needle aspiration (FNA) can be performed, potentially eliminating the need for surgery. CT scans are used for treatment planning for radiation therapy (RT). Baseline laboratory tests include complete blood count (CBC), creatinine level, PSA (if not yet done), and alkaline phosphatase level, and preoperative studies are performed if surgery is being considered (see Tables 14.2 and 14.3).

Prognostic Factors at the Time of Diagnosis

- Stage (Table 14.2 and 14.3)
- Grade (GS)

TABLE 14.2. *Staging of prostate cancer: tumor–node–metastasis (TNM) system*

T1 Tumor not palpable or visible by imaging
  T1a Tumor incidental finding in ≤5% of tissue resected (TURP)
  T1b Tumor incidental finding in >5% of tissue resected (TURP)
  T1c Tumor identified by needle biopsy alone (after PSA is found to be elevated)
T2 Tumor confined to the prostate
  T2a Tumor involves half of a lobe or less
  T2b Tumor involves more than half of a lobe, but not both lobes
  T2c Tumor involves both lobes
T3 Tumor extends through the prostatic capsule
  T3a Extracapsular extension (unilateral or bilateral)
  T3b Tumor invades the seminal vesicle(s)
T4 Tumor is fixed or invades adjacent structures other than seminal vesicles: bladder neck,
    external sphincter, rectum, levator muscles, and/or pelvic wall
N0 No regional lymph node metastasis
N1 Metastases in regional lymph node(s)
M0 No distant metastases
M1 Distant metastases (M1a, nonregional LN; M1b, bone(s); M1c, other).

Stage grouping

I	T1a	N0	M0	Any GS
II	T1a	N0	M0	GS 2, 3, or 4
	T1b,c	N0	M0	Any GS
	T1/2	N0	M0	Any GS
III	T3	N0	M0	Any GS
IV	T4	N0	M0	Any GS
	Any T	N1	M0	Any GS
	Any T	Any N	M1	Any GS

TURP, transurethral resection of the prostate; PSA, prostate-specific antigen.

- PSA level
- DNA ploidy in stage C or D1 patients (diploid is better)
- Age
- Serum alkaline phosphatase level.

TREATMENT

Surgery

Radical Prostatectomy

RP is performed by the perineal or retropubic approach. Pelvic lymph node dissection may be performed at the time of RP, although it may not be necessary in patients with T1c disease whose PSA is <10 ng per mL and GS is <7; the results will alter therapeutic decision less than 1% of the time in these patients. For patients at high risk of developing positive lymph nodes, pelvic laparoscopic lymph node dissection can be performed initially.

The formula for predicting percentage chance of positive pelvic lymph nodes is

$$\text{\% Positive pelvic LN} = 2/3 \times \text{PSA} + (\text{GS} - 6) \times 10 \tag{14.1}$$

Nerve-sparing Radical Prostatectomy

This is an appropriate procedure for men with small-volume disease in an attempt to conserve potency. However, after nerve-sparing RP, the rates of impotency that have been reported in the community are much higher than the rates in the original reports from certain tertiary

TABLE 14.3. *Modified Jewett system*

A: Clinically undetectable tumor confined to the prostate gland/incidental at prostate surgery
   A1: Well differentiated, focal involvement
   A2: Moderately or poorly differentiated, involves multiple foci of the gland
B: Tumor confined to the prostate gland
   B0: Nonpalpable, PSA detected
   B1: Single nodule in one lobe of the prostate
   B2: More extensive involvement of one lobe or both lobes
C: Tumor localized to the periprostatic area but extending through the prostatic capsule or involving the seminal vesicles
   C1: Clinical extracapsular extension
   C2: Extracapsular tumor producing bladder outlet or ureteral obstruction
D: Metastatic disease
   D0: Clinically localized disease with persistently elevated acid phosphatase
   D1: Regional lymph nodes only
   D2: Distant lymph nodes, metastases to bone or visceral organs
   D3: D2 patients who relapse after adequate endocrine therapy

PSA, prostate-specific antigen.

referral centers. Talcott et al. (6) reported data on 94 patients who underwent RP and who were observed before surgery and for up to 12 months after surgery. Nearly 80% of the men who had bilateral nerve-sparing surgery reported erections inadequate for sexual intercourse at 12 months after surgery, compared with 33% of such instances before surgery. Unilateral nerve-sparing surgery provided no benefit in potency. These numbers are significantly lower than those published previously in several retrospective studies. Studies have shown that diagnosis at a younger age and the absence of capsular penetration or seminal vesicle invasion correlate with a greater likelihood of conservation of potency after surgery.

Incontinence rates vary among single-institution experiences, and various definitions of incontinence make interpretation of studies difficult. In one prospective study evaluating urinary control at 3, 12, and 24 months after RP, it was reported that 58%, 35%, and 42% of patients, respectively, wore pads in their underwear, and 24%, 11%, and 15% of patients, respectively, reported "a lot" of urine leakage or escalating symptoms.

The Prostate Cancer Outcomes Study reported on the quality of life of patients following either surgery or RT. As one might expect, for patients with normal baseline function, surgery was associated with (a) an inferior urinary outcome score (approximately a 30-point decrease on a 100-point scale) compared with RT (less than 5-point decrease), (b) a better bowel score (less than 5-point decrease) compared with RT (about a 10-point decrease), and (c) slightly worse sexual function score (about a 40-point decrease) compared with RT (about a 30-point decrease), with all comparisons being statistically significant.

Neoadjuvant Therapy

The role of neoadjuvant hormonal therapy before RP is still under investigation. A recent randomized trial compared neoadjuvant treatment with 3 versus 8 months of leuprolide plus flutamide for clinically confined CaP (7). The proportion of men with negative margins and organ-confined disease was significantly higher in the group receiving 8 months of neoadjuvant hormonal therapy. Although there was a trend in the neoadjuvant group toward a delay in biochemical recurrence, it is too early in this study to determine survival. Thus, in general, neoadjuvant hormonal therapy prior to RP should be used only in the context of a clinical trial.

Extracapsular extension or positive margins in the surgical specimen portends a high incidence of disease recurrence, and such patients can be considered for clinical trials involving postoperative radiation, chemotherapy, or hormonal treatment. Radiation may delay disease recurrence, but it has yet to show a convincing impact on survival.

After surgery, a detectable PSA level indicates a relapse, either local or systemic, although PSA increase may be slow and not necessarily indicate immediate treatment. In a study of nearly 2,000 men whose PSA was measured every 3 months after surgery, the median time for the development of metastases after detection of an elevated PSA (>0.2 ng per mL) was 8 years (8). PSA doubling time and GS were predictive of time to metastases.

Surgical Complications

Complications include immediate morbidity or mortality (2%) from surgery, impotence (35% to 60%), urinary incontinence (10% to 30%, depending on the definition), urinary stricture, and fecal incontinence (approximately 5%, with the retropubic approach, to 18%, with the perineal approach).

Radiation Therapy

External Beam

The traditional four-field box arrangement is used, with approximately 70 Gy given over 7 to 8 weeks. Prophylactic radiation of pelvic lymph nodes along with neoadjuvant and concurrent ADT has been shown to increase progression-free survival in patients when compared with those who do not receive whole pelvis radiation or short-term adjuvant ADT [Radiation Therapy Oncology Group (RTOG) 9413].

Ten-year cause-specific survival rates with RT:

- T1, 79%
- T2, 66%
- T3, 55%
- T4, 22%.

Adjuvant Treatment with Androgen-deprivation Therapy

There are compelling data that combining ADT with RT in patients at high risk for recurrent disease improves OS (see Table 14.4). One large trial conducted by the RTOG 8531 randomized 945 patients having either T3 or T1–2, and N1 to RT (prostate and pelvis) with either adjuvant gonadotropin-releasing hormone agonist (GnRH-A) therapy for an indefinite period or GnRH-A therapy at the time of relapse (9,10). The recently presented 10-year OS favored the hormone-treated group (53% versus 38%, $p < 0.0043$) (11).

In addition, the European Organization for Research and Treatment of Cancer (EORTC) performed a trial in 412 patients with poorly differentiated (WHO grade 3) or T3–4 cancers (13). Patients were randomized to receive radiation with or without concurrent and adjuvant GnRH-A therapy for 3 years, with the first month of GnRH-A therapy given with

TABLE 14.4. *Risk categories for posttherapy prostate-specific antigen failure (12)*

	Low	Intermediate	High
Stage	T1c, T2a	T2b	T2c
PSA	<10	10–20	>20
Gleason score	≤6	7	≥8
Qualifier	And	Or	Or
5-Year risk of biochemical failure	<25%	25%–50%	>50%

From Beer TM, Hough KM, Garzotto M, et al. Weekly high-dose calcitriol and docetaxel in advanced prostate cancer. Semin Oncol 2001;28(4):49–55, with permission.

an antiandrogen. The 5-year OS was 78% in the hormonal therapy group versus 62% in the radiation-alone therapy group ($p = 0.0002$) (14).

A subsequent trial (RTOG 9202) studied the use of neoadjuvant and concurrent hormonal therapy (GnRH-A with antiandrogen) with or without adjuvant GnRH-A therapy for 2 years in 1,554 patients who had a T stage of at least T2b (15). This trial demonstrated an OS advantage at 5 years (81% versus 71%, $p = 0.044$) in the subset of patients who had GS 8 to 10 tumors.

Another smaller randomized trial that stratified patients by biopsy-proven lymph node metastasis showed similar results, with improvement in median OS in the combined treatment arm seen only in the lymph node–positive tumor patients, further suggesting that patients who are at high risk for systemic disease benefit from ADT (16). Taken together, these trials provide strong evidence that patients at high risk for recurrence who are receiving definitive RT should be treated with long-term hormonal therapy.

Investigations are being initiated to test the addition of adjuvant chemotherapy in this setting.

3-D Conformational or High-dose Radiation Therapy

With careful treatment planning using 3-D conformational techniques, higher doses of radiation (up to 80 Gy over 7 to 8 weeks) can be delivered to the prostate while sparing normal tissue. This approach appears promising in that it may offer higher dosages to the tumor and thus greater efficacy and less toxicity to the surrounding structures.

Brachytherapy

Interstitial brachytherapy with radioactive palladium or iodine (I 125) seeds has been used for patients with T1 or T2 tumors. Initially, this approach required retropubic implantation (which required laparotomy), but over the last 10 years, CT and/or transrectal ultrasound have been used to guide seed placement, and the procedure is performed on an outpatient basis. Better definition of tumor volume and radiation dosimetry have made this technique more accurate. Initial results have been very promising; however, a randomized trial comparing brachytherapy to surgery had to be closed because of poor accrual.

External Beam and Brachytherapy

The use of combined external beam and brachytherapy has come into increasing use (17,18). A 10-year review of experience with this combination showed a biochemical (i.e., normal PSA) relapse-free survival of 79% in T3 tumors, suggesting a strong role for the combination in these lesions (19). However, there are no randomized trials comparing this combination with external beam or brachytherapy alone, and thus, this treatment approach remains investigational at this point.

Complications of Radiation Therapy

- Acute (during treatment) complications: cystitis, proctitis, enteritis, and fatigue.
- Long-term complications: impotence, incontinence (3%), frequent bowel movements (10%, more than with RP), and urethral stricture [RT is delayed by 4 weeks after transurethral resection of the prostate (TURP)].

Cryosurgery

Cryosurgery involves destruction of CaP cells through probes that subject the prostate tissue to freezing followed by thawing. Some believe that cryosurgery is a good option for men with high-grade tumors (Gleason 8 to 10), high PSA levels (20 to 40 ng per mL), or stage C tumors, who potentially do not respond well to RT or surgery. Cryosurgery is also an option for local recurrence of CaP. This technique is still in early development, and long-term efficacy is not fully established. Side effects include incontinence, impotence, and injury to the bladder outlet and rectal tissues.

Observation

In several European countries, observation of patients with CaP, particularly of low stage or low or moderate grade, is commonplace. Particularly with elderly patients, survival equivalent to aggressive treatment has been reported.

Hormonal Therapy

ADT is used most commonly for metastatic CaP, although it has been used in the treatment of localized disease and in the neoadjuvant, and adjuvant, settings with RT. Androgen blockade is achieved through bilateral surgical castration or depot injections of GnRH-A (e.g., leuprolide, goserelin, and buserelin), which offer equivalent efficacy. Combined androgen blockade can be achieved by adding an oral antiandrogenic agent (e.g., nilutamide, flutamide, and bicalutamide); however, this is controversial, and if a benefit does exist, it is small.

Tumor flare is possible with the use of GnRH-A, which initially causes an increase in luteinizing hormone (LH) and follicle-stimulating hormone (FSH). Because the CaP cells are androgen sensitive, this increase in testosterone-inducing hormones can exacerbate symptoms of CaP and can elevate PSA. Tumor flare can be prevented by the use of oral antiandrogens, which compete with androgens at the androgen receptor site, at low dose for several weeks before beginning therapy. There is a reduced risk of tumor flare with a lower volume of disease. Abarelix is a GnRH antagonist that also may be used in patients who are at high risk for complications associated with tumor flare. Because of the risk of potentially life-threatening allergic reactions, its use is limited to those who are have advanced, symptomatic CaP and who do not have other treatment options.

The use of estrogen [e.g. diethylstilbestrol (DES)] has fallen into disfavor because of its side-effect profile. Therapeutic doses were shown to induce a high frequency of cardiovascular complications and mortality in a population predisposed to cardiovascular disease.

Intermittent androgen ablation (IAA) is a recent approach to treating patients with hormone-sensitive CaP. This involves treatment with hormonal therapy for 2 to 3 months beyond "best response," followed by a discontinuation of hormonal therapy and restarting hormones at some predetermined point (e.g., based on the PSA value). IAA has the potential advantage of improved quality of life during the time the patient is not receiving hormonal therapy. The effects of these manipulations on a hormonally sensitive tumor, however, are unknown. A large randomized trial by the Southwestern Oncology Group (SWOG) is under way to evaluate the effects of these manipulations.

The rationale for continued androgen blockade, antiandrogen withdrawal, and additional hormonal therapy (e.g., ketoconazole and aminoglutethimide) are discussed in subsequent text about second-line hormonal therapy.

Dosages and Side Effects of Hormonal Therapy

- **Bilateral orchiectomy:** Side effects include tumor flare (see subsequent text), impotence, loss of libido, gynecomastia, hot flashes, and osteoporosis.
- **GnRH agonists:**
  1. Goserelin acetate (Zoladex), 3.6 mg s.c. every month or 10.8 mg s.c. every 3 months. Side effects are the same as with orchiectomy.

2. Leuprolide acetate (Lupron), 7.5 mg s.c. every month or 22.5 mg i.m. every 3 months, or 30 mg s.c. every 4 months. Comparable efficacy with long-acting formulations. Side effects are the same as with orchiectomy.
- **GnRH antagonist:**
  1. Abarelix (Plenaxis), 100 mg i.m. on days 1, 15, 29, and every 4 weeks thereafter. In addition to orchiectomy-like side effect, patients are at risk for allergic reactions and must be observed for 30 minutes after injection.
- **Oral antiandrogens:**
  1. *Flutamide (Eulexin), 250 mg PO t.i.d.* Side effects include diarrhea, nausea, breast tenderness, hepatotoxicity [liver enzymes levels must be monitored], loss of libido, and impotence.
  2. *Bicalutamide (Casodex), 50 mg daily.* Side effects include nausea, breast tenderness, hepatotoxicity (transaminases must be monitored), hot flashes, loss of libido, and impotence.
  3. *Nilutamide (Nilandron), 150 mg PO daily.* Side effects include pulmonary fibrosis (rare), visual field changes (i.e., night blindness or abnormal adaptation to darkness), hepatotoxicity (liver enzymes must be monitored), impotence, loss of libido, hot flashes, nausea, and disulfiram-like reaction.

Hot flashes from hormonal therapy can be treated with clonidine (0.1 mg per day), low-dose estrogens, or possibly antidepressants. Painful gynecomastia can be treated with external beam radiation (electron beam) therapy to the breasts.

Testosterone-lowering therapy causes a decrease in estradiol levels because of decreased peripheral aromatization. Because estradiol is needed to maintain bone density, osteoporosis is increasingly being diagnosed in patients who are receiving ADT (20). This side effect is most likely to occur with long duration of ADT and in men who have had baseline osteoporosis before starting anti-androgen therapy. In general, all men receiving ADT should receive vitamin D (400 to 800 IU) and calcium (1,200 to 1,500 mg) daily. Bone densitometry can be performed to assess the presence and/or severity of osteoporosis. Treatment with bisphosphonates should be considered in patients with low bone mineral density.

COMPARISON OF PRIMARY TREATMENT MODALITIES

Comparison of treatment modalities with respect to primary outcomes [OS and disease-free survival (DFS)] is difficult because of variability in study design, patient selection, and technique of each therapy. No satisfactory randomized trials comparing RT with RP have been conducted.

In general, comparing single-modality studies is difficult because of disparities in treatment groups; men receiving RT tend to be older and have more comorbid illnesses. A major problem is that men receiving RT would have had only clinical staging of their cancer, whereas many patients who undergo surgery would have had pathologic staging that may upstage their tumor, including the discovery of positive pelvic lymph nodes (metastatic disease). One way to compare the two modalities is by PSA and PSA-free survival (also called *biochemical relapse-free survival*), provided that the patients have reproducible PSA values on repeated measurement before their definitive, primary therapy.

In the "PSA era," RT and RP appear to have equivalent PSA-free survival in appropriately matched patients at 5 years, but differ in type and frequency of side effects. Brachytherapy appears to be promising, although most studies have been conducted in patients with early stage, low-grade disease only, who are thought to be the most appropriate patients for this treatment modality. One comparison of 3-D conformational RT with ^{125}I implants in comparable patients concluded that both treatment modalities had equivalent efficacy, with higher urinary complications in the brachytherapy group.

Continuing research in quality of life may allow more informed choices among the various treatment modalities.

INITIAL TREATMENT, BY STAGE

Treatment decisions should be made with regard to the patient's age and comorbid conditions (i.e., life expectancy) and preferences, as well as tumor-related factors (i.e., stage, grade, and PSA). Enrollment in clinical trials is appropriate at each stage of disease.

T1a

Observation is often appropriate for elderly patients with low-grade disease. Definitive treatment should be considered for high PSA levels or GS if life expectancy is long with (a) RT (external beam, 3-D, and brachytherapy) and (b) RP.

Localized Disease (T1b through T2c)

Two factors, in particular, are important in deciding whether to treat localized disease. These are (a) the probability of having organ-confined disease: normograms based on PSA, clinical stage and GS, and (b) the patient's overall life expectancy. Observation can be considered in selected patients.

For a long life expectancy and a reasonable chance of having organ-defined disease, RT (including 3-D/high dose or brachytherapy) or RP remains the standard of care. Surgery is usually reserved for patients younger than 70 years. For a short life expectancy, RT (external beam, 3-D, and brachytherapy), hormonal therapy, or deferring treatment until the presentation of symptoms is recommended.

Patients in whom surgery would pose a great risk (e.g., cardiovascular or pulmonary disease) should have RT (i.e., external beam, 3-D, or brachytherapy). Otherwise, patient preference should play a major role in deciding primary treatment choice, after informed discussions have occurred. Certain patients should be considered for neoadjuvant hormonal therapy in combination with RT (see earlier discussion). The role of neoadjuvant hormonal therapy in surgical patients remains investigational (see earlier).

If pelvic lymph nodes are found to be grossly positive at the time of surgery, prostatectomy should not be performed. A recently updated randomized trial (21) compared men with T1 or T2 lesions and microscopically positive lymph nodes. Men were randomized to immediate hormonal therapy (orchiectomy or goserelin) versus observation (with hormonal therapy started at the time of metastases or symptomatic local recurrences). The difference in OS at 10 years was 72.4% versus 49% ($p = 0.025$), favoring the immediate ADT group.

If the tumor is found to have extracapsular extension on the pathologic specimen, consideration can be given to enrolling in clinical trials using adjuvant RT, hormonal therapy, or a combination of the two. As yet, these strategies have unproven survival benefits.

There are insufficient data to claim a survival benefit for surgery versus radiation as a primary treatment modality.

Stage III (T3 N0 M0)

RP can be considered for well-differentiated tumors. Other patients should probably receive RT (external beam) with or without neoadjuvant hormonal therapy. Hormonal therapy alone (surgical castration or GnRH-A) is another option. Some patients are treated with brachytherapy followed by external beam RT, but results are preliminary at this point.

T3b, T3c, T4 N0

These patients are unlikely to be cured by surgery. Viable treatment options include hormonal therapy, RT alone, or RT with hormonal therapy. With node-positive disease, patients are considered metastatic at the time of diagnosis, and local therapy should be used primarily for symptom management. Observation is a viable option for this group of patients, given the side effects of hormonal therapy and RT and their primarily palliative role.

N + or M1

There are no conclusive data that RT or RP improves survival in patients who are node positive. Hormonal therapy remains the standard of care. Surgical castration or medical orchiectomy with GnRH-A offer equivalent efficacy. There is no proven survival benefit of maximal androgen blockade (surgical castration and oral antiandrogen) compared with surgical castration alone. A randomized study of leuprolide with or without flutamide alone showed a slight survival advantage (22); however, a similar study design that used orchiectomy instead of GnRH-A showed equivalent survival (23). In the trial with orchiectomy and flutamide versus flutamide alone, quality of life was shown to be reduced in the group receiving antiandrogen therapy in addition to castration (24). The reason for the discrepancy between the results of two trials is not completely known. A meta-analysis found an OS advantage for the combined blockade at 5 years, but not 2 years; however, the magnitude of the difference is of questionable clinical significance (25).

Another area of controversy is the use of delayed or immediate hormonal therapy in patients who are initially metastatic or in those in whom tumors recur. The Medical Research Council trial (26) randomized patients with locally advanced or asymptomatic metastatic CaP to immediate versus deferred orchiectomy and GnRH-A. A significant difference in survival was noted in the patients, especially in M0 patients. However, this study has often been criticized. The comprehensive, evidence-based review conducted by the Agency for Health Care Policy and Research (AHCPR) concluded that there is no evidence favoring immediate compared with deferred androgen suppression; however, many practitioners tend toward early antiandrogen therapy, and newer evidence favoring early antiandrogen therapy is beginning to mount. Again, quality-of-life issues should play a role in decision analysis.

ADJUVANT TREATMENT AFTER RADICAL PROSTATECTOMY WITH POSITIVE MARGINS OR LOCAL RELAPSE

RT after RP for patients with margin-positive disease has been either used soon after surgery (adjuvant) or delayed until PSA progression occurs (salvage). Not surprisingly, biochemical failure appears to be less likely when adjuvant RT is used. Higher biochemical failure rates were seen in patients with seminal vesicle involvement (adjuvant) and with a GS of 4 or 5, or PSA >2.0 ng per mL (salvage). Long-term follow-up is not available with this approach. A combination of RT and hormonal therapy after local relapse is also being examined. In addition, some patients with a negative metastatic workup and local recurrence after RT can be considered for salvage surgery; the evidence for this is even less defined.

FOLLOW-UP OF DEFINITIVELY TREATED PATIENTS

Patients treated with curative intent should have their PSA level ascertained at least every 6 months for 5 years and then annually. Annual DRE is appropriate to detect recurrences.

After treatment with RP, any reproducible, detectable PSA indicates a relapse. PSA failure after RT is defined as three consecutive increases in PSA levels. Treatment for patients who relapse after radiation has not been standardized; participation in clinical trials should be encouraged. Hormonal treatment and salvage surgery (if a metastatic workup is negative and if patient is in good health) are options.

Surveillance and PSA measurement may be optional for patients with a short life expectancy who are treated with observation alone. Treatment should be guided by symptoms. For patients with a longer life expectancy, annual DRE and PSA along with workup and treatment of symptoms are appropriate if watchful waiting is selected as the primary treatment.

For patients with metastatic disease, intensity and type of follow-up are determined by the degree of clinical progression; for patients who respond well to hormonal therapy, follow-up at 3 months (with PSA) is reasonable. Bone scans are indicated depending on clinical symptoms but should not be ordered routinely. Patients with bony metastases are at risk for spinal cord compression, and MRI should be ordered when signs or symptoms are suggestive of this complication.

It is important to note that there is interlaboratory variation in PSA levels.

RESPONSE CRITERION IN PROSTATE CANCER

In this chapter, PSA response rates (PRRs) are shown as percentage of patients with a PSA decline greater than 50%, which is a generally agreed upon criterion (27). Ranges of PRRs are given when available. Confidence intervals are not shown around the PRR but are, in general, wide. Because of differences in patient selection, it is difficult to compare clinical trials by PRRs alone. Quality of life is an extremely important consideration in treating patients with CaP and may be a primary consideration in the choice of chemotherapeutic agents for metastatic androgen-insensitive prostate cancer (AIPC). An important caveat, however, is that some agents (particularly cytostatic agents) may upregulate or downregulate PSA expression independent of their effect on cancer growth.

HORMONAL THERAPY FOR METASTATIC DISEASE

Metastatic prostate cancer tends to present at the spine or axial skeleton. Visceral metastases are uncommon, and brain metastases are even rarer. CaP cells usually respond to hormonal manipulations that block the production of androgen with durable remissions and significant palliation. Duration of response ranges from 12 to 18 months, with 20% of patients having a complete biochemical response at 5 years. However, ultimately, androgen-independent CaP cells emerge and lead to progression of disease.

The use of maximal androgen blockade is not currently considered as standard of care in the initial treatment of metastatic disease. In patients who are being treated with GnRH-A or who undergo surgical castration, the addition of an antiandrogen agent may produce positive responses in up to 30% to 40% of instances.

Antiandrogen Withdrawal

Once GnRH-A therapy is started for patients with metastatic disease, it should be continued for life. It has been shown that metastatic CaP can reactivate if testosterone levels are allowed to increase or if exogenous testosterone is administered, and anecdotal evidence has shown a worsening of disease in patients who discontinued GnRH-A. Approximately 20% of patients being treated by maximal androgen blockade have PRR upon discontinuation of the oral antiandrogen [range, 15% to 33% relative risk (RR)], although these declines in PSA levels are relatively short lived (median duration, 3 to 5 months). Decreased cancer-related anemia and decreased pain were also reported. Antiandrogen withdrawal response occurs within 4 to 6 weeks, depending on the half-life of the agent.

Second-line Hormonal Therapy

Even after androgen withdrawal has failed, some patients will benefit from switching to antiandrogens or initiating treatment with aminoglutethimide, ketoconazole, or glucocorticoids. A minimum of 1 month is required to assess patients for a response. A few patients are likely to respond, and responses are usually not long in duration, but these agents offer much less toxicity than chemotherapy.

Adrenal Androgen Inhibitors

Adrenal androgen inhibitors work by achieving a "medical adrenalectomy," which further decreases androgen production. Responses have been seen in patients after antiandrogen withdrawal. It is important to use steroid replacements in patients receiving adrenal androgen inhibitors; this is often started with hydrocortisone 20 mg every morning and 10 mg every evening but is increased to 20 mg PO b.i.d if patients show symptoms of glucocorticoid insufficiency (e.g., fatigue).

Adrenal Androgen Inhibitors: Regimens and Toxicities

Aminoglutethimide + hydrocortisone (RR = 49%) (28):

- Aminoglutethimide (Cytadren), 125 mg PO q.i.d., increasing to 250 mg q.i.d. + hydrocortisone, 20 mg PO b.i.d.
- Side effects: sedation, skin rashes, and fever
- Rarer side effects: ataxia, hypothyroidism, abnormal liver enzyme levels, and peripheral edema.

Ketoconazole + hydrocortisone (RR = 35% to 50%) (29):

- Ketoconazole (Nizoral), 200 mg PO t.i.d., increasing to 400 mg PO t.i.d. + hydrocortisone, 20 mg PO b.i.d.
- Side effects: impotence, pruritus, nail changes, adrenal insufficiency, nausea, emesis, and hepatotoxicity. Liver transaminases need to be monitored. (Ketoconazole is absorbed at an acidic pH; therefore, the concomitant use of H_2 blockers, antacids, or proton pump inhibitors should be avoided. Coating agents such as sucralfate may be substituted.)

Corticosteroids (RR = 18% to 22%) (30):

- Corticosteroids alone have been shown to improve pain in patients with symptomatic bone metastases.
- Prednisone, 5 mg PO every morning and 2.5 mg PO every evening, increasing to 5 mg PO b.i.d.; side effects are the same as for any medical use of prednisone.

CHEMOTHERAPY FOR ANDROGEN-INDEPENDENT PROSTATE CANCER

Patients have a median survival of 12 to 18 months after developing androgen-independent prostate cancer. Chemotherapy with docetaxel-containing regimens has only recently been shown to improve survival in patients with AIPC, with median OS of about 18 months (31,32). Participation in clinical trials of novel agents or combinations should be encouraged. Antiangiogenic agents and immunotherapy or tumor vaccines are undergoing studies in AIPC.

Estramustine phosphate (EMP, Emcyt) is a compound that combines estradiol and nitrogen mustard. It works by binding to microtubule-associated proteins. Many phase II trials of single-agent estramustine have been conducted. However, a synergistic effect appears to result when estramustine is combined with other agents that have activity against the microtubule proteins (e.g., vinblastine and the taxanes); therefore, estramustine is usually given in combination.

Docetaxel (Taxotere)/Estramustine (Emcyt) (PRR = 50%) (31):

- Improved median OS from 15 months (mitoxantrone/prednisone) to 18 months ($p = 0.008$) is observed.
- Estramustine, 280 mg PO t.i.d., is administered 1 hour before or 2 hours after meals, on days 1–5, with docetaxel, 60 mg per m^2 on day 2. Patients were dose escalated to 70 mg per m^2 if there was no grade 3 toxicity observed in cycle 1.
- Dexamethasone, 20 mg PO t.i.d. × 3 doses, is administered, starting the evening of day 1 of each cycle.

- Cycle is repeated every 21 days.
- Side effects are grade 3 toxicity: hematologic effect (20%), gastrointestinal effect (20%), cardiovascular effect (15%), infection (14%), flu-like syndrome (10%), and neurologic effect (7%).

Docetaxel (Taxotere) (PRR 45%) (32):

- Improved median OS from 16.5 months (mitoxantrone/prednisone) to 18.9 months ($p = 0.0005$) and improved quality of life [Functional Assessment of Cancer Therapy-Prostate (FACT-P) 22% versus 13%; $p = 0.009$] are observed.
- Docetaxel 75 mg per m^2 i.v. is given.
- Prednisone 5 mg is given twice daily.
- Cycle is repeated every 21 days.
- Side effects include grade 3 toxicity, granulocytopenia (32%), infection (5.7%), anemia (4.9%), and fatigue (4.5%), and any grade of toxicity, anemia (67%), neutropenia (41%), fluid retention (24%), sensory neuropathy (30%), nausea (41%), fatigue (53%), myalgia (15%), and alopecia (65%).

Docetaxel (Taxotere) + Calcitriol (PRR = 81%;ORR 53%) (12):

- Calcitriol 0.5 μg per kg PO in four divided doses was given over 4 hours on day 1.
- Docetaxel 36 mg per m^2 i.v. over 15 to 30 minutes was given on day 2.
- Dexamethasone 8 mg PO was given 12 hours and 1 hour before docetaxel infusion and 12 hours after docetaxel infusion.
- Treatment was repeated each week for 6 out of every 8 weeks.
- Therapy was held when platelet count was less than 75,000 or when absolute neutrophil count (ANC) was less than 1,000; docetaxel dose was reduced by 25% if ANC or platelet recovery was greater than 1 week.
- Patients were maintained on reduced calcium diets (400 to 500 mg daily).
- Side effects include grade 3 or greater toxicity with leukopenia (41%), neutropenia (24%), anemia (3%), hyperglycemia (24%), and peptic ulcer (11%).

Mitoxantrone (Novantrone) + Prednisone (PRR = 33%) (30,33):

- This regimen has been shown to improve quality of life, but not DFS or OS, in two randomized controlled trials versus steroids alone.
- Prednisone, 5 mg PO b.i.d, on day 1, + mitoxantrone, 12 mg per m^2 i.v., on day 21, delayed if not recovered hematologically.
- Mitoxantrone was stopped at a cumulative dose of 140 mg per m^2. Prochlorperazine was used as an antiemetic.
- Side effects: cardiac abnormalities in 6% of patients in the mitoxantrone arm only [2% with congestive heart failure (CHF)], neutropenic fever (1.1%), neutropenia (45%), thrombocytopenia (5%), nausea and vomiting (29%), and alopecia (26%); exacerbation of diabetes in one patient.
- Prednisone, 5 mg PO b.i.d., on day 1, + mitoxantrone, 12 mg per m^2 i.v., on day 21, delayed if not recovered hematologically.

SELECTED MANAGEMENT ISSUES

CNS metastases are relatively rare, but not unheard of, in CaP. Visceral metastases occur in about 20% of patients; most patients have symptoms related to bone metastases.

Bone Metastases

The use of RT to localized painful bone metastases has been shown to provide palliation. Usually, the painful vertebra and the two vertebrae superior and inferior to the lesion are treated with 3,000 cGy radiation in ten fractions. Pain relief occurs in approximately 80% of patients; side effects generally are limited to fatigue and anemia that is usually reversible. The spinal cord can tolerate radiation up to approximately 5,000 cGy, so re-treating these areas with a radiation of 2,000 cGy can sometimes be attempted, although with caution.

For widespread disease, hemibody irradiation has been used, as has the radioisotope strontium-89 (Metastron), a calcium analog that preferentially localizes in the tumor. Palliation of pain with strontium has been reported in up to 75% of cases and typically occurs after 1 to 3 weeks of treatment and may continue for several months. Toxicities of strontium include the potential for flare (15%) that is often associated with a later response and a reversible thrombocytopenia in 25% of patients that usually resolves by 3 months. Strontium can often be readministered. Samarium-153 lexidronam (Quadramet) is a newer radioisotope with treatment indications similar to those of strontium and a shorter half-life than strontium.

Bisphosphonates, agents that inhibit osteoclastic bone resorption, have been shown to decrease skeletal-related events in patients with advanced androgen-independent disease (34). Careful attention to pain control with narcotics and adjuncts should be maintained in patients with bone metastases.

Spinal Cord Compression

Spinal cord compression, an oncologic emergency, is common in patients with metastatic prostate cancer who have widespread bony metastases. This consists largely of vertebral column metastases impinging on the spinal cord.

More than 90% of patients have pain as an early sign; pain that is worsening is particularly disturbing. There may be pain in the involved spine, muscle weakness, or abnormalities in the neurologic examination. Signs that are often indicative of irreversible damage include weakness and/or sensory loss corresponding to the level of the spinal cord compression. Signs such as genitourinary or gastrointestinal dysfunction (e.g., urinary retention or constipation) or autonomic dysfunction are late signs, and spinal cord compression usually progresses rapidly at this point.

One should have a high index of suspicion for spinal cord compression in patients known to have osseous metastases in CaP, particularly with new signs or any symptoms related to spinal cord compression. Diagnosis requires a thorough history and physical examination, with special attention to the musculoskeletal and neurologic examinations. The standard for diagnosing and localizing epidural cord compression is an MRI, usually with gadolinium. A myelogram is still used in patients with contraindications to MRI (e.g., a pacemaker).

Steroids should be started (dexamethasone, 100 mg i.v., followed by 4 mg i.v. or PO, every 6 hours) as soon as history or neurologic examination suggests spinal cord compression. RT, given as 3,000 cGy in ten fractions to the involved vertebra and to the two superior and two inferior vertebrae, is the usual treatment modality, and early consultation with an radiation oncologist is warranted. Surgical resection of the vertebral body is generally used in patients who have had previous RT of the involved area if these patients require procedures for spinal stability or experience progression despite treatment with steroids and RT or if RT facilities are not locally available. It should also be considered in patients with a rapidly progressive neurologic deficit because the relief from RT is slower (by days) than from a surgical decompressive procedure. A recent randomized trial showed that patients subjected to decompressive surgical resection followed by radiation retained the ability to walk significantly longer than those treated with radiation alone. Neurologic or orthopedic surgeons should be consulted early in the diagnosis of spinal cord compression as well.

REFERENCES

1. Chu KC, Tarone RE, Freeman HP. Trends in prostate cancer mortality among black men and white men in the United States. *Cancer* 2003;97(6):1507–1516.
2. Thompson IM, Goodman PJ, Tangen CM, et al. The influence of finasteride on the development of prostate cancer. *N Engl J Med* 2003;349(3):215–224.

3. Albanes D, Heinonen OP, Taylor PR, et al. Alpha-tcopherol and beta-carotene supplements and lung cancer incidence in the alpha-tocopherol, beta-carotene cancer prevention study: effects of base-line characteristics and study compliance. *J Natl Cancer Inst* 1996;88(21):1560–1570.
4. Clark LC, Combs GF Jr, Turnbull BW, et al. Effects of selenium supplementation for cancer prevention in patients with carcinoma of the skin. A randomized controlled trial. Nutritional prevention of cancer study group. *JAMA* 1996;276(24):1957–1963.
5. This can be accessed via the internet: http://cancer.gov/select
6. Talcott JA, Rieker P, Clark JA, et al. Patient-reported symptoms after primary therapy for early prostate cancer: results of a prospective cohort study. *J Clin Oncol* 1998;16(1):275–283.
7. Gleave M, Goldenberg L, Chin JL, et al. Natural history of progression after PSA elevation following radical prostatectomy: update. *J Urol* 2003;169(4):A690.
8. Pound CR, Partin AW, Eisenberger MA, et al. Natural history of progression after PSA elevation following radical prostatectomy. *JAMA* 1999;281(17):1591–1597.
9. Pilepich MV, Caplan R, Byhardt RW, et al. Phase III trial of androgen suppression using goserelin in unfavorable-prognosis carcinoma of the prostate treated with definitive radiotherapy: report of Radiation Therapy Oncology Group Protocol 85-31. *J Clin Oncol* 1997;15(3):1013–1021.
10. Lawton CA, Winter K, Murray K, et al. Updated results of the phase III Radiation Therapy Oncology Group (RTOG) trial 85-31 evaluating the potential benefit of androgen suppression following standard radiation therapy for unfavorable prognosis carcinoma of the prostate. *Int J Radiat Oncol Biol Phys* 2001;49(4):937–946.
11. Pilepich MV, Winter K, Lawton C, et al. Phase III trial of androgen suppression adjuvant to definitive radiotherapy. Long term results of RTOG study 85-31. *Proc Am Soc Clin Oncol* 2003;22:381. Abstract 1530.
12. Beer TM, Hough KM, Garzotto M, et al. Weekly high-dose calcitriol and docetaxel in advanced prostate cancer. *Semin Oncol* 2001;28(4):49–55.
13. Bolla M, Gonzalez D, Warde P, et al. Improved survival in patients with locally advanced prostate cancer treated with radiotherapy and goserelin. *N Engl J Med* 1997;337(5):295–300.
14. Bolla M, Collette L, Blank L, et al. Long-term results with immediate androgen suppression and external irradiation in patients with locally advanced prostate cancer (an EORTC study): a phase III randomised trial. *Lancet* 2002;360(9327):103–108.
15. Hanks GE, Pajak TF, Porter A, et al. Radiation Therapy Oncology Group. Phase III trial of long-term adjuvant androgen deprivation after neoadjuvant hormonal cytoreduction and radiotherapy in locally advanced carcinoma of the prostate: the radiation therapy oncology group protocol 92-02. *J Clin Oncol* 2003;21(21):3972–3978.
16. Granfors T, Modig H, Damber JE, et al. Combined orchiectomy and external radiotherapy versus radiotherapy alone for nonmetastatic prostate cancer with or without pelvic lymph node involvement: a prospective randomized study. *J Urol* 1998;159(6):2030–2034.
17. Dattoli M, Wallner K, True L, et al. Long-term outcomes after treatment with external beam radiation therapy and palladium 103 for patients with higher risk prostate carcinoma – influence of prostatic acid phosphatase. *Cancer* 2003;97(4):979–983.
18. Critz FA, Williams WH, Levinson AK, et al. Simultaneous irradiation for prostate cancer: intermediate results with modern techniques. *J Urol* 2000;164(3 Pt 1):738–741.
19. Kovacs G, Galalae R, Loch T, et al. Prostate preservation by combined external beam and HDR brachytherapy in nodal negative prostate cancer. *Strahlenther Onkol* 1999;175:87–88.
20. Daniell HW. Osteoporosis after orchiectomy for prostate cancer. *J Urol* 1997;157(2):439–444.
21. Messing E, Manola J, Sarosdy M, et al. Immediate hormonal therapy compared with observation after radical prostatectomy and pelvic lymphadenectomy in men with node positive prostate cancer: results at 10 years of EST 3886. *J Urol* 2003;169(4):1480.
22. Crawford ED, Eisenberger MA, McLeod DG, et al. A controlled trial of leuprolide with and without flutamide in prostatic carcinoma. *N Engl J Med* 1989;321(7):419–424.
23. Eisenberger MA, Blumenstein BA, Crawford ED, et al. Bilateral orchiectomy with or without flutamide for metastatic prostate cancer. *N Engl J Med* 1998;339(15):1036–1042.
24. Moinpour CM, Savage MJ, Troxel A, et al. Quality of life in advanced prostate cancer: results of a randomized therapeutic trial. *J Natl Cancer Inst* 1998;90(20):1537–1544.
25. Agency for Health Care Policy and Research. Relative effectiveness and cost-effectiveness of methods of androgen suppression in the treatment of advanced prostatic cancer (AHCPR Publication No 99-E012). 1999. http://www.ahrq.gov/clinic/epcsums/prossumm.htm

26. Adib RS, Anderson JB, Ashken MH, et al. Immediate versus deferred treatment for advanced pro-statics cancer: initial results of the Medical Research Council trial. *Br J Urol* 1997;79(2):235–246.
27. Bubley GJ, Carducci M, Dahut W, et al. Eligibility and response guidelines for phase II clinical tri-als in androgen-independent prostate cancer: recommendations from the Prostate-Specific Antigen Working Group. *J Clin Oncol* 1999;17(11):3461–3467.
28. Sartor O, Cooper M, Weinberger M. Surprising activity of flutamide withdrawal, when combined with aminoglutethimide, in treatment of hormone-refractory prostate-cancer. *J Natl Cancer Inst* 1994;86(6):463, 222.
29. Small EJ, Baron A, Bok R. Simultaneous antiandrogen withdrawal and treatment with ketoconazole and hydrocortisone in patients with advanced prostate carcinoma. *Cancer* 1997;80(9):1755–1759.
30. Tannock IF, Osoba D, Stockler MR, et al. Chemotherapy with mitoxantrone plus prednisone or prednisone alone for symptomatic hormone-resistant prostate cancer: a Canadian randomized trial with palliative end points. *J Clin Oncol* 1996;14(6):1756–1764.
31. Petrylak D, Tangen C, Hussain M, et al. SWOG 99-16: randomized phase III trial of docetaxel/estra-mustine versus mitoxantrone/prednisone in men with androgen-independent prostate cancer. *Proc Am Soc Clin Oncol* 2004;23:2.
32. Eisenberger M, De Wit R, Berry W, et al. A multicenter phase III comparison of docetaxel + prednisone and mitoxantrone + prednisone in patient with hormone refractory prostate cancer. *Proc Am Soc Clin Oncol* 2004;23:2.
33. Kantoff PW, Halabi S, Conaway M, et al. Hydrocortisone with or without mitoxantrone in men with hormone-refractory prostate cancer: results of the Cancer and Leukemia Group B 9182 study. *J Clin Oncol* 1999;17(8):2506–2513.
34. Saad F, Gleason DM, Murray R, et al. A randomized, placebo-controlled trial of zoledronic acid in patients with hormone-refractory metastatic prostate carcinoma. *J Natl Cancer Inst* 2002;94(19):1458–1468.

15

Bladder Cancer

Manish Agrawal and William L. Dahut

Medical Oncology Clinical Research Unit, Center for Cancer Research, National Cancer Institute, National Institutes of Health, Bethesda, Maryland

EPIDEMIOLOGY

In 2003, approximately 57,400 patients were estimated to have developed bladder cancer, and 12,500 patients were estimated to have died from it. Bladder cancer is a disease of the elderly; most people diagnosed with this disease are older than 60 years, and it is the second most prevalent cancer in men 60 years of age or older. The incidence of bladder cancer is more common in men than in women (3:1) and more common in whites than in blacks (2:1).

ETIOLOGY

- **Cigarette smoking:** The most common cause of bladder cancer is cigarette smoking; smokers have twice the risk of developing bladder cancer than do nonsmokers. There is a strong correlation between the amount and duration of cigarette smoking and bladder cancer.
- **Occupational exposures:** Occupational exposures to chemical carcinogens are associated with an increased risk of bladder cancer. In particular, workers exposed to arylamines in the dye, paint, rubber, and leather industries are at an increased risk. Truck, taxi, and bus drivers along with hairdressers are other workers whose occupations have been recently implicated as risk factors.
- **Analgesics:** The abuse of analgesics, in particular, phenacetin, is associated with an increased risk of urothelial cancers, with the greatest risk for the renal pelvis.
- **Treatment-related risks:** Treatment-related risks include pelvic radiation (for cervical, ovarian, and prostate cancer) and treatment with cyclophosphamide.
- **Chronic infections:** Chronic infection due to *Schistosoma haematobium* causes squamous metaplasia and increases the risk of squamous cell carcinoma (SCC) in endemic areas such as Egypt.
- **Others:** Other less-established and more controversial risk factors include drinking water, artifical sweeteners, coffee consumption, and chronic cystitis.

PATHOLOGY

Transitional Cell Carcinoma (TCC) accounts for 90% to 95% of all bladder tumors found in the United States. Five percent to 10% of bladder tumors are SCC, and 1% to 2% are adenocarcinomas. Carcinoma *in situ* (CIS) usually presents as diffuse urothelial involvement in patients with superficial bladder tumors. CIS increases the risk for subsequent invasive disease and recurrence regardless of whether it occurs alone or in association with superficial bladder tumors.

CLINICAL FEATURES

Painless gross or microscopic hematuria is seen in 85% of patients. Symptoms of bladder irritability are seen in 20% of patients. Patients with invasive disease may have flank pain because of ureteral obstruction, bladder mass, or lower extremity edema. Constitutional symptoms such as weight loss, abdominal pain, or bone pain may be present in patients with advanced disease.

DIAGNOSIS AND STAGING WORKUP

- The diagnostic workup of a patient with suspected bladder cancer includes intravenous pyelography, urinary cytologic studies, and cystoscopy with full evaluation of the bladder mucosa and urethra.
- Computerized tomography (CT) scan of the abdomen and pelvis is performed to detect local extension and involvement of abdominal lymph nodes. A chest x-ray is used as an initial screening tool for detecting pulmonary metastases.
- A bone scan is recommended for patients with an elevated alkaline phosphatase level or bone pain.

STAGING

The staging of bladder cancer (Fig. 15.1 and Table 15.1) is the most important independent prognostic variable for progression and overall survival. Bladder cancers are divided into

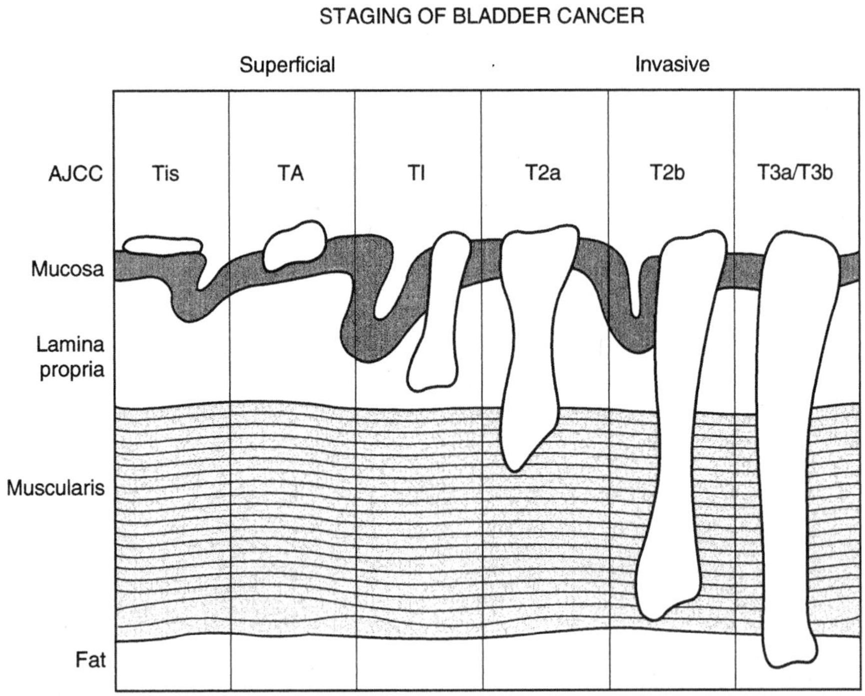

FIG. 15.1. Clinical staging of carcinoma of the bladder.

TABLE 15.1. *Tumor–node–metastasis (TNM) staging of bladder cancer*

Primary tumor (T)

The suffix "m" should be added to the appropriate T category to indicate multiple lesions. The suffix "is" may be added to any T to indicate the presence of associated carcinoma *in situ*

TX: Primary tumor cannot be assessed

T0: No evidence of primary tumor

Ta: Noninvasive papillary carcinoma

Tis: Carcinoma *in situ*: "flat tumor"

T1: Tumor invades subepithelial connective tissue

T2: Tumor invades muscle

   T2a: Tumor invades superficial muscle (inner half)

   T2b: Tumor invades deep muscle (outer half)

T3: Tumor invades perivesical tissue

   T3a: microscopically

   T3b: macroscopically (extravesical mass)

T4: Tumor invades any of the following: prostate, uterus, vagina, pelvic wall, or abdominal wall

   T4a: Tumor invades the prostate, uterus, vagina

   T4b: Tumor invades the pelvic wall and abdominal wall

Regional lymph nodes (N)

Regional lymph nodes are those within the true pelvis; all others are distant lymph nodes

NX: Regional lymph nodes cannot be assessed

N0: No regional lymph node metastasis

N1: Metastasis in a single lymph node, ≤2 cm in greatest dimension

N2: Metastasis in a single lymph node, >2 cm but = 5 cm in greatest dimension; or multiple lymph nodes, none >5 cm in greatest dimension

N3: Metastasis in a single lymph node >5 cm in greatest dimension

Distant metastasis (M)

MX: Distant metastasis cannot be assessed

M0: No distant metastasis

M1: Distant metastasis

Stage grouping

Stage 0a: Ta N0 M0

Stage 0is: Tis N0 M0

Stage I: T1 N0 M0

Stage II: T2a N0 M0 or T2b N0 M0

Stage III: T3a N0 M0 or T3b N0 M0 or T4a N0 M0

Stage IV: T4b N0 M0 or any T N1–N3 M0 or any T Any N M1

superficial and invasive cancers. Superficial bladder cancers are tumors that involve only the mucosa (Ta) or submucosa (T1) and flat CIS (Tis) and account for 75% of bladder cancers. Most superfical bladder cancers recur within 6 to 12 months, with the same stage, but 10% to 15% of patients can develop invasive or metastatic disease.

Invasive bladder cancers are tumors that invade the muscularis propria, perivesical tissues, or adjacent structures. Patients with muscle-invasive disease have a 50% likelihood of having occult distant metastases at the time of diagnosis. The usual sites of metastases are pelvic lymph nodes, liver, lung, bone, adrenal glands, and intestine.

PROGNOSIS

- The major prognostic factors are the tumor stage at the time of diagnosis and degree of differentiation of the tumor.
- Five-year relative survival rates for patients with superficial, muscle-invasive, and metastatic bladder cancer are 95%, 50%, and 6%, respectively.
- Old age, expression of p53, aneuploidy, tumor multifocality, and palpable mass are other adverse prognostic factors.

Treatment

Carcinoma In Situ

Transurethral resection (TUR) followed by intravesical bacille Calmette-Guérin (BCG) therapy is the most common treatment for CIS of the bladder (Fig. 15.2). It produces complete response rate in 70% to 80% of patients and a 5-year disease-free survival in more than 75% of patients. Intravesical chemotherapeutic agents such as thiotepa, doxorubicin, gemcitabine, and mitomycin produce complete response rates in 30% to 50% of patients and a 5-year disease-free survival in 20% to 40% of patients.

Superficial Bladder Cancer

- The treatment of superficial bladder cancer has two goals: to eradicate existing disease and provide prophylaxis against tumor recurrence.
- TUR is the primary therapy for superficial bladder cancer. Approximately 80% of these patients survive for 5 years if treated with TUR alone, but in 70% to 80% of these patients, tumor recurrence develops within 12 months.
- Adjuvant intravesical therapy permits high local drug concentrations to be achieved within the bladder, potentially destroying the remaining cancer cells. In high-risk patients, the tumor recurrence rate is decreased to about 20% with adjuvant intravesical BCG therapy.

Muscle-invasive Bladder Cancer

- Radical cystectomy with bilateral pelvic lymph node dissection is the standard therapy for muscle-invasive bladder cancer. In men, the surgery involves radical cystoprostatectomy, and a total urethrectomy is indicated if there is involvement of the prostatic urethra. In women, radical cystectomy involves wide excision of the bladder, urethra, uterus, adnexa, and anterior vaginal wall.
- Recent studies have shown that bladder-sparing options, which include aggressive TUR in combination with radiotherapy and chemotherapy, can be considered in select patients with T2 or T3a disease without compromising survival; however, this approach remains investigational.
- External beam radiotherapy with or without radiation-sensitizing agents such as cisplatin or 5-fluorouracil is an option for poor surgical candidates. Randomized trials have not shown any benefit for preoperative radiotherapy followed by radical cystectomy over radical cystectomy alone.
- There is no accepted standard of care for postoperative chemotherapy in the treatment of muscle-invasive bladder cancer. Several randomized trials have shown conflicting results, with some showing a survival advantage with adjuvant chemotherapy and others reporting no benefit. The negative trials have been criticized for being insufficiently powered, for using suboptimal chemotherapy, and for premature closure. Randomized controlled trials are under way—European Organization for Research and Treatment of Cancer (EORTC), The Cancer and Leukemia Group B (CALGB), Eastern Cooperative Oncology Group (ECOG)—to address this question, and eligible patients should be encouraged to enter these

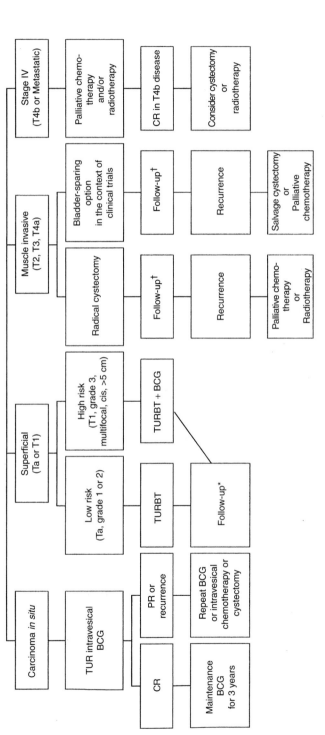

FIG. 15.2. Treatment of bladder cancer. *Cytoscopy and urine cytology q3mo × 2 years, followed by q6mo × 2 years, and then yearly for life. †Computerized tomography scan q6mo, intravenous pyelogram or ultrasound q12mo, cytoscopy and urine cytology q3mo × 1 year and then q6mo, serum creatinine and liver function test, and vitamin B₁₂ q3–6mo.

TABLE 15.2. *Combination chemotherapy regimens in advanced urothelial carcinoma*

Regimen	Treatment description	Cycle duration	Comments	Reference
CISCA	Cyclophosphamide, 650 mg/m² i.v. d 1 (total dose/cycle, 650 mg/m²) Doxorubicin, 50 mg/m² i.v. d 2 (total dose/cycle, 50 mg/m²) Cisplatin, 100 mg/m² i.v. d 2 (total dose/cycle, 100 mg/m²)	21–28 d		6, 7
CMV	Methotrexate, 30 mg/m² i.v. d 1 and 8 (total dose/cycle, 60 mg/m²) Vinblastine, 4 mg/m² i.v. d 1 and 8 (total dose/cycle, 8 mg/m²) Cisplatin, 100 mg/m² i.v. infusion over 4 h on d 2, ≥12 h, after methotrexate and vinblastine (total dose/cycle, 100 mg/m²)	21 d		8
Docetaxel + cisplatin[a]	Docetaxel, 75 mg/m² slow i.v. infusion over 1 h, d 1 (total dose/cycle, 75 mg/m²) Cisplatin, 75 mg/m² i.v. d 1 (total dose/cycle, 75 mg/m²)	21 d		9
Gemcitabine + cisplatin	Gemcitabine, 1,000 mg/m² i.v. d 1, 8, and 15 (total dose/cycle, 3,000 mg/m²) Cisplatin, 75 mg/m² i.v. d 1 (total dose/cycle, 75 mg/m²)	28 d		10
ITP[a]	Ifosfamide, 1,500 mg/m²/d i.v. for d 1–3 (total dose/cycle, 4,500 mg/m²) Mesna, 300 mg/m² i.v., 30 min before ifosfamide, and then Mesna, 300 mg/m² i.v. 4 and 8 h after ifosfamide, Mesna, 600 mg/m² PO 4 and 8 h after ifosfamide Paclitaxel, 200 mg/m² i.v. infusion over 3 h, d 1 (total dose/cycle, 200 mg/m²)	28 d	Regimen includes primary hematopoietic growth factor support with filgrastim, 5 µg/kg or per d, s.c.	11
M-VAC	Cisplatin, 70 mg/m² i.v. d 1 (total dose/cycle, 70 mg/m²) Methotrexate, 30 mg/m² i.v. d 1, 15, and 22 (total dose/cycle, 90 mg/m²) Vinblastine, 3 mg/m² i.v. d 2, 15, and 22 (total dose/cycle, 9 mg/m²) Doxorubicin, 30 mg/m² i.v. d 2 (total dose/cycle, 30 mg/m²) Cisplatin, 70 mg/m² i.v. d 2 (total dose/cycle, 70 mg/m²)	28 d	Withhold methotrexate and vinblastine on d 15 and 22 if WBC count is <2.5 × 10³/µL and platelets <100 × 10³/µL	4, 5
Paclitaxel + carboplatin[a]	Paclitaxel, 200 mg/m² i.v. infusion over 3 h, d 1 (total dose/cycle, 200 mg/m²) Carboplatin i.v. after paclitaxel; dosage is calculated by the Calvert formula to achieve a target AUC of 5 mg/mL/min (Calvert reference)[b]	21 d		12

AUC, graphically represented area under the plasma concentration versus time curve for carboplatin; GFR, glomerular filtration rate. In clinical application, urinary creatinine clearance during 24 h approximates the GFR; i.v., intravenously; PO, orally; s.c., subcutaneously; WBC, white blood cell.

[a]Antineoplastic regimen included primary prophylaxis with antihistamines and corticosteroids against hypersensitivity reactions before taxoid (paclitaxel or docetaxel) administration.

[b]Calvert formula: Total dose (mg) = [Target AUC (mg/mL/min)] × [GFR (mL/min) + 25].

Adapted from Calvert AH, Newell DR, Gumbrell LA, et al. Carboplatin dosage: prospective evaluation of a simple formula based on renal function. *J Clin Oncol* 1989;7:1748–1756, with permission.

important trials. Outside the context of a clinical trial, physicians and patients must discuss and evaluate the decision for adjuvant chemotherapy depending on the clinical scenario.
- Neadjuvant chemotherapy has been studied in numerous randomized clinical trials with conflicting results. The largest trial was of 975 patients conducted by the Medical Research Council and the EORTC. Patients were randomized to three cycles of neoajuvant CMV (cisplatin, methotrexate, and vinblastine) or to no chemotherapy, followed by management of the primary lesion with surgery or radiation or both. The 3-year survival benefit was 5.5% for the treatment arm but did not reach statistical significance because the trial was powered to detect a 10% increase in survival. A U.S. Intergroup trial (SWOG-8710) randomized 317 patients to neoajuvant M-VAC (methotrexate, vinblastine, doxorubicin, cisplatin) versus no chemotherapy and found an improvement in overall survival in the chemotherapy arm (77 months versus 46 months). Three other trials (Italian Bladder Tumor Study Group, Nordic-164, Nordic 2) did not find any benefit to neoadjuvant chemotherapy in their preliminary report. On the basis of the two large trials, there is an emerging opinion that in select patients, there may be a benefit to neoadjuvant chemotherapy. Eligible patients should be enrolled in clinical trials, and outside of clinical trials, each clinical situation should be evaluated individually.

Stage IV Bladder Cancer

- Cisplatin, methotrexate, paclitaxel, docetaxel, and gemcitabine are the most active single agents in treatment of bladder cancer, with response rates of 30% to 45%.
- Combination chemotherapy with the M-VAC regimen has been shown in randomized trials to be superior to single-agent cisplatin (1) and the three-drug regimen CISCA (cyclophosphamide, cisplatin, and doxorubicin) (2) (Tables 15.2 and 15.3). M-VAC has a response rate of 40% to 72%. The major drawback of using the M-VAC regimen is that it is associated with significant toxicity including neutropenia, sepsis, mucositis, and renal failure.
- More recently, the combination of gemcitabine plus cisplatin was compared to M-VAC in a randomized trial of 405 patients with stage IV TCC bladder cancer. The response rate, time to treatment failure, and median survival were similar for both regimens. However, there was less toxicity with the cisplatin plus gemcitabine arm in comparison to the M-VAC arm.
- Alternative treatment regimens incorporating docetaxel, gemcitabine, and paclitaxel as first-line agents are being actively studied and have shown response rates of 40% to 70%, with potentially less toxicity (Table 15.4) in phase II studies.

TABLE 15.3. *Randomized trials in patients with advanced urothelial carcinoma*

Randomized trial	Overall response rate	Median survival
M-VAC vs. cisplatin (1)	39% vs. 12%	12.5 mo vs. 8.2 mo
M-VAC vs. CISCA (2)	65% vs. 46%	48 wk vs. 36 wk
M-VAC vs. cisplatin (3) + gemcitabine	46% vs. 49%	13.8 mo vs. 14.8 mo

TABLE 15.4. *Newer agents in untreated advanced urothelial carcinoma patients*

Phase II trials	No. of evaluable patients	Overall response rate (%)
Docetaxel + cisplatin (4)	25	60
Gemcitabine + paclitaxel (5)	54	54
Ifosfamide + paclitaxel + cisplatin (6)	44	68
Paclitaxel + carboplatin (7)	35	51.5
Paclitaxel + cisplatin + Gemcitabine (8)	49	78

REFERENCES

1. Loehrer PJ Sr, Einhorn LH, Elson PJ, et al. A randomized comparison of cisplatin alone or in combination with methotrexate, vinblastine, and doxorubicin in patients with metastatic urothelial carcinoma: a cooperative group study [published erratum appears in *J Clin Oncol* 1993;11:384]. *J Clin Oncol* 1992;10:1066–1073.
2. Logothetis CJ, Dexeus FH, Finn L, et al. A prospective randomized trial comparing MVAC and CISCA chemotherapy for patients with metastatic urothelial tumors. *J Clin Oncol* 1990;8:1050–1055.
3. von der Maase H, Hansen SW, Roberts JT, et al. Gemcitabine and cisplatin versus methotrexate, vinblastine, doxorubicin, and cisplatin in advanced or metastatic bladder cancer: results of a large, randomized, multinational, multicenter, phase III study. *J Clin Oncol* 2000;18(17):3068–3077.
4. Sengelov L, Kamby C, Lund B, et al. Docetaxel and cisplatin in metastatic urothelial cancer: a phase II study. *J Clin Oncol* 1998;16:3392–3397.
5. Meluch AA, Greco FA, Burris HA, et al. Paclitaxel and gemcitabine chemotherapy for advanced transitional-cell carcinoma of the urothelial tract: a phase II trial of the Minnie pearl cancer research network. *J Clin Oncol* 2001;19(12):3018–3024.
6. Bajorin DF, McCaffrey JA, Hilton S, et al. Ifosfamide, paclitaxel, and cisplatin for patients with advanced transitional-cell carcinoma of the urothelial tract: final report of a phase II trial evaluating two dosing schedules. *Cancer* 2000;88(7):1671–1678.
7. Redman BG, Smith DC, Flaherty L, et al. Phase II trial of paclitaxel and carboplatin in the treatment of advanced urothelial carcinoma. *J Clin Oncol* 1998;16:1844–1848.
8. Bellmunt J, Guillem V, Paz-Ares L, et al. Spanish Oncology Genitourinary Group. Phase I-II study of paclitaxel, cisplatin, and gemcitabine in advanced transitional-cell carcinoma of the urothelium. *J Clin Oncol* 2000;18(18):3247–3255.

SUGGESTED READINGS

Advanced Bladder Cancer Meta-analysis Collaboration. Neoadjuvant chemotherapy in invasive bladder cancer: a systematic review and meta-analysis. *Lancet* 2003;361(9373):1927–1934.
Grossman HB, Natale RB, Tangen CM, et al. Neoadjuvant chemotherapy plus cystectomy compared with cystectomy alone for locally advanced bladder cancer. *N Engl J Med* 2003;349:859–866.
Harker WG, Meyers FJ, Freiha FS, et al. Cisplatin, methotrexate, and vinblastine (CMV): an effective chemotherapy regimen for metastatic transitional cell carcinoma of the urinary tract: a Northern California Oncology Group study. *J Clin Oncol* 1985;3:1463–1470.
Levin RM, Crawford DE. Bladder, renal pelvis, and ureters. In: Haskell CM, ed. *Cancer treatment*, 4th ed. Philadelphia, PA: WB Saunders, 1995:567–588.
Logothetis CJ, Dexeus FH, Chong C, et al. Cisplatin, cyclophosphamide and doxorubicin chemotherapy for unresectable urothelial tumors: the MD Anderson experience. *J Urol* 1989;141:33–37.
NCCN. Urothelial cancer practice guidelines. http://www.nccn.org/professionals/physician_gls/default.asp, 2004
Sher HI, Shipley WU, Herr HW. Cancer of the bladder. In: DeVita VT Jr, Hellman S, Rosenberg SA, eds. *Cancer: principles and practice of oncology*, 5th ed. New York: Lippincott–Raven Publishers, 1997:1300–1322.
Sternberg CN, Yagoda A, Scher HI, et al. Preliminary results of M-VAC (methotrexate, vinblastine, doxorubicin and cisplatin) for transitional cell carcinoma of the urothelium. *J Urol* 1985;133:403–407.

16

Testicular Carcinoma

Avi S. Retter* and Barnett S. Kramer†

Medical Oncology Clinical Research Unit, National Cancer Institute, National Institutes of Health, Bethesda, Maryland; and †Office of Disease Prevention, National Institutes of Health, Bethesda, Maryland

The opinions expressed in this chapter represent those of the authors and do not necessarily represent official positions or opinions of the U.S. government or of the U.S. Department of Health and Human Services.

Testicular cancer is rare (less than 1% of all tumors) but represents one of the most frequently occurring malignancies in young men. In most cases, the reproductive organs are the sites of the primary tumors; these tumors usually arise from the malignant transformation of primordial germ cells. Testicular cancer is highly curable, and life expectancy of affected individuals is long. Consequently, careful long-term follow-up of survivors is required. Not only oncologists but also primary care providers are likely to observe an increasing number of successfully treated patients in their practice. For these patients, careful monitoring for recurrent disease and therapy-related long-term sequelae is imperative.

CLINICAL FEATURES

Epidemiology

- For 2003, 7,600 new cases of testicular cancer and 400 deaths from this cancer were estimated.
- Testicular cancer accounts for 1% of all malignancies in men.
- Incidence in whites is greater than that in African Americans.
- Peak frequency is in early adulthood (greatest incidence is between the age of 20 and 35 years).
- Testicular cancer is uncommon after the age of 40.

Risk Factors

- Undescended (cryptorchid) testes (intraabdominal testes are at higher risk than inguinal testes)—in cryptorchidism, the contralateral normally descended testicle is also at high risk
- Testicular cancer in contralateral testis
- Klinefelter syndrome (increased risk of mediastinal germ cell tumors)
- HIV positivity.

History and Signs and Physical Examination

- Asymptomatic nodule or swelling
- Testicular mass, feeling of heaviness, pain, and/or hardness

- Patients with advanced disease may experience back or abdominal pain (due to retroperitoneal adenopathy), weight loss, gynecomastia [due to elevated β-human chorionic gonadotropin (β-HCG)], supraclavicular lymphadenopathy, superior vena cava syndrome (due to mediastinal disease), urinary obstruction, dyspnea and hemoptysis (secondary to extensive pulmonary metastases), and headaches or seizures (due to brain metastases) or bone pain (due to bone metastases).

DIFFERENTIAL DIAGNOSIS

- Epididymitis (may coexist with germ cell tumors)
- Hydrocele, varicocele, spermatocele, or orchitis
- Lymphoma
- Leukemia
- Metastasis from prostate cancer, melanoma, and lung cancer
- Tuberculosis, gumma, or other infections.

DIAGNOSTIC

Goals

- Any testicular mass requires prompt evaluation to exclude testicular carcinoma.
- Testicular cancer is highly curable (85% of cases).
- Histologic determination of tumor type and stage have prognostic and therapeutic significance.

Evaluation

The diagnostic workup for testicular carcinoma is outlined in Fig. 16.1.

Imaging

- **Ultrasound:** Ultrasound detects the presence of testicular parenchymal abnormality in the ipsilateral as well as the contralateral testes.
- **Radiographic studies:** Standard two-view chest radiograph rules out pulmonary metastases.
- **Computerized tomography (CT):** CT scans of chest, abdomen, and pelvis establish the extent of disease dissemination.
- **Magnetic resonance imaging (MRI):** MRI is used especially when results of the physical examination and testicular ultrasound are equivocal. Brain MRI in the setting of central nervous system (CNS) symptoms suggestive of brain metastases (e.g. headache, neurological deficit, seizure).
- **Positron emission tomography (PET) scan:** The exact role for PET scan in the diagnostic and follow-up process in germ cell tumors is evolving.

Laboratory

Serum α-Fetoprotein

- Serum α-fetoprotein (AFP) has a half-life of approximately 5 to 7 days.
- It is commonly excreted by embryonal cell cancers or yolk sac elements.
- It is not produced by pure seminoma, and its detection implies the presence of nonseminomatous elements (primary or metastatic site).

Serum β-Human Chorionic Gonadotropin

- The half-life of β-HCG is approximately 24 hours.
- It may be biologically active, causing enhanced estrogen production by the testes and consequent gynecomastia.

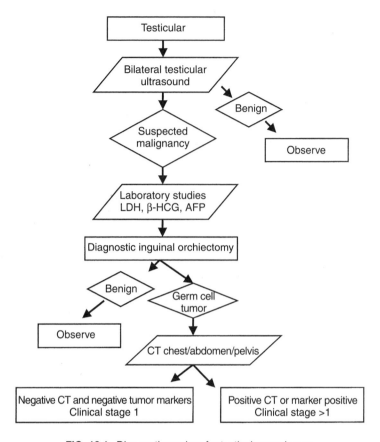

FIG. 16.1. Diagnostic workup for testicular carcinoma.

- It is secreted by syncytiotrophoblastic giant cells and chorionic elements.
- It is present in choriocarcinomas.
- It may occasionally be modestly elevated in pure seminomas.

Serum Lactate Dehydrogenase

- Serum lactate dehydrogenase (LDH) is a nonspecific tumor marker but is independently useful as a prognostic factor.
- It can reflect tumor burden and growth rate.

PATHOLOGIC EVALUATION

High inguinal orchiectomy with complete removal of the testis and spermatic cord through the inguinal ring is the procedure of choice for pathologic evaluation of suspected testicular tumors. Transcrotal testicular biopsy is not recommended because of concerns about local and nodal dissemination of tumor, although empirical evidence supporting this notion is weak.

- Germ cell tumors display an array of histopathology (see Table 16.1).
- Placental alkaline phosphatase (PLAP)–positive midline tumors of uncertain histogenesis, which are negative for low–molecular-weight keratins on immunohistochemical study, are

TABLE 16.1. *Histopathologic characteristics of germ cell tumors*

Tumor type	Pathologic feature
Germ cell tumors (95%)	**Seminomas** (40%–50%)
Single cell-type tumors (60%)	Primordial germ cell
Combination tumors (40%)	**Nonseminomas** (50%–60%)
	Embryonal cell tumors
	Yolk sac tumors
	Teratomas
	Choriocarcinomas
Tumors of gonadal stroma (1%–2%)	Leydig cell
	Sertoli cell
	Primitive gonadal structures
Gonadoblastoma (1%)	Germinal cell + stromal cell

suggestive of seminomas. Those tumors that express low–molecular-weight keratins are usually embryonal carcinomas.

- Germ cell tumors usually are hyperdiploid.
- Loss of heterozygosity is often demonstrated in early stage disease and is not associated with progression of disease.
- Eighty percent of cases have an isochromosome of the short arm of chromosome 12 [i(12p)], implicating one or more genes on 12p in the malignant transformation of primordial germ cells.

STAGING

Tables 16.2 and 16.3 contain thetumor–node–metastasis (TNM) classification and staging criteria of the American Joint Committee for Cancer (AJCC).

PROGNOSIS

Table 16.4 outlines the international consensus risk classification for germ cell tumors, and Table 16.5 discusses the expected survival.

THERAPY

Treatment Modalities According to Histology and Stage

Testicular cancer is highly treatable and can be broadly divided into seminoma and nonseminoma types (see Figs. 16.1 to 16.5). Seminomas are better cured by both radiation and chemotherapy (see Table 16.6). For patients with seminoma (all stages combined), the cure rate exceeds 90%. For those patients with low-stage disease, the cure rate approaches 100%. The management of tumors that contain a mixture of seminoma and nonseminoma components should be the same as that of nonseminomas. Tumors that appear to have a seminoma histology with elevated serum levels of AFP should be treated as nonseminomas. Elevation of only the β subunit of HCG is found in approximately 10% of patients with pure seminoma. Patients with brain metastasis should receive whole brain radiotherapy in addition to chemotherapy.

- A randomized study has shown similar overall survival and time-to-treatment failure results for BEP (bleomycin, etoposide, and cisplatin) and PVB (cisplatin, vinblastine, and bleomycin) regimens. Another randomized study has shown similar results for BEP and VIP (etoposide, ifosfamide, and cisplatin) regimens.
- BEP causes fewer instances of paresthesias, abdominal cramps, and myalgias than does PVB.

TABLE 16.2. *American Joint Committee on Cancer (AJCC) TNM classification and staging*

Primary tumor (pT)   (The extent of primary tumor is classified after radical orchiectomy)

pTX: Primary tumor cannot be assessed (if no radical orchiectomy has been performed)

pT0: No evidence of primary tumor (e.g., histologic scar in testis)

pTis: Intratubular germ cell neoplasia (carcinoma *in situ*)

pT1: Tumor limited to testis and epididymis without lymphatic or vascular invasion; tumor may invade into the tunica albuginea but not the tunica vaginalis testis

pT2: Tumor limited to testis and epididymis with vascular or lymphatic invasion, or tumor extending through the tunica albuginea with involvement of the tunica vaginalis testis

pT3: Tumor invades the spermatic cord with or without vascular or lymphatic invasion

pT4: Tumor invades the scrotum with or without vascular or lymphatic invasion

Regional lymph nodes (N)

NX: Regional lymph nodes cannot be assessed

N0: No regional lymph node metastasis

N1: Metastasis in a single lymph node, ≤2 cm in greatest dimension, or multiple lymph nodes, none >2 cm in greatest dimension

N2: Metastasis in a single lymph node, >2 cm but ≤5 cm in greatest dimension; or multiple lymph nodes, any one mass >2 cm but none >5 cm in greatest dimension

N3: Metastasis in a lymph node >5 cm in greatest dimension

Pathologic lymph nodes (pN)

pNX: Regional lymph nodes can not be assessed

pN0: No regional lymph node metastasis

pN1: Metastasis with a lymph node mass 2 cm or less in greatest dimension and ≤5 nodes positive, none >2 cm in greatest dimension

pN2: Metastasis with a lymph node mass >2 cm but not >5 cm in greatest dimension; or more than 5 nodes positive, none >5 cm; or evidence of extra nodal extension of tumor

pN3: Metastasis with a lymph node more than 5 cm in greatest dimension

Distant metastasis (M)

MX: Presence of distant metastasis cannot be assessed

M0: No distant metastasis

M1: Distant metastasis

M1a: Nonregional nodal or pulmonary metastasis

M1b: Distant metastasis other than to nonregional nodes and lungs

Serum tumor markers (S)

	LDH		β-HCG (mIU/mL)		AFP (ng/mL)
SX	Marker studies not available or not performed				
S0	NL		NL		NL
S1	<1.5 × ULN	and	<5,000	and	<1,000
S2	1.5–10 × ULN	or	5,000–50,000	or	1,000–10,000
S3	>10 × ULN	or	>50,000	or	>10,000

LDH, lactate dehydrogenase; HCG, human chorionic gonadotropin; AFP, α-fetoprotein; NL, normal limits; ULN, upper limit of normal.

• VIP has more hematologic (myelosuppressive) toxicity than BEP.
• A randomized study showed that four cycles of EP (etoposide and cisplatin) were equivalent to three cycles of BEP in patients with good- and intermediate-risk disease. However, four cycles of BEP is the standard of care for initial treatment of poor-risk disease.

TABLE 16.3. *American Joint Committee for Cancer stage groupings*

Stage 0	pTis N0 M0 S0
Stage I	pT1–4 N0 M0 SX
Stage IA	pT1 N0 M0 S0
Stage IB	pT2–4 N0 M0 S0
Stage IS	Any pT/Tx N0 M0 S1–3
Stage II	Any pT/Tx N1–3 M0 SX
Stage IIA	Any pT/Tx N1 M0 S0–1
Stage IIB	Any pT/Tx N2 M0 S0–1
Stage IIC	Any pT/Tx N3 M0 S0–1
Stage III	Any pT/Tx any N M1 SX
Stage IIIA	Any pT/Tx any N M1a S0–1
Stage IIIB	Any pT/Tx N1–3 M0 S2
	Any pT/Tx any N M1a S2
Stage IIIC	Any pT/Tx N1–3 M0 S3
	Any pT/Tx any N M1a S3
	Any pT/Tx any N M1b any S

TABLE 16.4. *International Consensus Risk Classification for germ cell tumors*

Prognosis	Nonseminoma	Seminoma
Good	Testis/retroperitoneal primary and no nonpulmonary visceral metastases and AFP <1,000 μg/mL HCG <5,000 IU/L (1,000 μg/mL) LDH <1.5 × ULN	Any primary site and no nonpulmonary visceral metastases and AFP <1,000 μg/mL, any concentration of HCG any concentration of LDH
Intermediate	Testis/retroperitoneal primary and no nonpulmonary visceral metastases and AFP ≥1,000 and ≤10,000 μg/mL or HCG ≥5,000 IU/L and ≤50,000 IU/L or LDH ≥1.5 × NL and ≤10 × NL	Any primary site and nonpulmonary visceral metastases and AFP <1,000 μg/mL Any concentration of HCG Any concentration of LDH
Poor	Mediastinal primary or nonpulmonary visceral metastases or AFP >10,000 μg/mL or HCG >50,000 IU/L (10,000 μg/mL) or >10 × ULN	None of the patients are classified as poor prognosis

AFP, α-fetoprotein; HCG, human chorionic gonadotropin; LDH, lactate dehydrogenase; ULN, upper limit of normal; NL, normal limit.

TABLE 16.5. *Expected survival*

	5-yr progression-free survival (%)		5-yr overall survival (%)	
Prognosis	Seminoma	Nonseminoma	Seminoma	Nonseminoma
Good	82	89	86	92
Intermediate	67	75	72	80
Poor[a]	—	41	—	48

[a]There is no poor prognosis category for seminoma.

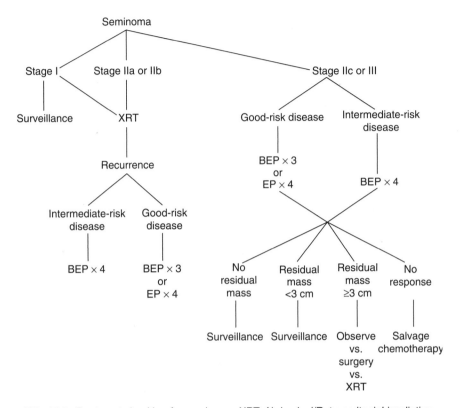

FIG. 16.2. Treatment algorithm for seminoma. XRT, Abdominal/Retroperitenial irradiation.

Follow-up

Appropriate surveillance of patients with testicular cancer is essential and should be determined by the tumor's histology, stage, and treatment (see Tables 16.7 and 16.8).

Salvage Therapy

- Salvage therapy is usually given to patients who fail to achieve an initial complete response.
- VIP is commonly used as an initial salvage therapy.
- High-dose chemotherapy with autologous bone marrow or peripheral stem cell support is investigational and may represent a therapeutic option for selected patients.

Therapy-related Toxicity

Fertility

- Approximately 25% of patients have oligospermia or sperm abnormalities before therapy.
- Almost all patients become oligospermic during chemotherapy.
- Sperm banking should be recommended for all patients desiring to father children after therapy; however, many patients recover sperm production after completion of therapy and can father children.
- Children of treated patients do not appear to have an increased risk of congenital malformations.

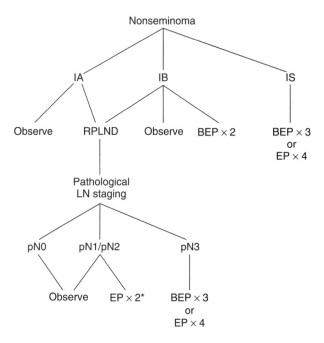

FIG. 16.3. Treatment algorithm for nonseminoma: stages IA, IB, and IS. *Some would give BEP × 2.

Pulmonary Toxicity

- Pulmonary toxicity is associated with bleomycin.
- The toxicities are rarely fatal when total cumulative doses of bleomycin are less than 400 units.
- Bleomycin should be discontinued if early signs of pulmonary toxicity develop.
- Asymptomatic decreases in pulmonary function are frequent and are usually reversible after the completion of chemotherapy.
- Routine use of pulmonary function tests (PFTs) [e.g., diffusing capacity of lung for carbon monoxide (DLCO)] is rarely indicated and should be reserved for patients with signs and symptoms of pulmonary toxicity (e.g., dry rales on physical examination and shortness of breath or dyspnea on exertion).
- Patients should be questioned about their smoking history and current smokers should be encouraged to stop.
- If deemed medically necessary, supplemental oxygen should be used with caution by minimizing exposure and by using low fraction of inspired oxygen (F_{IO_2}) settings.
- If fluids are indicated, i.v. colloids rather than crystalloids are preferred.

Nephrotoxicity

- Minor decreases in creatinine clearance can occur with platinum-based regimens, but these appear to remain stable in the long term without clinically significant deterioration.

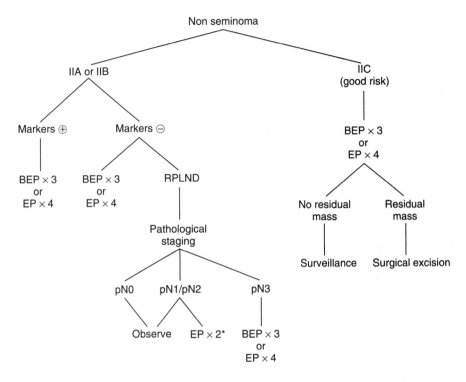

FIG. 16.4. Treatment algorithm for nonseminoma: stages IIA, IIB, and IIC (high-risk disease). *Some would give BEP × 2.

Neurologic

- Hearing deficits occur with cisplatin-based regimens, but they generally occur at sound frequencies higher than the range of conversational tones; for most patients, routine monitoring for hearing deficit is not indicated, and use of hearing aids after therapy is rarely needed.

Cardiovascular

Cardiovascular events include:

- Angina, myocardial infarction, and sudden cardiac death
- Hypertension
- Raynaud phenomenon
- Hypercholesterolemia.

Secondary Malignancies

- Secondary malignancies are associated with use of alkylating agents (e.g., cisplatin), etoposide, and radiation.

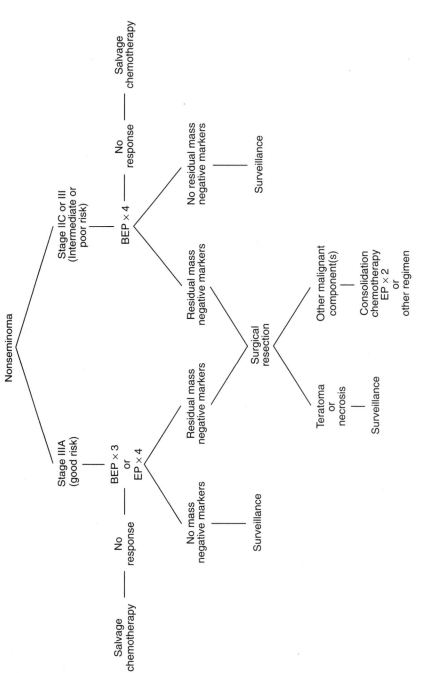

FIG. 16.5. Treatment algorithm for nonseminoma: stages IIC (intermediate and poor-risk disease) and III.

TABLE 16.6. *Commonly used chemotherapeutic regimens*

BEP	Bleomycin, 30 units i.v. weekly on days 2, 9, and 16	Two to four cycles
	Etoposide, 100 mg/m^2 i.v. daily $\times$ 5 d	administered
	Cisplatin, 20 mg/m^2 i.v. daily $\times$ 5 d	at 21-d intervals
EP	Etoposide, 100 mg/m^2 i.v. daily $\times$ 5 d	Four cycles administered
	Cisplatin, 20 mg/m^2 i.v. daily $\times$ 5 d	at 21-d intervals
VIP	VePesid (etoposide) 75 mg/m^2 i.v. daily $\times$ 5 d	
	Ifosfamide 1.2 g/m^2 i.v. daily $\times$ 5 d	
	Platinol (cisplatin) 20 mg/m^2 i.v. daily $\times$ 5 d	
	Mesna 400 mg i.v. bolus prior to first ifosfamide dose then 1.2 g/m^2 i.v. infused continuously daily for 5 d	
VeIP	Vinblastine, 0.11 mg/kg wk 1 and 2	Three to four cycles
	Ifosfamide, 1.2 g/m^2 i.v. daily $\times$ 5 d	administered
	Mesna 400 mg i.v. bolus prior to first ifosfamide dose then	at 21-d intervals
	1.2 g/m^2 i.v. infused continuously daily for 5 d,	
	Cisplatin, 20 mg/m^2 i.v. daily $\times$ 5 d	
PVB	Cisplatin, 20 mg/m^2 i.v. daily $\times$ 5 d	Three cycles administered
	Vinblastine, 0.11 mg/kg wk 1 and 2	at 21-d intervals
	Bleomycin, 30 units i.v. weekly on d 2, 9, 16	

TABLE 16.7. *Surveillance for seminoma[a]*

(a) Stage IA, IB, IS (postradiation)

Yr	H & P, CXR, markers (monthly interval)	ABD/pelvic CT (monthly interval)
1	3	12
2	4	12
3–5	6	12 (only 3rd yr)

(b) Stage IIA, IIB (postradiation) or stage IIC, III (postchemotherapy)

Yr	H & P, CXR, markers (monthly interval)	ABD/pelvic CT
1	2	After fourth mo and every 3 mo until stable
2	3	
3	4	
4	6	
5+	12	

H&P, history and physical; CXR, chest x-ray; ABD, abdomen.
[a]These are National Comprehensive Cancer Network (NCCN) guidelines. However, there is considerable interinstitutional variation in the standard of follow-up care, with little evidence that different schedules lead to different outcomes.

TABLE 16.8. *Surveillance for nonseminoma[a]*

(a) Observation/surveillance for stage IA, IB nonseminoma

Yr	H & P, CXR, markers (monthly interval)	ABD/pelvic CT (monthly interval)
1	1–2	3–4
2	2	3–4
3	3	4
4	4	6
5	6	12
6+	12	12

(b) Surveillance after complete response to chemotherapy and/or retroperitoneal lymph node dissection (RPLND) in nonseminoma

Yr	H & P, CXR, markers (monthly interval)	ABD/pelvic CT (monthly interval)
1	1–2	6
2	2	6
3	3	12
4	4	12
5	6	12
6+	12	12

H&P, history and physical; CXR, chest x-ray; ABD, abdomen.
[a]These are National Comprehensive Cancer Network (NCCN) guidelines. However, there is considerable interinstitutional variation in the standard of follow-up care, with little evidence that different schedules lead to different outcomes.

- Secondary leukemias are primarily of myeloid lineage and are associated with etoposide-containing regimens; these are often characterized by an 11q23 translocation and usually occur within several years after therapy.
- Cancers of the stomach, the bladder, and possibly the pancreas are associated with radiation therapy, which is often used in the management of pure seminomatous germ cell cancers; these are often limited to the radiation portal and may have a latency period of a decade or more.

SUGGESTED READINGS

American Cancer Society. *Cancer facts and figures 2003.* Atlanta, GA: American Cancer Society, 2003.
Baniel J, Foster RS, Gonin R, et al. Late relapse of testicular cancer. *J Clin Oncol* 1995;13:1170–1176.
Bosl GJ, Chaganti RSK. The use of tumor-markers in germ-cell malignancies. *Hematol Oncol Clin North Am* 1994;8:573–587.
Bosl GJ, Motzer RJ. Testicular germ-cell cancer. *N Engl J Med* 1997;337:242–253.
Bosl GJ, Steinfeld J, Barjorin DF, et al. Cancer of the testis. In: DeVita VT, Hellman S, Rosenberg SA, eds. *Cancer: principles and practice of oncology,* 5th ed. Philadelphia, PA: Lippincott–Raven Publishers, 1997:1397–1425.
Einhorn LH. Testicular cancer: an oncological success story. *Clin Cancer Res* 1997;3:2630–2632.
Einhorn LH, Donohue JP. Advanced testicular cancer: update for urologists. *J Urol* 1998;160:1964–1969.
Fox EP, Loehrer PJ. Chemotherapy for advanced testicular cancer. *Hematol Oncol Clin North Am* 1991;5:1173–1187.

Harland SJ, Cook PA, Fossa SD, et al. Intratubular germ cell neoplasia of the contralateral testis in testicular cancer: defining a high risk group. *J Urol* 1998;160:1353–1357.

Huddart RA, Norman A, Shahidi M, et al. Cardiovascular disease as a long-term complication of treatment for testicular cancer. *J Clin Oncol* 2003;21:1513–1523.

Lehne G, Johansen B, Fossa SD. Long-term follow-up of pulmonary function in patients cured from testicular cancer with combination chemotherapy including bleomycin. *Br J Cancer* 1993;68:555–558.

Mead GM. Testicular cancer: staging, treatment and outcome. *Eur J Cancer* 1997;33:6.

Mead GM, Stenning SP, Cook P, et al. International germ cell consensus classification: a prognostic factor-erased staging system for metastatic germ cell cancers. *J Clin Oncol* 1997;15:594–603.

Miller KD, Loehrer PJ, Gonin R, et al. Chemotherapy with vinblastine, ifosfamide, and cisplatin in recurrent seminoma. *J Clin Oncol* 1997;15:1427–1431.

Murty VS, Bosl GJ, Houldsworth J, et al. Allelic loss and somatic differentiation in human male germ-cell tumors. *Oncogene* 1994;9:2245–2251.

Osanto S, Bukman A, Vanhoek F, et al. Long-term effects of chemotherapy in patients with testicular cancer. *J Clin Oncol* 1992;10:574–579.

Stephenson WT, Poirier SM, Rubin L, et al. Evaluation of reproductive capacity in germ-cell tumor patients following treatment with cisplatin, etoposide, and bleomycin. *J Clin Oncol* 1995;13:2278–2280.

Travis LB, Curtis RE, Storm H, et al. Risk of second malignant neoplasms among long-term survivors of testicular cancer. *J Natl Cancer Inst* 1997;89:1429–1439.

Vanbasten JP, Koops HS, Sleijfer DT, et al. Current concepts about testicular cancer. *Eur J Surg Oncol* 1997;23:354–360.

SECTION 6

Gynecologic

17

Ovarian Cancer

Eddie Reed* and Ramin Altaha[†]

*Mary Babb Randolph Cancer Center, Robert C. Byrd Health Sciences Center, West Virginia University, Morgantown, West Virginia; [†]Section of Hematology/Oncology, Robert C. Byrd Health Sciences Center, West Virginia University, Morgantown, West Virginia

Ovarian cancer is divided into three broad histologic categories: epithelial carcinomas, germ cell tumors, and stromal cell tumors. Approximately 90% of all cases of ovarian cancer are of the epithelial variety. This chapter is devoted to epithelial ovarian carcinoma, except for the section on fallopian tube carcinoma and extraovarian peritoneal carcinoma. The number of estimated new cases of ovarian cancer in 2003 was 25,400 in the United States, the estimated number of deaths from this disease totaled 14,300. Ovarian cancer represents approximately 25% of the total number of cancer cases involving the female genital tract. However, unlike cervical cancer or endometrial cancer, the most ovarian cancer cases present as stage III or stage IV. The overall survival rate had improved from approximately 35% in the 1970s, to more than 50% in the 1990s. This decrease is believed to have resulted from the introduction of platinum-based therapy for management of this disease. Further improvements in survival have been observed with the introduction of paclitaxel and other agents that have been recently approved for use in this disease by the U.S. Food and Drug Administration (FDA). Some reports suggest that the introduction of cisplatin and carboplatin into chemotherapeutic regimens not only resulted in improved survival statistics but may also be associated with emerging patterns of metastatic spread suggestive of more aggressive disease.

TUMOR MARKERS

The best tumor marker for this disease is CA125. CA125 is a high–molecular-weight glycoprotein that is elevated in up to 50% of stage I tumors and elevated in 80% to 90% of stage II, III, or IV tumors. Minor elevations in CA125 levels are not specific for ovarian cancer and can be seen in endometriosis, benign tumors, fibroids, and in pregnant or postpartum women. In addition, moderate elevations in CA125 levels can be seen in other adenocarcinomas such as breast cancer and endometrial cancer. However, CA125 levels greater than 2,000, with the appropriate clinical history, should be considered to represent epithelial ovarian cancer until proved otherwise.

Once the diagnosis of ovarian cancer has been made, CA125 is useful in following the disease. It is a useful surrogate for tumor response but does not predict complete response. A persistently rising CA125 following disease response is representative of tumor recurrence. Some reports suggest that CA125 plus transvaginal ultrasound may be effective in screening for previously undiagnosed disease. Other biochemical entities have been suggested as possible markers for previously undiagnosed ovarian cancer. They include OVX-1, lysophosphatidic acid, and an advanced proteomic analysis method performed on patient plasma.

SCREENING

The National Cancer Institute (NCI) recommends screening for ovarian cancer in women with known genetic syndromes associated with this disease and for women with a particularly strong family history of the disease regardless of the presence of a recognized genetic syndrome. A recent study randomized 20,000 women without a family history of ovarian cancer to screening and to no screening. CA125 was the first screening test, followed by ultrasound for patients with an elevated CA125. There was no difference between the two groups in the ability to detect early stage disease nor was there any difference in the number of deaths from ovarian cancer. Therefore, routine screening of women without a family history of ovarian cancer is not recommended.

RISK FACTORS AND PREVENTION

Ovarian cancer risk increases with age and with a family history of ovarian cancer. Although most cases of ovarian cancer occur in women without any known risk factors, there are several genetic syndromes that are strongly associated with this disease. These syndromes include the hereditary breast and ovarian cancer syndromes associated with BRCA1 and BRCA2 and with the hereditary nonpolyposis colorectal cancer syndrome (Lynch II syndrome). In each of these genetic syndromes, variable penetrance has been observed.

Recent studies show that prophylactic total abdominal hysterectomy and bilateral salpingo-oophorectomy (TAH/BSO), can be effective in reducing the predicted occurrence of ovarian cancer in women with BRCA1 or BRCA2 mutations. In addition, studies suggest that oral contraceptives may have a preventive effect on this disease, which appears to increase with the duration of contraceptive use. It should be noted that the newer, low-estrogen formulations have not yet proved to have the same protective effect. Other maneuvers that are associated with a reduction in the number of ovulations (i.e., pregnancy, nursing after pregnancy, etc.) appear to have protective effects as well.

PATHOLOGY

Epithelial histologies account for about 90% of all ovarian cancers. These include the histologies of serous, mucinous, endometrioid, transitional, and clear cells. Among these cell types, clear cell appears to have a consistently worse prognosis. Tumors of low malignant potential (borderline tumors) may exist within each of the above five histologic types. Mixed Müllerian tumor is probably of epithelial origin and is also associated with clinical resistance to therapy.

Generally, any of the aforementioned tumor histologies may be well differentiated, moderately differentiated, or poorly differentiated. Clinical prognosis worsens with poorly differentiated cells. Rarely, a tumor may clearly be an ovarian cancer but may be sufficiently undifferentiated so that it cannot be assigned to any of the six cell types noted.

The germ cell tumors are classified as dysgerminoma, endodermal sinus tumor, malignant teratoma, embryonal carcinoma, or primary choriocarcinoma. Stromal tumors are mesenchymal in origin and consist of granulosa tumors or Sertoli-Leydig cell tumors.

DIAGNOSIS AND WORKUP

Clinically, the nature of the three broad classes of tumors is directly related to the clinical presenting symptoms of the disease. Tumors of epithelial histology tend to present in the advanced stage (i.e., III or IV) and are associated with abdominal discomfort, low back pain, bloating, and abdominal distension. Germ cell tumors tend to behave clinically in a manner similar to that of germ cell tumors in men. Sertoli-Leydig cell tumors produce virilization in affected individuals. Granulosa cell tumors may cause precocious puberty in premenarchal women, amenorrhea in women of reproductive age, and vaginal bleeding in postmenopausal women.

A small percentage of women of reproductive age in whom surgery is performed for a pelvic mass will have a malignant tumor, with the likelihood of the malignancy increasing with age. Approximately 50% of the postmenopausal women in whom surgery is performed for a pelvic mass will have a malignant neoplasm. Preoperative workup of a patient suspected to have an ovarian mass may include any or all of the following: blood chemistries, liver function tests (LFTs), renal function tests, complete blood counts (CBCs), ultrasonography, CA125, computerized tomography (CT) scan of the abdomen and pelvis, α-fetoprotein, and β-human chorionic gonadotropin (β-HCG). Additional studies may be performed, as appropriate. A summary of the suggested preoperative workup is given in Table 17.1.

Surgery should be performed by a gynecologic oncologist or a surgical oncologist—preferably the former. The Gynecologic Oncology Group (GOG) has defined the appropriate surgical procedure for ovarian cancer and has insisted that surgical protocol should be followed in every patient undergoing surgery for this disease. The prognostic importance of maximal surgical debulking has been demonstrated in multiple studies over the last 4 decades.

Favorable prognostic factors include younger age at the time of diagnosis (younger than 65 years), good performance status, cell type other than clear cell, stage I or II disease, well-differentiated tumor, diploid tumors, no overexpression of HER2, low vascular endothelial growth factor (VEGF) expression, and optimal tumor debulking during surgery to <1 cm for any single lesion. Patients with germline mutations of BRCA1 may have better survival after chemotherapy. Unfavorable prognostic factors include clear cell histology, high tumor grade, increased VEGF or other markers of increased angiogenesis, elevated postoperative CA125 level, stage III or IV disease, residual tumor masses >3 cm after surgery, and aneuploidy.

STAGING

Ovarian cancer may exist in stage I, II, III, or IV. This determination can be made only after appropriate abdominopelvic surgery. Stage IV disease can sometimes be diagnosed without invasion of the abdominopelvic space. However, recent studies show that tumor debulking favorably affects prognosis, even in stage IV disease. Current Federation Internationale de Gynecogie et d'Obstetrique (FIGO) staging criteria are listed in Table 17.2.

Stage I disease is confined to one or both ovaries. Malignant ascites, but no implants, may be present on the abdominopelvic wall. Stage II involves one or both ovaries, with extension to the pelvic viscera. As in the case of stage I disease, there may be malignant ascites, but no implants on the abdominopelvic wall. Stage III disease is associated with implants on the abdominopelvic wall or the serosal surface of the liver or involves the small bowel or omentum.

TABLE 17.1. *The workup for patients suspected of having an ovarian malignancy*

Personal and family history and physical examination
Liver function tests, BUN, creatinine, LDH
CBC with platelets, PT, PTT, INR
Tumor markers (CA125, AFP, and β-HCG)
CT scan of abdomen and pelvis, and CXR. CT of chest if CXR is abnormal.
Radiographic tests of unclear utility: MRI of abdomen and pelvis, PET scan

BUN, blood urea nitrogen; LDH, lactate dehydrogenase; CBC, complete blood count; PT, prothrombin time; PTT, partial thromboplastin time; INR, international normalized ratio; AFP, α-fetoprotein; HCG, human chorionic gonadotropin; CT, computerized tomography; CXR, chest x-ray; MRI, magnetic resonance imaging; PET, positron emission tomography.
　Consider possible abnormal hormone secretion syndromes.
　Consider possible concurrent malignancies from other sites.
　Consider possible metastases to the ovary, from other sites (breast, colon, etc.).

TABLE 17.2. *Federation Internationale de Gynecogie et d'Obstetrique (FIGO) staging of ovarian cancer*

Stage I	**Growth limited to one or both ovaries**
IA	Growth limited to one ovary; no ascites; no tumor on the external surfaces; capsule intact
IB	Growth limited to both ovaries; no ascites; no tumor on the external surfaces; capsule intact
IC	Tumor either stage IA or IB but with tumor on the surface of one or both ovaries; capsule ruptured; ascites present containing malignant cells; or positive peritoneal washings
Stage II	**Growth involving one or both ovaries with pelvic extension**
IIA	Extension and/or metastases to the uterus and/or fallopian tubes
IIB	Extension to other pelvic organs
IIC	Tumor either stage IIA or IIB but with tumor on the surface of one or both ovaries; capsule(s) ruptured; ascites present containing malignant cells; or positive peritoneal washings
Stage III	**Tumor involving one or both ovaries with peritoneal implants outside the pelvis and/or positive retroperitoneal or inguinal nodes: metastases to the surface of the liver equals stage III; tumor is limited to the true pelvis but with histologically verified malignant extension to the small bowel or omentum**
IIIA	Tumor grossly limited to the true pelvis with negative nodes but with histologically confirmed microscopic seeding of abdominal peritoneal surfaces
IIIB	Tumor of one or both ovaries; histologically confirmed implants of abdominal peritoneal surfaces, none >2 cm in diameter; node negative
IIIC	Abdominal implants >2 cm in diameter and/or positive retroperitoneal or inguinal nodes
Stage IV	**Growth involving one or both ovaries and with distant metastases; if pleural effusion is present, there must be positive cytologic test results to allot a case to stage IV; parenchymal liver metastasis equals stage IV**

Stage IV disease shows metastasis to parenchymal liver, lung, the pleural cavity, or other demonstrated metastases outside the abdominopelvic space.

TREATMENT OF OVARIAN CANCER

Surgery

Upon initial presentation, surgery is the primary tool in the treatment and staging of the disease. When surgeons follow the specific surgical protocol designed by the GOG, the disease can be definitively staged. Stage I disease with favorable prognostic features can be treated by surgery alone. Stage II disease with favorable prognostic features can be treated by surgery followed by a limited course of platinum-based chemotherapy (three to four cycles). For the initial presentation of the disease, all other settings of ovarian cancer of epithelial histology require appropriate surgery followed by at least six cycles of paclitaxel and carboplatin. Currently, there is debate over the potential value of following this regimen with two or more additional cycles of paclitaxel as a single agent.

The primary goal of ovarian cancer surgery is to remove all visible disease, if possible. Retrospective analyses show that patients with no visible disease after surgery, as a group, show significant recovery, followed by patients with visible disease of <1 cm, and then by patients with 2 to 3 cm disease, and finally by patients with bulky residual disease. This underscores the importance of the surgery being performed by a skilled, experienced individual. There are subsets of patients who appear to benefit from "interval debulking," and patients who benefit from "secondary debulking." Detailed discussion of these considerations is beyond the scope of this chapter.

Second-look laparotomy is no longer commonly used in this disease. Second-look laparoscopy is frequently used to assess the success of systemic chemotherapy. The purpose of either procedure is to determine whether the active disease continues to exist in the abdominopelvic space, and, if so, how extensive that disease might be. A second-look procedure should be utilized if clinical decision making will be influenced by this approach. If not, one should question the wisdom of exposing a patient to the surgical risk, however small that risk might be.

In tumors of low malignant potential, surgery may be the only treatment modality used for some individuals. In some cases, the disease may grow very slowly after the initial debulking procedure, thereby necessitating repeat surgery (without intervening chemotherapy) many years later. With use of this approach, a patient can be spared the toxicity of systemic chemotherapy in a setting in which cure is not feasible.

For stromal cell tumors too, surgery can be the only treatment approach for some individuals. However, chemotherapy with etoposide and carboplatin (with or without doxorubicin) may be required for persons with poor prognostic features.

x-Irradiation

There is a strong indication in the literature that external beam radiation therapy is clinically active in ovarian cancer. This is true for all stages of disease. However, this approach is used more extensively in Canada and Europe than in the United States. External beam radiation therapy appears to be potentially curative in early stage disease in some subsets of patients. However, long-term toxicity from x-irradiation tends to limit treatment options in patients who may have disease recurrence later on. Intraperitoneal P 32 was in common use several decades ago but is not routinely used presently.

External beam x-irradiation is useful for several manifestations of this illness. Metastases to the brain, although uncommon, are no longer considered rare. Gamma-knife approaches, IMRT (intensity modulated radiation therapy), and standard whole brain XRT (radiotherapy), are all effective in controlling metastatic disease. The use of any one of the approaches will depend on the clinical setting and the technology available. On occasion, large lesions in the pelvis or metastases to bone (unusual) will respond readily to XRT.

Chemotherapy for the Initial Disease Presentation

The following treatments are the standards of care for stage III or stage IV disease. After appropriate surgery, six cycles of carboplatin should be administered at an area under the exposure-time curve (AUC) of 5 or 6; with paclitaxel at 175 mg per m^2 given every 21 days. Current studies are investigating other approaches to the treatment of the initial presentation of advanced stage disease. Those approaches include neoadjuvant chemotherapy with surgical debulking after the first two to three cycles, the addition of two to four cycles of paclitaxel after the initial six chemotherapy treatments, other chemotherapy "doublets" for which there is demonstrated activity in this disease, and three-drug therapy for patients with a particularly poor prognosis (i.e., cisplatin, paclitaxel, and cytoxan). Several published regimens for the initial systemic therapy of this disease are given in Table 17.3.

On the basis of the current literature, each patient should be given an initial treatment regimen with platinum (carboplatin or cisplatin) and paclitaxel unless there is a specific medical reason to do otherwise (e.g., hypersensitivity to either drug). Generally, carboplatin is less toxic and better tolerated than cisplatin, and these two drugs show equal efficacy in this disease. Carboplatin dosing should be based on the Calvert formula for calculating AUC; milligram dosage of carboplatin = AUC $\times$ (GFR + 25), where GFR is glomerular filtration rate. At our institution, the carboplatin infusion is delivered over 1 hour and the paclitaxel infusion is delivered over 3 hours. Paclitaxel is always delivered first. For carboplatin and cisplatin, toxicity has been loosely correlated with the duration of the infusion, with shorter infusion times being associated with increased toxicities.

TABLE 17.3. *Chemotherapy regimens for the initial therapy of ovarian cancer*

Carboplatin plus paclitaxel	Standard therapy; should be considered first; Paclitaxel 175 mg/m^2/dose; one 3-hr i.v. infusion followed by carboplatin AUC = 5 or 6, one 1-hr i.v. infusion; repeat this regimen q21d for six cycles
Carboplatin plus cyclophosphamide	Should be considered in patients who are hypersensitive to paclitaxel; Carboplatin AUC = 5 or 6; or, carboplatin 400 mg/m^2/dose, one 1-hr i.v. infusion; cyclophosphamide 1,000 mg/m^2/dose; one 1-hr i.v. infusion; repeat this regimen q21d for six cycles
Doxorubicin plus cyclophosphamide	For consideration in patients who are hypersensitive to paclitaxel and platinum agents; Doxorubicin 40 mg/m^2/dose, one 1-hr i.v. infusion; Cyclophosphamide 1,000 mg/m^2/dose, one 1-hr i.v. infusion; Repeat this regimen q21d for six cycles
Cisplatin plus paclitaxel plus Cyclophosphamide	For consideration in poor prognosis patients as defined in Kohn EC, Sarosy G, Davis P, et al. *Gyn Oncol* 1996:62:181–191; Cyclophosphamide 750 mg/m^2/dose, one 1-hr i.v. infusion; Paclitaxel 250 mg/m^2/dose, one 24-hr i.v. infusion; Cisplatin 75 mg/m^2/dose, one 1-hr i.v. infusion; G-CSF 10 μg/kg/dose, s.c., daily $\times$ 8, starting the day after the cisplatin dose; Drugs given in this order; repeat q21–28 d depending on WBC recovery

AUC, area under the exposure-time curve; G-CSF, granulocyte colony stimulating factor; WBC, white blood cell.

Occasionally, patients will have hypersensitivity to paclitaxel and/or to platinum with the very first treatment doses. Several desensitization regimens have been published, and these generally meet with variable success. A regimen used in the past that might be considered in such patients is doxorubicin (or liposomal doxorubicin) plus cytoxan.

Chemotherapy for Recurrent or Persistent Disease

A number of agents have demonstrated substantial activity in recurrent and/or persistent ovarian cancer of epithelial histology. The more common currently used regimens include liposomal doxorubicin, topotecan, gemcitabine, taxotere, 5-fluorouracil, oral etoposide, weekly paclitaxel, tamoxifen, and hexamethylmelamine. These regimens are detailed in the Table 17.4. This list is not exhaustive. Although single agent therapy is usually recommended in the treatment of recurrent disease, one may chose to utilize any of the several published drug combinations.

The first step for patients with recurrent or persistent disease is to determine whether the patient's disease is platinum sensitive or platinum resistant. Generally, if a patient has persistent or progressive disease while receiving cisplatin- or carboplatin-based therapy, the disease should be considered platinum resistant. In addition, if the patient appears to respond but has disease recurrence or progression within 6 months of the most recent dose of platinum, the disease should be considered platinum resistant. If disease recurs more than 1 year after the most recent dose of platinum, the disease may be considered to be platinum sensitive. Data suggest that the likelihood of a second clinical response to retreatment with platinum is more than 70% in patients who have been given their last platinum dose more than 2 years prior to the retreatment. Furthermore, data suggest that this principle may hold true for paclitaxel in this disease.

Recurrent ovarian cancer is now considered a chronic disease by most medical and gynecologic oncologists. This is because this illness will usually respond to a series of different treatment regimens over time, commonly resulting in a 5- to 10-year time frame of disease persistence with

TABLE 17.4. *Chemotherapy regimens for the therapy of recurrent or persistent ovarian cancer*

Cisplatin or carboplatin	Use only for platinum-sensitive disease, as discussed in the text; Carboplatin AUC = 5 or 6 or carboplatin 400 mg/m^2/dose, one 1-hr i.v. infusion; q28 d
	Cisplatin 60 mg/m^2/dose or 75 mg/m^2/dose, one 1-hr i.v. infusion; q21–28d;
	Vigorous i.v. hydration is important with both drugs, and particularly so with cisplatin
5-Fluorouracil plus leucovorin	Leucovorin 500 mg/m^2/dose, i.v. over 30 min, followed 1 hr later by 5-FU at 375 mg/m^2/dose;
	i.v. bolus; repeat daily for five consecutive days; repeat this regimen q21–28d depending on WBC recovery; reduce to daily × 4, for grade >3 toxicity
Gemcitabine	1,000 mg/m^2/dose i.v. over 30 min, on d 1 and d 8; Repeat q21d depending on WBC recovery;
Hexamethylmelamine	Several different regimens are commonly used; 260 mg/m^2/day, PO, divided into 4 doses, after meals; each day for 14 consecutive d; then 7 or 14 d off; Repeat q21 or 28 d
Liposomal doxorubicin	40 mg/m^2 or 50 mg/m^2/dose, one 1-hr i.v. infusion; repeat q21 d
Oral etoposide (VP16)	Several different regimens are commonly used; 100 mg/dose, PO, daily, × 14 d, followed by 7 or 14 d off; repeat q21 or 28 d
Tamoxifen	20 mg/dose, PO, b.i.d, continuously
Taxotere	70 mg/m^2 or 80 mg/m^2/dose; one 1-hr i.v. infusion; repeat q21d
Topotecan	1.5 mg/m^2/dose; i.v., daily × 5; do not exceed 7.5 mg/m^2 total dose/cycle; Repeat q21d
Weekly paclitaxel	70 mg/m^2/dose or 80 mg/m^2/dose, one 1-hr i.v. infusion, weekly; 3 wk on, 1 wk off; Repeat q28d

WBC, white blood cell.

good quality of life. Accomplishing this, however, requires skillful utilization of currently accepted principles of clinical drug resistance and the treatment approaches used to counter drug resistance.

For example, a patient who receives initial therapy with carboplatin and paclitaxel may experience a clinical complete remission initially and exhibit disease recurrence several years later. In such instances, retreatment with carboplatin and paclitaxel would be appropriate. One can expect a likelihood of more than 70% that the disease will respond again. When the disease becomes platinum resistant, a non–cross-resistant medication such as liposomal doxorubicin must be used for treatment.

Once resistance develops to this new agent, the patient should be treated with an agent that is non–cross-resistant with any of the previous three medications, such as gemcitabine. The next regimen used might be topotecan, probably followed by oral VP16, and so on. With use of this type of approach, the disease can be controlled in some patients for several years, with acceptable toxicity and with good quality of life. For patients with disease recurrence but few or no symptoms, the use of tamoxifen at 20 mg PO b.i.d. should be considered. This can be done for biochemical recurrence of the CA125 only or for radiographic recurrence of disease without physical symptoms.

Common Toxicities from Treatment

Table 17.5 lists a range of toxicities that commonly occur with chemotherapy treatment regimens for ovarian cancer. With the exception of thrombocytopenia, the myelosuppression caused

TABLE 17.5. *Common toxicities from the treatment of epithelial ovarian cancer*

Myelosuppression	Associated with all the agents listed in this chapter, except tamoxifen
	All three lineages affected; persistent thrombocytopenia is associated with the platinum compounds
Nausea and vomiting	Preventive treatment is very important; delayed nausea and vomiting is very common
	Steroids, HT3 inhibitor, and substance P inhibitor all are recommended for routine use with platinum-containing regimens
Renal dysfunction	Seen with cisplatin and with carboplatin; usually more clinical significant with cisplatin
	Serum creatinine may be normal, in the face of a markedly reduced creatinine clearance; this is important because the use of other renally cleared drugs may be needed (antibiotics, etc.);
	Platinum-related renal insufficiency is nonoliguric; vigilance is required
Neurotoxicity	Clinically occurs before detectable changes on EMG/NCTs; stocking-and-glove distribution;
	Usually progressive with repeated platinum doses, and can become severe; cisplatin is more likely to cause this problem than carboplatin
Fatigue/weakness	May be related to anemia but is a frequent side effect of several newer agents including gemcitabine, topotecan, irofulven, and others
Altered sexual function	Common side effect; seldom discussed spontaneously by the patient; can be an underlying contributing factor to family disruption, and clinical reactive depression;
	Usually is a combined function of surgery, and effect of neuroactive anticancer agent (platinum, etc.)
Clinical depression	Common side effect; many patients will request a medication for this; sometimes a severe problem
Rare toxicities	Acute hypersensitivity to paclitaxel; acute hypersensitivity to cisplatin/carboplatin (usually after six–eight cycles of therapy, when it occurs);
	Desensitization is occasionally appropriate and can be successful. On most occasions, switch to another agent right away

by these regimens can be readily treated with currently approved cytokines, such as granulocyte colony stimulating factor (G-CSF) and erythropoietin. Nausea and vomiting should be approached in a preventative manner. Aggressive preventive antinausea therapy should be used for platinum-containing regimens. Once nausea and vomiting are well established in a patient, it is usually very difficult to control.

Renal dysfunction is frequently underestimated in patients who have received either cisplatin or carboplatin in the past. Substantial reductions in creatinine clearance can coexist with a normal blood urea nitrogen (BUN) and serum creatinine after substantial doses of either agent. Neurotoxicity is common, and mild, when currently accepted doses of carboplatin and/or paclitaxel are used. When severe neurotoxicity develops (grade 3 or greater), this can be very difficult to manage and tends to resolve slowly. Drug-induced fatigue (as opposed to anemia-related fatigue) is a frequently overlooked side effect and should be considered when symptoms develop.

Altered sexual function is a frequent, but not frequently discussed, clinical problem. This may contribute to family discord, and clinical depression, in some situations. This problem is currently understudied. Rare but severe side effects (using current treatment and supportive regimens) include hypersensitivity to paclitaxel and/or platinum compounds and acute leukemia.

Experimental Therapy

Generally, patients should be encouraged to participate in controlled clinical trials approved by the NCI and/or the FDA. Cooperative groups such as the GOG routinely conduct phase III trials for individuals who are diagnosed for the first time. It is through carefully performed clinical phase III trials that improvements on current treatment approaches can be made. For all patients beyond their initial diagnosis, efforts should be made to identify phase III or phase II clinical trials that are appropriate. Phase I clinical trials are reasonable treatment options for some patients.

Experimental therapies that are being tested, or have recently been tested, include gene therapy approaches, high-dose chemotherapy with bone marrow transplantation, antiangiogenesis therapies, immunotherapies, efforts to reverse resistance to standard drugs, novel combinations of drugs, and novel small molecules. Generally, high-dose chemotherapy with bone marrow transplantation is not currently recommended in this disease. In addition, intraperitoneal therapy, once considered to have great promise, is currently not in general use.

FALLOPIAN TUBE CARCINOMA AND EXTRAOVARIAN PERITONEAL CARCINOMA

These are two variants of adenocarcinoma that occur in women, which clinically behave and respond to therapy in a manner similar to epithelial ovarian cancer. The staging process is very similar to ovarian cancer for both malignancies, and the treatment approaches are identical, stage for stage.

SUPPORTIVE CARE

Among those clinical situations that may occur as a direct result of uncontrolled disease, bowel obstruction and urinary tract obstruction are the most troublesome. In the setting of the initial presentation of the illness, every effort should be made to surgically relieve this problem and should be immediately followed by systemic therapy. In recurrent or persistent disease, if there is a strong likelihood of clinical drug sensitivity, surgical remedy of either problem should again be attempted immediately.

As stated previously, nausea and vomiting should be treated preventively. Clinical depression can sometimes interfere with a patient's adherence to therapy and should be taken seriously. Participation of the patient in cancer support groups can sometimes be very helpful to the affected individual, and this can be of assistance to the health care provider.

SUGGESTED READINGS

Berek JS. Epithelial ovarian cancer. In: Berek JS, Hacker NF, eds. *Practical gynecologic oncology*, 3rd ed. Philadelphia, PA: Lippincott Williams & Wilkins, 2000:457–522.

Calvert AH, Newell DR, Gumbrell LA, et al. Carboplatin dosage; prospect of evaluation of a simple formula based on renal function. *J Clin Oncol* 1989;7:1748–1756.

Cornelison TL, Reed E. Nephrotoxicity and hydration management for cisplatin, carboplatin, and ormaplatin: a review. *Gynecol Oncol* 1993;50:147–158.

Hoskins WJ, McGuire WP, Brady MF, et al. The effect of diameter of largest residual disease on survival after primary cytoreductive surgery in patients with suboptimal residual epithelial ovarian carcinoma. *Am J Obstet Gynecol* 1994;170:974–979.

Jacobs I, Skates SJ, MacDonald N, et al. Screening for ovarian cancer: a pilot randomized controlled trial. *Lancet* 1999;353:1207–1210.

Kohn EC, Sarosy G, Davis P, et al. A phase I/II study of dose-intense paclitaxel with cisplatin and cyclophosphamide as initial therapy of poor-prognosis advanced-stage epithelial ovarian cancer. *Gynecol Oncol* 1996;62:181–191.

Link C, Bicher A, Kohn E, et al. Flexible G-CSF dosing in ovarian cancer patients receiving dose intense taxol therapy. *Blood* 1994;83:1188–1192.

McGuire WP, Hoskins WJ, Brady MF, et al. Taxol and cisplatin improve outcome in patients with advanced ovarian cancer as compared to cytoxan/cisplatin. *N Engl J Med* 1996;334:1–6.

Ozols RF, Bundy BN, Greer BE et al, Gynecologic Oncology Group. Phase III trial of carboplatin and paclitaxel compared with cisplatin and paclitaxel in patients with optimally resected stage III ovarian cancer: a Gynecologic Oncology Group study. *J Clin Oncol* 2003;21:3194–3200.

Ozols RF, Schwartz PE, Eifel PJ. Ovarian cancer, fallopian tube carcinoma, and peritoneal carcinoma. In: DeVita VT Jr, Hellman S, Rosenberg SA, eds. *Cancer principles and practice of oncology*, 6th ed. Philadelphia, PA: Lippincott Williams & Wilkins, 2001:1597–1532.

Reed E. Cisplatin and analogs. In: Chabner BA, Longo D, eds. *Cancer chemotherapy and biotherapy principles and practice*, Chapter 15, 3rd ed. Philadelphia, PA: Lippincott Williams & Wilkins, 2001: 447–465.

Reed E, Evans MK. Acute leukemia following cisplatin-based chemotherapy in a patient with ovarian cancer. *J Natl Cancer Inst* 1990;82:431–432.

Reed E, Jacob J. Carboplatin and renal dysfunction. *Ann Intern Med* 1989;110:409.

Reed E, Zerbe CS, Brawley OW, et al. Analysis of autopsy evaluations of ovarian cancer patients treated at the National Cancer Institute, 1972-1988. *Am J Clin Oncol* 2000;28:107–116.

Sarosy G, Reed E. Autologous stem cell transplantation in ovarian cancer: is more better? *Ann Intern Med* 2000;133:555–556.

18

Endometrial Cancer

Christina M. Annunziata* and Michael J. Birrer†

*Medical Oncology Clinical Research Unit, National Cancer Institute, National Institutes of Health, Bethesda, Maryland; and †Department of Cell and Cancer Biology, National Cancer Institute, National Institutes of Health, Rockville, Maryland

EPIDEMIOLOGY

- Endometrial cancer is the most common pelvic gynecologic malignancy in women (6% of all cancers in women).
- In 2002, 39,300 new cases were diagnosed (the incidence of endometrial cancer was 22 cases per 100,000 population in the 1980s and has been constant since then).
- An estimated 6,400 deaths due to this malignancy are predicted yearly (accounting for 2% of all cancer deaths).
- The mortality rate has continued to decline since 1989, likely because of increased awareness of symptoms (abnormal vaginal bleeding).
- Mortality is twice as high in African American women than in white women. However, the incidence is 1.4 times higher in white women than in African American women.
- Peak incidence is in the sixth and seventh decades of life (5% of cases are diagnosed before the age of 40; 20% to 25% of patients are diagnosed before menopause).

RISK FACTORS

- Endogenous estrogen excess
- Polycystic ovary disease
- Anovulatory menstrual cycles
- Obesity: being overweight by more than 20 to 50 lb increases the risk threefold and being overweight by more than 50 lb increases the risk 10-fold
- Granulosa cell tumor of the ovary (or other estrogen-secreting tumors)
- Advanced liver disease
- Endogenous prolonged estrogen exposure: early menarche and late menopause; menopause in women older than 52 years increases the risk by 2.4-fold.
- Irregular menses, infertility, and nulliparity: nulliparous women have twice the risk of developing uterine cancer compared to women with one child and thrice the risk when compared to women who give birth to five or more children
- Exogenous unopposed estrogen sources, including tamoxifen (TAM), a weak estrogen that increases the relative risk (RR) of developing endometrial cancer to 2.3
- Type 2 diabetes mellitus (DM), possibly related to the effects of hyperinsulinemia
- Hypertension

- Family history: history of endometrial cancer in a first-degree relative increases the risk by threefold, and history of a colorectal cancer in a first-degree relative increases the risk of an endometrial cancer by twofold
- Personal history of breast, ovarian, or colorectal cancer; personal or family history consistent with hereditary nonpolyposis colorectal cancer (HNPCC) (Lynch II syndrome).

PROTECTIVE FACTORS

- Oral contraceptives: There is a 50% decrease in RR when oral contraceptives are used for at least 12 months. This protection lasts for at least 10 years after discontinuation.
- Cigarette smoking: There appears to be a modest protective role of cigarette smoking. However, this is strongly outweighed by the significant increased risk of lung cancer and other major health hazards.

DIAGNOSIS AND SCREENING

- Routine screening for endometrial cancer is not required in asymptomatic women.
- Women taking TAM should have a gynecologic evaluation according to the same guidelines as for women who are not taking this drug. Endometrial biopsy should be done when the patient is symptomatic (vaginal bleeding or spotting).

Signs and Symptoms

- Abnormal vaginal bleeding is a common symptom of endometrial cancer (seen in approximately 90% of cases). Premenopausal women with prolonged and/or heavy menses, or intermenstrual spotting, should undergo endometrial biopsy. All postmenopausal women with vaginal bleeding should be evaluated for endometrial cancer (20% of these patients will ultimately be diagnosed with the malignancy). Biopsy is also recommended in women taking estrogen therapy for menopausal symptoms who may have withdrawal bleeding.
- Asymptomatic patients with abnormal glandular tissue on Papanicolaou smear should be evaluated for endometrial cancer (approximately 10% of uterine cancer cases are detected by a Papanicolaou smear). Papanicolaou smear, however, is not an adequate tool for detection of endometrial malignancy.
- Palpable, locally advanced tumor detected on pelvic examination is suggestive of endometrial cancer.
- Signs and symptoms of advanced disease (manifestation in <10% of cases) include bowel obstruction, jaundice, ascites, pain.

Procedures

- Endocervical curettage and outpatient endometrial biopsy is a common procedure.
- Papanicolaou smear is of limited value (see previous text).
- Fractional curettage under anesthesia is a method that involves scraping of the endocervical canal, followed by the walls of the uterus in a set sequence. It is the standard procedure for the diagnosis of endometrial cancer that is used in symptomatic women with negative or inadequate endometrial biopsy.
- Available data on transvaginal ultrasound suggest a correlation between endometrial stripe thickness, as seen on ultrasound, and subsequent risk of endometrial cancer. Less than a 4 to 5 mm "cutoff" of endometrial stripe has been used as a diagnostic criterion; however, occasional cases of endometrial cancer could still be missed. Therefore, there is no general agreement on the cutoff thickness of endometrial stripe for recommending endometrial biopsy. Patients taking TAM have thicker endometrium than their counterparts who do not take TAM.

HISTOLOGY

- Endometrioid (75% to 80%)
- Uterine papillary serous (5% to 10%)
- Clear cell (1% to 5%)
- Mucinous (1%)
- Squamous cell (<1%)
- Mixed mesodermal (10%)
- Undifferentiated.

Endometrial carcinoma may also be divided into two types (I and II) according to its dependence on estrogen:

Type I (estrogen related): It is the more common type of endometrial carcinoma, is associated with DM and obesity, and tends to have better prognosis [more differentiated; more favorable histologic subtypes such as endometrioid, mucinous, and secretory carcinoma; higher incidence of superficial invasion, lower grade, and lower stage; higher progesterone receptor (PgR) levels; and younger patients].

Type II (unrelated to estrogen stimulation and endometrial hyperplasia): This type is less common; it usually has a short duration of symptoms, poor differentiation, deep myometrial invasion, poor prognosis, and more aggressive histology (serous, clear cell).

Adenomatous hyperplasia is an estrogen-dependent lesion, which could be seen along with type I but not type II endometrial carcinoma.

PRETHERAPY EVALUATION

- Physical examination
- Chest x-ray (CXR)
- Urinary imaging studies (i.v. pyelogram or renal scan), cystoscopy, and proctoscopy (very rarely done)
- Routine blood and urine studies
- Routine age-appropriate health maintenance; if HNPCC is suspected, colonoscopy should be performed before planning treatment
- Evaluation of specific symptoms or physical examination findings, as indicated
- Routine use of ultrasound, computerized tomography (CT) scan, and magnetic resonance imaging (MRI) are NOT recommended, and bone scan rarely adds useful information.

STAGING

- Staging for endometrial carcinoma is surgical (see Table 18.1) and is based on information from hysterectomy, bilateral salpingo-oophorectomy (BSO), peritoneal cytology, and pelvic and periaortic lymph node (LN) dissection.
- Endometrial cancer distribution by stage is as follows:

  Stage I: 73%
  Stage II: 12%
  Stage III: 12%
  Stage IV: 3%.

PROGNOSTIC FACTORS

Uterine

- Histologic type
- Histologic differentiation

TABLE 18.1. *Staging for endometrial cancer: 1988*

Stage IA G123	Tumor limited to endometrium
Stage IB G123	Invasion to <50% of the myometrium
Stage IC G123	Invasion to >50% of the myometrium
Stage IIA G123	Endocervical glandular involvement only
Stage IIB G123	Cervical stromal invasion
Stage IIIA G123	Tumor invades serosa and/or adnexa, and/or positive peritoneal cytology
Stage IIIB G123	Vaginal metastases
Stage IIIC G123	Metastases to pelvic and/or paraaortic lymph nodes
Stage IVA G123	Tumor invasion of bladder and/or bowel mucosa
Stage IVB	Distant metastases including intraabdominal and/or inguinal lymph nodes

Histopathology: Degree of differentiation
  Cases of carcinoma of the corpus should be classified (or graded) according to the degree of histologic differentiation, as follows:
  G1: 5% of a nonsquamous or nonmorular solid growth pattern
  G2: 6% of 50% of a nonsquamous or nonmorular solid growth pattern
  G3: >50% of a nonsquamous or nonmorular solid growth pattern

Notes on pathologic gradings
1. Notable nuclear atypia, inappropriate for the architectural grade, raises the grade of a grade 1 or grade 2 tumor by 1.
2. In serious adenocarcinomas, clear cell adenocarcinomas, and squamous cell carcinomas nuclear grading takes precedence.
3. Adenocarcinomas with squamous differentiation are graded according to the nuclear grade of the glandular component.

Rules related to staging
1. Because corpus cancer is now staged surgically, procedures previously used for determination of stages are no longer applicable, such as the findings from fractional dilation and curettage to differentiate between stage I and II.
2. It is appreciated that there may be a small number of patients with corpus cancer who will be treated primarily with radiation therapy. If that is the case, the clinical staging adopted by FIGO in 1971 should still apply, but designation of that staging system would be noted.
3. Ideally, width of the myometrium should be measured along with the width of tumor invasion.

FIGO, Federation Internationale de Gynecogie et d'Obstetrique.
From DiSaia PJ, Creasman WT. *Clinical gynecologic oncology*, 5th ed. St. Louis: Mosby, 1997:140–141, with permission.

- Stage of disease: 5-year survival (%) distribution by stage is as follows: I: 86%; II: 66%; III: 44%; and IV: 16%
- Myometrial invasion
- Vascular space invasion (rate of disease recurrence seen is approximately 25%).

Extrauterine

- Positive peritoneal cytology (rate of disease recurrence seen is approximately 15%)
- LN metastasis: involvement of pelvic LN or peritoneal metastases poses approximately 25% risk for disease recurrence, whereas metastasis to periaortic LN increases this risk to 40%
- Adnexal metastasis (approximately 15% recurrence risk)
- Tumor hormone–receptor status: the presence of estrogen receptor (ER)/PgR and their levels were found to be inversely proportional to histologic grade and was associated with a longer survival
- Tumor size: tumors larger than 2 cm have worse prognosis
- Molecular factors include deoxyribonucleic acid (DNA) ploidy and p53 overexpression (however, most studies are small and use different techniques and cutoff values; further standardization is needed before conclusions can be drawn).

MANAGEMENT

- **Endometrial hyperplasia:** Total abdominal hysterectomy (TAH) or BSO is the treatment of choice for patients with persistent endometrial hyperplasia after the failure of adequate therapy with progestin.
- **Endometrial carcinoma:** Therapy should be individualized.

Low Risk: Stage IA, IB (or IC with Grade 1 Histology)

TAH/BSO (selected pelvic LN may be removed): This is considered adequate for patients with well-differentiated or moderately differentiated tumors, with negative peritoneal cytology (if no peritoneal fluid is found during surgery, peritoneal washing with normal saline should be done), with no vascular space invasion, and with less than 50% myometrial invasion.

Intermediate Risk: Stage II, Grade 1

1. **TAH/BSO combined with paraaortic and selective pelvic LN sampling or dissection:** If there are no medical or technical contraindications (e.g., morbid obesity), this should be done in patients with
   a. tumors involving more than 50% of outer myometrium
   b. tumor presence in cervical isthmus
   c. adnexal and other extrauterine metastases
   d. serous, clear cell, undifferentiated, or squamous histology and
   e. LN enlargement (visible or palpable).
2. **Adjuvant (postoperative) total pelvic irradiation:** This method is used for tumors with deep myometrial invasion, grade 2 or 3 histology, vascular space invasion, and/or cervical involvement. Radiation doses of 45 to 50 Gy of standard fractionation and daily treatments of multiple fields with small-bowel protection are applied.

Special Considerations

- Low-risk patients who are not surgical candidates can be treated with radiation therapy alone; however, this may achieve a lower cure rate than surgery.
- Combined surgery and external radiation has a higher complication rate than either treatment alone (e.g., bowel complications, 4%). Therefore, special attention should be given to appropriate patient selection and choice of surgical techniques [e.g., fewer complications are seen with retroperitoneal approach, as well as with LN sampling versus LN dissection (trials comparing conventional TAH/BSO and pelvic and periaortic LN dissection versus laparoscopic pelvic and periaortic LN dissection, BSO, and vaginal hysterectomy are ongoing)].
- Pelvic surgery has an increased risk for thrombophlebitis in the pelvis and lower extremities; hence, low-dose heparin or Venodyne boots should be used in these patients.
- In case of papillary serous tumor histology, because of the higher rate of vaginal, pelvic, and upper abdominal recurrences seen with this histology, treatment recommendations include whole-abdominal irradiation for up to 30-Gy dose and additional treatments to reach a pelvic dose of 50 Gy. A vaginal cylinder or colpostats can be used to give an additional surface dose of 40-Gy radiation (a 5-year survival of 50% was documented with this approach).

High risk: Stage IB (or Beyond) Grade 3, Stage IC (or Beyond) Grade 2, or Any Stage III

- **Hysterectomy, BSO, and periaortic LN sampling, followed by postoperative radiation:** The radiation therapy is administered as an external beam to a dose of 45 to 50 Gy along with vaginal irradiation with vaginal cylinder or colpostats to bring the vaginal surface dose to 80 to 90 Gy (5-year disease-free survival of 80% and locoregional control of 90% were seen with this treatment). Whole-abdominal radiation should be considered for high-risk patients with positive peritoneal washings or micrometastases in the upper abdomen.

- **Preoperative intracavitary radiation plus external-beam radiation:** This method is a combination of preoperative intracavitary radiation (consisting of uterine tandem and vaginal colpostat insertions with a standard Fletcher applicator delivering 20 to 25 Gy to a point A) and external-beam radiation (dose of 40 to 45 Gy with standard fractionation delivered to multiple fields). In patients with extensive cervical involvement precluding initial hysterectomy, the external-beam radiation should be followed in 4 to 6 weeks by hysterectomy and BSO with periaortic LN sampling (this approach can provide 5-year disease-free survival of 70% to 80%).
- **Adjuvant chemotherapy:** This method is not routinely recommended because of insufficient data. It should be given only in the setting of a clinical trial.

Special Considerations for High-risk Patients

- Women with isolated ovarian metastasis form a subgroup with a relatively better prognosis. However, some believe that this represents double primary tumors rather than true metastasis from primary endometrial cancer. Five-year disease-free survival ranges between 60% and 82% (depending on the histologic grade of tumor and the depth of myometrial invasion). The pelvic radiation doses of 45 to 50 Gy are given in standard fractionation, with vaginal boost with cylinder or colpostats adding 30 to 35 Gy to the vaginal surface.
- If tumor extends to the pelvic wall, patients would be considered inoperable and should be treated with radiation.
- When parametrial extension is present, preoperative radiation (external and intracavitary) is applied.
- If the pelvic and/or paraaortic LNs are involved in the tumor, patients should be treated with extended-field radiation (encompassing pelvic and periaortic regions) by using 45- to 50-Gy doses, and they may be included as candidates for clinical trials on radiation and/or chemotherapy because they are at higher risk for recurrence (see previous text).
- Patients who are not candidates for either surgery or radiation are treated with progestational agents (see subsequent text).

Stage IV and Recurrent Disease

- Therapy recommendations depend on the sites of metastasis or recurrent disease and the disease-related symptoms. All patients should be considered for clinical trials.
- **Pelvic exenteration:** This method can be considered for patients with disease extending only to the bladder or rectum (tumor tissue should be checked for ER and PgR levels) and for isolated central recurrence after irradiation (some long-term survivals have been reported).
- **Radiation** (palliative): Radiation is applied for localized recurrences, for example, pelvic LN (external-beam radiation together with brachytherapy boost), paraaortic LN, or distant metastases.
- In isolated vaginal recurrence (if not previously given), irradiation may be curative.
- **Hormonal therapy:** This therapy produces responses in 15% to 30% of patients and is associated with improved survival (two times longer survival than those seen in nonresponders). On average, responses last for 1 year. Hormone-receptor levels and degree of tumor differentiation correlate well with responses.

Drugs and Regimens Most Frequently Used in Uterine Cancer

Hormonal Therapy

- Medroxyprogesterone acetate (Depo-Provera), 400 to 1,000 mg i.m. weekly for 6 weeks, and then monthly
- Oral medroxyprogesterone (Provera), approximately 150 mg PO daily

- Megestrol acetate (Megace), 40 to 80 mg PO four times daily
- Tamoxifen, 20 mg PO daily, with or without a progestin
- The use of aromatase inhibitors (e.g., anastrozole, letrozole) is under investigation for the treatment of endometrial carcinoma.

Chemotherapy

- No standard chemotherapeutic regimen is available.
- Chemotherapeutic use is restricted to stage IV or recurrent disease or to nonresponders to hormonal therapy.
- On average, duration of responses is around 4 months, and survival is for 9 months.
- The most active single agents are doxorubicin [35% to 40% odds ratio (OR)], cisplatin (36% OR), and paclitaxel (36% OR).
- Chemotherapy can be used in conjunction with hormonal therapy.
- Several combination regimens have been tried including carboplatin and paclitaxel; carboplatin, methotrexate, 5-fluorouracil, and medroxyprogesterone; melphalan, 5-fluorouracil, and medroxyprogesterone; cisplatin, doxorubicin, etoposide, and medroxyprogesterone; each regimen produced better response rates than historic controls, but no phase III studies have shown improvement in survival to date.

ESTROGEN-REPLACEMENT THERAPY

In patients with endometrial cancer, estrogen-replacement therapy remains controversial.

POSTTHERAPY SURVEILLANCE (SUGGESTED)

The following posttherapy surveillances have been suggested for endometrial cancer:

- Physical examination, CA125 measurement, and vaginal cytology every 3 to 6 months for 2 years, and then annually.
- Most recurrences are seen in the first 3 years after primary therapy.

SUGGESTED READINGS

American Joint Committee on Cancer. *AJCC cancer staging manual*, 6th ed. Springer-Verlag, New York 2002.

Hoskins WJ, Perez CA, Young RC. *Principles and practices of gynecologic therapy*, 3rd ed. Lippincott Williams and Wilkins, Philadelphia, 2000.

NCCN practice guidelines in clinical oncology, Uterine Cancer, version1. 2002. found at http://www.nccn.org/professionals/physician_gls/f_guidelines. © National Comprehensive Cancer Network, Inc. 2001, 2002, 2003, 2004, 2005. NCCN and NATIONAL COMPREHENSIVE CANCER NETWORK are registered trademarks of National Comprehensive Cancer Network, Inc.

NCI-Pdq Pahe at http://cancer.gov/search/clinical_trials/results_clinicaltrials.aspx 2003.

Chen L-M and Berek JS. (1) Clinical features and diagnosis of endometrial cancer; (2) Staging and treatment of endometrial cancer. UpToDate online, version11.2, 2003 Portions©1990-2000 click2learn.com, Inc. All rights reserved. http://www.uptodateonline.com/application/

19

Cervical Cancer

Edwin M. Posadas and Herbert L. Kotz

Medical Oncology Clinical Research Unit, National Cancer Institute, National Institutes of Health, Bethesda, Maryland

EPIDEMIOLOGY

Worldwide

- Cervical cancer is one of the most common cancers affecting women (6% of all female malignancies) (1).
- More than 371,100 new cases are diagnosed each year (1).
- An estimated 190,000 women die each year as a consequence of this disease (1).
- It is currently the third leading cause of cancer death in women.

United States

- Cervical cancer is the third most common cancer of the female reproductive tract.
- Although the introduction of Papanicolaou smear screening has reduced the incidence and mortality of invasive cancer by almost 75% over the last 50 years, 10,000 to 15,000 new cases and 3,500 to 5,000 deaths are still occurring annually for the last 10 to 15 years.
- More than 12,000 new cases and 4,100 deaths were expected in 2003 (2).
- Only about one third of women at risk for cervical cancer receive appropriate screening.
- The lifetime risk for developing cervical cancer is 0.88%; the lifetime risk of dying from the disease is 0.29%.
- The incidence of cervical carcinoma is higher among women with a history of sexually transmitted diseases [e.g., human papillomavirus (HPV) infection and herpes simplex virus (HSV) infection].

RISK FACTORS

Human Papillomavirus

- Women who have never had HPV infection and those who developed HPV infection earlier are not at risk for cervical cancer. However, more than 99% of all cervical cancers harbor the HPV DNA (deoxyribonucleic acid) (3,4,5).
- More than 200 types of HPV have been recognized on the basis of DNA sequence (3,6). More than 50 distinct HPV types are known to infect the genital tract, and at least 20 types have been associated with cancer (7).
- HPV types 6, 11, 42, 43, and 44 are viruses of "low oncogenic potential" and are associated with benign cervical lesions.

- HPV types 16, 18, 31, 33, 34, 35, 39, 45, 51, 52, 56, 58, 59, 66, and 68 to 70 are viruses of "high oncogenic potential" that are associated with high-grade cervical intraepithelial neoplasia (CIN 2, 3 and carcinoma *in situ*) (3).
- Some of the high-risk types of HPV are found more often in squamous intraepithelial lesions than in cancer and are called intermediate risk types.
- The oncogenic effect appears to be mediated by E6 and E7 proteins of the high-risk HPV subtypes. The E6 and E7 proteins have been shown to inactivate tumor-suppressor genes p53 and pRb, respectively, with subsequent loss of the cell-cycle regulatory mechanism, leading to malignant transformation.
- The current clinical data shows no evidence that determining whether an invasive cervical cancer harbors HPV influences clinical outcome or management. Therefore, routine HPV type is not recommended except in a clinical trial setting. For patients with CIN, the presence of high-risk HPV serotypes increases the risk of invasive disease.

Demographic Factors

- Race: Higher incidence among Latin American, African American, and Native American women
- Socioeconomic status: More prevalent in lower socioeconomic classes
- Education: Higher incidence among undereducated
- Age: More common in older women.

Personal or Sexual Factors

- Sexual partners: History of more than six sexual partners increases the relative risk (RR) for developing cervical cancer to 2.2 times the background incidence. Women married to a man whose previous partner had had cervical cancer have a threefold increase in the risk for developing the disease. History of genital warts increases the incidence by 18-fold. Penile cancer in a male sexual partner places a woman at higher risk for cervical cancer.
- If the age at first intercourse is before 18 years, the RR is 1.6.
- Smoking increases RR to 1.7.
- Using oral contraceptive for more than 10 years results in an RR of 2.2.
- Human immunodeficiency virus (HIV)–positive women have an RR of 2.5 [standardized incidence ratio = 12.5 (8)].

Medical and Gynecologic Factors

- Parity: Incidence of cervical cancer is more common among multiparous women (RR =1.5 to 5.0).
- Papanicolaou (Pap) smear: Prior abnormal Pap smear or documented dysplasia is associated with an increased risk.
- Immunosuppression: Renal transplantation (RR = 5.7) and HIV infection increase the risk [acquired immunodeficiency syndrome (AIDS) in HIV-positive women with cervical cancer is defined according to the Centers for Disease Control and Prevention (CDC) criteria from 1993].

SCREENING (9)

- The American College of Obstetricians and Gynecologists recommendations are as follows:
  - Women should begin screening 3 years after the onset of sexual activity or at 21 years, whichever is earlier.
  - Screening should end at age of 70, or earlier if a woman has had a complete hysterectomy.

- In addition, women should have a negative test result yearly on a liquid-based Pap test every 2 years until the age of 30. Then, if they have had three normal test results consecutively, they can continue screening at a frequency of every 2 to 3 years.
  - Alternatively, a combination of cytology and DNA testing can be performed. If both are negative, testing need not be repeated for at least 3 years.
- Cervical cytology should be described using the 2001 Bethesda System, detailing specimen adequacy and interpretation.
- Interpretation is divided into nonmalignant findings and epithelial cell abnormalities including atypia, low-grade and high-grade intraepithelial lesions, and squamous cell carcinoma (see Table 19.1).

PRECURSOR LESIONS

- Mild, moderate, and severe dysplasias are also known as CIN I, II, and III.
- Most mild-to-moderate dysplasias are more likely to regress than progress. The rate of progression of mild dysplasia to severe dysplasia is 1% per year, whereas the risk of progression of moderate dysplasia to severe dysplasia is 16% within 2 years and 25% within 5 years (6).
- CIN III, if left untreated, will progress to invasive cancer over a period of 20 years in more than 12% of cases.

SIGNS AND SYMPTOMS

- Abnormal vaginal bleeding (i.e., postcoital, intermenstrual, and menorrhagia) is usually the first manifestation.
- Vaginal discharge (serosanguineous or yellowish, sometimes foul smelling) usually represents a more advanced lesion.
- Fatigue and other anemia-related symptoms are seen in patients with chronic bleeding.
- Pain in the lumbosacral or gluteal area suggest the possibility of hydronephrosis or involvement of iliac or periaortic lymph nodes (LN), extending to the lumbar roots or causing hydronephrosis.
- Urinary or rectal symptoms (hematuria, rectal bleeding, etc.) can be seen with bladder or rectal involvement.
- Leg edema (persistent, unilateral or bilateral) results from lymphatic and venous blockage caused by extensive pelvic wall disease.
- Leg pain, edema, and hydronephrosis are characteristic of advanced stage disease (IIIB).

PHYSICAL EXAMINATION

- Can be normal
- Most frequent findings include visible cervical lesion or abnormal bimanual pelvic examination.

DIAGNOSTIC WORKUP

- History
- Physical examination (including bimanual pelvic and rectal examinations).

Diagnostic Procedures

- Pap smear, if no gross lesion
- Colposcopically directed biopsy
- Conization (subclinical tumor)
- Punch biopsies (edge of gross tumor)

TABLE 19.1. *The 2001 Bethesda System*

Specimen adequacy
- Satisfactory for evaluation (note presence/absence of endocervical/transformation zone component)
- Unsatisfactory for evaluation (specify reason)
  - Specimen rejected/not processed (specify reason)
  - Specimen processed and examined, but unsatisfactory for evaluation of epithelial abnormality because of (specify reason)

General categorization (Optional)
- Negative for intraepithelial lesions or malignancy
- Epithelial cell abnormality
- Other

Interpretation/Result
- Negative for intraepithelial lesion or malignancy
  - Organisms
    - *Trichomonas vaginalis*
    - Fungal organisms morphologically consistent with *Candida* species
    - Shift in flora suggestive of bacterial vaginosis
    - Bacteria morphologically consistent with *Actinomyces* species
    - Cellular changes consistent with herpes simplex virus
  - Other nonneoplastic findings (optional to report; list not comprehensive)
    - Reactive cellular changes associated with
      - Inflammation (includes typical repair)
      - Radiation
      - Intrauterine contraceptive device
    - Glandular cells status posthysterectomy
    - Atrophy
- Epithelial cell abnormalities
  - Squamous cell
    - Atypical squamous cell (ASC)
      - Of undetermined significance (ASC-US)
      - Cannot exclude HSIL (ASC-H)
    - Low-grade squamous intraepithelial lesion (LSIL)
      - Encompassing
        - Human papillomavirus
        - Mild dysplasia
        - Cervical intraepithelial neoplasia 1(CIN 1)
    - High-grade squamous intraepithelial neoplasia (HSIL)
      - Encompassing moderate and severe dysplasia, carcinoma *in situ*
      - CIN 2 and CIN 3
    - Squamous cell carcinoma
  - Glandular cell
    - Atypical glandular cells (AGC) (specify endocervical, endometrial or not otherwise specified)
    - AGC, favor neoplastic (specify endocervical or not otherwise specified)
    - Endocervical adenocarcinoma *in situ* (AIS)
    - Adenocarcinoma
- Other (list not comprehensive)
  - Endometrial cells in a woman 40 yr old or more

Automated review and ancillary testing (include as appropriate)
Educational notes and suggestions (optional)

From Solomon D, Davey D, Kurman R, et al. The 2001 Bethesda System: terminology for reporting results of cervical cytology. *JAMA* 2002;287(16):2114–2189, with permission.

- Dilation and curettage
- Cystoscopy and rectosigmoidoscopy (stages IIB, III, IVA) if there are symptoms referable to the bladder, colon, or rectum.

Radiologic Studies

- Chest x-ray (CXR)
- Intravenous pyelography or computerized tomography (CT) scan with i.v. contrast
- Barium enema (stage III, IVA, and earlier stages if there are symptoms referable to colon or rectum)
- Magnetic resonance imaging (MRI), if required, for better disease evaluation
- CT and MRI are not used for staging.

Laboratory Studies

- Complete blood count
- Blood chemistries
- Urinalysis.

HISTOLOGY

Cervical carcinoma originates at the squamous–columnar junction of the cervix (transformation zone). Of cervical cancers, 80% to 85% are of squamous cell histology. The remaining 15% to 20% are mostly adenocarcinomas or adenosquamous carcinomas.

STAGING

- In contrast to other gynecologic malignancies, cervical cancer is a clinically staged disease (see Table 19.2).
- Laparoscopy, lymphangiography, and major surgical procedures cannot be used for the purpose of staging.
- Surgical staging is more accurate than clinical staging; however, there is no evidence that it will improve the overall survival (OS). Therefore, surgical staging should be done only as part of a clinical trial.

PROGNOSTIC FACTORS

- On the basis of the experience of the Gynecologic Oncology Group (GOG) (where paraaortic LN staging was obligatory), multivariate analysis showed paraaortic LN involvement as the most important negative prognostic factor, followed by pelvic LN involvement, larger tumor size, younger age, and advanced stage.
- Lymph–vascular invasion and tumor grade is a significant prognostic factor.
- It remains controversial whether adenocarcinoma of the cervix carries a worse prognosis than does squamous cell cancer.
- Five-year survival (%) depends on the stage: 0: 95% to 100%; I: 80%; II: 60%; III: 30%; and IV: 5%.

MODE OF SPREAD

- Cervical cancer is a locally progressive and destructive tumor with the following spread pattern.
- Local spread: into vaginal mucosa or endomyometrium, or direct extension into adjacent structures or parametria.
- Lymphatic spread: pelvic and paraaortic LNs are most commonly involved.
- Hematogenous spread: most common sites are lung, liver, and bone.

TABLE 19.2. *International Federation of Gynecology and Obstetrics (FIGO)*
staging of carcinoma of the cervix (1994)

Stage			Definition
0			Carcinoma *in situ*
			Confined to cervix
	IA		microscopic evidence of cancer
		IA1	measured stromal invasion no greater than 3.0 mm in depth and extension no wider than 7.0 mm
		IA2	measured stromal invasion greater than 3.0 mm and no greater than 5.0, with an extension no wider than 7.0 mm
	IB		clinically visible lesion limited to cervix uteri
		IB1	clinically visible lesions no greater than 4.0 cm
		IB2	clinically visible lesions greater than 4.0 cm
II			Carcinoma invades beyond the uterus but not to pelvic wall or to lower third of vagina
	IIA		no obvious parametrial involvement
	IIB		obvious parametrial involvement
III			Extension to pelvic wall
	IIIA		Tumor involves lower third of vagina, with no extension to the pelvic wall
	IIIB		Extension to the pelvic wall and/or hydronephrosis or nonfunctioning kidney
IV			Extension beyond the true pelvis or has clinically involved the mucosa of the bladder or rectum
	IVA		Spread to adjacent organs
	IVB		Spread to distant organs

From International Gederation of Gynecology and Obstetrics. Benedet JL, Odicino F, Maisonneneuve P, et al. Carcinoma of the cervix uteri. *J Epidemiol Biostat* 2001; 6(1):5–44, with permission.

MANAGEMENT

Stage 0 (Carcinoma *In Situ*)

- Noninvasive lesions can be eradicated by electrocautery, cryotherapy, or laser therapy.
- Loop electrosurgical excision procedure (LEEP) allows excision of the entire transformation zone of the cervix with a low-voltage diathermy loop. It has the advantage of being a one-step diagnostic and therapeutic option.
- In select situations, LEEP may be an acceptable alternative to cold-knife conization because it is a quick, outpatient procedure requiring only local anesthesia. However, current data do not support LEEP as an adequate replacement for conization for all clinical situations.
- Because of limited series, the diagnosis and management of preinvasive and microinvasive adenocarcinomas remains unsettled (10).

Invasive Cervical Cancer

- Treatment in each stage may vary, depending on the size of the tumor.
- Results from five recently reported randomized phase III trials demonstrated an OS advantage for cisplatin-based chemotherapy given concurrently with radiation therapy. These trials have demonstrated a 30% to 50% overall reduction in risk of death in patients with International Federation of Gynecology and Obstetrics (FIGO) stage IB2 to IVA and in patients with FIGO I to IIA with poor prognostic factors (i.e., pelvic LN involvement, parametrial disease, and positive surgical margins). Therefore, cisplatin-based chemoradiation is the current standard of care for patients with more advanced disease requiring radiation therapy.
- Various regimens and schedules (cisplatin every week or every 3 weeks) have been used for concurrent cisplatin-based chemotherapy and radiation.

- Some regimens use cisplatin as a single agent, once weekly, 40 mg per m^2 i.v. (maximum of 70 mg) for six doses concurrent with radiation.
- In published studies of combination chemotherapy (e.g., 5-fluorouracil/cisplatin) with concomitant radiation, cisplatin doses of 50 to 75 mg per m^2 have been given on various schedules (11). 5-FU has been administered as a 96-hour continuous infusion at doses of 1,000 to 4,000 mg/m^2/day at varying intervals.

Stage IA1

- For patients without lymphovascular invasion who have completed childbearing, a simple hysterectomy is indicated.
- For those who wish to preserve fertility, a conization with negative margins is adequate therapy.

Stage IA2, IB1, IB2, IIA

1. Radical trachelectomy (a fertility-preserving radical surgery) may be an option for small-volume early-stage disease (12).
2. Radical hysterectomy with bilateral pelvic LN dissection is another option. Paraaortic LN sampling is included in patients with positive pelvic nodes, clinically enlarged nodes, or for patients with larger volume disease.
3. Radiation therapy, external beam pelvic irradiation followed by intracavitary applications, can also be considered.
   - Higher central doses of radiation can be delivered with the combination of external beam radiation and intracavitary irradiation than with the external radiation therapy alone. This combination method leads to an improved pelvic control and survival.
   - The use of HDR (high-dose rate, 200 to 300 cGy per minute) versus LDR (Low-dose rate, 50 to 60 cGy per hour) brachytherapy is still controversial. The relative benefits of each are under evaluation.
   - Radioactive isotopes (e.g., cesium 137) are introduced into the uterine cavity and vaginal fornices with special applicators (the most commonly used applicator is the Fletcher–Suit intrauterine tandem and vaginal ovoid).
   - The important issues that must be addressed in delivering radiation for therapy of cervical cancer are the maximum bladder and rectal doses and the dose delivered to the two standard pelvic points: A and B.
   - Point A is located 2 cm cephalad and 2 cm lateral to the cervical os. Anatomically, it correlates with the medial parametrium or lateral cervix, the point where the ureter and uterine artery cross.
   - Point B is located 5 cm lateral to the center of the pelvis at the same level as point A. Anatomically, it correlates to the obturator LN or lateral parametrium.
   - Typical doses of external radiation are 40 to 50 Gy, followed by 40 to 50 Gy to point A with brachytherapy for a total dose of 80 to 90 Gy to point A. Depending on the extent of disease, a parametrial boost of a total dose of 60 Gy may be applied to point B, with external beam radiation and brachytherapy.
   - Surgery and radiation are equivalent treatment options for stages IB and IIA, with identical 5-year OS and disease-free survival (DFS). Expected cure rate is 75% to 80% (85% to 90% in small-volume disease).
   - The choice of surgery versus radiation depends on many factors including size of the tumor, age of the patient, availability of local expertise, and presence of other comorbid conditions. Consideration must also be given to younger women wishing to preserve ovarian function.
   - Pelvic inflammatory disease, inflammatory bowel disease, and pelvic kidney are relative contraindications to pelvic radiation.

- For patients with stage IB2 disease treated with radiation alone, pelvic control and survival are both lower in comparison to those with nonbulky tumors. For bulky tumors, pelvic control and survival are 57% and 40%, respectively. For tumors smaller than 4 cm, these values are 93% and 82%, respectively.
- Postradiation surgery may be a consideration in patients with residual tumor confined to the cervix or in patients with suboptimal brachytherapy because of vaginal anatomy.
- A study by the Radiation Therapy Oncology Group (RTOG) revealed an 11% 10-year survival advantage for patients with IB2, IIA, and IIB disease treated with prophylactic paraaortic nodal and pelvic wall radiation compared to those treated with pelvic irradiation alone (11).

4. Postoperative pelvic chemoradiation after radical hysterectomy and bilateral pelvic LN dissection are applied to patients with negative pelvic nodes who are at risk for pelvic failure [primary tumor >4 cm, outer third cervical stromal invasion, lymph–vascular space invasion, and close vaginal margins (<0.5 cm)]. This provides reduced recurrence rate and improved survival.
   - This approach is recommended for patients with positive pelvic nodes or positive surgical margins (13).
   - Radiation doses used are 45 to 50 Gy by external pelvic radiation, with boosts given to specific sites (as needed) with external beam, intracavitary, or interstitial radiation.

Special Considerations

- Recent studies have clearly demonstrated the deleterious effect of anemia on the results of radiotherapy. There is both increased local recurrence and decreased survival when hemoglobin is <12 g per dL during radiation therapy. The best method of optimization of the hemoglobin is being studied.
- Patients with suspected or confirmed paraaortic nodal disease should receive extended-field radiation encompassing pelvic and paraaortic areas. RTOG 79-20 demonstrated a survival advantage in stage IB2, IIA, and IIB disease with addition of external beam paraaortic radiation over external beam pelvic irradiation alone (14). Some patients with small-volume disease in paraaortic LNs and controllable pelvic disease can potentially be cured. However, in gross paraaortic disease, the role of radiation is limited because tolerance of surrounding organs (i.e., bowel, kidney, and spinal cord) precludes the delivery of adequately high radiation doses. For this reason, preradiation removal of grossly involved nodes should be considered.
- Toxicity from paraaortic LN radiation is greater than that from pelvic radiation alone but is seen mostly in patients with prior abdominopelvic surgery.
- Different surgical techniques alter the rate of complications secondary to paraaortic lymph node irradiation (e.g., extraperitoneal LN sampling by incision or by laparoscopy leads to fewer postradiation complications than those seen in the transperitoneal approach).

Stages IIB, III, IVA

The role of surgery as a curative treatment decreases when tumor spreads beyond the cervix and vaginal fornices. Patients presenting with tumors at these stages are treated with the following options:

- Chemoradiation: single-agent weekly cisplatin is the most commonly utilized chemosensitizer. Other agents have been proposed, but they are still in the clinical trial stage.
- Radiation therapy: for patients without paraaortic LN involvement, external beam pelvic radiation of 45 to 50 Gy followed by brachytherapy with 40 to 50 Gy to point A for a total dose of 80 to 90 Gy (applies to stages IB2 to IVA). Patients with paraaortic LNs involved will benefit from extended-field radiation covering the paraaortic area.

Special Considerations

The multivariate analysis determined that the therapeutic factors associated with improved pelvic tumor control and survival in cervical cancer patients were use of intracavitary radiation, total dose of more than 8,500 cGy to point A (advanced stage only), use of chemosensitizers, and overall treatment time less than 8 weeks.

Stage IVB

Radiation or chemoradiation are used for palliation of central disease or distant metastases.

Palliative Chemotherapy

- No standard chemotherapy regimen has been shown to produce prolonged complete remissions.
- All patients are appropriate candidates for clinical trials.
- The most active single agents include
  1. Cisplatin, 50 mg per m^2 (usual dose as a single agent or in combination regimens), i.v. once every 3 weeks for a maximum of six cycles. A response rate of 18% to 31% has been documented. Higher doses (e.g., 100 mg per m^2 i.v. once every 3 weeks) produce higher response rates, but toxicity is greater, and response duration, survival, and progression-free survival were similar to those seen with the 50-mg per m^2 dose.
  2. Carboplatin has a 15% response rate. It has less nephrotoxicity and neurotoxicity than cisplatin; thus, carboplatin may be considered an alternative to cisplatin in select patients.
  3. Ifosfamide has a 16% to 33% response rate in advanced disease and 15% response rate in recurrent disease.
  4. Paclitaxel has 17% to 25% response rate (depending upon dose).
  5. Irinotecan provides 13% to 21% response rate.
     The GOG executed a randomized phase III trial (GOG 169) comparing the combination of cisplatin and taxol to cisplatin alone. The response rates and progression-free survival were better with the combination, but OS increased by only 1 month.
- Responses to chemotherapy are of brief duration.
- Benefit of chemotherapy with or without radiation versus best supportive care in this group of patients has not yet been established.

Recurrent Disease

- A 10% to 20% recurrence rate has been reported following primary surgery or radiotherapy in patients with stage IB to IIA disease with negative nodes, whereas up to 70% of patients with more advanced stage disease with or without positive nodes will exhibit recurrences (15). As the volume of primary disease site increases, the proportion of local recurrence in the pelvis as the only site of treatment failure is greater than the proportion developing distant metastases.
- No standard therapy is available for recurrent disease outside previous surgical or radiation field.
- Radiation can be combined with cisplatin.
- It is used for recurrence in the pelvis after radical surgery.
- From 40% to 50% of these patients may be cured.
- Pelvic exenteration (resection of the bladder, rectum, vagina, uterus/cervix):
  1. This is used for centrally located, recurrent disease after irradiation.
  2. From 32% to 62% 5-year survival can be achieved in select patients.
  3. Reconstruction is possible; continent urinary conduit, rectal anastomosis, and myocutaneous graft are performed for neovagina.

4. High-dose intraoperative radiation therapy combined with surgical resection is offered by some centers for patients whose tumors extend close to the pelvic sidewalls.
- Chemotherapy is palliative, not curative. The chemotherapeutic agents tested are listed under the section Palliative Chemotherapy for stage IVB (it provides low response rates, short response duration, and low OS).
  1. Cisplatin is the single most active agent with a response rate of 20% to 30% and a median survival of 7 months (15). However, even with GOG studies, the response rate varies between 17% and 31% depending on the sites of disease and patient characteristics.

TREATMENT OF CERVICAL CANCER IN PREGNANCY

- Cervical cancer is the most common gynecologic malignancy associated with pregnancy, ranging from 1 in 1,200 to 1 in 2,200 pregnancies.
- No therapy is warranted for preinvasive lesion; colposcopy is recommended to rule out invasive cancer.
- Conization is reserved for suspicion of microinvasion or for persistent cytologic evidence of invasive cancer in the absence of colposcopic confirmation. Definitive management of dysplasia is usually postponed until the postpartum period.
- Treatment of invasive cancer depends on the tumor stage and gestational age. If cancer is diagnosed before fetal maturity, immediate appropriate cancer therapy for the relevant stage is recommended. However, with close surveillance, delay of therapy to achieve fetal maturity is a reasonable option for patients with IA and early IB disease (16). For more advanced disease, there is a paucity of data to justify a delay of therapy. If diagnosis is made in the final trimester, treatment may be delayed. When acceptable fetal maturity is reached, a classical caesarean section is done prior to definitive treatment (17).

TREATMENT OF CERVICAL CANCER IN HUMAN IMMUNODEFICIENCY VIRUS–INFECTED WOMEN

- The women infected with the HIV virus have more aggressive and more advanced disease with poorer prognosis than do the HIV-negative cervical cancer patients.
- The same standard therapy is used for preinvasive lesions and invasive cervical cancer in HIV-positive as in HIV-negative patients.
- Response to therapy in patients with HIV infection is usually worse than in those with no HIV infection.
- Data from Africa show that cervical cancer is the most common AIDS-defining neoplasm in women.
- HIV alters the natural history of HPV infections, with decreased regression rates and more rapid progression to high-grade and invasive lesions (18).

FOLLOW-UP AFTER PRIMARY THERAPY

Optimal posttreatment surveillance has not been determined. Eighty percent to 90% of tumors recur in the first 2 years following therapy. Therefore, most oncologists schedule follow-up visits frequently, for example, every 3 to 4 months for 1 year, every 4 months for the next year, every 6 months for 3 years, and then annually to detect any potentially curable recurrences.

PREVENTION

With advances in vaccine research, much attention has been paid to the field of vaccination against the etiologic pathogen for cervical cancer—HPV. In 2002, the efficacy of vaccination was demonstrated in a population of HPV-16–negative women immunized against HPV-16.

Following therapy, they showed lower rates not only of HPV-16 infection but also of HPV-16 associated intraepithelial neoplasias (19). Public health groups and statisticians have postulated that vaccination in conjunction with screening may be both an economic and effective way to prevent invasive cervical cancers (20).

REFERENCES

1. Committee on Practice Bulletins-Gynecology, ACOG Practice Bulletin. Diagnosis and treatment of cervical carcinomas, number 35. *Obstet Gynecol*, 2002;99(5 Pt 1):855–867.
2. Jemal A, Murray T, Samuels A, et al. Cancer statistics, 2003. *CA Cancer J Clin* 2003;53(1):5–26.
3. Murthy NS, Mathew A. Risk factors for pre-cancerous lesions of the cervix. *Eur J Cancer Prev* 2000;9(1):5–14.
4. Wright JD, Herzog TJ. Human papillomavirus: emerging trends in detection and management. *Curr Womens Health Rep* 2002;2(4):259–265.
5. Bosch F, Manos M, Munoz N, et al. Prevalence of human papillomavirus in cervical cancer: a worldwide perspective. International biological study on cervical cancer (IBSCC) Study Group. *J Natl Cancer Inst Cancer Spectrum* 1995;87(11):796–802.
6. Burd EM. Human papillomavirus and cervical cancer. *Clin Microbiol Rev* 2003;16(1):1–17.
7. Einstein MH, Goldberg GL. Human papillomavirus and cervical neoplasia. *Cancer Invest* 2002; 20(7-8):1080–1085.
8. Serraino D, Carrieri P, Pradier C, et al. Risk of invasive cervical cancer among women with, or at risk for, HIV infection. *Int J Cancer* 1999;82(3):334–337.
9. Saslow D, Runowicz CD, Solomon D, et al. American Cancer Society guideline for the early detection of cervical neoplasia and cancer. *CA Cancer J Clin* 2002;52(6):342–362.
10. Krivak TC, Rose GS, McBroom JW, et al. Cervical adenocarcinoma in situ: a systematic review of therapeutic options and predictors of persistent or recurrent disease. *Obstet Gynecol Surv* 2001;56(9):567–575.
11. Grigsby PW. Cervical cancer: combined modality therapy. Cancer J 2001;7(Suppl. 1):S47–S50.
12. Krauss T, Huschmand NA, Viereck V, et al. New developments in the treatment of cervical cancer. *Onkologie* 2001;24(4):340–345.
13. Grigsby PW, Herzog TJ. Current management of patients with invasive cervical carcinoma. *Clin Obstet Gynecol* 2001;44(3):531–537.
14. Rotman M, Pajak TF, Choi K, et al. Prophylactic extended-field irradiation of para-aortic lymph nodes in stages IIB and bulky IB and IIA cervical carcinomas. Ten-year treatment results of RTOG 79-20. *JAMA* 1995;274(5):387–393.
15. Friedlander M. Guidelines for the treatment of recurrent and metastatic cervical cancer. *Oncologist* 2002;7(4):342–347.
16. Nguyen C, Montz FJ, Bristow RE. Management of stage I cervical cancer in pregnancy. *Obstet Gynecol Surv* 2000;55(10):633–643.
17. McDonald SD, Faught W, Gruslin A. Cervical cancer during pregnancy. *J Obstet Gynaecol Can* 2002;24(6):491–498.
18. Clarke B, Chetty R. Postmodern cancer: the role of human immunodeficiency virus in uterine cervical cancer. *Mol Pathol* 2002;55(1):19–24.
19. Koutsky LA, Ault KA, Wheeler CM, et al. A controlled trial of a human papillomavirus type 16 vaccine. *N Engl J Med* 2002;347(21):1645–1651.
20. Kulasingam SL, Myers ER. Potential health and economic impact of adding a human papillomavirus vaccine to screening programs. *JAMA* 2003;290(6):781–789.

20

Vulvar Cancer

Christina M. Annunziata* and Michael J. Birrer†

*Medical Oncology Clinical Research Unit, National Cancer Institute, National Institutes of Health, Bethesda, Maryland; and †Department of Cell and Cancer Biology, National Cancer Institute, National Institutes of Health, Rockville, Maryland

EPIDEMIOLOGY

- Vulvar cancer accounts for 4% of all female genital malignancies; 4,000 new cases were projected for 2003.
- It is most frequent in women between 65 and 75 years old, and is occasionally diagnosed in women younger than 40 years.

ETIOLOGY AND RISK FACTORS

- The etiology remains unclear and potentially involves two distinct diseases associated with
  1. human papillomavirus (HPV) DNA, especially type 16, found in 80% of intraepithelial lesions and in 10% to 15% of invasive vulvar cancers (especially squamous cell)
  2. chronic inflammation: venereal or granulomatous lesions, Lichen sclerosus (coexists with up to 25% of vulvar cancers), and Paget disease (preinvasive, see below).
- Vulvar intraepithelial neoplasia (VIN), especially high grade (VIN III), increases risk for development of vulvar cancer.
- Classic risk factors such as hypertension, diabetes mellitus, and obesity most probably represent conditions associated with aging and are not truly independent risk factors for this malignancy.

HISTOLOGY

Squamous cell carcinomas (SCCs) constitute more than 90% of cases, and melanomas constitute less than 10% of cases. The remainder are adenocarcinoma, basal cell carcinoma, verrucous carcinoma, sarcoma, and other rare tumors.

VULVAR SQUAMOUS CELL CARCINOMA

Vulvar SCC is commonly indolent, with slow extension and late metastases. Signs and symptoms in order of decreasing frequency are pruritus, mass, pain, bleeding, ulceration, dysuria, and discharge.

Diagnostic Workup

- Biopsy, cystoscopy, proctoscopy, chest x-ray (CXR), and i.v. urography, if needed, based on the extent of disease
- Suspected bladder or rectal involvement must be biopsied.

Indications for Excisional Biopsy of Vulvar Lesions

- Any gross lesion
- Red, white, dark brown, or black skin patches
- Areas firm to palpation
- Pruritic, tingling, or bleeding lesions
- Any nevi in the genital tract
- Enlarged or thickened areas of Bartholin glands, especially in postmenopausal women.

Location and Metastatic Spread Pattern of Vulvar Squamous Cell Carcinoma

- Vulvar squamous cell carcinoma is found on the labia majora in 50% of cases and on the labia minora in 15% to 20%; the remainder of these cancers are on the clitoris and perineum.
- The carcinoma tends to grow locally, with subsequent spread to inguinal, femoral, and pelvic lymph nodes (LNs). Hematogenous spread usually takes place after LN involvement.

Staging

- Vulvar cancer is a surgically staged disease (see Table 20.1).

Prognostic Factors and Survival (True for Most Histologies)

- Survival depends on stage, LN involvement, depth of invasion, structures involved, and tumor location.
- Survival is most dependent on the pathologic status of the inguinal LNs and on the size of the primary lesion (lesions <2-cm in greatest dimension, inguinal LN(−), show 98% 5-year survival; lesions of any size, three or more unilateral LN(+) or two or more bilateral LN(+), show 29% 5-year survival).
- LN metastases are related to tumor size, clinical stage, and depth of invasion.

Management

Stage 0

The following therapeutic approaches are equally effective:

1. Wide local excision, laser beam therapy, or combination of the two
2. Skinning vulvectomy with or without grafting.

In some cases, a 5% 5-fluorouracil (5-FU) cream can be used [response rate (RR) is 50% to 60%], but it is not the first choice of therapy.

Recurrences are seen regardless of type of procedure used for initial treatment (most common sites are perianal skin, presacral area, and clitoral hood).

Stage I

- Less than 1-mm invasion: *wide local excision*
- From 1-mm to 5-mm invasion: *modified radical vulvectomy with ipsilateral superficial inguinal lymphadenectomy* for lesions located laterally, and *bilateral node dissection* for centrally placed lesions. Sentinel LN biopsy is an emerging technique in early stage vulvar cancer and may obviate the need for full nodal dissections in many women.

TABLE 20.1. *Staging*

TNM		Staging (FIGO) 1988	
T Primary tumor			
Tis	Preinvasive carcinoma (carcinoma *in situ*)	Stage 0 Tis	Carcinoma *in situ*; intraepithelial carcinoma
T1	Tumor confined to the vulva and/or *perineum*—2 cm or less in diameter	Stage I	Tumor confined to the vulva and/or *perineum*—2 cm or less in greatest dimension. *No nodal metastases*
			T1 N0 M0
T2	Tumor confined to the vulva and/or *perineum*—more than 2 cm in diameter	Stage II	Tumor confined to the vulva and/or *perineum*—more than 2 cm in greatest dimension. *No nodal metastases*
			T2 N0 M0
T3	Tumor of any size, with adjacent spread to the urethra, vagina, anus, or all of these	Stage III	Tumor of any size with the following: (a) adjacent spread to the lower urethra, the vagina, the anus, and/or (b) *unilateral regional lymph node metastases*
			T3 N0 M0
			T3 N1 M0
T4	Tumor of any size infiltrating the bladder mucosa or the rectal mucosa or both, including the upper part of the urethral mucosa or fixed to the anus	Stage IVA	Tumor invades any of the following: upper urethra, bladder mucosa, pelvic bone, and/or *bilateral regional lymph node metastases*
			T1 N1 M0
			T1 N2 M0
			T2 N2 M0
			T3 N2 M0
			T4 any N M0
N Regional lymph nodes		Stage IVB any T, any N, M1	Any distant metastases, including pelvic lymph nodes
N0	No nodes palpable		
N1	*Unilateral regional lymph node metastases*		
N2	*Bilateral regional lymph node metastases*		
M Distant metastases			
M0	No distant metastases		
M1	Distant metastases *(including pelvic lymph node metastases)*		

Italicized words indicate changes from the pre-1988 definitions.
From Creasman WT. New gynecologic cancer staging. *Obstet Gynecol* 1990;75(2):287–288, with permission.

- Poor surgical candidates can be treated with radiation therapy, achieving long-term survival.
- Surgical complications include mortality (2% to 5%), wound breakdown or infection, sepsis, thromboembolism, chronic leg lymphedema (use of separate incision for the groin LN dissection reduces wound breakdown and leg edema), urinary tract infection, stress urinary incontinence, and poor sexual function.

Stage II

Modified radical vulvectomy and bilateral inguinal lymphadenectomy can be used if at least 1 cm of negative margins can be achieved with preservation of midline structures.

Stages III and IV

The management of stage III and IV disease is shown in Fig. 20.1. Special considerations:

- Management of positive groin nodes: one LN requires no further therapy, whereas two or more LNs can be treated with groin and pelvic radiation therapy (based on data from GOG randomized trial in which improved survival was documented with this therapy as compared to pelvic LN dissection).
- Suggested doses of localized adjuvant radiation are 45 to 50 Gy.
- Neoadjuvant chemoradiation can be used in stage III and IV disease to improve the operability of the tumor. Recent GOG trials have been successful with the use of cisplatin and 5-FU concurrently with radiation.
- Patients with inoperable disease can achieve long-term survival with radical radiation therapy.
- When radiation is given as primary definitive treatment, it is suggested that the addition of 5-FU with cisplatin or mitomycin C be considered.

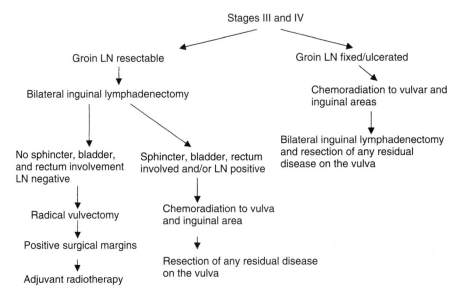

FIG. 20.1. Management algorithm for stages III and IV disease. (From DiSaia PJ, Creasman WT. Clinical gynecologic oncology, 5th ed. St. Louis: Mosby, 1997:222, with permission.)

- Radiation fraction size of less than or equal to 180 cGy has been proven to minimize the radiation complication rate (i.e., late fibrosis, atrophy, telangiectasia, and necrosis). Total doses of 54 to 65 Gy should be used.

Recurrent and Metastatic Disease

- Treatment and outcome depend on site and extent of recurrence.
- *Local recurrence* can be treated with wide local reexcision with or without radiation (5-year survival of 56% if regional LNs are negative). In cases with small localized recurrence, radiation with or without 5-FU can be curative.
- Another option is radical vulvectomy and pelvic exenteration.
- *Groin nodes* can be subjected to radiation and surgery.
- *Distant recurrence*: no standard systemic chemotherapy is available for metastatic disease. These patients are appropriate candidates for clinical trials. Agents such as cisplatin, methotrexate, cyclophosphamide, bleomycin, and mitomycin C have shown a partial RR of only 10% to 15%, and they are of short duration a (few months). Trials evaluating the efficacy of paclitaxel in vulvar cancer are ongoing.

VERRUCOUS CARCINOMA

- Verrucous carcinoma is very rare and can be confused with condyloma acuminátum because of exophytic growth pattern.
- It is locally destructive and rarely metastasizes.
- It is associated with HPV type 6.
- The main treatment is surgery; LN dissection is of questionable value unless LNs are obviously involved. Radiation is contraindicated because it is not effective and can potentially lead to more aggressive behavior.

PAGET DISEASE

- Paget disease is characterized by preinvasive lesions.
- The most frequent symptoms include pruritus, tenderness, or vulvar lesions (i.e., hyperemic, well-demarcated, thickened lesions, with areas of induration and excoriation).
- Paget disease can be associated with underlying adenocarcinoma of the vulva (1% to 2%). These patients should be treated the same way as are patients with other vulvar malignancies.

MALIGNANT MELANOMA

- Malignant melanoma is a rare tumor (5% of all melanoma cases).
- Most melanomas are located on the labia minora and clitoris.
- Prognosis depends on the size of the lesion and on the depth of invasion.
- Staging of malignant melanoma is the same as for skin melanoma.
- The suggested therapy is radical vulvectomy with inguinal and pelvic lymphadenectomy (lately the tendency is for a more conservative approach). For most well-demarcated lesions, 2-cm margins are suggested for thin (up to 7 mm) lesions and 3- to 4-cm margins are suggested for thicker lesions.

BARTHOLIN GLAND

Adenocarcinoma

- Adenocarcinoma of the Bartholin gland is a very rare tumor (1% of all vulvar malignancies).
- Its peak incidence is in women in their mid-60s.

- Enlargement of the Bartholin gland area in postmenopausal women requires evaluation for malignancy.
- The therapy includes radical vulvectomy with wide excision to achieve adequate margins and inguinal lymphadenectomy.

Adenoid Cystic Carcinoma

- Adenoid cystic carcinoma is a very rare tumor.
- It is characterized by frequent local recurrences and very slow progression.
- The recommended therapy is wide local excision with ipsilateral inguinal lymphadenectomy.

Basal Cell Carcinoma

- The natural history and therapeutic approach for basal cell carcinoma are similar to those for primary tumors seen in other sites (i.e., wide local excision).

ACKNOWLEDGMENT

We would like to thank Dr. Helen Frederickson for her critical review of this chapter.

SUGGESTED READINGS

DiSaia PJ, Creasman WT. *Clinical gynecologic oncology*, 5th ed. St. Louis: Mosby, 1997.

Moore RG, DePasquale SE, Steinhoff MM, et al. Sentinel node identification and the ability to detect metastatic tumor to inguinal lymph nodes in squamous cell cancer of the vulva. *Gynecol Oncol* 2003; 89(3):475–479.

Montana GS, Thomas GM, Moore DH, et al. Preoperative chemo-radiation for carcinoma of the vulva with N2/N3 nodes: a gynecologic oncology group study. *Int J Radiat Oncol Biol Phys* 2000;48(4): 1007–1013.

Nash JD, Curry S. Vulvar cancer. *Surg Oncol Clin North Am* 1998;7(2):335–346.

NCI-PDQ Page. at: http://cancernet.nci.nih.gov/clinpdq/soa/Cervical_cancer_Physician.html, 2003.

SECTION 7

Musculoskeletal

21

Sarcomas and Malignancies of the Bone

Patrick J. Mansky* and Lee Helman†

National Center for Complementary and Alternative Medicine, National Institutes of Health, Bethesda, Maryland and †Pediatric Oncology, Center for Cancer Research, National Cancer Institute, National Institutes of Health, Bethesda, Maryland

Malignancies of the soft tissue (6.1%) and bones (4.7%) account for more than 10% of newly diagnosed cancers in children, adolescents, and young adults. Fortunately, benign musculoskeletal neoplasms are 100 times more common than malignant soft-tissue tumors. Median age at diagnosis of rhabdomyosarcoma (RMS) is 5 years, with a male preponderance. Osteosarcomas account for approximately 60% of malignant bone tumors in the first two decades of life. Most of the remaining bone malignancies in children and adolescents are Ewing sarcomas and the histologically similar and genetically identical peripheral primitive neuroectodermal tumors (PNETs). Together, these tumors are often called the Ewing family of tumors (EFT). Chondrosarcomas are seen in older adults. Identification of specific, recurrent genetic alterations in RMS and Ewing sarcoma has improved diagnosis by clarifying pathogenesis. Better supportive care and systematic application of effective multimodality treatment have dramatically improved survival during the last 30 years (see Fig. 21.1 and Table 21.1).

RHABDOMYOSARCOMA

Clinical Presentation

RMS has been encountered in almost all anatomic sites. It is associated with development of a mass and signs and symptoms typically related to the anatomic location (see Fig. 21.2):

- *Orbit:* proptosis
- *Nasopharynx:* nasal discharge and obstruction
- *Basal skull and posterior orbit:* cranial nerve palsies and visual loss
- *Parameninges:* headache and meningism
- *Genitourinary tract*: vaginal polyp and vaginal discharge (vaginal or uterine tumors)
- *Bladder or prostate tumor, pelvis:* urinary obstruction
- *Genital:* paratesticular scrotal mass.

Pathophysiology

RMSs are of mesenchymal origin, characterized by myogenic differentiation. They are histologically distinguished into two main forms, embryonal (80%) and alveolar (15% to 20%)

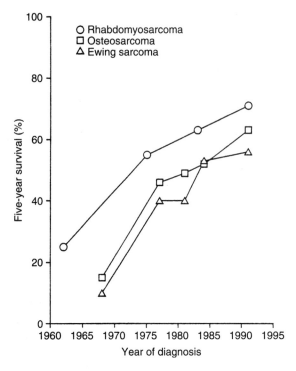

FIG. 21.1. Five-year survival rates among children and adolescents with rhabdomyosarcoma, with osteosarcoma, and with Ewing sarcoma. (From Arndt CAS, Crist WM. Common musculoskeletal tumors of childhood and adolescence. *N Engl J Med* 1999;342:342–352, with permission.)

subtypes, with characteristic genetic differences (see Table 21.2 and Fig. 21.3). Botryoid RMS and spindle cell sarcoma are both morphologic variants of embryonal RMS.

An increased risk for the development of RMS has been associated with a number of environmental and genetic factors (see Table 21.3).

Diagnosis

Diagnostic Radiology

A comprehensive staging of evaluation of extent of disease includes the following:

1. *Tumor localization*
   • Computerized tomography (CT) and magnetic resonance imaging (MRI).
2. *Assessment of metastatic spread*
   • CT of chest and lungs
   • Technetium bone scan for bone or bone marrow involvement.

Biopsy and Pathologic Diagnosis

Open biopsy is the preferred approach for tissue diagnosis and should be undertaken at an oncology center, where diagnostic material can be optimally used and the initial surgical

TABLE 21.1. *Outcome of therapy for musculoskeletal tumors of childhood and adolescence*

Type of tumor	Commonly used agents	Duration of therapy (mo)	Long-term survival (%)	Additional treatment
Rhabdomyosarcoma				
Low-risk group (those with group I or II embryonal tumors at sites with a favorable outcome or group III orbital tumors)	Vincristine, dactinomycin	8–12	90–95	Resection of primary tumor for all tumors except orbital tumors; irradiation of group II or III tumors
Intermediate-risk group	Vincristine, dactinomycin, cyclophosphamide	8–12	70–80	Irradiation of primary tumor and metastases, if present
High-risk group [all those with metastases (group IV) except patients younger than 10 years who have embryonal tumors]	Vincristine, dactinomycin, and cyclophosphamide; new agents; high-dose therapy with hematopoietic stem-cell transplantation	8–12	20	Irradiation of primary tumor and all metastatic lesions
Osteosarcoma				
Localized to limb	Doxorubicin, high-dose methotrexate, ifosfamide, and cisplatin	8–12	58–76	Surgery for control of tumor
Metastatic	Doxorubicin, methotrexate, ifosfamide, cisplatin	8–12	14–50	Resection of primary tumor and metastases needed for cure
Ewing sarcoma				
Localized	Vincristine, doxorubicin, cyclophosphamide, dactinomycin, etoposide-ifosfamide	8–12	50–70	Surgery, radiation therapy, or both for local control of tumor
Metastatic	Vincristine, doxorubicin, cyclophosphamide, dactinomycin, etoposide-ifosfamide; high-dose therapy with hematopoietic stem-cell transplantation	8–12	19–30	Surgery, radiation therapy, or both for local control of tumor

The estimated rates of survival at 3–5 years without the need for re-treatment (progression-free or relapse-free survival) are shown.

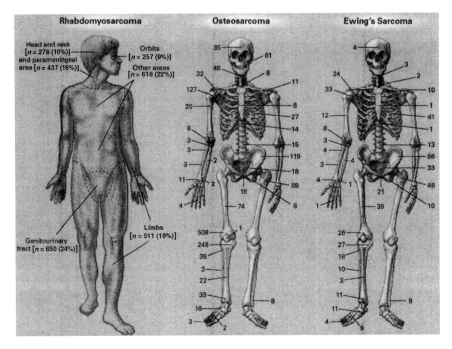

FIG. 21.2. Primary sites of rhabdomyosarcoma, osteosarcoma, and Ewing sarcoma. The numbers of patients with primary tumors at specific sites are shown.

approach can be determined by a multidisciplinary team responsible for the patient's subsequent treatment. Needle biopsy may restrict access to fresh and frozen tissue for cytogenetic and molecular genetic investigations.

1. *Tumor characterization*
   - Histopathology
     - Immunohistochemistry: desmin and myoD1
   - Genetic characterization of tumor
     - Reverse transcriptase-polymerase chain reaction (RT-PCR) for presence of PAX/FKHR translocation
     - Cytogenetics.

TABLE 21.2. *Histologically distinguished subtypes of rhabdomyosarcomas*

Embryonal RMS
- Characteristic loss of heterogenicity (LOH) 11p15.5 (IGH-II gene)
- Hyperdiploid DNA

Alveolar RMS
- Characteristic translocations
  1. PAX3/FKHR t(2,13)(q35;q14)
  2. PAX7/FKHR t(1;13)(p36;q14)
- Tetraploid DNA

RMS, rhabdomyosarcomas; DNA, deoxyribonucleic acid.

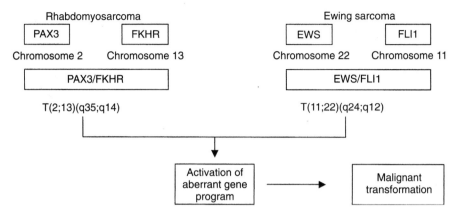

FIG. 21.3. Molecular pathogenetic mechanisms in rhabdomyosarcoma and Ewing sarcoma.

2. *Metastatic spread*
   - Cerebrospinal fluid polymerase chain reaction (CSF PCR) for PAX/FKHR translocation
   - Bone marrow aspirate cytology
   - Bone marrow biopsy for histochemistry and PCR.

Treatment Strategies Overview

The diversity of primary sites, the distinctive surgical and radiation therapies for each primary site, the subsequent site-specific rehabilitation, and the potential treatment-related sequelae underscore the importance of treating children and young adults with RMS in the context of a clinical trial at a major medical center with appropriate experience in all therapeutic modalities (see Table 21.4).

Surgery

Local tumor control is the cornerstone of therapy, especially for patients with nonmetastatic disease. Primary tumor resection should be undertaken only if there is no evidence of

TABLE 21.3. *Associated risk factors for rhabdomyosarcoma*

Genetic	Familial cancer risk
	Germline mutant p53
	Congenital abnormalities
	Neurofibromatosis type I
	Li-Fraumeni syndrome
	Risk of breast cancer in female relatives[a]
Environmental parental habits	Smoking
	Recreational drugs
	Occupational chemical exposure
	Fetal alcohol syndrome

[a]Link between rhabdomyosarcoma and risk of breast cancer in a female relative plays an important role in cancer surveillance in at-risk families.

TABLE 21.4. Treatment options, local control, and potential toxicity in rhabdomyosarcoma

Treatments	Local control	Sequelae			
		Sterility	Kidneys	On growth	Esthetics
1. Orbit					
Radical surgery then VA ± C	++	−	−	±	±
Biopsy then radiation + V ± C	++	±	−	++	++
Biopsy then IVA/VAC	±	±	±	−	−
No complete remission:					
Radical surgery	−	−	−	++	++
or Radiotherapy	−	−	−	++	++
2. Paratesticular					
Surgery + VA	±	−	−	−	−
Surgery + VAC/IVA	++	±	±	−	−
3. Limbs					
Surgery + VA	±	−	−	−	±
Surgery + IVA	++	±	±	−	±
4. Vagina					
IVA/VAC, complete remission followed by monitoring	±	±	±	−	−
IVA followed by elective surgery or interstitial radiation	++	±	±	±	±
5. Bladder/prostate					
Radical surgery then IVA/VAC with or without selective radiotherapy	++	++	++	++	++
IVA/VAC followed by local surgery	±	±	±	−	±
No complete remission, radiation	±	−	−	−	−
6. Thorax, abdomen, pelvis					
IVA/VAC then selective radiation, then IVA/VAC	−	++	±	±	±
IVA/VAC, CR with or without surgery followed by IVA/VAC	±	±	±	±	−
7. Parameningeal					
IVA/VAC followed by extensively early radiation, then IVA/VAC	++	±	±	++	−
IVA/VAC, followed by delayed limited radiation and then by IVA/VAC	±	±	±	±	−
8. Nonparameningeal head and neck					
Radical surgery followed by VA	++	−	−	−	++
Biopsy then IVA/VAC, followed by CR	±	±	±	−	−
Or non-CR and radiation	−	−	−	++	±
Or non-CR and surgery	−	−	−	−	±

VA, vincristine–actinomycin D; C, cyclophosphamide; V, vincristine; IVA, ifosfamide–vincristine–actinomycin D; VAC, vincristine–actinomycin D-cyclophosphamide; CR, complete remission. ++, Yes; ±, possibly; −, No.

lymph node or metastatic disease and if the tumor can be excised with good margins without functional impairment or mutilation. Surgery has a small role or no role in the primary management of orbital tumors and only a limited role in the local control of head and neck tumors. However, to avoid pelvic irradiation in very young children, the morbidity of radical surgery necessary to achieve local control may be accepted.

Radiation Therapy

Radiation therapy is recommended for patients with the following characteristics after initial surgical resection or chemotherapy:

1. *Completely resected tumor* (clinical group I)
   - unfavorable histology (alveolar RMS)
2. *Microscopic residual disease* (clinical group II)
   - radiation therapy to 4,100 cGy
3. *Gross residual disease* (clinical group III)
   - radiation therapy to 5,040 cGy.

Treatment volume:

- Volume is determined by the extent of disease at diagnosis prior to resection and chemotherapy.
- Radiation field should extend 2-cm beyond tumor margin.
- Whole-brain irradiation of 2,340 to 3,060 cGy is given for parameningeal disease with intracranial extension.

Chemotherapy

It has long been recognized that neoadjuvant combination, multiagent chemotherapy given for extensive (primarily unresectable) tumors could reduce the extent of subsequent surgery or radiation therapy. Figure 21.4 provides an outline of this multidisciplinary approach for osteosarcoma.

OSTEOSARCOMA

Osteosarcoma is a primary bone malignancy with a peak incidence during the pubescent growth spurt (from 15 to 19 years) in the metaphyses of the most rapidly growing bones. Risk factors are listed in Table 21.5.

Clinical Presentation

- Bone pain
- Swelling
- Most often, mass in area of metaphyseal bones of femur or tibia.

Diagnosis and Staging

Diagnostic Radiology

1. *Assessment of tumor*
   - Destruction of bone visualized on plain radiograph, with a consequent loss of normal trabeculae and the appearance of radiolucent areas
   - New bone formation
   - Lytic or sclerotic appearance
   - "Sunburst sign": periosteal elevation by tumor penetrating the cortical bone.

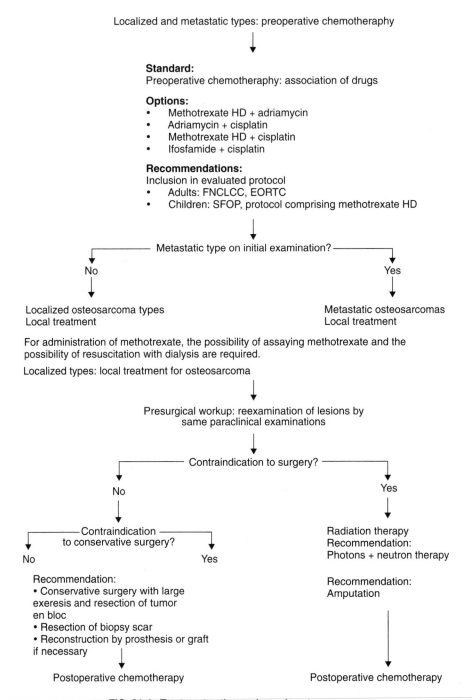

Localized and metastatic types: preoperative chemotheraphy

Standard:
Preoperative chemotheraphy: association of drugs

Options:
- Methotrexate HD + adriamycin
- Adriamycin + cisplatin
- Methotrexate HD + cisplatin
- Ifosfamide + cisplatin

Recommendations:
Inclusion in evaluated protocol
- Adults: FNCLCC, EORTC
- Children: SFOP, protocol comprising methotrexate HD

Metastatic type on initial examination?

No → Localized osteosarcoma types / Local treatment

Yes → Metastatic osteosarcomas / Local treatment

For administration of methotrexate, the possibility of assaying methotrexate and the possibility of resuscitation with dialysis are required.

Localized types: local treatment for osteosarcoma

Presurgical workup: reexamination of lesions by same paraclinical examinations

Contraindication to surgery?

No

Yes → Radiation therapy
Recommendation:
Photons + neutron therapy

Recommendation:
Amputation

Contraindication to conservative surgery?

No

Yes

Recommendation:
- Conservative surgery with large exeresis and resection of tumor en bloc
- Resection of biopsy scar
- Reconstruction by prosthesis or graft if necessary

Postoperative chemotherapy

Postoperative chemotherapy

FIG. 21.4. Treatment options schema in osteosarcoma.

TABLE 21.5. *Risk factors for osteosarcoma*

Familial cancer	Li-Fraumeni syndrome
Secondary osteosarcoma	Irradiated bones
	Bilateral retinoblastoma (independent of therapy modality)
Loss of tumor-suppressor genes	p53 and Rb (retinoblastoma)

  2. *Determination of extent of disease*
  - MRI to assess primary tumor boundaries of entire long bone area (T1 weighted), including search for skip lesions
  - Technetium bone scan.
  3. *Metastatic spread (15% to 20%)*
  - Technetium bone scan
  - CT chest/lungs.

Biopsy and Laboratory Investigations

Histologic diagnosis depends on the presence of a frankly malignant sarcomatous stroma associated with the production of tumor osteoid. It is highly recommended that if the surgeon suspects a primary malignant bone lesion after a preliminary assessment with history, physical examination, and plain radiographs, all invasive procedures, especially the placement and technique of biopsy, should be done by an experienced orthopedic oncologist.

Generous amounts of fresh and frozen tissue should be available to perform various prognostic assays including measurement of tumor DNA content, molecular genetic evaluations, and P-glycoprotein estimation. Serum lactate dehydrogenase (LDH) levels are also powerful prognostic factors and may be elevated in 30% of patients without metastases.

Treatment Strategies

Almost all patients with osteosarcoma have subclinical micrometastatic disease. Thus, treatment requires surgical ablation of the primary tumor (amputation or limb-sparing resection) and treatment of micrometastatic disease with chemotherapy (see Figs. 21.4 to 21.7).

Chemotherapy

Most patients receive neoadjuvant and adjuvant therapy.

  1. *Neoadjuvant chemotherapy*
  - Evaluation of bone marrow, cardiac liver, and renal function
  - Initiation early after completion of biopsy and staging studies
  - Duration: 9 to 12 weeks.
  2. *Adjuvant chemotherapy*
  - Evaluation of extent of tumor necrosis in surgical specimen for prognostic purposes (predictor of disease-free and overall survival)
  - Initiation early after definitive surgery of primary tumor
  - Duration: 35 to 40 weeks.

Surgery

Both amputation and limb-salvage operations incorporate the basic principle of wide *en bloc* excision of the tumor and biopsy site through normal tissue planes, leaving a cuff of normal tissue around the periphery of the tumor. Limb-sparing surgery is now the preferred approach

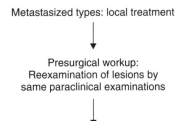

Metastasized types: local treatment

Presurgical workup:
Reexamination of lesions by
same paraclinical examinations

Standard surgery of primary tumor and metastases

Recommendations:

• Conservative surgery with large exeresis and resection
  of tumor en bloc
• Resection of biopsy scar
• Amputation must remain the exception
• Surgery of metastases according to localization

Postoperative chemotherapy

FIG. 21.5. Treatment options in metastatic osteosarcoma.

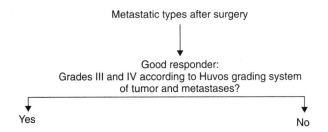

Metastatic types after surgery

Good responder:
Grades III and IV according to Huvos grading system
of tumor and metastases?

Yes

No

Standard:
Postoperative chemotherapy:
Same protocol as in preoperative

Standard:
Postoperative chemotherapy:
Other drugs effective in
osteosarcoma

Options:
If methotrexate and adriamycin in preoperative:
• Ifosfamide + VP16 or
• Ifosfamide + cisplatin

Recommendation:
Protocol evaluated:
• Adults: FNCLCC, EORTC
• Children: SFOP
• Adults and children: phase II trial

FIG. 21.6. Treatment options in postoperative metastatic osteosarcoma.

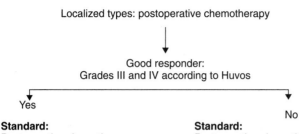

Localized types: postoperative chemotherapy

Good responder:
Grades III and IV according to Huvos

Yes

Standard:
Postoperative chemotherapy:
Same protocol as in preoperative

No

Standard:
Postoperative chemotherapy:
Other drugs effective in osteosarcoma

Options:
If methotrexate and adriamycin in preoperative:
• Ifosfamide + VP16 or
• Ifosfamide + cisplatin

Recommendation:
Protocol evaluated:
• Adults: FNCLCC, EORTC
• Children: SFOP

FIG. 21.7. Treatment options in postoperative localized osteosarcoma.

for most (70% to 90%) patients with osteosarcoma because it achieves a better functional outcome. Reconstruction uses allografts, customized endoprosthetic devices, modular endoprosthetic devices, or combinations of these methods. This requires a multidisciplinary team and close cooperation between the chemotherapist and orthopedic oncologist.

Follow-up

Patients with osteosarcomas should be monitored frequently for metastases with radiographic studies for at least 5 years after completion of therapy. Most first recurrences appear asymptomatically in the lungs. All patients with recurrent disease should be approached with curative intent because durable salvage has been reported in 10% to 20% of such patients.

EWING FAMILY OF TUMORS

The EFT include Ewing sarcoma of the bone, PNETs, Askin–Rosai tumor (PNET of the chest wall), and extraosseous Ewing (EOE) sarcoma. Studies using immunohistochemical markers, cytogenetics, and tissue culture indicate that these tumors are all derived from the same primordial stem cell and are distinguished only by the degree of neural differentiation. Epidemiologically, it is remarkable that there is a low incidence in black and Chinese populations. Nearly 12% of patients with Ewing sarcoma also have associated urogenital anomalies such as cryptorchidism, hypospadias, and ureteral duplication. Ewing sarcoma accounts for 10% to 15% of all malignant bone tumors; peak incidence is between 10 and 15 years of age.

Clinical Presentation

• Persistent and increasing pain, local swelling, and functional impairment of affected area (see Table 21.6)
• Fever
• Associated neurologic symptoms include paraplegia and peripheral nerve abnormalities

TABLE 21.6. *Clinical presentation of osteosarcoma and Ewing family of tumors*

	Osteosarcoma	EFT
Tumor localization	Metaphyseal bone	Diaphyseal/flat bones
Radiographic characteristics	Periosteal elevation with new bone formation: "sun burst"	Patchy bone destruction: "moth eaten" Periosteal lamellation: "onion skin"
Associated signs	Soft-tissue swelling	Soft-tissue swelling, pleural effusion

EFT, Ewing family of tumors.

- Uncommon symptoms include
  1. lymph node involvement
  2. meningeal spread
  3. central nervous system (CNS) disease.

Diagnosis and Staging

Diagnostic Radiology

1. *Evaluation of primary tumor*
   - CT and MRI of primary lesion
2. *Metastatic spread (20%)*
   - CT scan of the chest and lungs
   - Technetium bone scan for tumor extent and bone marrow involvement.

Approximately 20% of patients have visible metastases at diagnosis. Of these patients, about 50% have lung metastases and about 40% have multiple-bone involvement and diffuse bone marrow involvement.

Biopsy and Laboratory Investigations

Open biopsy is the preferred approach for tissue diagnosis and should be undertaken at an oncology center, where the diagnostic material can be optimally used and the initial surgical approach can be determined by a multidisciplinary team responsible for the patient's subsequent treatment. Needle biopsy may restrict access to fresh and frozen tissue for cytogenetic and molecular genetic investigations.

1. *Serology*
   - LDH: prognostic indicator reflecting disease burden
2. *Histopathologic evaluation*
   - "Small blue round cell tumor"
   - Immunohistochemistry: NSE, vimentin, S-100, HBA-71
3. *Cytogenetics/molecular genetics*
   - t(11;22)(q24;q12) in 85% of tumors
   - RT PCR of EWS/FLI transcripts.

The t(11;22)(q24;q12) translocation results in the formation of a chimeric gene between *EWS* (Ewing sarcoma gene), a novel putative RNA-binding gene located on chromosome 22q12, and *FLI1,* a member of the erythroblastosis virus–transforming sequence (ETS) family

Treatment Schema

iii c eee a	iii c eee a	iii c eee a	SR RAD	V Dac		V Dac	V	V Dac	Dac	I E	C A
0	3	6	9	11		15		17		20	23
I E	C A	I E	C A	C A							
26	29	32	35	41	138	44					

Induction (week 0–6)
i = ifosfamide 2 g/m^2/day × 3
e = etoposide 150 mg/m^2/day × 3
c = cyclophosphamide 1.5 g/m^2 day 5
a = doxorubicin 45 mg/m^2 day 5

Local control (weeks 9–17)
SR = surgical resection
V = vincristine 1.5 mg/m^2
Dac = dactinomycin 1.5 mg/m^2
RAD = start radiotherapy

Maintenance (week 20–44)
I = ifosfamide 2 g/m^2/day × 5
E = etoposide 150 mg/m^2/day × 5
C = cyclophosphamide 1.0 OR 1.5 g/m^2/day × 2
A = doxorubicin 60 mg/m^2 continous infusion
    over 24 hours

FIG. 21.8. Dose-intensive chemotherapy for children with Ewing family of tumors. (From Marina NM, Pappo AS, Parham DM, et al. Chemotherapy dose-intensification for pediatric patients with Ewing family of tumors and desmoplastic small round cell tumors: a feasibility study at St. Jude Children's Research Hospital. *J Clin Oncol* 1999;17:180–190, with permission.)

of transcription factors located on chromosome 11q24, and has been fully characterized at the molecular genetic level. RT PCR of the fusion transcripts from the tumor can identify patients with favorable prognosis with localized primary tumors.

Treatment Strategies

Almost all patients with apparently localized disease at diagnosis have subclinical micrometastatic disease. Hence, a multidisciplinary approach including local disease control with surgery and/or radiation as well as systemic chemotherapy is indicated (see Fig. 21.8).

Surgery

Generally, surgery is the preferred approach if the lesion is resectable. Radiation therapy is used for patients who do not have a surgical option that preserves function and for patients whose tumors have been excised but with inadequate margins.

Radiation Therapy

The Intergroup Ewing's Sarcoma Study (IESS) recommendations include the following:

- For gross residual disease: 4,500 cGy plus a 1,080-cGy boost to tumor site.
- For microscopic residual disease: 4,500 cGy plus 5,400-cGy boost.
- For pulmonary metastasis: whole-lung radiation of 1,200 to 1,500 cGy even if complete resolution of pulmonary metastatic disease is possible with chemotherapy.
- For metastatic sites of disease in bone and soft tissues: 4,500 to 5,600 cGy.

Radiation therapy should be delivered in a setting in which stringent planning techniques are applied by those experienced in the treatment of EFT.

Chemotherapy

The two most effective agents are cyclophosphamide and doxorubicin, but vincristine and dactinomycin are also active. Recently, dose-intensification studies using ifosfamide and etoposide have shown significant promise. Prognosis was poor before the advent of effective multiagent chemotherapy (5-year survival of 10% to 20%, despite good local control) and continues to be dismal in patients with metastatic disease (one recent study reported a 3-year event-free survival of only 26.7% ± 13.2%).

FUTURE DIRECTIONS

Better understanding of the molecular pathogenesis of these tumors by characterization of chromosomal translocations associated with RMS and Ewing sarcoma can lead to novel therapeutic strategies. Some current investigational approaches include biologic response modifiers; cell cycle signaling pathway inhibitors; vaccines designed to elicit T-cell immunity, with specificity for tumor-specific fusion peptides; and antibody targeting of immunotoxins to tumor cells.

SUGGESTED READINGS

Arndt CAS, Crist WM. Common musculoskeletal tumors of childhood and adolescence. *N Engl J Med* 1999;342:342–352.
Ginsberg JP, Woo S, Johnson ME. Ewing's sarcoma family of tumors. In: Pizzo PA, Poplack DG, eds. *Principles and practice of pediatric oncology*. Philadelphia, PA: Lippincott–Raven Publishers, 2002: 973–1016.

Link PM, Gebhardt MC, Meyers PA. Osteosarcoma. In: Pizzo PA, Poplack DG, eds. *Principles and practice of pediatric oncology*. Philadelphia, PA: Lippincott–Raven Publishers, 2002:1051–1089.

Marina NM, Pappo AS, Parham DM, et al. Chemotherapy dose-intensification for pediatric patients with Ewing's family of tumors and desmoplastic small round cell tumors: a feasibility study at St. Jude Children's Research Hospital. *J Clin Oncol*1999;17:180–190.

NCNN. Pediatric osteosarcoma practice guidelines. *Oncology*1996;10:1799–1806.

PDQR Cancer Information Summaries. http://cancernet.nci.nih.gov/pdq/pdq_treatment.shtml 2005.

Philip T, Blay JY, Brunat-Mentigny M, et al. Standards, options and recommendations (SOR) for diagnosis, treatment and follow-up of osteosarcoma [French]. *Bull Cancer*1999;86:159–176.

Pinkerton CR. *Clinical challenges in pediatric oncology*. Oxford: ISIS Medical Media, 1999:117–134, 143–156.

Sommelet D, Pinkerton R, Brunat-Mentigny M, et al. Standards, options and recommendations (SOR) for clinical care of rhabdomyosarcoma (RMS) and other soft tissue sarcoma in children [French]. *Bull Cancer*1998;85:1015–1042.

Wexler LH, Christ WM, Helman LJ. Rhabdomyosarcoma and undifferentiated sarcomas. In: Pizzo PA, Poplack DG, eds. *Principles and practice of pediatric oncology*. Philadelphia, PA: Lippincott–Raven Publishers, 2002:939–971.

SECTION 8

Skin Cancer

22

Skin Cancers and Melanoma

Upendra P. Hegde* and Barry Gause†

Division of Hematology/Oncology, University of Connecticut Health Center, Farmington, Connecticut; and †Medical Oncology Clinical Research Unit, National Cancer Institute, National Institutes of Health, Bethesda, Maryland

The skin is the largest organ of the human body. It is embryologically derived from the neuroectoderm and the mesoderm. It consists of three layers: epidermis, dermis, and subcutis. Skin cancers can arise from various cell types and structures in various layers of the skin (1). The exposure of the skin to the environment has a special relevance because a wide variety of carcinogens can interact directly with the genetic components of skin cells. Such exposure has increased the incidence of skin cancers. The cells of origin in various types of skin cancers are outlined in Tables 22.1 and 22.2. The skin cancers are best divided into melanoma and nonmelanoma.

MELANOMA

Melanoma is a skin tumor that originates from the melanocyte, which is derived from the neural crest, and migrates during embryogenesis predominantly to the skin and less commonly to other tissues, such as the meninges, the ocular choroid, the mucosa of the respiratory tract, the gastrointestinal tract, and the genitourinary tract, where melanoma is rarely encountered.

Epidemiology

- Melanoma ranks as the seventh leading type of cancer in the United States.
- Its incidence in women is increasing faster than that of any other cancer except lung cancer.
- The incidence of melanoma is 10 times greater in whites than in the African Americans. The incidence in U.S. whites is 10 per 100,000 population, although some geographic areas have higher rates.

TABLE 22.1. *Cells of epidermis and respective tumor type*

Cells of epidermis	Tumor type	Incidence (%)
Melanocyte	Melanoma	5–7
Epidermal basal cell	Basal cell carcinoma	60
Keratinocyte	Squamous cell carcinoma	30
Merkel cell	Merkel cell tumor	1–2
Langerhans cell	Histiocytosis X	<1
Appendage cells	Appendageal tumors	<1

TABLE 22.2. *Cells of dermis and respective tumor type*

Cells of dermis	Tumor type	Incidence (%)
Fibroblast	Benign and malignant fibrous histiocytic tumors	<1
Mast cell	Mast cell tumor	<1
Vasculature	Angioma and angiosarcoma	<1
	Lymphangioma	<1

- In 2004, it was estimated that 55,100 new cases of cutaneous melanoma would have been diagnosed in the United States, with 7,910 deaths.
- Australia has the highest incidence of melanoma in the world, approximately 17 cases per 100,000 per year.
- In the year 2000, the estimated lifetime risk of melanoma in American whites was 1 person in 75.

Etiology

- Sunlight exposure: ultraviolet B rays
  1. Intermittent intense exposure
  2. Exposure at a young age
  3. Individuals with propensity for sunburns and poor tanners
  4. Individuals with fair skin, blue eyes, blonde or red hair
- Age: Higher incidence in young and middle-aged adults (except lentigo maligna melanoma on sun-exposed surfaces in the elderly)
- Sex: Slightly more common in female subjects than in male subjects
- Ethnicity: Higher incidence in northern Europeans than in eastern and southern Europeans
- Familial melanoma: One in ten patients with melanoma has a family history of melanoma.

Following are the characteristic features of familial melanoma:

1. Multiple melanomas
2. Melanoma at young age
3. Melanoma often associated with dysplastic nevi
4. Locus for melanoma or the dysplastic nevus resides in the distal portion of the short arm of chromosome 1
5. Other genetic loci are possible, which include chromosome 9 (loss of 9p21).

Precursor lesions of melanoma:

- Dysplastic nevi
- Congenital nevi
- Acquired melanocytic nevi.

Risk Factors for Melanoma

- Xeroderma pigmentosum
- Familial atypical mole melanoma syndrome (FAMMS)
- Numerous acquired melanocytic nevi
- Dysplastic nevi
- Giant congenital nevus
- Prior melanoma
- Sun exposure/sun-sensitive phenotype

TABLE 22.3. *Differences between acquired melanocytic and dysplastic nevus*

Acquired melanocytic nevus	Dysplastic nevus
Develops in early childhood through fourth decade	Develops throughout life
<5 mm in diameter, sharp borders, evenly pigmented	>6–8 mm in diameter, irregular borders, variegated pigment, and topographic asymmetry
If >100 in number, risk of melanoma increases by 10 times	Presence of dysplastic nevus increases the risk of melanoma

- Immunosuppression
- Melanoma in a first-degree relative
- Freckling.

Differences between acquired melanocytic nevus and dysplastic nevus are listed in Table 22.3 and Fig. 22.1.

Common Chromosomal Abnormalities in Malignant Melanoma

Early chromosomal abnormalities:

- Loss of 10q
- Loss of 9p.

Late chromosomal abnormalities:

- Deletion of 6q
- Loss of terminal part of 1p
- Duplication of chromosome 7
- Deletion of 11q23.

Clinicohistologic Types of Melanoma

The measurement of melanoma cells in the dermis and subcutaneous fat has been defined in a reproducible manner by two groups: Clark et al. (2) and Breslow (3) (see Table 22.4). Clark et al. subdivided the invasion of the papillary dermis into a deep group, in which melanoma cells accumulate at the junction of the papillary and reticular dermis, and a superficial group, in which these cells do not accumulate (see Fig. 22.2).

Breslow measured the thickness of melanoma lesions by using an ocular micrometer, which measured the vertical depth of penetration from the granular layer of the epidermis or from the base of the ulcer to the deepest identifiable contiguous melanoma cell (Breslow thickness), and showed it to be a more reproducible and accurate prognostic parameter than the Clark method of microstaging.

Clark Method of Microstaging (Level of Invasion)

CLARK LEVEL

I Melanoma limited to the epidermis
II Invasive melanoma with superficial infiltration to the papillary dermis
III Melanoma extending to the superficial vascular plexus in the dermis
IV Primary melanoma involving the reticular dermis
V Melanoma involving the subcutaneous fat.

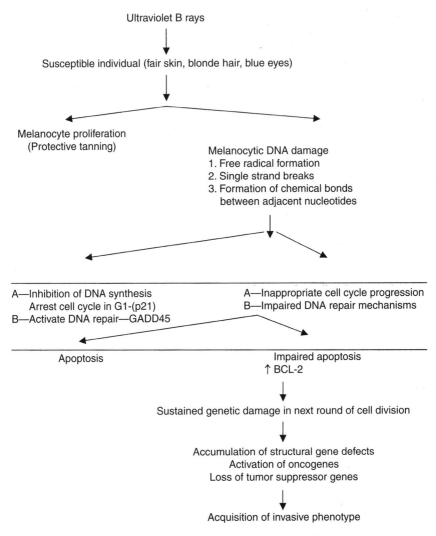

FIG. 22.1. Model of ultraviolet B light mediated pathogenesis of cutaneous melanoma.

Salient features of the new cancer staging system for cutaneous melanoma by the American Joint Committee for Cancer (2001)

1. The new version retains the anatomic compartmentalization: Stages I and II represent localized melanoma to skin, stage III represents metastasis to the regional lymph node/s, and stage IV represents distal metastasis.
2. T-category thresholds of melanoma thickness are defined by even integers (i.e., 1.0, 2.0, and 4.0 mm).
3. Thick melanoma (>4 mm in thickness) is assigned to stage II.

TABLE 22.4. *Revised American Joint Committee for Cancer staging system for cutaneous melanoma (2001) (4)*

Melanoma TNM Classification		
T classification	Thickness	Ulceration status
T1	≤ 1.0 mm	a: without ulceration and level II/III b: with ulceration or Clark level IV/V
T2	1.01–2.0 mm	a: without ulceration b: with ulceration
T3	2.01–4.0 mm	a: without ulceration b: with ulceration
T4	>4.0 mm	a without ulceration b: with ulceration
N classification	**No. of metastatic nodes**	**Nodal metastatic mass**
N1	1 node	a: micrometastases[a] b: macrometastases[b]
N2	2–3 nodes	a: micrometastases[a] b: macrometastases[b] c: in-transit met(s)/satellite(s) without metastatic nodes
N3	4 or more metastatic nodes, or matted nodes, or in-transit met(s)/satellite(s) with metastatic node(s)	
M classification	**Site**	**Serum lactate dehydrogenase**
M1a	Distant skin, subcutaneous, or nodal mets	Normal
M1b	Lung metastases	Normal
M1c	All other visceral metastases Any distant metastases	Normal Elevated

Proposed stage groupings for cutaneous melanoma

	Clinical staging[c]			Pathologic staging[d]		
	T	N	M	T	N	M
0	Tis	N0	M0	Tis	N0	M0
IA	T1a	N0	M0	T1a	N0	M0
IB	T1b	N0	M0	T1b	N0	M0
	T2a	N0	M0	T2a	N0	M0
IIA	T2b	N0	M0	T2b	N0	M0
	T3a	N0	M0	T3a	N0	M0
IIB	T3b	N0	M0	T3b	N0	M0
	T4a	N0	M0	T4a	N0	M0
IIC	T4b	N0	M0	T4b	N0	M0
III [e]	Any T	N1	M0	—	—	—
		N2		—	—	—
		N3		—	—	—
IIIA	—	—	—	T1–4a	N1a	M0
				T1–4a	N2a	M0

continued on next page

TABLE 22.4. *Continued*

IIIB	—	—	—	T1–4b	N1a	M0
				T1–4b	N2a	M0
				T1–4a	N1b	M0
				T1–4a	N2b	M0
				T1–4a/b	N2c	M0
IIIC	—	—	—	T1–4b	N1b	M0
				T1–4b	N2b	M0
				Any T	N3	M0
IV	Any T	Any N	Any M1	Any T	Any N	Any M1

The AJCC Melanoma Database consisted of a total of 30,450 melanoma patients, of which 17,600 patients (58%) had information available for all of the factors required for the proposed TNM classification and stage grouping.

[a]Micrometastases are diagnosed after sentinel or elective lymphadenectomy.

[b]Macrometastases are defined as clinically detectable nodal metastases confirmed by therapeutic lymphadenectomy or when nodal metastases exhibit gross extracapsular extension.

[c]Clinical staging includes microstaging of the primary melanoma and clinical/radiologic evaluation for metastasis. By convention, it should be used after complete excision of the primary melanoma, with clinical assessment for regional and distant metastasis.

[d]Pathologic staging includes microstaging of the primary melanoma and pathologic information about the regional lymph nodes after partial or complete lymphadenectomy. Pathologic stage 0 or stage IA patients are the exception; they do not require pathologic evaluation of their lymph nodes.

[e]There is no stage III subgroup for clinical staging.

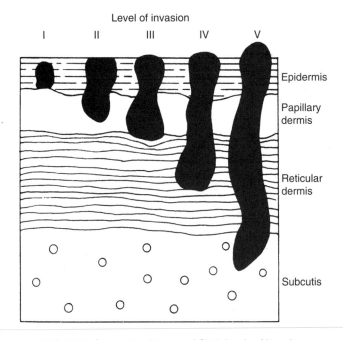

FIG. 22.2. Schematic diagram of Clark levels of invasion.

4. The level of invasion as described by Wallace Clark is an independent predictive feature for thin (T1) melanoma but not for thicker lesions (5).
5. Melanoma ulceration, defined as the absence of an intact epidermis overlying a major portion of the primary melanoma on the basis of microscopic examination of the histologic sections, predisposes patients to a high risk for metastasis.
6. The new staging system incorporates the pathologic information obtained after lymphatic mapping and sentinel lymph adenectomy that is included in the definition of clinical and pathologic staging.
7. When patients present with multiple primary melanomas, the T-category staging is based on the melanoma with the worst prognostic features.
8. Stage III melanoma patients include those with regional metastasis either in the regional lymph nodes or in the intralymphatic metastases, manifesting as either satellite or in-transit metastases.
9. There are four major determinants of outcome for pathologic stage III melanoma:
   - Number of metastatic lymph nodes: N1 = one metastatic lymph node, N2 = 2 to 3 metastatic lymph nodes, and N3 = 4 or more metastatic lymph nodes
   - Tumor burden in the lymph node is either (a) microscopic or (b) macroscopic
   - Presence or absence of ulceration of the primary tumor and
   - Presence or absence of satellite or in-transit metastases.
10. Size of the metastatic lymph node does not demonstrate independent prognostic value.
11. The presence of clinical or microscopic satellite metastases around a primary melanoma as well as in-transit metastases between the primary melanoma and the regional lymph nodes represent intralymphatic metastases and portend a poor prognosis. In addition, patients with a combination of satellites and in-transit metastases plus nodal metastases have a worse outcome than patients who experience either event alone.
12. In patients with distant metastases, the site(s) of metastases and elevated serum levels of lactate dehydrogenase (LDH) are used to delineate the M categories into three groups: M1a, M1b, and M1c, with 1-year survival rates ranging from 41% to 59%. There are no subgroups of stage IV disease because the survival differences between the M categories are small.

Prognostic Factors

The prognostic factors of melanoma are listed in Table 22.5 and Fig. 22.3.

TABLE 22.5. *Prognostic factors*

Good prognostic factors	Poor prognostic factors
1. Tumor involving an extremity	Melanoma of the skin of the trunk, head, and neck
2. Thin tumor	Thick tumor
3. No ulceration of tumor	Tumor ulceration present
4. Radial growth pattern	Nodular histology
5. Early stage (stage I and II)	Late stage at presentation (stage III and IV)
6. Absence of foci of regression and satellites of the tumor in the reticular dermis and subcutaneous fat	Presence of foci of regression and/or tumor satellites in reticular dermis and subcutaneous fat
7. Absence of vascular and/or lymphatic invasion	Presence of vascular and/or lymphatic invasion
8. Low tumor cell mitotic rate	High tumor cell mitotic rate

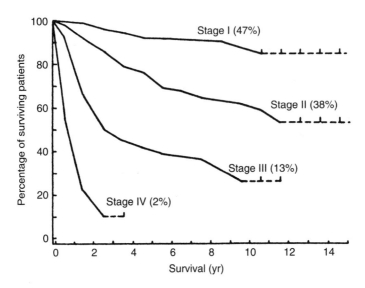

FIG. 22.3. Fifteen-year survival results for more than 4,000 melanoma patients treated at the University of Alabama at Birmingham and the Sydney Melanoma Unit, staged according to the American Joint Committee on Cancer four-stage system. Distribution of patients is shown in parentheses. Note that patients with clinically localized melanoma (stage I in the original three-stage system) are divided into two stages according to tumor thickness and histologic level of invasion (designated stages I and II). (From Ketcham AS, Moffat FL, Balch CM. Classification and staging. In: Balch C, ed. *Cutaneous melanoma.* 2nd ed. Philadelphia: JB Lippincott, 1992:213–220, with permission.)

Clinical Features of Malignant Melanoma

Cutaneous melanoma can occur anywhere in the body. The most common sites are the lower extremities in the women and the trunk in men. The classic signs include a pigmented skin lesion that demonstrates a change in color or variegated color, a change in lesion size, and irregular borders. Progressive lesions show nodularity and ulceration or bleeding, with or without pruritus.

Most lesions are pigmented, although less than 1% of lesions lack pigment and are called *amelanotic melanomas.*

Diagnosis

The types of skin biopsies used in the diagnosis of malignant melanoma are listed in Tables 22.6 and 22.7.

Prognosis

Most melanomas are diagnosed in the early stages and are thin. More than 95% of thin melanomas are curable, and approximately 85% of stage I and II melanomas are cured. The prognosis is inversely proportional to the stage of the cancer, and only 40% to 50% of persons with stage III melanoma live for 5 years. Less than 5% of patients with stage IV melanoma live for 5 years (6).

TABLE 22.6. *Diagnosis of melanoma*

Immunohistologic tests for the diagnosis of malignant melanoma

Antigen	Result
S-100 protein	+
Cytokeratin	−
Premelanosomal protein (HMB-45)	+
Vimentin	+
Nerve growth factor receptor	+
Tyrosinase-related protein-1 (MEL-5)	+

TABLE 22.7. *Types of skin biopsy for melanoma diagnosis*

Types of skin biopsy	Characteristics
Excisional skin biopsy	1. Completely removes the tumor. Curative if the tumor is small, and tumor-free margins of 2 mm could be obtained. 2. May not be feasible because of anatomic or cosmetic restraints constraints.
Incisional skin biopsy	1. Performed if a tumor is large. 2. For flat lesions, the darkest area should be sampled. If the lesion is raised, the thickest area should be sampled.

Shave biopsy—contraindicated in melanoma because it may not yield adequate deep specimen for accurate microstaging.

TABLE 22.8. *Relationship between microstage of primary melanoma, incidence of regional lymph node metastases, and long-term survival in patients from John Wayne Cancer Institute*

	Microstage	Patient number	Lymph node metastases (%)	10-Year survival (%)
Breslow thickness	<0.75 MM	768	8.3	97
	0.76–1.5 MM	802	20.2	87
	1.51–3.99 MM	765	36.6	67
	≥4 MM	205	40.0	40
Clark level	I/II	622	9.2	97
	III	1,046	23.9	85
	IV	785	35.0	68
	V	87	38.0	46

Table 22.8 shows a graph depicting the survival in relation to the stage of the melanoma.

Management

The algorithm for the management of primary melanoma is reviewed in Fig. 22.4.

Prevention:

- Patients should be educated about the risk factors for developing melanoma—ultraviolet light (intense mid-day sun between 11 AM and 1 PM). Use of sunblock [sun protection factor (SPF) >15] and light clothing should be encouraged.
- Patients should be educated about clinical features of melanoma and precursor lesions and should be taught to perform self-examination of the skin.

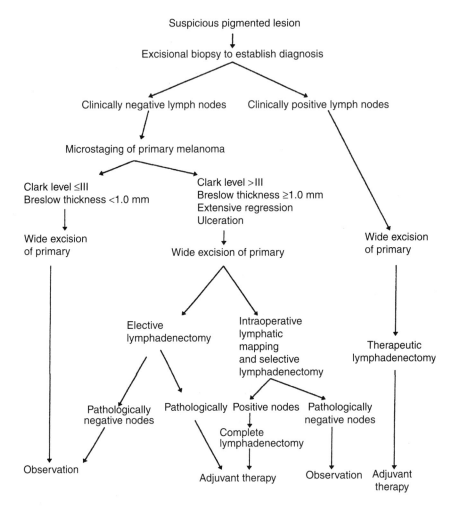

FIG. 22.4. Algorithm for the management of primary melanoma (American Joint Committee for Cancer stage I/II) (7).

- Close surveillance is required in high-risk patients.
  - Digital photographs are used for comparing the multiple pigmented skin lesions and for assessing any changes as described previously, as in dysplastic nevus syndrome.
  - Dermoscopy (epiluminescence microscopy) is a technique used to visualize a variety of structures in pigmented lesions that are not discernible to the naked eye. Lotion or mineral oil is applied to the surface of the lesion to make the epidermis more transparent. Examination of the lesion with a 10 × ocular scope, a microscope ocular eyepiece (held upside down), or a dermatoscope (available from surgical supply houses) then reveals several features that are helpful in differentiating between benign and malignant pigmented lesions. This technique provides additional criteria for the diagnosis of melanoma.

General principles and issues in treatment:

- Surgical excision is the primary treatment for melanoma.
- Regional lymph node dissection for metastasis is performed before any distant spread of the tumor occurs.
- Adjuvant radiation therapy after lymph node dissection is used in selected instances.
- Isolated limb perfusion with chemotherapy is given in selected instances.
- Interferon-α is provided as adjuvant therapy in patients with high-risk resected cutaneous melanomas.
- Multiple options in metastatic melanoma include single-agent chemotherapy such as oral temozolomide, combination chemotherapy, biologic therapy such as high-dose interleukin-2 (IL-2), interferon-α, and chemobiotherapy. Radiation therapy may be used in select instances such as in patients who present with brain metastasis or as an adjuvant to surgery in head and neck melanoma or in postlymphadenectomy lymph node basins with extracapsular spread of metastatic melanoma.
- Newer experimental immunotherapy includes vaccines.

Surgical Management of Primary Melanoma

Principle: Complete surgical excision of the primary melanoma, confirmed by comprehensive histologic examination of the entire excised specimen, forms the basis for surgical treatment of primary melanoma (8).

Risk of local recurrence is not significantly associated with the extent of surgical margin of excision (see Table 22.9).

Ocular Melanoma

Early and limited-stage ocular melanomas are usually managed by close observation. Various methods of treatment include radiation therapy, photoradiation, cryotherapy, ultrasonic hyperthermia, local resection, and enucleation.

Indications for enucleation of the eye in ocular melanoma:

- Tumor growing in a blind eye
- Melanoma involving more than half of the iris
- Tumor involving the anterior chamber of the eye or extraocular extension
- Failure of previous local therapy.

Lymph Node Dissection

Invasion of the lymphatics by a vertically growing melanoma causes the tumor to lodge in the local lymph node basin. The tumor, uninterrupted at this lymph node basin, may spread to deeper lymphatics or hematogenously to systemic organs. This principle forms the rationale for complete surgical resection of the tumor from the lymph node basin before the tumor spreads to distant organs, and is considered a potentially curative procedure.

TABLE 22.9. *Recommended margin of surgical excision based upon pathologic stage of primary cutaneous melanoma*

Pathologic stage	Thickness	Margin of excision
ptis	Melanoma *in situ*	5 mm
pT1 and pT2	0–1.5 mm	1 cm
pT3	>1.5–4 mm	1–2 cm
pT4	>4 mm	2–3 cm

From Chapman PB, Einhorn LH, Meyers ML, et al. Phase III multicenter randomized trial of the Dartmouth regimen versus dacarbazine in patients with metastatic melanoma. *J Clin Oncol* 1999;17:2745–2751, with permission.

TABLE 22.10. *Lymph node dissection*

Advantages	Disadvantages
Helps eradicate occult lymph node metastasis	Overtreatment in 50%–60% patients
Correctly stages the tumor	Invasive procedure
Efficacy proved in melanoma of thickness between 1.1 and 2 mm in patients younger than 60 yr	Morbidity of the procedure

Lymph node dissection can be classified as follows (see Table 22.10):

- Elective: Lymph node dissection is said to be elective when the lymph nodes that are not clinically palpable are dissected from the lymph node basin because of the high suspicion that the melanoma has spread to the lymph nodes without evidence of distant spread.
- Therapeutic: When the lymph nodes are clinically palpable and are suspected to be involved without distant organ spread, the dissection is therapeutic.
- Delayed: When initially nonpalpable lymph nodes appear to enlarge over a close follow-up period without distant organ spread, the dissection is considered delayed.

Sentinel Lymph Node Dissection

Characteristics of a sentinel lymph node are as follows:

- First lymph node in the lymph node basin to which the primary melanoma drains.
- Lymph node at the greatest risk for metastasis.
- Histology of sentinel node reflects the histology of all lymph nodes in the basin.
- Easily accessible.
- If the lymph node is negative for metastasis, it spares the patient major surgical morbidity.

Surgical Approach to Obtain a Sentinel Lymph Node

Preoperative lymphoscintigraphy uses vital blue dye and provides a road map of the lymph node basin. Intraoperative lymphoscintigraphy uses radiocolloid injection around the primary tumor, and a gamma camera detects the radioactivity from the involved lymph node, thereby acting as a navigator to the involved lymph node. The combination of vital blue dye and technetium-labeled sulfur colloid identifies the sentinel lymph node in 94% of cases (9).

Isolated Limb Perfusion

Principle: To deliver maximally tolerated chemotherapy doses to a regionally confined tumor area while limiting systemic toxicity. Hyperthermia and oxygenation of the circulation potentiate the tumoricidal effects of the chemotherapeutic agents. Chemotherapeutic agents used in this method of treatment are

- melphalan
- thiotepa (response rate, 50% to 60%)
- mechlorethamine
- one of the above agents along with tumor necrosis factor and interferon-α (response rate, 91%).

Isolated limb perfusion is described in Table 22.11.

TABLE 22.11. *Isolated limb perfusion*

Advantages	Disadvantages
1. Local control of the disease	1. Expensive
2. Resolution of edema, bleeding, or ulceration	2. Invasive
3. Relieves pain	3. May cause ischemia of the limb, peripheral neuropathy, and bone marrow suppression

Indications for isolated limb perfusion:

- Adjuvant to lymph node dissection
- Recurrent melanoma of extremity (10)
- Bulky symptomatic melanoma of the extremity, with bleeding, ulceration, or edema.

Role of radiation therapy for melanoma treatment in the adjuvant setting:

Although melanoma is generally considered as a "radioresistant tumor," radiation therapy has been found to be of clinical benefit after surgical lymph node resection in the following instances:

- Head and neck melanomas (11)
- Multiple large lymph nodes
- Extracapsular spread
- Local recurrence in a previously dissected lymph node basin
- Parotid gland lymph nodes
- Desmoplastic melanoma with neurotropism
- Brain metastasis of melanoma.

Studies by Skibber et al. (12) suggested that external radiation to the brain after surgical resection of the solitary brain metastasis with malignant melanoma has survival benefit.

Biologic Agents in Malignant Melanoma

Interferon-α was the first recombinant cytokine that was investigated in phase I/II trials, in the metastatic setting, on the basis of its antiproliferative as well as immunomodulatory effects.

- The response rate in metastatic melanoma was approximately 16%.
- One third of these responses were complete responses.
- Responses could be observed up to 6 months after the therapy was initiated.
- Up to one third of the responses were durable.
- Patients with frequent interruptions due to side effects of interferon therapy did less well than those patients without interruptions.
- Patients with small-volume tumors did better than those with large-volume tumors.

Interferon in Metastatic Melanoma

The study by Falkson et al. (13) showed a response rate of 53% and a median survival of 17.6 months with interferon-α 2b along with dacarbazine compared to a response rate of 20% and a median survival of 9.6% months with dacarbazine alone. These results were not reproducible by the European Organization for the Research and Treatment of Cancer (EORTC) studies.

Interferon in the Adjuvant Setting in Malignant Melanoma

Principle: There is a high incidence of relapse among patients with stage III melanoma after therapeutic or elective lymph node dissection and in those with thick melanoma lesions (>4 mm). The effect of interferon on disease-free survival has been evaluated in this setting (see Table 22.12) (14).

TABLE 22.12. *Use of adjuvant interferon*

Study group (accrual)	Treatment regimen	Outcomes analysis
ECOG E1684 (287 patients with stage IIB or stage III malignant melanoma AJCC stage)	Interferon α-2b, 20 million units/m²/dose i.v., 5 d/wk × 4 wk (total dose/wk, 100 million units/m²), *followed by*	Favored interferon therapy overall survival, 0.047
	Interferon α-2b, 10 million units/m² s.c., three times/wk for 48 wk (total dose/wk, 30 million units/m²) vs. Observation	Relapse-free survival, *p* = 0.004 Significant toxicity of interferon observed.
ECOG 1690 (642 patients)	Interferon α-2b, 20 million units/m²/dose i.v., 5 d/wk × 4 wk (total dose/wk, 100 million units/m²), *followed by* Interferon α-2b, 10 million units/m² s.c., three times/wk for 48 wk (total dose/wk, 30 million units/m²) vs. Low-dose interferon: Interferon α-2b, 3 million units/m² s.c., three times/wk for 104 wk (total dose/wk, 9 million units/m²) vs. Observation	Survival benefit for high-dose interferon • Relapse-free survival *p* = 0.05 in both node-positive & node-negative patients • greatest in those with 2–3 nodes (*p* = 0.02) • No overall 5-yr survival benefit
ECOG E 1697 (1,444 patients AJCC stage II A) The aim is to know the impact of interferon on relapse-free survival and overall survival in the adjuvant setting in stage IIA disease	Interferon α-2b, 20 million units/m²/dose i.v., 5 d/wk × 4 wk (total dose/wk, 100 million units/m²), *OR* Observation	Ongoing
UKCCCR Study (1,000 patients AJCC stage II or III)	Interferon α-2a, 3 million units/m² s.c., three times/wk for 2 yr (total dose/wk, 9 million units/m²), *OR* Observation	Ongoing

continued on next page

TABLE 22.12. *Continued*

EORTC study (18-952) (1,000 patients AJCC stage II or III disease) for interferon in adjuvant setting. The goal is to see the impact of the two lower doses and subcutaneously administered interferon on the disease	Interferon α-2b, 10-million units/m²/dose s.c. 5 d/wk for 4 wk (total dose/wk, 50 million units/m²), *followed by* Interferon α-2b, 10 million units/m² s.c., three times/wk for 1 yr (total dose/wk, 30 million units/m²), *OR* Interferon α-2b, 5 million units/m² s.c., three times/wk for 2 yr (total dose/wk, 15 million units/m²)	Ongoing

ECOG, Eastern Cooperative Oncology Group; AJCC, American Joint Committee for Cancer; UKCCCR, The UK Coordinating Committee on Cancer Research; EORTC, European Organization for the Research and Treatment of Cancer; i.v. intravenous; s.c., subcutaneous; vs., versus.
Adapted from Kirkwood JM, Strawderman MH, Ernstoff MS, et al. Interferon α-2b adjuvant therapy of high risk resected cutaneous melanoma: the Eastern Cooperative Oncology Group trial EST 1684. *J Clin Oncol* 1996;14:7–17, with permission.

Interleukin-2 Therapy for Metastatic Melanoma

IL-2, first identified as a T-cell growth factor in 1976, is produced primarily by T-helper cells. It is a 15-kD glycoprotein and interacts with IL-2 receptors expressed on activated T cells, resulting in proliferation and differentiation of both B and T cells and of cytotoxic cells, and stimulates the cascade of cytokines including various interleukins, interferons, and tumor necrosis factors. The antitumor effects of IL-2 are mediated by its ability to cause proliferation of natural killer cells (NKs), lymphokine-activated killer cells (LAKs), and other cytotoxic cells.

IL-2 Doses and Administration Methods: The U.S. Food and Drug Administration (FDA)–approved dosage for treatment of metastatic melanoma is 600,000 IU per kg administered as a bolus over 15 minutes every 8 hours for a maximum of 14 doses. Following a rest period of about 5 to 9 days, the regimen is repeated if tolerated by the patient. Imaging studies are repeated at the end of two courses, and if tumor responses or disease stabilization is documented, the treatment is repeated, with periodic assessment of disease response. The overall response rate is about 16% and a complete response rate of 6%, and responses have been noted in all the disease sites (15,16). Patients who achieved complete responses had the highest chances of achieving prolonged disease-free survival. Patients with good baseline performance status and chemonaive status were most likely to respond to the high-dose IL-2 treatment.

The toxicity profile of IL-2 is dose, route, and administration dependent. Common toxicity profile involves gastrointestinal system (i.e., nausea and vomiting), cardiovascular system (i.e., hypotension or arrhythmias), lung (i.e., hypoxemia and pleural effusions), kidneys (i.e., azotemia), and central nervous system (i.e., confusion and delirium) in addition to fever and fluid retention, most of which are the manifestations of the capillary leak syndrome. Toxicity is accentuated in patients with baseline pulmonary, cardiac, and metabolic disease. Highly skilled nursing and selection of the right patients for high-dose IL-2 have significantly reduced mortality in patients treated with high-dose IL-2. Because high-dose IL-2 therapy causes significant toxicity, it is also administered either subcutaneously or as a continuous intravenous infusion at 9 to 18 million IU/m²/day for 4 to 5 days, and dosages up to 24 million IU/m²/day in patients not eligible for high dose of IL-2. Although total response rates as high as 16.8% have been reported, complete responses are lower than those reported with high-dose IL-2.

Combination IL-2 regimens: Preclinical data have suggested synergistic immunologic effects of combining IL-2 with interferon-α and chemotherapeutic agents. These observations have resulted in combinations of IL-2 and interferons that did not show a significant advantage in *in vivo* studies. Concurrent or sequential combination of chemotherapeutic agents with IL-2 and/or interferon-α (biochemotherapy) produces less toxicity than high-dose IL-2 and shows mixed results, with overall responses ranging from 25.3% to 50% (17). Presently, the use of biochemotherapy is experimental until the final results of a large intergroup study comparing biochemotherapy and chemotherapy in metastatic melanoma are reported.

CONCLUSIONS

- High-dose interferon remains the most active adjuvant agent evaluated to date for high-risk melanoma.
- It prolongs the relapse-free survival, but its impact on overall survival is less clear.

A summary of the management options of melanoma in advanced tumor stage is found in Table 22.13. Chemotherapy agents and their response rates in metastatic melanoma are listed in Table 22.14. Combination chemotherapy in metastatic melanoma is described in Table 22.15.

A recent phase III multicenter randomized trial of dacarbazine alone versus the Dartmouth regimen (i.e., cisplatin, carmustine, dacarbazine, and tamoxifen) in patients with metastatic melanoma failed to show a statistical difference in survival or tumor response in patients with melanoma (EORTC study) (18).

Combination of chemotherapy regimen and biologic therapy (Biochemotherapy): Rationale

- Anticancer effects of the combination therapy are additive or synergistic
- There are different mechanisms of action for different regimens
- Nonoverlapping toxicity
- No cross resistance
- There is a suggestion that biologic agents may produce long-term survivals.

Combination chemotherapy with biologic agents is described in Table 22.16.

TABLE 22.13. *Management options*

Management	Metastatic site	Comments
Combination chemotherapy	Systemic metastasis	Palliative in nature, dacarbazine is the drug of choice
Surgical resection	Brain, soft tissue, lung, or liver	Isolated single legion
Radiation therapy	Brain, bone, or symptomatic systemic metastasis	Treatment of symptomatic lesions
Combination chemotherapy + biologic therapy (interleukin-2 and/or interferon α)	Systemic metastatic disease	Promising and effective. Regression of visceral metastasis is seen with possible survival advantage
Immunotherapies	Systemic metastatic disease Experimental	Experimental

TABLE 22.14. *Chemotherapy agents and response rates*

Chemotherapeutic agent	Response rates (%)
Dacarbazine	15–25
Temozolomide (DTIC analog)	21
Nitrosoureas	10–20
Cisplatin	
Carboplatin	
Vinca alkaloids	15–25
Vincristine	
Vinblastine	
Vindesine	
Taxoids	18
Paclitaxel	
Docetaxel	
Piritrexim	23

DTIC, dacarbazine.

TABLE 22.15. *Description of chemotherapy regimens*

Chemotherapy regimens	Treatment description	Response rates (%)
CBDT, the "Dartmouth regimen"*	Cisplatin, 25 mg/m^2/d i.v. for 3 d, d 1–3 (total dose/cycle, 75 mg/m^2) Carmustine, 150 mg/m^2 i.v. d 1 on every odd-numbered cycle (i.e., every 43 d) (total dose every two cycles, 150 mg/m^2) Dacarbazine, 220 mg/m^2/d i.v. for 3 d, d 1–3 (total dose/cycle, 660 mg/m^2) Tamoxifen, 10 mg twice daily PO during the therapy Cycle repeated every 21 d	19–55
CVD (MD Anderson Cancer Center)[†]	Cisplatin, 20 mg/m^2/d i.v. for 4 d, d 2–5 (total dose/cycle, 80 mg/m^2) Vinblastine, 1.6 mg/m^2/d i.v. for 5 d, d 1–5 (total dose/cycle, 8 mg/m^2) Dacarbazine, 800 mg/m^2 i.v. on d 1 (total dose/cycle, 800 mg/m^2) Cycle repeats every 21 d	

*From Del Prete SA, Maurer LH, O'Donnell I, et al. Combination chemotherapy with cisplatin, carmustine, dacarbazine, and tamoxifen in metastatic melanoma. *Cancer Treat Rep* 1984;68: 1403–1405, with permission.

[†]From Legha SS, Ring S, Papadopoulos N, et al. A prospective evaluation of a triple-drug regimen containing cisplatin, vinblastine, and dacarbazine (CVD) for metastatic melanoma. Cancer 1989;64:2024–2029.

Vaccine Therapy in Malignant Melanoma

Immunization principally involves recognition of tumor-specific peptide by cytotoxic T cells when presented by antigen-presenting cells bound to major histocompatibility complex (MHC) molecules. A number of tumor-associated peptide antigens are purified and either administered intradermally with an immune adjuvant (19) or the peptide is "pulsed" onto

TABLE 22.16. *Combination chemotherapy with biologic agents*

Treatment	Response rates (%)
Dacarbazine, 1,000 mg/m^2 as a continuous infusion over 24 h (total dose/cycle, 1,000 mg/m^2) Recombinant interleukin-2, administered i.v. over 30 min on an outpatient basis on days 15–19 and d 22–26. The dose of interleukin-2 was 24 MIU/m^2 for 10 doses, d 1–5 and 8–12 (total dose/cycle, 240 MIU/m^2) Dacarbazine was repeated once every 28 d and supportive treatment given during this protocol	22
Dacarbazine, 200 mg/m^2 i.v. for 5 d, start every wk 4 Interferon α-2b, 15 MU/m^2 i.v. daily for 5 d/wk for 3 wk, and thereafter, 10 MU/m^2 s.c. 3 times/wk. Cycle repeats every 28 d	53
Cisplatin, 100 mg/m^2 i.v. on d 1 (total dose/cycle, 100 mg/m^2) Interferon α-2a, 10 MU/d s.c. on d 1–5 (total dose/cycle, 50 MU) Interleukin-2 given as continuous infusion for 6 d (d 3–8) in a decrescendo schedule, starting on d 3 with 18 MU/m^2 every 6 h, followed by 18 MU/m^2 every 12 h, 18 MU/m^2 every 24 h, and a maintenance dose of 4.5 MU/m^2 every 24 h for 72 h (total dose/cycle, 139.5 MU/m^2). Cycle repeats every 28 d	33 (overall response rate)
CVD regimen	64 (overall response rate)
Cisplatin, 20 mg/m^2/d i.v. for 4 d, d 2–5 (total dose/cycle, 80 mg/m^2) Vinblastine, 1.6 mg/m^2/d i.v. for 5 d, d 1–5 (total dose/cycle, 8 mg/m^2) Dacarbazine, 800 mg/m^2 i.v. on d 1 (total dose/cycle, 8 mg/m^2) *PLUS* Interleukin-2, 9 million units/m^2/d continuous i.v. infusion for 4 d, d 6–9 (total dose/cycle, 36 million units/m^2) Interferon α, 5 million units/m^2/dose s.c. for 5 d, d 6–10 (total dose/cycle, 25 million units/m^2) Note: The therapy schedule with the biologic agents either immediately precedes or follows the CVD regimen. Cycle repeats every 21 d	
Cisplatin, 25 mg/m^2 i.v. 2-h infusion on d 1–3 and 22–25 (total dose/cycle, 175 mg/m^2) Carmustine, 150 mg/m^2 i.v. 1-h infusion on d 1 (total dose/cycle, 150 mg/m^2) Dacarbazine, 220 mg/m^2 i.v. 2-h infusion on d 1–3 and 22–25 (total dose/cycle, 1,540 mg/m^2) Tamoxifen, 10-mg tablet PO b.i.d. for 6 wk and begin on d 1 Interleukin-2, 1.5 million units/m^2 administered i.v. every 8 h, starting d 4 for 15 doses, d 4–8 and 17–21 (total dose/cycle, 45 million units/m^2) *PLUS* Interferon α-2b, 6 million units/m^2/d s.c. for 10 d, d 4–8 and 17–21 (total dose/cycle, 60 million units/m^2). Cycle repeats every 6 wk	55

MIU, million international units; MU, million units.

autologous antigen-presenting cells, and the combination is injected intradermally (20). DiFronzo et al. (21) have used polyvalent melanoma vaccine derived from the melanoma cell cultures in patients with AJCC stage II melanoma and have reported enhanced humoral immune response to correlate with improved disease-free survival and overall survival. The seminal observation that heat-shock proteins isolated from cancer cells of mice and rats elicited specific immunity to the cancers from which they were derived led to the discovery that heat-shock proteins are associated with peptides, including antigenic tumor-specific peptides, and elicit potent tumor-specific T-cell immunity when injected back. Preliminary phase I and II studies of heat-shock proteins purified from the autologous melanoma tumors in humans have shown clinically relevant significant tumor-specific immune responses (22). A multiinstitutional phase III study is ongoing to elucidate the clinical significance of heat-shock protein vaccine derived from the autologous tumor cells. Other approaches include gene therapy for appropriate peptide expression in the antigen-presenting cells, which then process the peptide intracellularly and bind tightly to the appropriate human leukocyte antigen (HLA) molecule for presentation to cytotoxic T cells.

Some of the melanoma-associated antigen epitopes are listed in Table 22.17. Various studies are in progress, and final results are awaited.

NONMELANOMA SKIN CANCER

There are two major types of nonmelanoma skin cancers: basal cell carcinoma and squamous cell carcinoma. Together they account for nearly one third of all the cancers in the United States.

Basal Cell Carcinoma

- Basal cell carcinoma is the most common cancer in the U.S. white population.
- It accounts for 77% of 77,000 new cases of nonmelanoma skin cancers seen in the United States.

Common clinical presentations of basal cell carcinoma include the following:

- Shiny skin, colored pink, with translucent papule with telangiectasia
- Nodular variant consists of nodule with central depression and rolled margins and may bleed from trauma. Usual location is head and neck area
- Pigmented basal cell carcinoma: Nodular with brown to black pigment.
- Sclerosing or morphea-type basal cell carcinoma: Yellowish, infiltrated, with indistinct borders, may not be diagnosed for a long time. Mohs surgery may be appropriate for treatment.
- Other less common presentations include hyperkeratotic type carcinoma: Usually involves head and neck area, exhibits sessile growth on the lower trunk, is multicentric on face with ulcer and scar tissues, and is of the giant exophytic type and the cystic type that presents as a blue–gray nodule on the face.

Squamous Cell Carcinoma

Squamous cell carcinoma involving the skin has the following characteristics:

- Usually found in elderly white men with sun-damaged skin
- Common sites include back of the hand, forearm, face, and neck; single or multiple lesions
- Firm, indurated, expanding nodule, often at the site of actinic keratosis
- The nodule may be ulcerated, and regional lymph nodes may be enlarged.

TABLE 22.17. *Melanoma-associated antigen epitopes*

Antigen	HLA restriction	Cellular location
MAGE-1	A1/Cw 1601	Cytoplasm
MAGE-3	A1/A2	Cytoplasm
MART1/Mela-A	A2	Cytoplasm
Tyrosinase	A2/A24	Melanosomal

Squamous cell carcinoma of a mucocutaneous site:

- Elderly men with chronic history of smoking, alcohol use, or chewing tobacco or betel nut
- Common sites include mouth and lower lip
- Lesions usually start as an erosion or a nodule that ulcerates.

Other sites include the following:

- Sole of the foot, verrucous form
- Male genitalia: human papillomavirus (HPV) related, underlying condylomata of Buschke–Lowenstein (see Table 22.18).

Table 22.19 lists the comparative features of basal and squamous cell carcinomas of the skin.

Diagnosis of Nonmelanoma Skin Cancer

History should include duration of the lesion, symptoms like pain/itching, and recent changes of the surface:

- History of sun exposure, and recreational and occupational history
- Ethnic background and the type of the skin
- History of radiation exposure, arsenic exposure, chronic ulcer/burn scar, or osteomyelitis.

TABLE 22.18. *Premalignant lesions of the epidermis*

Actinic keratosis
Chemical keratosis: arsenic, tar, polycyclic aromatic
   hydrocarbons, thermal keratosis
Radiation dermatitis
Bowen disease
Erythroplasia of Queyrat
Bowenoid papulosis
Epidermodysplasia verruciformis
Leukoplakia
Keratoacanthoma

TABLE 22.19. *Features of basal and squamous cell carcinomas of skin*

Characteristics	Basal cell carcinoma	Squamous cell carcinoma
Incidence	Most common cancer of the skin in whites	Next most common skin cancer in whites
Cell of origin	Basal cells of epidermis and hair follicles	Epidermal keratinocytes
Site of tumor	Sun-exposed areas of head and neck, ear, and extremities	Sun-exposed areas of head, neck, face, forearm, and dorsum of the hand
Ethnic background	Fair skin	Fair skin
Sun exposure	Continuous cumulative exposure	Continuous cumulative exposure
Male/female ratio	Common in men	Common in men
Growth and prognosis	Slow growing and good prognosis	Slow growing and good prognosis
Mucosal origin	None	Involves lip and mouth

Complete skin examination includes the following:

- Examination of scalp, ears, palms, soles, interdigital areas, and mucous membranes.
- Evaluation of the extent of sun damage to skin (i.e., solar elastosis, scaling, erythema, telangiectasia, and solar lentigines).

The skin should be evaluated for enlargement of the locoregional and distant metastases. Skin biopsy should be performed, either excisional when the tumor is small, or incisional when the tumor is large. A shave biopsy with a scalpel may be used in noduloulcerative, cystic, or superficial type.

Treatment Principles

- Surgery is the primary mode of treatment.
- Excision of the tumor with negative margins of approximately 4 to 6 mm is sufficient.
- The procedure is performed under local anesthesia.
- Locally draining nodes are examined and removed only if they are enlarged.
- Plastic surgery may be needed to close the defects produced by excision of the tumor.
- Mohs surgery: This is a progressive excision technique that allows excision of the tumor until the negative margins are achieved. Mohs micrographic surgery uses the fresh-tissue technique with the use of frozen section and is less time-consuming than the original surgery.

Role of Radiation Therapy

Radiation therapy delivers x-rays at a total dose of 2,000 to 3,000 cGy that penetrate up to 2 to 5 mm, where most of the basal cell and squamous cell carcinomas infiltrate. The total dose is divided into multiple fractions, usually over 3 to 4 weeks, to reduce side effects (see Table 22.20).

Various other types of treatments are listed in Table 22.21.

Other Cancers of the Skin

Merkel cell carcinoma arises from the neoplastic proliferation of the Merkel cells.

TABLE 22.20. *Radiation therapy*

Radiation therapy in nonmelanoma skin cancer	
Advantages	Common side effects
Most skin tumors are radiosensitive	Loss of hair follicles and sweat glands
Indicated for skin cancer in elderly patients who have high risk for surgery and large and bulky tumors	Skin atrophy and telangiectasia
Tumors located on the nose, eye, lip, eyelid, and inner and outer canthi of the eye as well as skin cancer along the embryonal fusion planes	Radiation dermatitis
Cure rate for squamous cell carcinoma and basal cell carcinoma are >90%	Radiation-induced precancerous lesions of the skin

TABLE 22.21. *Other types of treatment*

Treatment method	Characteristic features
1. Curettage and electrodesiccation preceded by a shave biopsy	Advantages Useful to treat basal cell carcinoma, superficial squamous cell carcinoma, Bowen disease, and keratoacanthoma actinic keratosis Cure rates in selected patients, 77%–97% Disadvantages Not suitable for tumors in high-risk areas, histologically aggressive tumors, or morphea-type tumors
2. Cryotherapy kills tumor cells by freezing Liquid nitrogen (−195.5°C) causes tissue necrosis	Advantages Suitable for small tumors of the eyelids, nose, chest, back, or morphea-type basal cell carcinoma Simple procedure; no anesthesia necessary Disadvantages Cannot be used in patients with Raynaud phenomenon or tumors >3 cm in diameter
3. Fluorouracil cream, 1% or 5%, applied topically to cover the lesions twice daily for a few weeks. An inflammatory response id desired; if it does not occur, the drug concentration or frequency of applications or treatment duration should be increased. Typical treatment duration is 2–6 wk longer	Advantages Suitable for basal cell carcinoma on the face and extremities, and on superficial tumors Disadvantages Photosensitivity, allergic reactions, and not useful in other cancers of skin. Occlusive dressings may increase the incidence of inflammatory reactions in adjacent normal skin. Porous gauze dressings may be used to cover application sites.
4. Fluorouracil plus 2,4-dinitrochlorobenzene	Selected cases of Bowen disease and *in situ* epidermoid cancer.
5. Combination chemotherapy fluorouracil plus cisplatin	As a palliative treatment in metastatic skin cancer when surgery is not curative.

Characteristics of the Merkel cell:

- Arises from the neural crest cells and is a member of the amine precursor uptake and decarboxylation (APUD) cell system
- Situated in the basal layer of the epidermis and hair follicles
- Important for tactile sensations in lower animals
- Functions as a mechanoreceptor in humans.

Characteristics of Merkel cell tumor:

- Rare tumor seen in elderly whites with sun-exposure history
- Involves skin of the head and neck and found less commonly in the extremities and genitals

- Presents as intracutaneous bluish, firm, and nontender nodule about 0.5 to 1 cm
- Histologically, a small round cell tumor, containing neurosecretory cytoplasmic granules
- Neuron-specific enolasepositive and anticytokeratin antibody, CAM 5.2, positive
- Differential diagnosis includes small cell carcinoma of lung and lymphoma
- Early spread by lymphatics and hematogenously to the distant site
- Surgical excision is the primary treatment, and radiation is used in the adjuvant setting.

Tumors arising from the skin appendages, pilosebaceous complex:

- Hair follicle
- Sebaceous gland
- Arrector pili muscle
- Apocrine sweat gland.

Most of these tumors are benign, and carcinomas are rare.
Significance: Of interest to dermatopathologist.

REFERENCES

1. Santa Cruz DJ, Hurt MA In: Steinberg SS, ed. *Diagnostic surgical pathology*, 2nd ed., Vol. 1. New York: Raven Press, 1999: 57–101.
2. Clark WH Jr, From L, Bernadino EA, et al. The histogenesis and biologic behavior of primary human malignant melanomas of skin. *Cancer Res* 1969;29:705.
3. Breslow A. Thickness, cross-sectional areas and depth of invasion in the prognosis of cutaneous melanoma. *Ann Surg* 1970;172:902.
4. Balch CM, Buzaid AC, Soong S-J, et al. Final version of the American Joint Committee on Cancer staging system for cutaneous melanoma. *J Clin Oncol* 2001;19:3655–3648.
5. Balch CM, Soong S-J, Gershenwald JE, et al. Prognostic factors analysis of 17,600 melanoma patients: Validation of the American Joint Committee on Cancer melanoma staging system. *J Clin Oncol* 2001;19:3622–3634.
6. Balch CM, Reintgen DS, Kirkwood JM, et al. Cutaneous melanoma. In: De Vita VT Jr, Hellman S, Rosenberg SA, eds. *Cancer: principles and practice of oncology*, 5th ed. Philadelphia, PA: Lippincott-Raven Publishers, 1997:1947–1994.
7. Morton DL, Essner R, Kirkwood JM, et al. Malignant melanoma. In: Holland JF, Frei E, Bast RC Jr, et al., eds. *Cancer medicine*, 4th ed. Baltimore, MD: Williams & Wilkins, 1997.
8. McCarthy WH, Shaw HM. The surgical treatment of primary melanoma. *Hematol Oncol Clin North Am* 1988;12:797–805.
9. Morton DL. Sentinel lymphadenectomy for patients with clinical stage I melanoma. *J Surg Oncol* 1997;66:267–269.
10. Ghussen F, Nage IK, Groth W, et al. Hyperthermic perfusion with chemotherapy and melanoma of the extremities. *World J Surg* 1989;13:598.
11. Ang KK, Byers RM, Peters LJ, et al. Regional radiotherapy as adjuvant for head and neck malignant melanoma: preliminary results. *Arch Otolaryngol Head Neck Surg* 1990;116:9.
12. Skibber JM, Soong S-J, Aushin AC, et al. Cranial irradiation after surgical excision of brain metastasis in melanoma patients. *Ann Surg Oncol* 1996;3:118–123.
13. Falkson JM. Improved results with the addition of interferon alpha-2b to dacarbazine in the treatment of patients with metastatic malignant melanoma. *J Clin Oncol* 1991;9:1403–1408.
14. Grobb JJ, Dreno B, Salmoniere P, et al. Randomized trial of interferon alpha-2a as adjuvant therapy in resected primary melanoma thicker than 1.5 mm without clinically detectable node metastasis. *Lancet* 1998;351:1905–1910.
15. Rosenberg SA, Yang JC, Topalian SL, et al. Treatment of 283 consecutive patients with metastatic melanoma or renal cell cancer using high-dose bolus interleukin 2. *JAMA* 1994;271:907–913.
16. Atkins MB, Lotze MT, Kutcher JP, et al. High-dose recombinant interleukin-2 therapy for patients with metastatic melanoma: analysis of 270 patients between 1985 and1993. *J Clin Oncol* 1999;17: 2105–2116.
17. Legha SS, Ring S, Bedikian A, et al. Treatment of metastatic melanoma with combined chemotherapy containing cisplatin, vinblastine, dacarbazine (CVD) and biotherapy using interleukin 2 and interferon alpha. *Ann Oncol* 1996;7:827–835.

18. Chapman PB, Einhorn LH, Meyers ML, et al. Phase III multicenter randomized trial of the Dart-mouth regimen versus dacarbazine in patients with metastatic melanoma. *J Clin Oncol* 1999;17:2745–2751.
19. Rosenberg SA, Yang JC, Schwartzentruber DJ, et al. Immunologic and therapeutic evaluation of a syn-thetic peptide vaccine for the treatment of patients with metastatic melanoma. *Nat Med* 1998;4:321–327.
20. Mukherji B, Chakraborty NG, Sporn JR, et al. Induction of peptide antigen reactive cytolytic T cells following immunization with MAGE-1 peptide pulsed autologous antigen presenting cells. *Proc Natl Acad Sci USA* 1995;92:8078–8082.
21. DiFronzo LA, Gupta RK, Essner R, et al. Enhanced humoral immune response correlates with improved disease-free and overall survival in American Joint Committee on Cancer stage II melanoma patients receiving adjuvant polyvalent vaccine. *J Clin Oncol* 2002;1:3242–3248.
22. Belli F, Testori A, Rivoltini L, et al. Vaccination of metastatic melanoma patients with autologous tumor-derived heat shock protein gp96-peptide complexes: clinical and immunologic findings. *J Clin Oncol* 2002;20:4169–4180.

SECTION 9

Hematologic Malignancies

23

Acute Leukemias

Michael Craig*, Jame Abraham†, and Brian P. Monahan‡

Section of Hematology/Oncology, West Virginia University, Morgantown, West Virginia; †Mary Babb Randolph Cancer Center, West Virginia University, Morgantown, West Virginia; and ‡Department of Hematology and Medical Oncology, Uniformed Services, University of the Health Sciences, Bethesda, Maryland

Acute leukemia represents a very aggressive, malignant transformation of an early hematologic precursor. The malignant clone is arrested in an immature, blast form; proliferates abnormally; and no longer has the ability to undergo maturation. In contrast, the chronic leukemias are characterized by resistance to apoptosis and by accumulation of nonfunctional cells. Accumulation of the blasts within the bone marrow results in progressive hematopoietic failure, with associated infection, anemia, and thrombocytopenia. It is these complications that often prompt evaluation in newly diagnosed patients.

Acute leukemia continues to present a grave diagnosis because of its rapid clinical course. Patients require aggressive and urgent evaluation and treatment initiation. As a general rule, treatment is expected to improve quality of life and prolong survival. Unfortunately, many patients present at an advanced age and with comorbid conditions, making cytotoxic treatment difficult. Elderly or unwell patients who are given the best supportive care survive only for a few months.

The immature, clonally proliferating cells that form blasts may be derived from myeloid or lymphoid cell lines. Transformation of granulocyte, RBC, or platelet (myeloid) precursors results in acute myelogenous leukemia (AML). Acute lymphoblastic leukemia (ALL) originates from B or T lymphocytes. This general division has implications for different treatment and diagnostic approaches. It is the first step in classifying the leukemic process occurring in the patient.

EPIDEMIOLOGY

- Estimated new cases in the United States in 2003 were 10,500 for AML and 3,600 for ALL (age-adjusted estimates).
- AML accounts for 7,800 deaths and ALL accounts for 1,400 deaths annually in the United States (age-adjusted estimates).
- The risk of developing AML increases with advanced age, the median age being 60 to 69.
- Seventy-five percent of newly diagnosed patients with AML are older than 60.
- AML is the most common leukemia in adults (80% of cases).
- ALL is more common in children; 60% of cases are found in patients younger than 20 years.
- A small decrease and a plateau in the incidence of new cases has been observed since 1995.

TABLE 23.1. *Risk factors for acute leukemia*

Exposure: ionizing radiation, benzene, cytotoxic drugs, alkylating agents, cigarette smoking, ethanol use by the mother

Acquired disorders: myelodysplastic syndrome, paroxysmal nocturnal hemoglobinuria, polycythemia vera, chronic myelogenous leukemia, myeloproliferative disorders, idiopathic myelofibrosis, aplastic anemia, eosinophilic fasciitis, myeloma, primary mediastinal germ cell tumor (residual teratoma elements evolve into myeloid progenitors that evolve into AML years later)

Genetic predisposition: Down syndrome, Fanconi anemia, Diamond-Blackfan anemia, Kostmann syndrome, Klinefelter syndrome, Chromosome 21q disorder, Wiskott-Aldrich syndrome, ataxia-telangiectasia, dyskeratosis congenita, combined immunodeficiency syndrome, von Recklinghausen disease, neurofibromatosis 1, Shwachman syndrome

Familial: nonidentical sibling (1:800), monozygotic twin (1:5), first-degree relative (three times increased risk).

Infection: human T-cell leukemia virus and T-cell ALL

AML, acute myelogenous leukemia; ALL, acute lymphoblastic leukemia.

RISK FACTORS

Most patients will have no identifiable risk for developing leukemia. Table 23.1 lists the conditions that are identified with an increased risk for developing acute leukemia. Most studies have evaluated the relationship between the risk factors and AML. The conditions that are most associated with AML are chronic benzene exposure, exposure to ionizing radiation, and previous chemotherapy. In the case of chronic lymphocytic leukemia (CLL), the herbicide from the Vietnam War era, Agent Orange, has been associated with at least compensable risk.

Ionizing Radiation Exposure Explored in Atomic Bomb Survivors

- Ionizing radiations have a latency period of 5 to 20 years and a peak period of 5 to 9 years in atomic bomb survivors.
- They exhibit a 20- to 30-fold increased risk of AML and chronic myelogenous leukemia (CML).

Chemotherapy

- Therapy-related AML may account for 10% to 20% of new cases.
- It is reported in Hodgkin and non-Hodgkin lymphoma; breast, small cell, germ cell, and ovarian tumors; as well as in patients who have received high-dose therapy.
- Leukemia associated with alkylating agents may be associated with cytogenetic changes of chromosomes 5, 7, and 13. Often there is a multiyear latent-phase myelodysplastic syndrome preceding the development of AML.
- Topoisomerase II agents, often with an abnormal chromosome 11q23 in the blasts, can rapidly evolve after initial therapy. Usually, these are preceded by only a brief myelodysplastic state rapidly evolving to AML.
- Previous high-dose therapy with autologous transplant leads to a cumulative risk of 2.6% by 5 years, especially with total body irradiation (TBI)–containing regimens.

CLINICAL SIGNS AND SYMPTOMS

1. Ineffective hematopoiesis—results from marrow infiltration by the malignant cells
   - Anemia: pallor, fatigue, and shortness of breath
   - Thrombocytopenia: epistaxis, petechiae, and easy bruising
   - Neutropenia: fever and pyogenic infection.

2. Infiltration of other organs
   - Skin: leukemia cutis in 10%
   - Gum hypertrophy: especially in monocytic leukemia (AML M5)
   - Granulocytic sarcoma: localized tumor composed of blast cells; it imparts poorer prognosis; these sarcomas are occasionally extramedullary leukemia masses associated with 8;21 translocation
   - Liver, spleen, and lymph nodes: common in ALL, occasionally in monocytic leukemia (AML M5)
   - Thymic mass: present in 15% of ALL in adults
   - Testicular infiltration: also a site of relapse for ALL
   - Retinal involvement: may occur in ALL.
3. Central nervous system (CNS) and meningeal involvement
   - Five percent to 10% of cases at diagnosis, mainly ALL, inv(16) [French–American–British (FAB) M4Eo], and high blast count
   - Analysis and prophylaxis are given in ALL to decrease CNS relapse
   - Symptoms: headache and cranial nerve palsy, but mostly asymptomatic.
4. Disseminated intravascular coagulation (DIC) and bleeding
   - Very common with promyelocytic leukemia t(15;17); mechanism is related to tissue factor release by granules and fibrinolysis; it worsens with cytotoxic treatment and improves with all-trans retinoic acid (ATRA)
   - Can be present in AML inv(16) or monocytic leukemia or can be related to sepsis.
5. Leukostasis
   - Occurs with elevated blast count; 25% of patients with ALL present with white blood cell (WBC) count greater than 50,000
   - Symptoms result from capillary plugging by leukemic cells; it is associated with large nondeformable blasts in AML and ALL and is rarely seen in CLL
   - Common signs: dyspnea, headache, confusion, and hypoxia
   - Initial treatment includes leukapheresis, aggressive hydration, and chemotherapy to rapidly lower the circulating blast percentage with drugs (e.g., oral hydroxyurea or intravenous cyclophosphamide)
   - Transfusions should be avoided because these may increase viscosity
   - Leukapheresis is repeated daily in conjunction with chemotherapy until the blast count is less than 50,000.

DIAGNOSTIC EVALUATION

- History and physical examination are an essential part of diagnosis of acute leukemia.
- Complete blood count (CBC) and differential, manual examination of peripheral smear, and peripheral blood flow cytometry are considered when circulating blasts are sufficiently abundant to establish a diagnosis without need for bone marrow biopsy.
- Coagulation tests include prothrombin time (PT), partial thromboplastin time (PTT), D-dimer, and fibrinogen.
- Electrolytes with calcium, magnesium, phosphorus, and uric acid. Low glucose, potassium, and Po_2 (partial pressure of oxygen) can occur with delay in analysis of high blast count.
- Bone marrow biopsy and aspirate (with analysis for morphology), cytogenetics, flow cytometry, and cytochemical stains (Sudan black, myeloperoxidase, acid phosphatase, and specific and nonspecific esterase) are used for diagnosis.
- Human leukocyte antigen (HLA) testing of patients who are transplant candidates—the test is performed before the patient becomes cytopenic. Specimen requirements are minimal when DNA-based HLA typing is performed.
- Hepatitis B and C, cytomegalovirus, herpes simplex virus, human T-cell leukemia virus, and human immunodeficiency virus antibody titers are obtained.

- Typing and screening of blood products of patients with their consent: Blood product selection should prospectively consider the allogeneic transplant candidacy needs of cytomegalovirus CMV conversion reduction and irradiation to incapacitate donor lymphocytes from contaminating products.
- Pregnancy test (β-human chorionic gonadotropin).
- Electrocardiogram (ECG) and analysis of cardiac ejection fraction should be done prior to treatment with anthracyclines.
- Lumbar puncture—performed when signs and symptoms of ALL or monocytic leukemia are present. Low platelets should be corrected. The procedure may be performed after reduction of peripheral blast count to avoid inoculation of blasts into uninvolved cerebrospinal fluid (CSF). Obtain cell count, opening pressure, protein level, and submit cytocentrifuge specimen for cytology.
- Central venous access should be obtained using dual-lumen tunnel catheter or triple-lumen line. An implanted port-type catheter is not recommended. Coagulation abnormalities should be corrected if present. It is often possible to initiate induction therapy with normal peripheral veins and await subsidence of coagulopathy to reduce risk of procedural complications.
- Supplemental testing of fluorescent *in situ* hybridization (FISH) assay for 15;17 translocation is performed when acute promyelocytic leukemia (APL) is suspected, and BCR-ABL test is performed when *de novo* CML or blast crisis transformation is suspected to be critical. Cytogenetic analysis of blasts will contribute dramatically to subsequent preferred management.

INITIAL MANAGEMENT

The initial management of acute leukemia involves the following:

- Hydration with i.v. fluids, 1,500 to 2,000 mL per day.
- Tumor lysis prophylaxis should be started.
- Blood product support suggestions for prophylactic transfusions are hemoglobin level less than 8 and platelet level less than 10,000. Platelet trigger threshold can be higher in the context of fever or bleeding (less than 20,000 suggested), cryoprecipitate can be used if fibrinogen level is less than 100, and fresh frozen plasma (FFP) can be used for significantly elevated levels of PT and PTT. The minimum "safe" platelet level required to prevent spontaneous hemorrhage is not known. Additional platelet optimization strategies include avoidance of cyclooxygenase-2 (COX-2)–selective nonsteroidal antiinflammatory drug (NSAID), aspirin, and clopidogrel-like agents.
- WBC filter (if CMV-negative blood inventory is not available) should be used and blood products should be irradiated in those patients who are future allogeneic transplant candidates.
- Fever and neutropenia require blood and urine cultures, followed by treatment with appropriate antibiotics (see Chapter 36), and imaging.
- Therapeutic anticoagulation should be given with extreme caution in patients during periods of extreme thrombocytopenia. Adjustment of prophylactic platelet transfusion thresholds or anticoagulants is required.
- Suppression of menses
- Medroxyprogesterone (Provera) 10 mg daily or twice daily.

Tumor Lysis Syndrome

- Tumor lysis syndrome can be spontaneous or can be induced by chemotherapy.
- Risk factors include elevated uric acid, high WBC count, elevated lactate dehydrogenase (LDH), high tumor burden, and those factors that are already present spontaneously in tumor lysis at presentation.
- Laboratory tests indicate elevated creatinine, low calcium, high phosphorus, acidosis, and coagulopathy.

- The patients should be initiated on allopurinol 300 mg twice daily for 3 days, followed by once daily until risk is resolved.
- For hydration, alkalinizing fluids (0.5N saline with 50 mEq sodium bicarbonate 2,000 mL per day) should be considered.
- Rasburicase (Elitek) 0.15 mg per kg i.v. daily should be used for up to 5 days if the patient is in tumor lysis at presentation or has rising creatinine level or hyperuricemia during induction.
- Hemodialysis may be required in refractory cases or urgently in the setting of life-threatening hyperkalemia, or volume overload if oliguric (see Chapter 38).

CLASSIFICATION OF ACUTE MYELOGENOUS LEUKEMIA

There are two current systems to classify AML. One system has been suggested by the World Health Organization (WHO) and incorporates recurrent cytogenetic abnormalities and prognostic groups (see Table 23.2). Marrow blasts should make up 20% of the nucleated cells within the aspirate unless t(8;21) or inv(16) is present. The French-American-British (FAB) classification is also used and classifies AML into eight subtypes. The blasts may be characterized as myeloid lineage by the presence of Auer rods; a positive myeloperoxidase, Sudan black, or nonspecific esterase stain; and the immunophenotype shown by flow cytometry. Cell surface markers associated with myeloid cell lines include CD13, CD33, CD34, c-kit, and HLA-DR. Monocytic markers include CD64, CD11b, and CD14. CD41 (platelet glycophorin) is associated with megakaryocytic

TABLE 23.2. *The World Health Organization (WHO) and French–American–British (FAB) classification of myeloid leukemia*

AML with recurrent genetic abnormalities

- AML with t(8;21) (usually FAB M2)
- AML with abnormal bone marrow eosinophils and inv(16) or t(16;16) (usually FAB M4Eo)
- Acute promyelocytic leukemia with t(15;17) (FAB M3)
- AML with 11q23 abnormalities

AML with multilineage dysplasia

- Following MDS or myeloproliferative disorder
- Without prior MDS but with dysplasia in 50% cells in two cell lines

AML and MDS, therapy related

- Alkylating agent or radiation related
- Topoisomerase II related
- Others

AML not otherwise categorized

- AML minimally differentiated (FAB M0)
- AML without maturation (FAB M1)
- AML with maturation (FAB M2)
- Acute myelomonocytic leukemia (FAB M4)
- Acute monocytic leukemia (FAB M5)
- Acute erythroid leukemia (FAB M6)
- Acute megakaryocytic leukemia (FAB M7)
- Acute basophilic leukemia
- Acute panmyelosis with myelofibrosis
- Myeloid sarcoma

AML, acute myelogenous leukemia; MDS, myelodysplasia.

leukemia, and glycophorin A is present on erythroblasts. HLA-DR–negative blast phenotype is uniquely seen in APL and serves as a rapidly available test in confirming the suspicion of this subtype requiring a specific induction therapy.

CLASSIFICATION OF ACUTE LYMPHOBLASTIC LEUKEMIA

The WHO classification of ALL divides the disease into precursor B-cell, precursor T-cell, and Burkitt-cell leukemia. Immunophenotyping of B-lineage ALL reveals lymphoid markers (CD19, CD20, CD10, TdT, and immunoglobulin). T-cell markers include TdT, CD2, CD3, CD4, CD5, and CD7. Burkitt-cell leukemia is characterized by a translocation between chromosome 8 (the *c-myc* gene) and chromosome 14 (immunoglobulin heavy chain), or chromosome 2 or 22 (light chain) regions.

PROGNOSTIC GROUPS IN ACUTE MYELOGENOUS LEUKEMIA

Those patients who are older (older than 60) and those with an elevated blast count at diagnosis (>20,000) have a worse prognosis. Chemotherapy-related AML and prior history of myelodysplasia (MDS) imparts a lower chance of obtaining complete remission (CR) and long-term survival. A history of trisomy 21 may impart a good prognosis. Table 23.3 illustrates the prognostic groups according to cytogenetics.

PROGNOSTIC GROUPS IN ACUTE LYMPHOBLASTIC LEUKEMIA

As in AML, patients with ALL have a worse prognosis when presenting with advanced age or elevated WBC count. B-cell phenotypes have a worse prognosis than T-cell phenotypes. Burkitt-cell (mature B-cell) leukemia or lymphoma has an improved prognosis with intensive chemotherapy and CNS treatment; it usually has a translocation involving chromosome 8q24. Table 23.4 lists the prognostic groups according to cytogenetic analysis. The presence of

TABLE 23.3. *Cytogenetic risk groups in treated adult acute myelogenous leukemia (AML) cases*

Favorable risk (5-yr survival with therapy as high as 40%)

- t(15;17)
- inv(16), del(16q), t(16;16)
- t(8;21) with or without complex karyotype and del(9q)

Standard risk (5-yr survival with therapy approximately 20%)

- no cytogenetic abnormality identified (i.e., normal)
- all other cytogenetic abnormalities not associated with a specific prognosis

Poor risk (5-yr survival with therapy <10%)

- –5, –7
- inv(3) or t(3;3)
- t(9;22)
- 11q23 (MLL) abnormalities
- three or more abnormalities
- t(6;9)

From Grimwade D, Walker H, Harrison G, et al. The predictive value of hierarchical cytogenetic classification in older adults with acute myeloid leukemia (AML): analysis of 1065 patients entered into the United Kingdom Medical Research Council AML11 trial. *Blood* 2001;98:1312–1320, with permission.

TABLE 23.4. *Prognostic groups in adult acute lymphoblastic leukemia (ALL)*

Poor risk:

- t(9;22)
- t(4;11)
- Hypodiploid
- t(1;19)

Good risk:

- 8q24 translocations
- t(12;21)
- t(10;14)
- t(7;10)

t(9;22) (Philadelphia chromosome) is the most common abnormality in adults. It is present in 20% to 30% of patients with ALL and in up to 50% of patients in the B-cell lineage. Long-term survival is dismal in this group if treated by chemotherapy alone. (These adults are not treated with maintenance chemotherapy and are recommended to undergo allogeneic transplantation if they are a suitable candidate in first CR.)

TREATMENT INDUCTION IN ACUTE MYELOGENOUS LEUKEMIA [NON–t(15;17) ACUTE PROMYELOCYTIC LEUKEMIA]

The goal of induction chemotherapy is to obtain CR, which has been shown to correlate with improved survival. CR is the elimination of the malignant clone (marrow blasts <5%) and recovery of hematopoiesis [absolute neutrophil count (ANC) >1,000 to 1,500 and platelet count >100,000]. Patients typically have a leukemia cell burden of approximately 10×10^{15} that is reduced to approximately 10×10^{12} by induction. Additional intensive "consolidation" cycles of chemotherapy are given to further reduce this residual burden in the hope that host immune mechanisms can suppress the residual leukemia population, thereby leading to sustained CR. The general approach to induction chemotherapy for adults is shown in Table 23.5. Patients should be considered for clinical trials if available.

In general:

- Idarubicin may be the preferred anthracycline agent in AML.
- Addition of high-dose cytarabine (HDAC) or etoposide has been evaluated in published regimens for induction that may benefit some patients younger than 60. These additions have not been demonstrated to be conclusively superior to 3 days of anthracycline and 7 days of cytarabine alone. Multiple regimens are available; Table 23.6 shows a choice evaluated in a randomized trial.

TABLE 23.5. *Standard induction for acute myelogenous leukemia (AML)*

"7 + 3," 7 d of cytarabine and 3 d of anthracycline:
Cytarabine 100–200 mg/m² daily as continuous infusion × 7 d with
  Idarubicin 12 mg/m² daily bolus for 3 d

Or

Daunorubicin 45–60 mg/m² daily bolus for 3 d

Or

Mitoxantrone 12 mg/m² daily bolus for 3 d

TABLE 23.6. *Southwest Oncology Group (SWOG) regimen for HDAC induction*

Cytarabine 2 g/m^2 over 1 h q12h on d 1–6 (12 doses) and daunorubicin 45 mg/m^2/day bolus on d 7–9 (three doses)

- Bone marrow aspiration should be repeated at approximately 14 days. If residual blasts are present (>5%), induction chemotherapy should be repeated (consider "5 + 2" in Table 23.7). If significant disease is present (<40% to 50% reduction in disease volume), induction should be repeated or a change in the regimen to age-appropriate HDAC should be considered.
- Elderly (older than 65) patients may benefit from treatment. HDAC should be avoided because of excess CNS toxicity and commonly observed poor survival prospects regardless of therapy selection.

SUPPORTIVE CARE

- Infection is a major cause of morbidity and mortality. Prophylactic antibiotics and antifungals are often used during prolonged neutropenia with uncertain benefit. Broad-spectrum antimicrobials are used for neutropenic fever (see Chapter 36).
- Growth factors such as granulocyte colony stimulating factor (G-CSF) are associated with shortened length of neutropenia and are of demonstrated value in patients older than 65 years. Initiation of G-CSF, when employed, is delayed until after day 14, when bone marrow shows a satisfactory induction pattern. Growth factors may benefit most those with fever or infection.
- Dexamethasone eye drops are required during HDAC infusions to reduce risk of exfoliative keratitis.

TREATMENT—ACUTE MYELOGENOUS LEUKEMIA CONSOLIDATION, NON–t(15;17)

The consolidation options for those patients who enter CR are shown in Table 23.7. HDAC especially may benefit those patients with good-risk disease [t(8;21) or inv(16)]. Consolidation usually consists of two to four cycles (the minimum effective number is not known). Patients with preceding MDS or very poor risk cytogenetics may proceed to allogeneic transplantation.

TABLE 23.7. *Consolidation of acute myelogenous leukemia*

Age <60

- Cytarabine 3 mg/m^2 infused over 2 h, q12h on d 1, 3, and 5 (six doses).
- Creatinine 1.5–1.9 mg/dL: Decrease cytarabine 1.5 g/m^2 per dose.

Age >60

- "5 + 2:" Cytarabine 100 mg/m^2 daily as continuous infusion for 5 d and anthracycline agent (idarubicin 12 mg/m^2, daunorubicin 45–60 mg/m^2, or mitoxantrone 12 mg/m^2) bolus daily for 2 d.

Or

- If age of patient is 60–70, good performance status and renal function: Intermediate dose cytarabine 1 g/m^2 q12h on d 1, 3, 5.

TREATMENT—ACUTE PROMYELOCYTIC LEUKEMIA, t(15;17)

The t(15;17) brings together the retinoic acid receptor-α and the promyelocytic leukemia genes, allowing for transduction of a novel protein (PML-RAR). The protein plays a role in blocking differentiation of the promyelocyte, thereby allowing abnormal accumulation within the marrow space. Because characteristic translocation occurs in this subgroup of AML, therapy incorporates ATRA, which acts as a differentiating agent. Table 23.8 shows a treatment summary in APL.

Management notes:

- Time to attain remission may be more than 30 days and a bone marrow biopsy is not performed on day 14.
- PCR should be followed for PML-RAR: high-dose cytarabine should be considered if positive postconsolidation is present; also, levels should be followed during the maintenance phase. A return of the transcript to positive heralds relapse.
- APL syndrome (retinoic acid syndrome) consists of capillary leak and cytokine release resulting in fever, respiratory compromise (dyspnea and infiltrates), weight gain, renal dysfunction, effusions (pleural and pericardial), and hypotension. This syndrome occurs in 20% of patients during induction, often around day 7, and is associated with a rapidly rising neutrophil count. Treat with dexamethasone 10 mg i.v. b.i.d. Discontinuation of ATRA or use of leukocyte apheresis should be considered in severe cases. ATRA may be safely employed in maintenance phase therapy because the ATRA syndrome is limited to the induction-period neutrophilia.
- A similar syndrome, not involving ATRA, is seen with the use of arsenic trioxide.

Prognosis with APL is very good, with 90% of patients attaining a CR and 70% long-term disease-free survival. Those patients with WBC counts greater than 10,000 and platelets less than 40,000 at diagnosis may have increased risk of relapse.

Relapsed Disease:

1. Arsenic trioxide 0.15 mg/kg/day until second CR
   - Average of 35 days to remission
   - Daily electrolytes, ECG (prolonged QT interval) determinations, neuropathy assessment
   - Twenty-five percent of patients may develop APL syndrome similar to ATRA

TABLE 23.8. *Treatment of acute promyelocytic leukemia*

Induction

- ATRA 45 mg/m^2/d PO divided into two doses, daily until CR and
- Anthracycline: Idarubicin 12 mg/m^2 every alternate days for four doses (d 2, 4, 6, 8) or daunorubicin 50–60 mg/m^2 daily for 3 d.

Consolidation

- Alternating anthracycline/anthracenedione: Idarubicin 5 mg/m^2 daily for 5 d (first consolidation), then mitoxantrone 10 mg/m^2 daily for 6 d (second consolidation), followed by idarubicin 12 mg/m^2 times one dose (third consolidation)

Or

- 2 cycles of daunorubicin 50–60 mg/m^2 daily for 3 d

Maintenance (2 yr)

- ATRA 45 mg/m^2 daily for 15 d q3mo
- 6-MP 100 mg/m^2 daily
- MTX 10 mg/m^2 weekly

ATRA, all-trans retinoic acid; 6-MP, 6-mercaptopurine; MTX, methotrexate.

- Eighty-five percent of patients have achieved CR
- Arsenic trioxide may be followed by further cycles at a dose of 0.15 mg/kg/day for 25 doses.
2. Autologous transplant with PCR-negative harvest or allogeneic transplant should be considered.

TREATMENT OF RELAPSED OR REFRACTORY ACUTE MYELOGENOUS LEUKEMIA

Relapse of AML after initial CR is very common (60% to 80% of all cases). Relapse occurring within 6 months of induction or a patient never attaining remission with induction (refractory disease) complicates many induction attempts. The prognosis for long-term survival in this subset of patients is very poor with chemotherapy alone, and all patients who are able to tolerate the treatment should be evaluated for allogeneic transplantation. Other options are described in the following.

1. Gemtuzumab ozogamicin (Mylotarg)
   - Gemtuzumab ozogamicin is an anti-CD33 monoclonal antibody conjugated with calicheamicin.
   - The dosage is 9 mg per m^2 as 2-hour infusion on days 1 and 15.
   - It is approved for use in adults older than 60 years in first relapse.
   - Thirty percent of patients achieved CR (13% without complete platelet recovery).
   - Side effects include nausea, thrombocytopenia, and increase in liver enzyme levels.
   - WBC count should be reduced to less than 30,000 before treatment.
   - Gemtuzumab ozogamicin is not for patients who may undergo allogeneic transplantation due to increased risk of venoocclusive disease (VOD).
   - Overall treatment-related morbidity can be considered similar to that of conventional chemotherapy induction.
2. Reinduction with "7 + 3" or high-dose cytarabine
   - Reinduction may be an option for those patients who relapse more than 12 months after induction.
   - Remission rates are approximately 50%, although usually of shorter duration (<50% of the duration of the preceding remission).
3. FLAG: Fludarabine, Cytarabine, and G-CSF (can be combined with idarubicin or mitoxantrone)
   - CR is obtained in 55% of patients.
4. Liposomal daunorubicin and cytarabine combination is used at high dose.
   - CR is 29% and overall response rate is 40%.
5. Etoposide, mitoxantrone, ± cytarabine (EM or MEC)
6. In cases of isolated CNS relapse, it should be considered that systemic relapse almost always follows soon and that a systemic therapy is also required.

TREATMENT OF ACUTE LYMPHOCYTIC LEUKEMIA

General scheme: induction, consolidation, maintenance, and CNS treatment.

Several strategies exist for the treatment of adult ALL. Table 23.9 illustrates the Hyper-CVAD (cyclophosphamide, vincristine, doxorubicin, and dexamethasone) regimen employed in many North American centers. The Larson regimen reported by Cancer and Leukemia Group B (CALGB) Study 9111, shown in Table 23.10, is also commonly employed. Other options based on the Hoelzer and Linker regimen are available. Burkitt-cell leukemia (mature-B ALL, L3) is not included because of high resistance to typical induction chemotherapy. It can be treated with hyper-CVAD without maintenance therapy but requires aggressive CNS treatment to prevent relapse.

TABLE 23.9. *The hyper-CVAD and MTX/HIDAC regimen*

Cycle 1, 3, 5, 7

- Cyclophosphamide 300 mg/m^2 i.v. over 2 h q12h d 1–3 (six doses)
- Mesna 600 mg/m^2/d i.v. as continuous infusion d 1–3, complete 12 h post cyclophosphamide
- Vincristine 2 mg i.v. d 4, 11
- Doxorubicin 50 mg/m^2 i.v. d 4
- Dexamethasone 40 mg PO daily d 1–4 and 11–14
- G-CSF 10 μg/kg/d s.c. starting d 5

Cycle 2, 4, 6, 8

- Methotrexate 200 mg/m^2 i.v. over 2 h on d 1, followed by
- Methotrexate 800 mg/m^2 over 22 h on d 1
- Leucovorin 50 mg i.v. starting 12 h after methotrexate completed, followed by leucovorin 15 mg i.v. every 6 h × eight doses, dose adjusted on the basis of methotrexate levels as well. Meticulous monitoring of methotrexate levels is required to ensure appropriate leucovorin scheduling. Rapidly changing renal function during or shortly after the methotrexate infusion should prompt consideration for urgent measures to mitigate toxicity (higher leucovorin doses, infusion of investigational carboxypeptidase-G to cleave plasma methotrexate to inactive fragments).
- Cytarabine 3 g/m^2 i.v. over 2 h every 12 h on d 2 and 3 (four doses)
- Methylprednisolone 50 mg i.v. twice daily d 1–3
- G-CSF 10 μg/kg/d s.c. starting d 4

CNS Prophylaxis[a]

- Methotrexate 12 mg intrathecal (IT) d 2 of the course
- Cytarabine 100 mg IT d 8 of the course

Maintenance therapy[b] (POMP)

- 6-Mercaptopurine 50 mg PO three times daily
- Methotrexate 20 mg/m^2 PO, weekly
- Vincristine 2 mg i.v. monthly
- Prednisone 200 mg/d for 5 d each month

Dosage adjustments

- Vincristine reduced to 1 mg if bilirubin >2 mg/dL
- Doxorubicin decreased to 25% for bilirubin 2–3 mg/dL, decreased to 50% if bilirubin 3–4 mg/dL, and decreased 75% if bilirubin >4 mg/dL
- Methotrexate reduced to 25% if creatinine 1.5–2 mg/dL, reduce to 50% if creatinine >2 mg/dL
- HIDAC decreased to 1 g/m^2 if patient >60 yr, creatinine >2 mg/dL, or MTX level >20 μmol/L
- May need to decrease MTX/HIDAC doses for toxicity

G-CSF, granulocyte colony stimulating factor; CNS, central nervous system; POMP, 6-mercaptopurine–methotrexate–vincristine–prednisone; HIDAC, high-dose cytosine arabinoside; MTX/HIDAC, methotrexate/high-dose cytosine arabinoside.
[a]Dosing interval based on risk stratification (see text).
[b]Maintenance therapy was not given in Burkitt-cell leukemia/lymphoma.

SUPPORTIVE CARE

The regimens described previously incorporate growth factors to reduce neutropenia and allow more scheduled chemotherapy to proceed. All patients will require blood product support at some point during the treatment. Those patients treated with hyper-CVAD receive prophylactic antimicrobials (i.e., levofloxacin 500 mg daily, fluconazole 200 mg daily, and valacyclovir 500 mg daily). Prophylactic trimethoprim–sulfamethoxazole and valacyclovir 500 mg were given three times per week during the first 6 months of maintenance.

TABLE 23.10. *The Larson regimen*

Course I: Induction (4 wk).

- Cyclophosphamide 1,200 mg/m^2 i.v. d 1[a]
- Daunorubicin 45 mg/m^2 i.v. d 1–3[a]
- Vincristine 2 mg i.v. d 1, 8, 15, 22
- Prednisone 60 mg/m^2/d PO d 1–21[a]
- L-Asparaginase (*Escherichia coli*) 6,000 IU/m^2 s.c./i.m. d 5, 8, 11, 15, 18, 22
- G-CSF 5 µg/kg/d subcutaneously (s.c.) starting d 4

Course IIA (4 wk; repeat once for Course IIB)

- Methotrexate 15 mg intrathecal (IT) d 1
- Cyclophosphamide 1,000 mg/m^2 i.v. d 1
- 6-Mercaptopurine 60 mg/m^2/d PO d 1–14
- Cytarabine 75 mg/m^2/d s.c. d 1–4 and 8–11
- Vincristine 2 mg i.v. d 15 and 22 (two doses)
- L-Asparaginase (*E. coli*) 6,000 IU/m^2 s.c./i.m. d 15, 18, 22, 25 (four doses)
- G-CSF 5 µg/kg/d s.c. starting d 4.

Course III: CNS prophylaxis and interim maintenance (12 wk)

- IT Methotrexate 15 mg d 1, 8, 15, 22, 29
- Cranial irradiation 2,400 cGy (fractionated) d 1–12
- 6-Mercaptopurine 60 mg/m^2/d PO d 1–70
- Methotrexate 20 mg/m^2 PO d 36, 43, 50, 57, 64

Course IV: Late intensification (8 wk)

- Doxorubicin 30 mg/m^2 i.v. d 1, 8, 15
- Vincristine 2 mg i.v. d 1, 8, 15
- Dexamethasone 10 mg/m^2/d PO d 1–14
- Cyclophosphamide 1,000 mg/m^2 i.v. d 29
- 6-Thioguanine 60 mg/m^2/d PO d 29–42
- Cytarabine 75 mg/m^2/d s.c. d 29–32 and 36–39

Course V: Prolonged maintenance (until 24 mo from diagnosis)

- Vincristine 2 mg i.v. d 1 of every 4 wk
- Prednisone 60 mg/m^2/d PO d 1–5 of every 4 wk
- 6-Mercaptopurine 60 mg/m^2/d PO d 1–28
- Methotrexate 20 mg/m^2 PO d 1, 8, 15, 22

CNS, central nervous system.
[a]Dosage reductions for age >60 yr: cyclophosphamide 800 mg/m^2 d 1, daunorubicin 30 mg/m^2 i.v. d 1–3, and prednisone 60 mg/m^2/d PO d 1–7.

THERAPY FOR CENTRAL NERVOUS SYSTEM DISEASE

- CNS is a sanctuary site.
- CNS disease is diagnosed by the presence of neurologic deficits at diagnosis *or* by 5 or more blasts per microliter of CSF.
- Therapy for CNS disease is radiation (fractionated to 2,400 to 3,000 cGy) and intrathecal (IT) methotrexate (MTX) or cytarabine (Ara-C).
- Prophylaxis decreases CNS relapse from 30% to less than 5%. The prophylactic radiation and chemotherapy schedule intensity are dependent on the relapse risk.
- Radiation and IT MTX are equivalent to systemic high-dose chemotherapy and IT chemotherapy. There are potential late-term cognitive toxicities in treated subjects.
- In the hyper-CVAD regimen, patients with high-risk disease (i.e., LDH level >600, mature B-cell disease, or elevated proliferative index) receive 16 IT treatments, those with low-risk disease (no factors) receive 4 IT treatments, and those with unknown disease receive 8 IT doses.

TREATMENT OF RELAPSED ACUTE LYMPHOBLASTIC LEUKEMIA

Marrow is the most common site of relapse but relapse can occur in testes, eye, and CNS. Patients with late relapse (more than 1 year from induction) may respond to reinduction with the original regimen. Early relapse or refractory disease will require transplantation or changing treatment plan. Several options are available, including:

- high-dose cytarabine with idarubicin, mitoxantrone, or fludarabine
- dose escalation of imatinib [Philadelphia-positive (Ph-positive)]
- hyper-CVAD, if not given initially.

USE OF MONOCLONAL ANTIBODIES IN ACUTE LYMPHOBLASTIC LEUKEMIA

1. Rituximab (Rituxan)
   - Anti-CD20 chimeric murine–human monoclonal antibody
   - May have a role in addition to the previously noted regimens in front-line therapeutic combinations
   - Palliation in those patients who are not able to tolerate intensive regimens.
2. Alemtuzumab (Campath-1H)
   - Anti-CD52 chimeric monoclonal antibody employed in relapsed CLL
   - Limited experience in relapsed and refractory disease, but may have a role in palliation
   - Side effects include fever, rigor, nausea with infusion, and prolonged lymphopenia.
3. Gemtuzumab ozogamicin (Mylotarg)
   - Anti-CD33 monoclonal antibody conjugated with calicheamicin (dose listed in preceding text)
   - 30% of ALL patients may express CD33 (55% Ph-positive cases).

TRANSPLANTATION

Autologous Transplant

- Autologous transplant is a further consolidation for patients with poor-risk disease who have no donors for allogeneic transplant.
- It may be performed after intensive consolidation chemotherapy.
- It may be performed in older patients (as old as 60 to 70).
- It may increase disease-free survival.

Allogeneic Transplant

- Allogeneic transplant has the added benefit of "graft versus leukemia" effect.
- Its increased short-term toxicity may limit the ability to proceed with the transplantation.
- In the setting of unrelated donor searches, the prolonged time needed to identify a donor needs to be considered at the time of diagnosis.
- It is considered for all patients with relapsed or refractory disease, as it is the option that may yield long-term survival.
- It is performed in the first CR or early in the course for those patients with poor risk cytogenetics, t(9;21), or MDS, especially with a matched-related donor.
- It may be associated with increased failure-free survival.
- When transplanted in first CR, overall survival is 60%; it decreases to less than 35% when performed for patients with relapsed disease, and is lower than 10% for patients with refractory disease.
- Nonmyeloablative transplantation is being explored for those patients unable to proceed with ablative treatment secondary to age or illness.

PROGNOSIS AND SURVIVAL

Adults with acute leukemia remain at high risk for disease-related and treatment-related complications. In AML, the prognostic characteristics of the disease are associated with survival. High-risk AML is associated with 80% to 90% CR rate, and long-term disease-free survival is 60% to 70% in younger patients treated with HDAC. Poor-risk features are associated with only a 50% to 60% chance of obtaining a CR, and a high risk of relapse is observed in those patients who enter CR.

CR and long-term outcome have improved for adult patients with ALL who were receiving intensive courses of chemotherapy. With the Larson regimen, 85% obtained CR (39% older than 60 years). The hyper-CVAD course yielded a CR of 91% (79% for patients older than 60 years). Median duration of CR was 30 months with Larson regimen and was 33 months with hyper-CVAD. Five-year survival was approximately 40%.

SUGGESTED READINGS

Beutler E, Lichtman M, Coller B, et al., eds. *Williams hematology*, 6th ed. New York: McGraw-Hill, 2001.

Bloomfield C, Lawrence D, Byrd J, et al. Frequency of prolonged remission duration after high-dose cytarabine in acute myeloid leukemia varies by cytogenetic subtype. *Cancer Res* 1998;58:4173–4179.

Byrd J, Mrozek K, Dodge R, et al. Pretreatment cytogenetic abnormalities are predictive of induction success, cumulative incidence of relapse, and overall survival in adult patients with de novo acute myeloid leukemia: results from Cancer and Leukemia Group B (CALGB 8461). *Blood* 2002;100:4325–4336.

Cortes J, Estey E, O'Brien S, et al. High-dose liposomal daunorubicin and high-dose cytarabine combination in patients with refractory or relapsed acute myelogenous leukemia. Cancer 2001;92:7–14.

Estey E. Therapeutic options for acute myelogenous leukemia. *Cancer* 2001;92:1059–1073.

Ferrando A, Look AT. Clinical implications of recurring chromosomal and associated molecular abnormalities in acute lymphoblastic leukemia. *Semin Hematol* 2000;37:381–395.

Garcia-Manero G, Kantarjian HM. The hyper-CVAD regimen in adult acute lymphocytic leukemia. *Hematol Oncol Clin North Am* 2000;14:1381–1396.

Garcia-Manero G, Thomas D. Salvage therapy for refractory or relapsed acute lymphocytic leukemia. *Hematol Oncol Clin North Am* 2001;15:163–205.

Grimwade D, Walker H, Harrison G, et al. The predictive value of hierarchical cytogenetic classification in older adults with acute myeloid leukemia (AML): analysis of 1065 patients entered into the United Kingdom Medical Research Council AML11 trial. *Blood* 2001;98:1312–1320.

Hoelzer D, Gokbuget N, et al. Outcome of adult patients with T-lymphoblastic lymphoma treated according to protocols for acute lymphoblastic leukemia. *Blood* 2002;99:4379–4385.

Hoffman R, Benz E, Shattil S, et al., eds. *Hematology*, 3rd ed. New York: Churchill Livingstone, 2000.

Jaffe E, Harris N, Stein H, et al., eds. *World health organization classification tumors: pathology and genetics of tumours of haemotopoietic and lymphoid tissues*. Lyon: IARC Press, 2001.

Larson RA. Recent clinical trials in acute lymphoblastic leukemia by the Cancer and Leukemia Group B. *Hematol Oncol Clin North Am* 2000;14:1367–1379.

Larson RA, Dodge RK, Linker CA, et al. A randomized controlled trial of filgrastim during remission induction and consolidation chemotherapy for adults with acute lymphoblastic leukemia: CALGB Study 9111. *Blood* 1998;92:1556–1564.

Leone G, Voso MT, Sica S, et al. Therapy related leukemias: susceptibility, prevention, and treatment. *Leuk Lymphoma* 2001;41:255–276.

Maris M, Niederwieser D, Sandmaier B, et al. HLA-matched unrelated donor hematopoietic cell transplantation after nonmyeloablative conditioning for patients with hematologic malignancies. *Blood* 2003;102:2021–2030.

Montillo M, Mirto S, Petti MC, et al. Fludarabine, cytarabine, and G-CSF (FLAG) for the treatment of poor risk acute myeloid leukemia. *Am J Hematol* 1998;58:105–109.

Sievers EL, Larson RA, Stadmauer EA, et al. Efficacy and safety of gemtuzumab ozogamicin in patients with CD33-positive acute myeloid leukemia in first relapse. *J Clin Oncol* 2001;19:3244–3254.

Slovak ML, Kopecky KJ, Cassileth PA, et al. Karyotypic analysis predicts outcome of preremission and postremission therapy in adult acute myeloid leukemia: a Southwest Oncology Group/Eastern cooperative Oncology Group Study. *Blood* 2000;96:4075–4083.

Soignet SL, Frankel SR, Douer D, et al. United States multicenter trial of arsenic trioxide in relapsed acute promyelocytic leukemia. *J Clin Oncol* 2001;19:3852–3860.

Tallman M, Nabhan C, Feusner J, et al. Acute promyelocytic leukemia: evolving therapeutic strategies. *Blood* 2002;99:759–767.

Weick J, Kopecky K, Appelbaum F, et al. A randomized investigation of high-dose versus standard-dose cytosine arabinoside with daunorubicin in patients with previously untreated acute myeloid leukemia: a Southwest Oncology Group Study. *Blood* 1996;88:2841–2851.

24

Chronic Leukemias

Muzaffar H. Qazilbash and Michael J. Keating

M.D. Anderson Cancer Center, University of Texas, Houston, Texas

Chronic lymphocytic leukemia (CLL) accounts for more than one third of all leukemias, and because of its prevalence in hematologic practice, it is the focus of this chapter. Additional chronic leukemias discussed in this chapter include prolymphocytic leukemia (PLL) and hairy cell leukemia (HCL) (see Tables 24.1 and 24.2).

DIAGNOSIS

Various diagnostic criteria have been proposed for CLL; two of the most commonly used criteria are the guidelines of the National Cancer Institute–sponsored working group (NCI-WG) and of the International Workshop on Chronic Lymphocytic Leukemia (IWCLL). The NCI-WG guidelines require (a) an absolute lymphocytosis ($\geq 5 \times 10^3$ per μL), with cells having a morphologically mature appearance sustained for 4 weeks; (b) a normocellular or hypercellular bone marrow with lymphocyte count $\geq 30\%$; and (c) monoclonal B-cell phenotype expressing CD5, with a low-level surface immunoglobulin (Ig) expression. The IWCLL recommends similar criteria but requires a lymphocyte count of $\geq 10 \times 10^3$ per μL if facilities for obtaining phenotyping are not available.

STAGING AND PROGNOSIS

There are several staging methods for CLL. The three most commonly used staging methods are the Rai, modified Rai (see Table 24.3), and the Binet staging systems. Prognosis based on Rai staging system is outlined in Table 24.4.

TABLE 24.1. *Chronic lymphocytic leukemia*

CLL	Comments
Origin	B-cell malignancy (>95%)
Incidence	10,000 cases annually in the United States
Median age	55 yr
M:F	2:1
Etiology	No known causes; slight increased risk of CLL and B-cell malignancies in family members
Molecular	Accumulation of clonal lymphocytes, possibly a result of overexpression of bcl-2, which can interfere with apoptosis
Cytogenetic abnormalities	Trisomy 12; abnormalities in chromosomes 11 and 17; Deletion of 13q14

CLL, chronic lymphocytic leukemia.

TABLE 24.2. *Clinical and laboratory features*

	Comments
Symptoms	Fatigue, weight loss, fever in the absence of active infection, night sweats, unusually severe local reactions to insect bites, increased frequency of bacterial and viral infections
Physical examination	Lymphadenopathy and splenomegaly
Laboratory features	Lymphocytosis (5–500 × 10³/μL), appear as normal lymphocytes by light microscopy with presence of scant cytoplasm; presence of smudge cells (artifact of blood smear preparation); absolute neutrophil count can be low, normal, or increased; anemia or thrombocytopenia may be present
Bone marrow	Demonstrates nodular or diffuse infiltration of small- to medium-sized lymphocytes with mature features and normal myeloid components
Lymph nodes	Infiltrates of small- to medium-sized lymphocytes with condensed mature-appearing chromatin and an occasional nucleolus; larger lymphocytes with more prominent nucleoli are usually present and are termed prolymphocytes, can be clustered as pseudofollicles
Immunologic features	The hallmark is the coexpression of CD5, CD19, CD20, and CD23 surface antigens that are detected by flow cytometry

TABLE 24.3. *Staging*

Rai	Modified Rai	Criteria
0	Low risk	Lymphocytosis only (≥15 × 10³/μL in peripheral blood)
1	Intermediate risk	Lymphocytosis with enlarged nodes
2	Intermediate risk	Lymphocytosis with increased splenic or hepatic size
3	High risk	Lymphocytosis with anemia (Hb ≤11 g/dL)
4	High risk	Lymphocytosis with thrombocytopenia (≤100 × 10³/μL)

Hb, hemoglobin.

TABLE 24.4. *Prognosis*

Modified Rai stage	Median survival (yr)
Low risk	>10
Intermediate risk	7
High risk	3

A number of newly identified prognostic factors predict an inferior outcome. These factors include an elevated serum β-2-microglobulin level, high-soluble CD23 level, naive B cells that lack Ig gene hypermutation, and elevated CD38 level.

TREATMENT

CLL is clearly an indolent hematologic malignancy often not requiring treatment at diagnosis. In general, treatment is initiated after the occurrence of one of the following complications:

(a) significant and persistent fatigue; (b) weight loss; (c) fever without infection; (d) night sweats; (e) significant anemia (hemoglobin level <10 g per dL); (f) thrombocytopenia (platelet count $<50 \times 10^3$ μL); and (g) disfiguring or bulky lymphadenopathy and/or significant splenomegaly. Usually, the level of lymphocytosis is not an absolute indication for treatment. However, treatment is usually initiated for a lymphocytosis $>200 \times 10^3$ per μL.

Historically, the most common initial systemic therapies used are chlorambucil and fludarabine. Although none of the regimens have so far demonstrated a survival advantage, the overall survival in the management of CLL has improved over a number of years. Now that purine analogs and alkylating agent combinations have been demonstrated to be active, with suggestions of superior responses, new opportunities continue to appear. The role of monoclonal antibodies (MoAbs) and their integration into overall therapeutic plans is actively being explored. Table 24.5 describes several treatment options available for CLL and comments on each of these therapies.

Complications can occur as an intrinsic component of the disorder or as a result of therapy. Table 24.6 is a summary of such complications.

T-Cell Chronic Lymphocytic Leukemia

T-cell CLL occurs in 2% to 5% of patients with CLL. A large amount of variability exists in the clinical findings and clinical course. PLL is shown in Table 24.7 and HCL in Table 24.8.

TABLE 24.5. *Therapy*

Therapy	Comments
Chlorambucil	Well tolerated, can be administered daily (4–8 mg/d), or pulse intermittent schedule of 40–80 mg PO over 1–3 d q2–4wk; myelosuppression is the main toxicity
Cyclophosphamide	Not evaluated extensively as a single agent but used predominantly in combinations like CVP
Fludarabine	25 mg/m^2 i.v. daily for 5 d q4wk, consider precautions against tumor lysis during first cycle; cumulative toxicity includes myelosuppression and prolonged immunosuppression; response rate around 50% in previously treated patients and 70%–80% in untreated patients
Cladribine	0.1 mg/kg i.v. continuous infusion for 7 d q wk, or 0.14 mg/kg daily over 2 h for 5 d q4wk; response rate comparable to fludarabine, with shorter remission duration
Rituximab	A humanized chimeric antibody active against CD20; dose escalation improves the response rate in CLL (30%–50% in pretreated cases, 60%–80% in untreated cases)
Alemtuzumab	A humanized antibody that targets CD52, widely distributed on all lymphocytes; 33% response rate in previously treated patients
Fludarabine-based combinations	Fludarabine + cyclophosphamide + rituximab (FCR); early reports show higher complete and overall responses in untreated and previously treated patients
Allogeneic stem cell transplantation	Potentially curative therapy for patients with multiple relapses; nonmyeloablative approaches allow older patients and patients with comorbidities to undergo transplant; toxicities: graft versus host disease and opportunistic infections

CVP, cyclophosphamide–vincristine–prednisolone; CLL, chronic lymphocytic leukemia.

TABLE 24.6. *Complications*

Complication	Comments
Anemia	May be secondary to a suppressive effect of CLL or secondary to AIHA; AIHA may require high-dose prednisone and/or splenectomy for treatment
Thrombocytopenia	Also can be secondary to marrow suppression or can be of autoimmune nature
Granulocytopenia	Secondary to either CLL or chemotherapy
Hypogammaglobulinemia	Suggested by frequent sinopulmonary infections, CLL patients often have an inadequate humoral response to infections and immunizations; infections with encapsulated organisms and gram-negative bacteria constitute the major etiologies of mortality and morbidity in CLL
Pure red cell aplasia	Possibly caused by a suppressive effect of suppressor cytotoxic T cells; cyclosporine has been used successfully as treatment, with a reticulocyte response seen within 2 wk after starting therapy
Paraneoplastic pemphigus	Autoantibody-induced oral mucocutaneous lesions
Transformation	Transformation to more aggressive malignancies occurs in 10% of cases; these transformations include prolymphocytic, Richter syndrome (large B-cell lymphoma), ALL, and multiple myeloma

CLL, chronic lymphocytic leukemia; AIHA, autoimmune hemolytic anemia; ALL, acute lymphoblastic leukemia.

TABLE 24.7. *Prolymphocytic leukemia*

	Comments
Morphology	Large cells with abundant cytoplasm and prominent nucleolus within a convoluted nucleus with immature chromatin
Immunology	Mostly a B-cell neoplasm; high-density immunoglobulin, CD19, CD20, and CD22, with absence of CD5
Cytogenetics	t(11;14), which represents the translocation of the bcl-1 oncogene in proximity to the Ig heavy chain gene
Clinical findings	High blast counts with splenomegaly, usually lacking significant adenopathy, occurs as a terminal finding in up to 10% of CLL
Treatment	Fludarabine alone and in combination with cladribine, Rituximab, and allogeneic stem cell transplantation
T-cell PLL	20% of PLL cases, usually a more aggressive course than the B-cell form; expression of CD3, CD4, occasionally CD8, with rearrangement of the T-cell–receptor gene; reports of successful treatment with pentostatin, alemtuzumab, and allogeneic transplantation

Ig, immunoglobulin; CLL, chronic lymphocytic leukemia; PLL, prolymphocytic leukemia.

TABLE 24.8. *Hairy cell leukemia*

	Comments
Clinical findings	Male predominance, pancytopenia, splenomegaly, lymphadenopathy is uncommon, necrotizing vasculitis, opportunistic infections, lytic bone abnormalities
Morphology	Lymphocytes with cytoplasmic projections, TRAP-stain positive
Bone marrow	Aspiration frequently unsuccessful secondary to fibrosis; marrow biopsy reveals "hairy" cells and classic "fried-egg" appearance
Immunology	High-intensity sIg, CD19, 20, 21, 22, 11c, 25, PCA-1 and Bly7, and light and heavy chain Ig rearrangements
Treatment indications	Life-threatening infections, vasculitis, bony involvement, symptomatic splenomegaly, neutropenia (<0.5–1.0 × 10⁹/mL), anemia (Hb, <8–10 g/dL), thrombocytopenia (<50–100 × 10⁹/mL), leukocytosis with a significant number of hairy cells
Treatment	**First-line:** Cladribine provides a >95% response, given at 0.1 mg/kg/d by CI over 7 d; 2-deoxycoformycin produces response rates of 40%–80% and is administered at 4 mg/m² every other week for 3–6 mo **Second-line:** interferon-α produces a >70% response rate and is administered three times/wk s.c. at 2 million units/m²; splenectomy is currently reserved for those with thrombocytopenia and bleeding or those for whom systemic chemotherapy has failed **Promising:** BL22, anti-CD22 monoclonal antibody linked to pseudomonas exotoxin. 70% CR in cladribine-refractory patients

TRAP, tartrate-resistant acid phosphatase; sIg, surface membrane immunoglobulin; Hb, hemoglobin; CI, continuous infusion; CR, complete response.

SUGGESTED READINGS

Binet JL, Auquier A, Dighiero G, et al. A new prognostic classification of chronic lymphocytic leukemia derived from a multivariate survival analysis. *Cancer* 1981;48:198–206.

Byrd JC, Waselenko JK, Maneatis TJ, et al. Rituximab therapy in hematologic malignancy patients with circulating blood tumor cells: association with increased infusion-related side effects and rapid blood tumor clearance. *J Clin Oncol* 1999;17:791–795.

Cassileth PA, Cheuvart B, Spiers ASD, et al. Pentostatin induces durable remissions in hairy cell leukemia. *J Clin Oncol* 1991;9:243–246.

Chikkappa G, Pasquale D, Phillips PG, et al. Cyclosporin-a for the treatment of pure red cell aplasia in a patient with chronic lymphocytic leukemia. *Am J Hematol* 1987;26:179–189.

Estey EH, Kurzrock R, Kantarjian HM, et al. Treatment of hairy cell leukemia with 2-chlorodeoxyadenosine (2-CdA). *Blood* 1992;79:882–887.

Flandrin G, Sigaux F, Sebahoun G, et al. Hairy cell leukemia: clinical presentation and follow-up of 211 patients. *Semin Oncol* 1984;11:458–471.

Flinn IW, Byrd JC, Morrison C, et al. Fludarabine/cyclophosphamide with filgrastim support in patients with previously untreated indolent lymphoid malignancies. *Blood* 2000;96:71.

Golomb HM, Catovsky D, Golde DW. Hairy cell leukemia: a clinical review based on 71 cases. *Ann Intern Med* 1978;89:677–683.

Hamblin TJ, Davis Z, Gardiner A, et al. Unmutated Ig V(H) genes are associated with a more aggressive form of chronic lymphocytic leukemia. *Blood* 1999;94:1848–1854.

Harris NL, Jaffe ES, Stein H, et al. A revised European-American classification of lymphoid neoplasms: a proposal from the International Lymphoma Study Group. *Blood* 1994;84:1361–1392.

Huguley CM. Treatment of chronic lymphocytic leukemia. *Cancer Treat Rev* 1977;4:261–273.

International Workshop on Chronic Lymphocytic Leukemia. Chronic lymphocytic leukemia: recommendations for diagnosis, staging, and response criteria. *Ann Intern Med* 1989;110:236–238.

Juliusson G, Liliemark J. High complete remission rate from 2-chloro-2'-deoxyadenosine in previously treated patients with B-cell chronic lymphocytic leukemia: response predicted by rapid decrease of blood lymphocyte count. *J Clin Oncol* 1993;11:679–689.

Keating MJ, Flinn I, Jain V, et al. Therapeutic role of alemtuzumab (Campath-1H) in patients who have failed: results of a large international study. *Blood* 2002;99:3554–3556.

Keating MJ, Kantarjian H, Talpaz M, et al. Fludarabine: a new agent with major activity against chronic lymphocytic leukemia. *Blood* 1989;74:19–25.

O'Brien SM, Kantarjian H, Thomas DA, et al. Rituximab dose escalation trial in chronic lymphocytic leukemia. *J Clin Oncol* 2001;19:2165.

Piro LD, Carrera CJ, Carson DA, et al. Lasting remissions in hairy-cell leukemia induced by a single infusion of 2-chlorodeoxyadenosine. *N Engl J Med* 1990;322:1117–1121.

Rai KR, Sawitsky A, Cronkite EP, et al. Clinical staging of chronic lymphocytic leukemia. *Blood* 1975;46:219–234.

Raphael B, Anderson JW, Silber R, et al. Comparison of chlorambucil and prednisone versus cyclophosphamide, vincristine, and prednisone as initial treatment for chronic lymphocytic leukemia: long-term follow-up of an Eastern Cooperative Oncology Group randomized clinical trial. *J Clin Oncol* 1991;9:770–776.

Robertson LE, Pugh W, O'Brien S, et al. Richter's syndrome: a report on 39 patients. *J Clin Oncol* 1993;11:1985–1989.

Sawitsky A, Rai KR, Glidewell O, et al. Comparison of daily versus intermittent chlorambucil and prednisone therapy in the treatment of patients with chronic lymphocytic leukemia. *Blood* 1977;50:1049–1059.

25

Myeloid Leukemia

Muzaffar H. Qazilbash and Jorge E. Cortes

M.D. Anderson Cancer Center, University of Texas, Houston, Texas

EPIDEMIOLOGY

Every year, approximately 5,000 to 7,000 individuals are diagnosed with chronic myeloid leukemia (CML) in the United States. The annual incidence of CML is one to two cases per 100,000 individuals. The median age at presentation reported from large cohort studies is 45 to 55 years. More than 80% of patients are diagnosed in the chronic phase, often incidentally during routine tests. CML rarely occurs in children (2% to 3% of childhood leukemias).

PATHOPHYSIOLOGY

The hallmark of CML is the Philadelphia chromosome (Ph-chromosome), a reciprocal translocation between the long arms of chromosomes 9 and 22 [i.e., t(9;22)]. The translocation results in the transfer of the Abelson (ABL) gene to an area of chromosome 22 termed the breakpoint cluster region (BCR), producing the BCR-ABL fusion gene. This fusion gene gives rise to a chimeric protein, $p210^{BCR-ABL}$, with tyrosine kinase activity, which is believed to play a pathogenic role in this disease.

STAGING AND PROGNOSIS

CML typically progresses over time from its chronic phase to an accelerated phase and then to a blast phase (see Table 25.1).

1. Blast crisis: An abrupt transition to a blast phase is called blast crisis. Features of a blast crisis include fever, malaise, progressive and painful splenomegaly and/or hepatomegaly, bone pain, worsening anemia and thrombocytopenia, and thrombotic or bleeding complications.
2. Prognosis: The *chronic phase* typically lasts 3 to 4 years, with the annual rate of progression to a blast phase being 5% to 10% in the first 2 years and 20% in the subsequent years. The prognosis for patient in the chronic phase is 5 to 6 years, with some patients surviving as long as 10 years. For patients in the *accelerated phase*, survival is usually less than 1 year, and for *blast phase*, the survival is a few months. A shorter chronic phase may be predicted by characteristic features at diagnosis, such as older age, male sex, increased lactate dehydrogenase (LDH) level, multiple cytogenetic abnormalities, high percentage of immature myeloid cells, basophilia, eosinophilia, thrombocytosis, and anemia. A useful predictive model using these multiple risk factors is the Sokal risk index. A recently modified version of this index that predicts patients who do best with chemotherapy or interferon (IFN)-α is illustrated in Table 25.2.

TABLE 25.1. *Chronic myeloid leukemia stages and prognosis*

Stage	Features	Median survival
Chronic phase	<5% Blasts and promyelocytes in PB or BM	5–6 yr
Accelerated phase	Increasing symptoms such as fever or bone pain, progressive splenomegaly, >5% blasts and promyelocytes in PB or BM, worsening thrombocytopenia, cytogenetic clonal evolution, and >20% peripheral basophils	<1 yr
Blast phase	>30% blasts and promyelocytes in the PB and BM, with features of accelerated phase, as described earlier	<6 mo

PB, peripheral blood; BM, bone marrow.

DIAGNOSIS AND CLINICAL FEATURES

Symptoms

1. Patients in the early chronic phase may have no symptoms
2. Fatigue
3. Anorexia
4. Weight loss
5. Dyspnea on exertion.

Signs

The most common finding is splenomegaly; the spleen can be massive (in about 10% of patients, the spleen is not enlarged even on splenic scan).

Laboratory Studies

CML is characterized by the following laboratory studies:

1. Increased white blood cell (WBC) count (usually $>25 \times 10^3$ per μL)
2. Increased platelet count in approximately 50% of cases
3. Myeloid cells at all stages of maturation in the peripheral smear (the percentage of immature myeloid cells in the blood or bone marrow can indicate the phase of the disease, as described earlier)
4. Marked marrow myeloid hyperplasia
5. Leukocyte alkaline phosphatase (LAP) activity of CML neutrophils is markedly diminished from the 20% reactivity of normal neutrophils (or leukoerythroblastic reaction)

TABLE 25.2. *Modified Sokal risk index*

Risk category	Median survival
Low risk; score ≥780 (good responses with interferon-α)	98 mo
Intermediate risk; score ≤1,480	65 mo
High risk; score ≥1,480	

Score = [0.6666 × age (0 when age <50 yr; 1 otherwise) + 0.420 × spleen size (cm below costal margin) + 0.0584 × blasts (%) + 0.0413 × eosinophils (%) + 0.2039 × basophils (0 when basophils <3%; 1, otherwise) + 1.0956 × platelet count (0 when platelets <1,500 × 10⁹/L; 1, otherwise)] × 1,000.

6. Diagnosis is confirmed through detection of the t(9;22) abnormality on cytogenetic analysis or through the polymerase chain reaction (PCR) detection of the BCL-ABL fusion in WBCs from peripheral blood [about 10% of patients will be negative for the t(9;22) on standard karyotypic analysis].

Differential Diagnoses

1. Leukoerythroblastic reaction in response to infection or malignancy (see Table 26.1 in Chapter 26 for features to distinguish CML from other myeloproliferative disorders)
2. Chronic myelomonocytic leukemia (CMML)
3. Atypical CML
4. Idiopathic myelofibrosis
5. Essential thrombocytosis
6. Polycythemia rubra vera.

TREATMENT

The treatment options for CML can be divided into:

Definitive therapy

- Stem cell transplantation (SCT)
- IFN-α with or without cytarabine
- Imatinib mesylate

Nondefinitive Therapy

- Hydroxyurea
- Other experimental agents

Stem Cell Transplantation

Allogeneic SCT is curative in select patients with CML and is most effective when performed during the chronic phase of disease. Conventional myeloablative hematopoietic stem cell transplantation (HSCT) carries risks of morbidity and mortality from regimen-related toxicities; its use has been restricted to relatively young patients in good medical condition. In patients older than 50 years with a matched sibling donor, nonmyeloablative SCT has shown promising results in clinical trials. A matched unrelated donor (MUD) may be found in an additional 10% of patients without a matched related donor; however, MUD SCT has a significantly higher transplant-related mortality and morbidity. Allogeneic SCT is currently being studied as a curative option for patients with imatinib-resistant chronic phase or for consolidation after treatment with imatinib in patients with accelerated or blast phase CML.

As such, this remains the treatment of choice for patients younger than 50 years with a matched sibling donor (about 20% of patients). In patients older than 50 years with a matched donor and with comorbidities, nonmyeloablative SCT may be considered.

Imatinib Mesylate

Imatinib has revolutionized the treatment and prognosis of CML. Several studies in patients with chronic-phase CML have shown high rates of complete cytogenetic responses. The impact of such therapy on long-term prognosis awaits further maturation of the data. However, if the early results continue to persist, with long-term follow-up of the high rates of complete and durable cytogenetic responses as well as low transformation and mortality rates, and if no new unexpected frequent long-term imatinib toxicities arise, then imatinib will soon be established as the most effective treatment for CML (see Table 25.3).

TABLE 25.3. *Suggested regimens, toxicities, and response rates*

Drug	Treatment plan	Toxicity	Response rate
Hydroxyurea	Hydroxyurea, 500–2,000 mg PO daily	Leukopenia, anemia, thrombocytopenia, nausea, rash	90% hematologic remission; 34%–44% 5-yr survival
Interferon-α-2a/b	Interferon-α, 5 × 10⁶ Units/m²/d s.c.	Fever, myalgia, rashes, depression, leukopenia, anemia, thrombocytopenia	Complete hematologic response: 40%–80%; major cytogenetic responses[a], 30%–50%; median survival 60–90 mo
Imatinib mesylate	400 mg PO daily	Nausea, vomiting, diarrhea, skin rash, muscle cramps, LFT abnormalities, myelosuppression	Complete hematologic response: 95% major cytogenetic response[a]: 65% 2-yr PFS: 87%
HLA-matched sibling stem cell transplantation	Busulfan, 4 mg/kg/d in divided doses orally on d 7, 6, 5, and 4 cyclophosphamide, 60 mg/kg i.v. or TBI, 10 Gy with lung shielding and cyclophosphamide as above	Graft-vs.-host disease, infections, mycosis	50%–70% 5-yr survival
HLA-matched unrelated stem cell transplantation	Regimens differ from center to center	Graft-vs.-host disease, infections, mucositis	57% 5-yr survival reported by Seattle
Nonmyeloablative transplantation	Fludarabine-based or low-dose TBI based	Graft-vs.-host disease, infections, mucositis	2-year survival: 40%–85%

LFT, liver function test; HLA, human leukocyte antigen; TBI, total body irradiation.
[a]<34% Ph-positive metaphases on cytogenetic analyses.

Hydroxyurea

Hydroxyurea is an excellent debulking agent and allows for the rapid control of the blood count, inducing hematologic responses in 50% to 80% of patients. Cytogenetic responses are rare, and hydroxyurea does not appear to change the natural history of CML. Hydroxyurea is very effective in initial cytoreduction as an adjunct to other more definitive therapies and to control disease in preparation for allogeneic SCT. However, it should not be considered as a definitive therapy for CML.

Interferon-α with and without Chemotherapy

Single-agent IFN-α is active in CML. Response rates with single-agent IFN-α include a complete hematologic response (CHR) of 40% to 80%, a cytogenetic response of 15% to 58%, a major cytogenetic response (Ph of 35%) of 30% to 50%, and a complete cytogenetic response (Ph of 0%) of 5% to 25%. The median survival ranges from 60 to 90 months. Achieving a complete cytogenetic response is associated with 10-year survival rates of 70% to 80%.

Combining chemotherapy with IFN-α may allow a greater reduction in the burden of abnormal clonal cells: IFN-α in combination with cytarabine produces greater long-term survival and more major cytogenetic responses compared with IFN-α alone. However, a randomized trial comparing interferon-α and low-dose cytarabine to imatinib showed a statistically significant improvement in major and complete cytogenetic responses and freedom from progression to accelerated and blast phases in the imatinib group.

Treatment of Blast Phase Chronic Myelogenous Leukemia

Curative treatment is usually unsuccessful in this phase. Approximately 30% of cases with a blast phase having lymphoid features [terminal deoxynucleotidyl transferase (Tdt) or CD10 positive] may respond to regimens used for acute lymphoblastic leukemia. In a phase I and II study in 75 patients with blast phase CML, imatinib mesylate produced a response rate of 52% and a median survival of 6.5 months, both superior to the historic controls treated with standard cytarabine combinations.

SUGGESTED READINGS

Barrett J. Allogeneic stem cell transplantation for chronic myeloid leukemia. *Semin Hematol* 2003; 40(1):59–71.

Kantarjian HM, Cortes J, O'Brien S, et al. Imatinib mesylate (STI571) therapy for Philadelphia chromosome-positive chronic myelogenous leukemia in blast phase. *Blood* 2002;99(10):3547–3553.

O'Brien SG, Guilhot F, Larson RA et al., IRIS Investigators. Imatinib compared with interferon and low-dose cytarabine for newly diagnosed chronic-phase chronic myeloid leukemia. *N Engl J Med* 2003;348(11):994–1004.

Sawyers CL. Chronic myeloid leukemia. *N Engl J Med* 1999;340:1330–1339.

26

Chronic Myeloproliferative Diseases

Manish Monga* and Marcel P. Devetten†

*Department of Oncology, Wheeling Hospital, Wheeling, West Virginia; and
†Department of Medicine, University of Nebraska Medical Center, Omaha, Nebraska

The World Health Organization (WHO) designates seven conditions as myeloproliferative disorders (MPDs): BCR-ABL–positive chronic myeloid leukemia (CML); chronic neutrophilic leukemia; chronic eosinophilic leukemia/hypereosinophilic syndrome; idiopathic myelofibrosis (MF, also known as agnogenic myeloid metaplasia); polycythemia vera (PV); essential thrombocythemia (ET); and myeloproliferative disease, unclassifiable (see Fig. 26.1). CML is discussed in Chapter 25 because of its specific association with the Philadelphia chromosome translocation (*bcr-abl* tyrosine kinase), and because of its unique treatment paradigm of imatinib mesylate and interferon-α (INF-α). This chapter is limited to a discussion of the three major clinical entities: PV, ET, and MF. Although these are distinct clinical entities, they all share some of the same clinical and laboratory features: increased numbers of one or more circulating cell lines, hepatosplenomegaly, and clonal marrow hyperplasia without dysplasia. Diagnosis depends on exclusion of secondary causes of increased blood counts and on distinguishing between the various MPDs (prompted by the particular blood cell lineage that appears to be in excess, followed by identifying characteristic biochemical or cytogenetic abnormalities) (see Table 26.1). Treatment for PV, ET, and MF is generally directed toward minimizing morbidity and prolonging survival by preventing complications such as hemorrhage and thrombosis, in the case of PV and ET, and alleviating anemia and symptoms associated with the splenomegaly of MF. Because these are clonal disorders, there is a risk of transformation of PV, ET, and MF to acute leukemia. This risk is highest for MF; therefore, bone marrow transplantation is a potentially curative option that should be considered for this disease.

EPIDEMIOLOGY AND RISK FACTORS

Annual incidence per 100,000 population:

- 0.5 to 1.7 cases of PV
- Approximately 2.5 cases of ET
- Approximately 1.4 cases of MF.

Median age at diagnosis:

- 50 to 60 years for all three disorders.

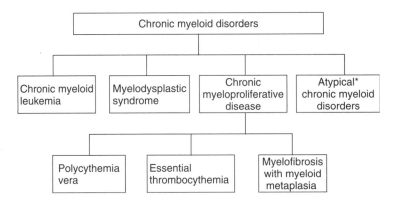

FIG. 26.1. Classification of the chronic myeloid disorders. *Atypical chronic myeloid diorders include chronic eosinophilic leukemia/hypereosinophilic syndrome, chronic neutrophilic leukemia, juvenile myelomonocytic leukmia, systemic cell disease, and a chronic myeloid process that shows characteristics of myelodysplastic syndrome and chronic myeloproliferative disorder.

TABLE 26.1. *Distinguishing features of the myeloproliferative disorders*

	CML	PV	ET	MF
Hematocrit	N or ↓	↑↑	N	↓
WBC count	↑↑↑	↑	N	↑ or ↓
Platelet count	↑ or ↓	↑	↑↑↑	↑ or
Splenomegaly	+++	+	+	+++
Cytogenetic abnormality	Ph chromosome	±	−	±
LAP score	↓	↑↑	N or ↑	N or ↑
Marrow fibrosis	±	± or ↓	±	+++ (Dry tap)
Marrow cellularity	↑↑↑ myeloid	↑↑	↑↑ megakaryocytes	N or ↓
Basophils ≥2%	+	±	±	Usually +

CML, chronic myeloid leukemia; PV, polycythemia vera; ET, essential thrombocytopenia; MF, myelofibrosis; N, normal; WBC, white blood cell; LAP, leukocyte alkaline phosphatase (see Chapter 25); MPD, myeloproliferative disease.

Risk Factors

Some studies have suggested radiation exposure or occupational exposure to solvents and glues as risk factors, but these have not been confirmed.

ETIOLOGY AND PATHOPHYSIOLOGY

Clonal Hematopoiesis

The etiology of these disorders remains unclear. PV and MF are disorders of an early stem cell or progenitor because blood lineages of all three disorders are derived from the same clone; however, careful clonal studies in patients with clinically diagnosed ET demonstrate clonal hematopoiesis in only about 50% of the cases. The detection of a clonal population has been shown to be associated with an increased risk for thrombotic complications. The marrow fibroblasts in MF are not derived from an abnormal clone. Because of clonal hematopoiesis, all the MPDs have a tendency to transform to acute leukemia, although the probability of this occurrence differs considerably among the disorders.

Growth Factor or Growth Factor–Receptor Mutations

Studies that have sought to implicate the involvement of erythropoietin (EPO) levels or erythropoietin receptor (EPO-R) in PV have thus far demonstrated the EPO-R involvement only in some cases of familial polycythemias. EPO levels tend to be low in PV. In contrast, thrombopoietin (TPO) levels can be high in ET, and molecular abnormalities of the *TPO* gene have been identified in certain families with an autosomal dominant form of hereditary thrombocytosis. Mutations of the TPO receptor have not been demonstrated in ET, but post-translational glycosylation impairment of the TPO receptor is common in PV. Increased levels of platelet-derived growth factor and other cytokines secreted by megakaryocytes and by platelets are believed to play a role in the marrow fibrosis of MF.

PROGNOSIS

Median Survivals

- Patients with PV have a median survival of 1.5 to 13 years. In a recent multicountry prospective study of 1,638 patients with PV, the 5-year event-free survival was 82%, with a relatively low risk of death from cardiovascular disease and a high risk of death from noncardiovascular causes (mainly hematologic transformations).
- The median survival is more than 10 years for patients with ET.
- For patients with MF, the median survival is 3 to 5 years.

Rate of Transformation to Acute Leukemia

- The rate of transformation of PV to acute leukemia is 1% to 5% [1.5% of patients treated with phlebotomy alone, 5.9% of patients treated with hydroxyurea (HU), 10% to 13.5% of those treated with chlorambucil or ^{32}P exhibit transformation of PV to acute leukemia].
- The rate of transformation for patients with ET is 3% to 5% (transformation to MF and acute leukemia).
- The rate of transformation for patients with MF is 10%.

The major cause of death in PV is thrombosis (i.e., cerebral, cardiac, pulmonary, and mesenteric), and the major causes of death in ET are thrombosis and hemorrhage.

Spent Phase

Both PV and ET may progress to a "spent phase," which resembles MF and which is characterized by cytopenia, splenomegaly, and marrow fibrosis.

Risk Factors for Thrombosis

- In PV, a hematocrit equal to and greater than 45% is a risk factor. Surgery should be avoided in patients until a hematocrit less than 45% has been maintained for more than 2 months.
- In ET, being older than 60 years and the presence of other cardiovascular risk factors (e.g., smoking and previous thrombosis) increases the risk for thrombosis.

In ET, an association between platelet count and thrombosis has not been established, but platelet cytoreduction on treatment with HU has been associated with a *reduced* risk.

Risk Factors for Hemorrhage

- In ET, a platelet count $>2 \times 10^6$ per μL is a risk factor for hemorrhage.

DIAGNOSIS AND CLINICAL FEATURES

Excluding Secondary Causes of Polycythemia or Thrombocytosis

In the absence of a disease-specific positive marker for PV, the Polycythemia Vera Study Group (PVSG), an international study group, has published the diagnostic criteria that include demonstration of increased red cell mass in the presence of normal hemoglobin oxygen saturation, supported by other diagnostic criteria such as splenomegaly, leukocytosis, thrombocytosis, elevated leukocyte alkaline phosphatase, and increased serum vitamin B_{12} levels. The application of these diagnostic criteria may exclude some cases of PV; therefore, an algorithmic approach using serum EPO and histologic characteristics of the bone marrow is useful in formulating a working diagnosis of PV (see Fig. 26.2). Karyotype abnormalities are infrequent and nonspecific in PV; they include trisomies of chromosomes 8 and 9 and deletions of long arms of chromosomes 13 and 20. PVSG has also established the diagnostic criteria for ET (see Table 26.2).

Distinguishing between the Myeloproliferative Disorders

All the MPDs can present because of incidentally noted abnormal blood counts (Table 26.1). Otherwise, PV can demonstrate symptoms of increased red blood cell (RBC) mass, such as headaches, vertigo, tinnitus, and blurred vision. A distinctive symptom in PV is pruritus aggravated by hot water. Cerebrovascular ischemia, digital ischemia, erythromelalgia, and spontaneous abortions resulting from arterial thrombosis are more commonly seen in patients with ET. Patients with MF may have symptoms related to anemia or may experience abdominal fullness or early satiety because of splenomegaly. Hypermetabolic symptoms such as weight loss and sweating can be seen in all types of MPDs. ET is diagnosed after excluding PV; MF is diagnosed after excluding PV and ET because marrow fibrosis can be a sequela of the other MPDs. The thrombotic episodes seen in all the MPDs can occur in unusual locations such as the hepatic vein (Budd–Chiari syndrome) and portal vein. Platelet function tests or bleeding times are of little use in diagnosing or in guiding the management of MPDs.

TREATMENT

Polycythemia Vera

Maintaining a hematocrit less than 45% dramatically decreases the incidence of thrombotic complications (in PV, 35% of initial thrombotic events are fatal). This is preferably achieved through phlebotomy; alternatives are myelosuppressive oral chemotherapy or IFN-α. Selection among these options is guided by data from the PVSG studies. A randomized study of 518 patients with PV has shown that treatment with low-dose aspirin (100 mg per day) lowers the risk of cardiovascular death, nonfatal myocardial infarction, and nonfatal stroke.

Polycythemia Vera Study Group Studies (Phlebotomy and Chemotherapy)

PVSG-01 randomized more than 400 patients to phlebotomy, chlorambucil, or ^{32}P. The thrombosis rate in patients treated with phlebotomy alone was significantly higher than that for those patients receiving myelosuppressive therapy with chlorambucil or ^{32}P. Median survival was more than 10 years in the groups treated with ^{32}P and phlebotomy, and was 9 years in the group treated with chlorambucil, with an excess of leukemic deaths in the group of patients treated with chlorambucil and ^{32}P. In PVSG-05, when aspirin, 325 mg three times a day, was given in addition to phlebotomy, the risk of life-threatening thrombosis did not decrease, but

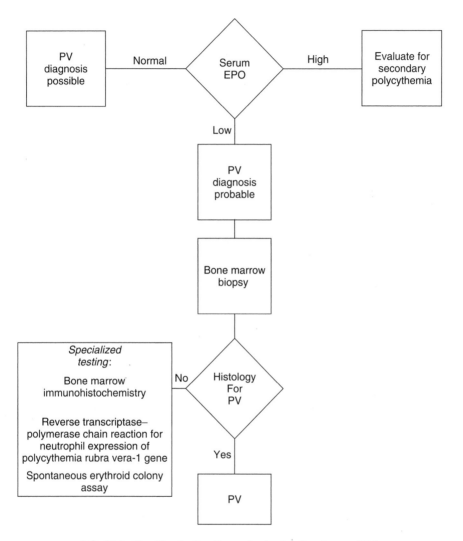

FIG. 26.2. Algorithm for the diagnosis of polycythemia vera (PV).

TABLE 26.2. *Diagnostic criteria for essential thrombocytopenia*

1. Platelets >600 × 10³/μL
2. Hct <40% or normal RBC mass
3. Stainable iron in marrow, or normal ferritin, or normal MCV
4. No Ph chromosome or *bcr-abl* rearrangement, or MDS-type cytogenetic abnormality
5. No marrow fibrosis or marrow fibrosis <1/3 of biopsy and no more than minimal splenomegaly and no leukoerythroblastic cells in the peripheral blood
6. No other cause for reactive thrombocytosis

Hct, hematocrit; MCV, mean corpuscular volume; Ph, Philadelphia; MDS, myelodysplastic syndrome.

hemorrhagic complications increased. PVSG-08 studied the nonalkylating myelosuppressive agent, HU, in the hope that this agent would not be associated with leukemic transformation, which was noted for ^{32}P and chlorambucil in PVSG-01. HU, with supplemental phlebotomy as needed, was found to have a significantly lower risk of thrombosis compared with phlebotomy alone. However, a statistically nonsignificant higher risk of transformation of PV to acute leukemia was observed in patients who were treated with HU alone.

A reasonable treatment strategy for PV is based on risk stratification:

- Low risk: Patients younger than 60 years, with no history of thrombocytosis and with platelet count <1,500 × 10^9 per L, are at low risk. Phlebotomy alone with or without low-dose aspirin should be recommended.
- Indeterminate risk: Patients younger than 60 years, with no history of thrombocytosis and with either a platelet count >1,500 × 10^9 per L or cardiovascular risk factors, are at intermediate risk. Phlebotomy alone is adequate therapy; use of low-dose aspirin is encouraged.
- High risk: Patients who are 60 years or older or with a positive history of thrombosis are at high risk. HU and low-dose aspirin are recommended therapies.
- Spent phase: Options to alleviate cytopenia associated with massive splenomegaly include HU, IFN-α, and EPO. Analgesia may be required for splenic infarct pain. It is difficult to treat cytopenia associated with marrow fibrosis and massive splenomegaly. Splenectomy can be followed by progressive hepatomegaly and can eventually transform to acute leukemia. In selected patients, allogeneic transplantation can be curative.
- Pruritus: Intractable pruritus responds to IFN-α in up to 81% of patients. In low-risk patients in whom IFN-α is not indicated, paroxetine, a selective serotonin reuptake inhibitor, can alleviate symptoms in most cases.
- Hyperuricemia: Allopurinol should be started before chemotherapy to decrease the risk of urate nephropathy (300 mg per day given orally; dose reduction needed in renal insufficiency).

Essential Thrombocythemia

Treatment in ET must be provided on the basis of the fact that life expectancy in this condition is nearly normal and that platelet reduction with HU may be associated with an increased risk for transformation to leukemia. Treatment is directed at preventing thrombosis and hemorrhage in those patients deemed to be at risk for these complications. These patients have a history of thrombosis, with associated cardiovascular risk factors such as smoking and age older than 60 years, and have a platelet count >2 × 10^6 per μL.

For platelet cytoreduction, see Table 26.3.

- A randomized trial of HU in 114 high-risk patients showed a significant reduction of thrombotic events in the treatment arm (3.6% versus 24%). The HU dose was adjusted to achieve a platelet count of <600 × 10^3 per μL. Anagrelide is a nonmutagenic orally active agent that produces selective platelet cytoreduction by interfering with megakaryocyte maturation. IFN-α can also effectively cause platelet cytoreduction. The study on HU has provided the precedent for a platelet count of 600 × 10^3 per μL as the therapeutic target with anagrelide or IFN-α therapy. Plateletpheresis is used as an emergency therapy when ongoing thrombosis cannot be adequately managed with chemotherapy and antithrombotic agents.
- Antiplatelet agents: Aspirin can exacerbate the bleeding tendency in patients with ET and other MPDs and should be used selectively. Low-dose aspirin (81 mg per day orally) may benefit patients with ET who have cerebral or digital ischemia. Erythromelalgia (painful nonischemic fingers and toes) responds to aspirin.

Myelofibrosis

- Palliative therapy: Palliative therapy for MF is directed toward alleviating anemia and painful splenomegaly. For anemia, androgens (oxymethalone, 1 to 5 mg/kg/day orally, may

TABLE 26.3. *Chemotherapeutic agents used in the therapy of the chronic myeloproliferative disorders*

Agent	Treatment plan	Indications	Toxicity
Hydroxyurea	Start with hydroxyurea, 1,000–2,000 mg PO daily. In PV, adjust to keep Hct <45% without producing thrombocytopenia or neutropenia Augment with phlebotomy if necessary In ET, adjust dose to maintain plt counts <600 × 10³/µL; long-term therapy is necessary	All PV pts >69 yr of age; younger patients with thrombosis, hemorrhage, severe pruritus, painful splenomegaly, or B symptoms. ET pts who require therapy (see text). MF pts requiring cytoreduction after splenectomy.	Increased risk of acute leukemic transformation or myelodysplastic syndrome with a chromosome 17p deletion; leg ulceration
Anagrelide	Anagrelide, 0.5–1 mg PO four times daily. Prolonged treatment is necessary	Generally used as a second-line agent for decreasing plt counts. Consider using as primary therapy for young pts with ET requiring therapy.	Fluid retention, congestive heart failure symptoms, postural hypotension, headaches, dizziness, nausea, and diarrhea
Interferon-α 2a/b	Start with interferon-α 2a/b 3 × 10⁶ Units s.c. three times/wk. Adjust the dose against response and adverse effects. Long-term treatment is necessary	Experimental therapy in PV (refer for clinical trials). Consider for young pts as an alternative to phlebotomy. A second-line plt-lowering agent in ET	Flu-like symptoms, altered mental status, and depression

Hct, hematocrit; PV, polycythemia vera; ET, essential thrombocytopenia; MF, myelofibrosis; plt, platelets; pts, patients; PO, oral administration; s.c., subcutaneous administration.

take 3 to 6 months to produce a response) produce responses in about 30% of patients. Transfusion support (with iron chelation when indicated) may be necessary. Splenectomy, as performed in experienced centers, is associated with an operative mortality of less than 10%, and in addition to alleviating pain, discomfort, and early satiety, it can improve anemia. Increasing white blood cell counts and platelet counts after splenectomy may necessitate HU therapy. IFN-α is an experimental therapy for MF.

- Curative therapy: Allogeneic transplantation should be considered for patients younger than 55 years who have MF; 5-year survivals with a related or an unrelated matched transplant are 54% and 48%, respectively, as determined by the European Group for Blood and Marrow Transplantation (EBMT). A recommendation for transplantation is not clear-cut in asymptomatic patients without cytogenetic abnormalities and no cytopenia because the median survival in this group is greater than 14 years with palliative therapy alone. Although the outcome with transplantation also is adversely affected by these features, poor prognostic features such as hemoglobin level <10 g per dL; white blood cell count <4×10^3 per µL or >30×10^3 per µL; more than 10% of circulating blasts, promyelocytes, or myelocytes; or abnormal cytogenetics should prompt consideration for transplantation. Pretransplantation splenectomy, although not necessary in every patient, is associated with faster engraftment and can be considered in those with massive splenomegaly. Marrow fibrosis is reversible with transplantation.

SUGGESTED READINGS

Berk PD, Goldberg JD, Donovoun PB, et al. Therapeutic recommendations in polycythemia vera based on Polycythemia Vera Study Group protocols. *Semin Hematol* 1986;23:132–143.

Cortelazzo S, Finazzi G, Ruggeri M, et al. Hydroxyurea for patients with essential thrombocythemia and a high risk for thrombosis. *N Engl J Med* 1995;332:1132–1136.

Fruchtman SM, Mack K, Kaplan ME, et al. From efficacy to safety: a polycythemia vera study group report on hydroxyurea in patient with polycythemia vera. *Semin Hematol* 1997;34:17–23.

Guardiola P, Anderson JE, Bandini G, et al. Allogeneic stem cell transplantation for agnogenic myeloid metaplasia: a European Group for Blood and Marrow Transplantation, Societe Francaise de Greffe de Moelle, Gruppo Italiano per il Trapianto del Midollo Osseo, and Fred Hutchinson Cancer Research Center collaborative study. *Blood* 1999;93:2831–2838.

Harris NL, Jaffe ES, Diebold J, et al. World Health Organization classification of neoplastic diseases of the hematopoietic and lymphoid tissues: report of the Clinical Advisory Committee meeting, Airlie House, Virginia, November 1997. *J Clin Oncol* 1999;17:3835–3849.

Kaplan ME, Mack K, Goldberg JD, et al. Long term management of polycythemia vera with hydroxyurea: a progress report. *Semin Hematol* 1986;23:167–171.

Landolfi R, Marchioli R, Kutti J, et al. Efficacy and safety of low-dose aspirin in polycythemia vera (ECLAP study). *Blood* 2003;102:5a.

Silver RT. Interferon-alpha: effects of long-term treatment for polycythemia vera. *Semin Hematol* 1997; 34:40–50.

Spivak J. Polycythemia vera: myths, mechanisms, and management. *Blood* 2002;100:4272–4290.

27

Multiple Myeloma

Sattva S. Neelapu* and Cynthia E. Dunbar†

*Department of Lymphoma and Myeloma, M.D. Anderson Cancer Center, University of Texas, Houston, Texas and †Hematology Branch, National Heart, Lung, and Blood Institute, National Institutes of Health, Bethesda, Maryland

EPIDEMIOLOGY

- In 2004, 15,270 new cases and 11,070 deaths from multiple myeloma (MM) were estimated in the United States.
- The incidence rate of myeloma is 5.5 per 100,000 population per year in the United States. Incidence among African Americans is twice that in whites and three times that in Asians and Pacific Islanders.
- The median age at diagnosis is 71 years.
- An increased incidence of myeloma in atomic bomb survivors implicates excessive radiation as a risk factor, but there is little evidence to implicate other environmental causes. Familial clustering has been reported in some cases.

PATHOPHYSIOLOGY

MM is characterized by the proliferation and accumulation of clonal plasma cells. The involvement of B cells is somewhat controversial, but the extent of somatic mutation in the complementarity-determining regions (the antigen-binding portions) of the variable gene segment suggests that the proliferation of the clone is antigen driven at some point, although the identity of the antigen or antigens is unknown (see Fig. 27.1). Five recurrent translocations involving the heavy chain locus on chromosome 14 have been identified and are present in approximately 40% of all myeloma tumors. Deletion of chromosome 13q is also common and portends a very poor prognosis. The clinical features of MM are a result of bone marrow infiltration by the malignant clone; damage from high levels of immunoglobulins or free light chains in the circulation or glomeruli; the secretion of osteoclast-activating factors such as RANKL (receptor activator of NF-κB ligand) and MIP-1 (macrophage inflammatory protein-1) with resultant bone damage; decreased production of the natural RANKL inhibitor OPG (osteoprotegerin); and impaired immunity, both cell mediated and humoral.

CLINICAL FEATURES

- Bone pain is present in 80% of patients with MM, and 70% of the patients develop pathologic fractures during the course of their disease. Any patient with spontaneous fractures, severe persistent bone pain, or unexplained severe osteoporosis should be evaluated for myeloma.

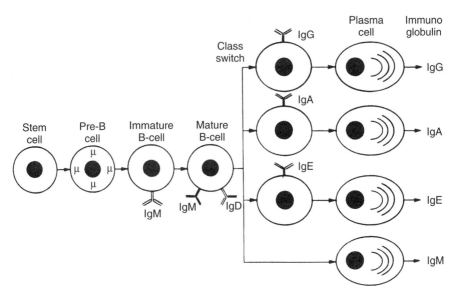

FIG. 27.1. Differentiation of B lymphocytes and plasma cells. A pleiotropic stem cell gives rise to the pre–B cell that has acquired the capacity to synthesize heavy chains (µ). The immature B cell can synthesize light chains so that a complete immunoglobulin M (IgM) molecule is formed and expressed on the cell surface. Mature B cells express both IgM and IgD on their surfaces. These cells can either mature into IgM-secreting plasmacytoid lymphocytes or undergo a class switch to express IgG, IgA, or IgE on their surfaces. The latter cells can undergo terminal differentiation into IgG- or IgE-secreting plasma cells. (From Stamatovannopoulos G, Nienhuis AW, Leder P, et al., eds. *The molecular basis of blood diseases.* Philadelphia: WB Saunders, 1987, with permission.)

- Other common clinical features include fatigue, normocytic normochromic anemia, and hypercalcemia (20%).
- Renal insufficiency is seen in at least 25% of patients at diagnosis and may be caused by hypercalcemia and related dehydration, light chain deposition in the tubules or glomeruli, or amyloid deposition. In some patients, amyloidosis can cause a nephrotic syndrome (<5%). Acquired Fanconi syndrome with glycosuria, phosphaturia, and aminoaciduria can occur.
- Infections are an important cause of morbidity and mortality in patients with MM.
- Hyperviscosity symptoms are rare except with immunoglobulin (Ig)A and IgG3 subtypes.

DIAGNOSIS

- Minimal criteria for the diagnosis of MM include:
  - (a) Bone marrow containing more than 10% plasma cells or histologic proof of a plasmacytoma along with the following criteria.
  - (b) An M protein in the serum (>3g per dL) or M protein in the urine or lytic bone lesions.
- An incidental detection of a serum M protein level of <3 g per dL in an asymptomatic patient with less than 10% bone marrow plasma cells and no other features of MM suggests the diagnosis of *monoclonal gammopathy of undetermined significance* (MGUS).

- In the asymptomatic patient, if the spike in serum M protein is >3 g per dL and if there are more than 10% bone marrow plasma cells but no other features of MM, *smoldering multiple myeloma* (SMM) is indicated.
- The diagnostic and staging work-up of MM should include a complete blood count with differential; levels of serum electrolytes, blood urea nitrogen, serum creatinine, calcium, phosphate, magnesium, uric acid, β_2-microglobulin, and lactate dehydrogenase; serum protein electrophoresis (SPEP) and immunofixation; 24-hour urine protein electrophoresis (UPEP) and immunofixation; quantitative immunoglobulins; 24-hour urine for Bence Jones reaction; at least a unilateral bone marrow aspirate and biopsy; and a radiographic skeletal survey. A nuclear medicine bone scan is not indicated because lytic lesions are not visualized on bone scans. Any patient with significant back pain should undergo a magnetic resonance imaging (MRI) of the spine to evaluate cord compression.
- An SPEP alone is inadequate because some myeloma clones secrete only light chains, which are rapidly cleared from the plasma to the urine (see Fig. 27.2).
- The circulating monoclonal protein is IgG in 50% of cases, IgA in 20%, light chain only (Bence Jones proteinemia) in 20%, IgD in 2%, and biclonal in 1%.

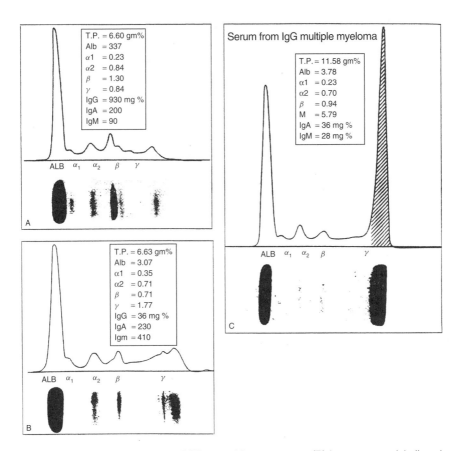

FIG. 27.2. Electrophoretic pattern of **(A)** normal human serum, **(B)** hypergammaglobulinemia, and **(C)** immunoglobulin G (IgG) multiple myeloma. (From Lee GR, Bithell TC, Foerster J, et al., eds. *Wintrobe's clinical hematology.* Philadelphia: Lea & Febiger, 1993, with permission.)

- Because bone marrow involvement may be focal rather than diffuse, repeated bone marrow sampling may be needed before diagnostic infiltrates of more than 10% plasma cells are identified.
- Radiologic changes include punched-out lytic lesions, osteoporosis, and fractures.

STAGING

The Durie–Salmon staging system for multiple myeloma is shown in Table 27.1.

PROGNOSIS

- The β_2-microglobulin level at diagnosis is the best single simple prognostic factor available for all patients with multiple myeloma. High levels of β_2-microglobulin predict poor prognosis.
- A high plasma-cell–labeling index also strongly predicts poor prognosis, but this test is not commonly available.
- Abnormalities in chromosome 13 detected by cytogenetic analysis predict poor outcome even with autologous or allogeneic transplantation.
- Median survival is less than 1 year in untreated patients and is 2 to 3 years with standard melphalan and prednisone (MP) regimen. More recent studies on unselected patients using autologous transplantation for those patients younger than 60 with good organ function and standard chemotherapy for other patients indicate that median survival has increased to 4 years or more for both groups.

TREATMENT

- **MGUS:** Patients with MGUS are monitored indefinitely without treatment because 20% to 25% of them will eventually progress to myeloma at a rate of approximately 1% per year.

TABLE 27.1. *Durie–Salmon (1) staging system for multiple myeloma*

Stage	Criteria	Myeloma cell mass ($\times 10^{12}$ cells/m^2)

I	All of the following:
	Hemoglobin >10 g/dL
	Serum calcium level ≤12 mg/dL (normal)
	Normal bone or solitary plasmacytoma on x-ray
	Low M-component production rate:
	  IgG <5 g/dL
	  IgA <3 g/dL
	  Bence Jones protein <4 g/24 h
		<0.6 (low)

II	Not fitting stage I or III	0.6–1.2 (intermediate)

III	One or more of the following:
	Hemoglobin <8.5 g/dL
	Serum calcium level >12 mg/dL
	Multiple lytic bone lesions on x-ray
	High M-component production rate:
	  IgG >7 g/dL
	  IgA >5 g/dL
	  Bence Jones protein >12 g/24 h
		>1.2 (high)

Subclassification
A: Serum creatinine <2 mg/dL
B: Serum creatinine >2 mg/dL

Checking serum or UPEP every 6 months along with watchful waiting for other symptoms is appropriate. Early intervention studies to date have shown no benefit for thalidomide or steroids.

- **SMM or stage I MM:** These patients can also be observed closely without therapy. Treatment is indicated when there is evidence of disease progression to stage II or higher stage MM (median time to progression is 2 years for SMM).
- **Solitary plasmacytoma:** These patients are treated with radiation therapy (solitary bone) and/or surgical removal (extraosseous plasmacytomas) of the affected area, followed by close monitoring of M protein because of the risk of overt MM.
- **Multiple myeloma:** To date, there is no clear curative therapy available for most MM patients. Patients may achieve a plateau phase with therapy, characterized by a stable M protein level and persistent bone marrow plasma cells, but by an absence of symptoms. The goal of standard therapy is to improve quality of life and to delay disease progression. With these objectives in mind, the choice of therapy (i.e., What intensity of therapy? When to start?) is guided by consideration of symptoms, prognosis, age, and performance status (see Fig. 27.3). Eligible patients should always be considered for enrollment in clinical trials that evaluate novel treatment strategies. The proposed criteria given by the European Group for Blood and Marrow Transplantation (EBMT) for evaluating disease response and progression in myeloma patients are outlined in Table 27.2 (2).

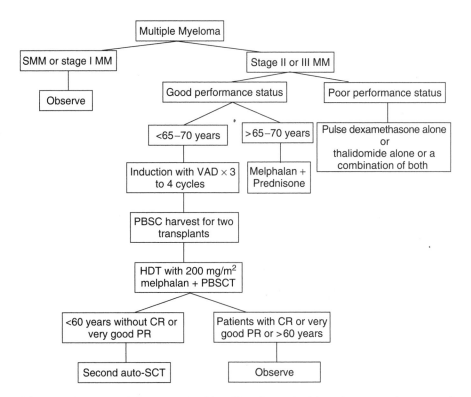

FIG. 27.3. A suggested treatment algorithm. All patients should receive supportive care and must be considered for bisphosphonate treatment and clinical trials.

TABLE 27.2. Criteria for evaluating response, relapse, and progression in myeloma patients (1)

Criteria	Complete response (CR)	Partial response (PR)	Minimal response (MR)	Relapse from CR	Progressive disease for patients not in CR
Serum M protein	Absent by immunofixation for 6 wk	≥50% Decrease for 6 wk	25%–49% Decrease for 6 wk	Reappearance by immunofixation or electrophoresis	>25% increase and absolute increase of ≥ 0.5 g/dL
Urinary M protein	Absent by immunofixation for 6 wk	≥90% Decrease in 24 h excretion or <200 mg/24 h for 6 wk	50%–89% Decrease in 24 h excretion for 6 wk	Reappearance by immunofixation or electrophoresis	>25% increase in 24 h excretion and absolute increase of ≥ 200 mg/24 h
Bone marrow plasma cells in aspirate and biopsy, if biopsy is performed	<5%	≥50% Decrease for nonsecretory myeloma for 6 wk	25%–49% Decrease for nonsecretory myeloma for 6 wk	≥5%	>25% increase and absolute increase of ≥10%
Lytic bone lesions	No change in size or number	No change in size or number	No change in size or number	Increase in size of bone lesions or new lytic lesions	Increase in size of bone lesions or new lytic lesions
Soft tissue plasmacytoma	Absent	≥50% Decrease	25%–49% Decrease	New soft tissue plasmacytoma	New soft tissue plasmacytoma
Hypercalcemia	N/A	N/A	N/A	Corrected serum calcium level >11.5 mg/dL	Corrected serum calcium level >11.5 mg/dL

From Blade J, Samson D, Reece D et al., European Group for Blood and Marrow Transplantation. Criteria for evaluating disease response and progression in patients with multiple myeloma treated by high-dose therapy and haemopoietic stem cell transplantation. Myeloma subcommittee of the EBMT. *Br J Haematol* 1998;102(5):1115–1123, with permission.

Initial Therapies

- *Cycles of pulse oral melphalan and prednisone* (MP) have been the standard treatment regimen for MM for many decades and may still be appropriate for patients for whom high-dose chemotherapy and autologous stem cell transplantation (HDC/auto SCT) are not being considered because of poor performance status or because the patients are older than 65 to 70 years (see Table 27.3) (3). MP should only be given for three to six cycles and should be discontinued once a plateau in the M protein level is reached in responding patients or after two cycles without response in nonresponding patients. More than six cycles of MP are associated with an increased risk of secondary myelodysplasia (MDS) or acute myelogenous leukemia (AML), the risk approaching 20% to 30% after 24 months of MP.

- Aggressive *combination chemotherapy* regimens containing vincristine, carmustine, melphalan, cyclophosphamide, and prednisone have somewhat higher initial response rates but offer no significant survival benefit compared to MP (4,5,8). At present, there are no indications for these regimens.

- Three to four cycles of infusional therapy with *vincristine, doxorubicin, and dexamethasone (VAD)* is commonly used as an induction regimen prior to autologous SCT because of the absence of myelotoxic agents (alkylating agents and nitrosoureas) in this combination (7). Response to VAD is more rapid than the response to MP, therefore it is also indicated in any patient with ongoing serious organ dysfunction due to high levels of paraprotein while instituting the therapy. Only two to three cycles are generally needed to reach a plateau.

- Dexamethasone accounts for almost 85% of the activity of VAD, and *high dose pulse dexamethasone alone* has been shown to induce an overall response rate of 43% in previously untreated myeloma patients (6). For this reason and because of reduced toxicity, high-dose pulse dexamethasone alone is a good alternative for VAD for pretransplantation induction therapy, especially in patients with very poor marrow function due to marrow replacement by tumor or in those patients receiving concurrent radiation therapy for a pathologic fracture.

- The addition of *thalidomide, bortezomib, or other newer agents* to initial treatment regimens is under investigation, but at present, no mature data are available on the efficacy of these agents in prolonging time to progression or survival. Thalidomide can be used alone or in combination with other initial therapies such as dexamethasone or VAD without detriment in terms of collecting adequate stem cells for autologous transplantation. *Thalidomide in combination with dexamethasone* as initial therapy for myeloma has been shown to yield a response rate of 64% (13).

- *Interferon-α* has been evaluated in many randomized trials either in combination with induction chemotherapy or as remission maintenance therapy following conventional chemotherapy (CC) in MM patients. Some of these trials have suggested benefit, whereas others have indicated no benefit. Meta-analyses of the randomized trials suggest small but significant improvement in the progression-free survival (PFS) as well as in overall survival, both when used in combination with induction chemotherapy and when given as remission maintenance therapy (20,21). However, these small benefits must be balanced against high treatment-related toxicity and cost.

- Two large randomized trials [InterGroupe Francophone du Myelome 90 (IFM 90) trial and the Medical Research Council Myeloma VII Trial] demonstrated that *high-dose therapy* (HDT) followed by *autologous SCT* significantly improves response rate and survival compared to CC in myeloma patients younger than 65 years with good performance status (see Table 27.4) (14,15). The IFM 95 randomized trial demonstrated that 200 mg per m^2 of melphalan is less toxic and at least as effective a conditioning regimen as total body irradiation of 8 Gy with 140 mg per m^2 melphalan before autologous SCT (22). Although SCT is commonly performed following three to four cycles of induction chemotherapy, a randomized trial comparing early versus late transplantation demonstrated that SCT can be delayed until relapse without compromising survival provided that the stem cells are harvested and cryopreserved early in the disease course. Therefore, the timing of SCT is based on patient preference and other clinical conditions (23).

TABLE 27.3. Chemotherapy regimens in multiple myeloma

Regimen	Treatment description	Cycle duration	Response rate	Reference
MP	Melphalan 10 mg/m² PO d 1–4 (total dose/cycle = 40 mg/m²) Prednisone 60 mg/m²/d PO d 1–4 (total dose/cycle = 240 mg/m²)	4–6 wk	53% in untreated patients	3–5
Pulse dexamethasone	Dexamethasone 40 mg/d PO d 1–4, 9–12, and 17–20 for odd cycles and d 1–4 for even cycles (total dose/cycle = 480 mg for odd cycles and 160 mg for even cycles)	28 d	43% in untreated patients	6
VAD	Vincristine 0.4 mg/m²/d continuous i.v. infusion d 1–4 (total dose/cycle = 1.6 mg/m²) Doxorubicin 9 mg/m²/d continuous i.v. infusion d 1–4 (total dose/cycle = 36 mg/m²) Dexamethasone 40 mg/d PO d 1–4, 9–12, and 17–20 for odd cycles and d 1–4 for even cycles (total dose/cycle = 480 mg for odd cycles and 160 mg for even cycles)	21 d	55%–84% in untreated patients	7
VMCP alternates with VBAP every 3 wk	Vincristine 1 mg/m² i.v. d 1 (total dose/cycle = 1 mg/m²) Melphalan 6 mg/m²/d PO d 1–4 (total dose/cycle = 24 mg/m²) Cyclophosphamide 125 mg/m²/d PO d 1–4 (total dose/cycle = 500 mg/m²) Prednisone 60 mg/m²/d PO d 1–4 (total dose/cycle = 240 mg/m²)	21 d	60% in untreated patients	4,5,8
VBAP	Vincristine 1 mg/m² i.v. d 1 (total dose/cycle = 1 mg/m²) Carmustine (BCNU) 30 mg/m² i.v. d 1 (total dose/cycle = 30 mg/m²) Doxorubicin 30 mg/m² i.v. d 1 (total dose/cycle = 30 mg/m²) Prednisone 100 mg/d PO d 1–4 (total dose/cycle = 400 mg)	21 d	60% in untreated patients	4,5,8
DCEP	Dexamethasone 40 mg/d PO d 1–4 (total dose/cycle = 160 mg)	4–6 wk	41% in refractory patients	9,10

continued on next page

TABLE 27.3 *Continued*

	Cyclophosphamide 400 mg/m^2/d continuous i.v. infusion d 1–4 (total dose/cycle = 1,600 mg/m^2) Etoposide 40 mg/m^2/d continuous i.v. infusion d 1–4 (total dose/cycle = 160 mg/m^2) Cisplatin 10 mg/m^2/d continuous i.v. infusion d 1–4 (total dose/cycle = 40 mg/m^2)		40% in refractory patients	11
DTPACE	Dexamethasone 40 mg/d PO d 1–4 (total dose/cycle = 160 mg) Thalidomide 400 mg/d PO daily at bedtime (continuous) Cisplatin 10 mg/m^2/d continuous i.v. infusion d 1–4 (total dose/cycle = 40 mg/m^2) Doxorubicin 10 mg/m^2/d continuous i.v. infusion d 1–4 (total dose/cycle = 40 mg/m^2) Cyclophosphamide 400 mg/m^2/d continuous i.v. infusion d 1–4 (total dose/cycle = 1,600 mg/m^2) Etoposide 40 mg/m^2/d continuous i.v. infusion d 1–4 (total dose/cycle = 160 mg/m^2)	4–6 wk		
Thalidomide	Thalidomide Start at 200 mg/d PO daily at bedtime for 2 wk; increase dose by 200 mg every 2 wk to a maximum of 800 mg/d	Continuous	32% in refractory patients	12
Thalidomide + dexamethasone	Dexamethasone 40 mg/d PO d 1–4, 9–12, and 17–20 for odd cycles and d 1–4 for even cycles Thalidomide 200 mg/d PO daily at bedtime	28 d	64% in untreated patients	13
Bortezomib	Bortezomib 1.3 mg/m^2/d i.v. on d 1, 4, 8, and 11 (total dose/cycle = 5.2 mg/m^2) Dexamethasone 20 mg/d PO on d 1, 2, 4, 5, 8, 9, 11, and 12 may be added for patients with suboptimal response	21 d	35% in refractory patients	14
HDT + AutoSCT	Conditioning regimen: Melphalan 200 mg/m^2 i.v. infusion over 30 min on d 2 (total dose/cycle = 200 mg/m^2) PBSC transplantation on day 0	N/A	>80% in untreated patients	15,16
Pamidronate	Pamidronate 90 mg i.v. infusion over 2 h (total dose/cycle = 90 mg)	Monthly	N/A	17
Zoledronic acid	Zoledronic acid 4 mg i.v. infusion over 15 min (total dose/cycle = 4 mg)	Monthly	N/A	18,19

SCT, stem cell transplantation; HDT, high dose therapy.

TABLE 27.4. *Conventional chemotherapy (CC) versus high-dose therapy (HDT) followed by autologous stem cell transplantation (SCT)*

Treatment	OR (CR + PR)	CR	Median overall survival	Median event-free survival
IFM 90 Trial (CC vs. HDT) (14)	57% vs. 81%	5% vs. 22%	44 vs. 57 mo	18 vs. 28 mo (EFS)
MRC7 Trial (CC vs. HDT) (15)	48% vs. 86%	8% vs. 44%	42 vs. 54 mo	20 vs. 32 mo (PFS)

OR, overall response; CR, complete response; PR, partial response; IFM, InterGroupe Francophone du Myelome; CC, conventional chemotherapy; HDT, high-dose therapy; EFS, event-free survival; MRC, Medical Research Council; PFS, progression free survival.

- The recently published IFM 94 trial established that *double transplantation* is superior to single autologous transplantation and should be considered as a treatment option, especially for patients younger than 60 years who do not have a very good partial response (defined as greater than 90% reduction in serum M protein level) after single transplantation (see Table 27.5) (24).
- *Allogeneic transplantation* may potentially benefit a small percentage of patients because of a powerful graft versus myeloma effect. However, myeloablative allotransplants were associated with high treatment-related mortality (TRM) of up to 50% because of severe graft versus host disease, opportunistic infections, and complications resulting from a second aggressive conditioning regimen in patients already surviving and relapsing following autologous transplantation.
- The recent experience with *nonmyeloablative allogeneic transplantation* suggests that the TRM could be reduced to less than 10% to 20%, but this strategy should currently be considered investigational (25). Nevertheless, up to 50% of patients relapse following allogeneic transplantation; therefore, at present, this option is far from ideal for most patients.
- The benefit of *posttransplantation maintenance therapy* with agents such as interferon-α, prednisone, and thalidomide has not been established and therefore should be used only in the context of a clinical trial.
- *Bisphosphonates* have become part of the standard armamentarium against MM and are generally thought to be beneficial in all patients with myeloma; however, randomized trials showing benefit in morbidity and time to progression exist only for patients with advanced myeloma and bone disease. Intravenous *pamidronate* given monthly reduced bone pain and the incidence of pathologic fractures and the need for surgery or irradiation to the bone in patients with Durie–Salmon stage III myeloma (17). A recent randomized trial demonstrated that *zoledronic acid* is safe and is as effective as pamidronate in reducing skeletal complications, in addition to having the advantage of a shorter administration time (18,19). The beneficial effects of the bisphosphonates may be a result of their effects on bone resorption as well as the direct antitumor effects and/or immune stimulation.

TABLE 27.5. *Single versus double autologous stem cell transplantation (SCT) [InterGroupe Francophone du Myelome (IFM) 95 Trial] (23)*

Treatment	OR (CR + PR) (%)	CR + very good PR (%)	Median overall survival (mo)	Median event-free survival (mo)	Treatment-related mortality
Single autoSCT	84	42	48	25	4%
Double autoSCT	88	50	58	30	6%

OR, overall response; CR, complete response; PR, partial response; SCT, stem cell transplantation.

SUPPORTIVE MEASURES

- Supportive measures in myeloma include adequate analgesia and/or local irradiation for bone pain, radiation or surgery for spinal cord compression, surgery for impending pathologic fractures, erythropoietin for anemia, treatment and prevention of hypercalcemia, avoidance of dehydration by a high fluid intake of around 3 L per day to maintain renal function, and dialysis if necessary. Intravenous immunoglobulin therapy may be beneficial for patients with recurrent life-threatening infections.

REFRACTORY OR RELAPSED DISEASE

- In a patient who progresses during MP or other initial therapy (refractory disease) or who relapses within 6 months of stopping induction therapy, *VAD* or *high-dose pulse dexamethasone* is a suitable second-line regimen (7,26). Other salvage regimens that have shown efficacy include *DCEP* and *DTPACE* (9–11).
- In a treatment-refractory patient with significant cytopenias, *pulse dexamethasone* alone can be considered (26).
- Oral *thalidomide* at doses of 200 to 800 mg per day has been reported to produce a decrease in myeloma protein in patients who are refractory to other therapies, including HDC (12). The overall response rate to thalidomide as a single agent in this group of patients was 32%. Thalidomide is not marrow suppressive; thus it can be used in patients with poor marrow function following transplantation or in combination with chemotherapy or irradiation. Side effects are rarely dangerous, but severe fatigue and neuropathies limit dose intensification. Thalidomide analogs with fewer side effects are under development.
- Recently, *bortezomib* (formerly known as PS-341), a member of a new class of anticancer drugs called *proteasome inhibitors*, has been shown to induce response rates of 35% in myeloma patients refractory to multiple lines of standard and high-dose regimens (including thalidomide) (14). Combinations of bortezomib with chemotherapy agents and/or thalidomide are currently being evaluated in clinical trials.

REFERENCES

1. Durie BG, Salmon SE. A clinical staging system for multiple myeloma. *Cancer* 1975;36:842–854.
2. Blade J, Samson D, Reece D, et al., European Group for Blood and Marrow Transplant. Criteria for evaluating disease response and progression in patients with multiple myeloma treated by high-dose therapy and haemopoietic stem cell transplantation. Myeloma subcommittee of the EBMT. *Br J Haematol* 1998;102(5):1115–1123.
3. Alexanian R, Haut A, Khan AU, et al. Treatment for multiple myeloma. Combination chemotherapy with different melphalan dose regimens. *JAMA* 1969;208(9):1680–1685.
4. Gregory WM, Richards MA, Malpas JS. Combination chemotherapy versus melphalan and prednisolone in the treatment of multiple myeloma: an overview of published trials. *J Clin Oncol* 1992; 10:334–342.
5. Myeloma Trialists' Collaborative Group. Combination chemotherapy versus melphalan plus prednisone as treatment for multiple myeloma: an overview of 6,633 patients from 27 randomized trials. *J Clin Oncol* 1998;16:3832–3842.
6. Alexanian R, Dimopoulos MA, Delasalle K, et al. Primary dexamethasone treatment of multiple myeloma. *Blood* 1992;80(4):887–890.
7. Barlogie B, Smith L, Alexanian R. Effective treatment of advanced multiple myeloma refractory to alkylating agents. *N Engl J Med* 1984;310(21):1353–1356.
8. Salmon SE, Haut A, Bonnet JD, et al. Alternating combination chemotherapy and levamisole improves survival in multiple myeloma: a Southwest Oncology Group Study. *J Clin Oncol* 1983; 1(8):453–461.
9. Munshi NC, Desikan KR, Jagannath S, et al. Dexamethasone, cyclophosphamide, etoposide and cis-platinum (DCEP), an effective regimen for relapse after high-dose chemotherapy and autologous transplantation. *Blood* 1996;88(Suppl. 1):2331a.

10. Lazzarino M, Corso A, Barbarano L, et al. DCEP (dexamethasone, cyclophosphamide, etoposide, and cisplatin) is an effective regimen for peripheral blood stem cell collection in multiple myeloma. *Bone Marrow Transplant* 2001;28(9):835–839.

11. Lee CK, Barlogie B, Munshi N, et al. DTPACE: an effective, novel combination chemotherapy with thalidomide for previously treated patients with myeloma. *J Clin Oncol* 2003;21(14):2732–2739.

12. Singhal S, Mehta J, Desikan R, et al. Antitumor activity of thalidomide in refractory multiple myeloma. *N Engl J Med* 1999;21:1565–1571.

13. Rajkumar SV, Hayman S, Gertz MA, et al. Combination therapy with thalidomide plus dexamethasone for newly diagnosed myeloma. *J Clin Oncol* 2002;20(21):4319–4323.

14. Richardson PG, Barlogie B, Berenson J, et al. A phase 2 study of bortezomib in relapsed, refractory myeloma. *N Engl J Med* 2003;348(26):2609–2617.

15. Attal M, Harousseau JL, Stoppa AM, et al. A prospective randomized trial of autologous bone marrow transplantation and chemotherapy in multiple myeloma. *N Engl J Med* 1996;335:91–97.

16. Child JA, Morgan GJ, Davies FE et al., Medical Research Council Adult Leukemia Working Party. High-dose chemotherapy with hematopoietic stem-cell rescue for multiple myeloma. *N Engl J Med* 2003;348(19):1875–1883.

17. Berenson J, Lichtenstein A, Porter L, et al. Efficacy of pamidronate in reducing skeletal events in patients with advanced multiple myeloma. *N Engl J Med* 1996;334:488–493.

18. Rosen LS, Gordon D, Kaminski M, et al. Long-term efficacy and safety of zoledronic acid compared with pamidronate disodium in the treatment of skeletal complications in patients with advanced multiple myeloma or breast carcinoma: a randomized, double-blind, multicenter, comparative trial. *Cancer* 2003;98(8):1735–1744.

19. Rosen LS, Gordon D, Kaminski M, et al. Zoledronic acid versus pamidronate in the treatment of skeletal metastases in patients with breast cancer or osteolytic lesions of multiple myeloma: a phase III, double-blind, comparative trial. *Cancer J* 2001;7(5):377–387.

20. Fritz E, Ludwig H. Interferon-alpha treatment in multiple myeloma: meta-analysis of 30 randomised trials among 3948 patients. *Ann Oncol* 2000;11(11):1427–1436.

21. Myeloma Trialists' Collaborative Group. Interferon as therapy for multiple myeloma: an individual patient data overview of 24 randomized trials and 4012 patients. *Br J Haematol* 2001;113(4):1020–1034.

22. Moreau P, Facon T, Attal M, et al., InterGroupe Francophone du Myelome. Comparison of 200 mg/m(2) melphalan and 8 Gy total body irradiation plus 140 mg/m(2) melphalan as conditioning regimens for peripheral blood stem cell transplantation in patients with newly diagnosed multiple myeloma: final analysis of the InterGroupe Francophone du Myelome 9502 randomized trial. *Blood* 2002;99(3):731–735.

23. Fermand JP, Ravaud P, Chevret S, et al. High-dose therapy and autologous peripheral blood stem cell transplantation in multiple myeloma: up-front or rescue treatment? Results of a multicenter sequential randomized clinical trial. *Blood* 1998;92(9):3131–3136.

24. Attal M, Harousseau JL, Facon T et al., InterGroupe Francophone du Myelome. Single versus double autologous stem-cell transplantation for multiple myeloma. *N Engl J Med* 2003;349(26):2495–2502.

25. Maloney DG, Molina AJ, Sahebi F, et al. Allografting with nonmyeloablative conditioning following cytoreductive autografts for the treatment of patients with multiple myeloma. *Blood* 2003;102(9): 3447–3454.

26. Alexanian R, Barlogie B, Dixon D. High-dose glucocorticoid treatment of resistant myeloma. *Ann Intern Med* 1986;105(1):8–11.

28

Non-Hodgkin Lymphoma

Martin E. Gutierrez[*], Richard F. Little[†], and Wyndham H. Wilson[†]

[*]*Medical Oncology Clinical Research Unit, National Cancer Institute, National Institutes of Health, Bethesda, Maryland and* [†]*Center for Cancer Research, National Cancer Institute, National Institutes of Health, Bethesda, Maryland*

The non-Hodgkin lymphomas (NHLs) are a group of entities that vary in clinical behavior and morphologic appearance. The various types of NHLs are thought to represent neoplastic lymphoid cells that are arrested at different stages of normal differentiation. On the basis of their natural history, NHLs can be clinically classified as indolent, aggressive, or highly aggressive.

EPIDEMIOLOGY

Over the last 20 years, the incidence of NHL has been steadily increasing at approximately 4% per year, which represents 55,000 new cases annually. Mortality has shown similar increases. Approximately one third of the increase has been attributed to a combination of improved diagnosis and immunosuppressive therapy, and to the AIDS epidemic. A slight decrease in the incidence of AIDS-related NHL (ARL) has been noted since 1996, but the incidence in other groups of other NHLs has continued to increase.

PATHOPHYSIOLOGY

Cytogenetics, gene rearrangement, and oncoproteins are important molecular markers of the histologic subtype, histogenesis, and mechanisms of lymphomagenesis. Tumor clonality may be assessed by immunoglobulin (Ig) gene rearrangement in B cells and by T-cell–receptor (TCR) rearrangement in T cells. Cytogenetics and/or oncogene rearrangement by polymerase chain reaction (PCR) may also be useful to assess clonality. However, the absence of evidence for clonality does not exclude the presence of a malignant lymphoid process, whereas the presence of its evidence does not necessarily confirm a malignant lymphoid process (see Tables 28.1 and 28.2).

A major known risk factor for NHL appears to be an abnormality in immune function (either immunodeficiency or dysregulation), as seen in human immunodeficiency virus (HIV) infection, iatrogenic immune suppression, congenital immune deficiencies (i.e., Wiskott-Aldrich syndrome and X-linked lymphoproliferative disorder), and autoimmune diseases. Infectious agents have also been implicated as risk factors; Epstein–Barr virus (EBV) is associated with African Burkitt lymphoma and AIDS-related diffuse large B-cell lymphomas (DLBCLs); Kaposi sarcoma–associated herpesvirus (KSHV, also known as human herpesvirus-8 or

TABLE 28.1. *Molecular characteristics of B-cell lymphomas*

Histology	Cytogenetics	Oncogene/protein	Ig gene rearrangements	
			Heavy	κ λ
CLL/SLL[a]	Trisomy 12; deletions of 13q14 and 11q22–23	—	+	+
Lymphoplasmacytoid lymphoma/Waldenström macroglobulinemia	t(9;14)	PAX-5 gene	+	+
Follicular center cell Grade I/II/IIIa[b]	t(14;18)	Bcl-2	+	—
Marginal zone[c]	Trisomy 3 t(11;18)	—	+	
Mantle cell lymphoma	t(11;14)	Bcl–1/Cyclin D1	+	—
Diffuse large B-cell[d]	t(14;18); 3q27; 17p	Bcl-2; Bcl-6; p53	+	+
Primary mediastinal large cell	Gains 9p	REL gene; MAL gene overexpression	+	+
Lymphoblastic lymphoma/leukemia	t(9;22) t(12;21) t(1;19)	BCR/ABL TEL/AML1 PBX/E2A	+	±
Burkitt lymphoma	t(8;14)(q24;q32) t(2;8)(11p; q24) t(8;22)(q24;q11)	c-myc	+ +	+

CLL, chronic lymphocytic leukemia; SLL, small lymphocytic lymphoma.
[a]Trisomy 12 is seen in 30% of cases and abnormalities in 13q are present in 25% of patients.
[b]t(14;18) is present in 75% to 95% of FCC NHL.
[c]Cytogenetic abnormalities have been seen in extranodal MZ NHL.
[d]Bcl-2 rearrangements up to 30% and Bcl-6 up to 45% of cases of DLBCL.

TABLE 28.2. *Molecular characteristics of T-cell lymphomas*

Histology	Cytogenetics	Oncoprotein	TCR gene rearrangements
T-CLL/T-PLL	Inv14(q11;q32), Trisomy 8q	Bcl-3	+
Mycosis fungoides	—	—	+
Peripheral T-cell lymphoma unspecified	—	—	±
Angioimmunoblastic T-cell lymphoma[a]	Trisomy 3 or 5, EBV +	—	+
ATLL	HTLV-1 integration +	—	+
Enteropathy T cell	–EBV–	—	β+
Hepatosplenic γ/δ	—	—	δγ+
Systemic ALCL[b,c]	t(2;5)	Alk+	+
Precursor T-lymphoblastic Lymphoma/leukemia	Variable t(7;9)	Tcl-4	Variable

TCR, T-cell–receptor; CLL, chronic lymphocytic leukemia; PLL, prolymphocytic leukemia; ATLL, adult T-cell lymphoma/leukemia; EBV, Epstein–Barr virus; ALCL, anaplastic large-cell lymphoma.
[a]TCR gene rearrangement is present in 75% and IgH in 10%.
[b]TCR gene rearrangement in 60% +.
[c]Alk: ALK gene.

HHV-8) is etiologically linked to primary effusion lymphomas and multicentric Castleman disease; and human retroviruses such as human T-cell lymphoma virus 1 (HTLV-1) are the etiologies of adult T-cell leukemia/lymphoma. Infectious agents have also been implicated through stimulating B-cell clones, such as hepatitis C virus and splenic marginal zone (MZ) lymphoma, *Helicobacter pylori* and gastric MZ lymphomas, and possibly, *Chlamydia* and ocular MZ lymphomas. Environmental and occupational exposures, especially organic compounds (organophosphate insecticides), have been etiologically linked to lymphoma.

Staging for Non-Hodgkin Lymphoma

- Staging evaluation of NHL should include history and physical examination and clinical laboratory assessment of organ function. In addition, viral serology for HIV (in aggressive NHL), HTLV-1, and hepatitis B and C viruses needs to be considered if indicated by risk or by lymphoma subtype.
- Routine blood tests including lactate dehydrogenase (LDH) should be performed.
- T-cell subset analysis (e.g., CD4 cell count) should be done if the patient is HIV positive.
- In young men with an isolated mediastinal mass, where the differential diagnosis includes mediastinal germ cell tumor, determination of serum α-fetoprotein or β-human chorionic gonadotropin can be useful.
- Radiologic evaluation should include chest x-ray and computerized tomographic scans of chest, abdomen, and pelvis. Positron emission tomography (PET) scans are useful for identifying sites of disease and for assessing responses. Gallium scans, although used in the past, are less sensitive and less specific than PET.

Staging procedures:

- Bone marrow (BM) biopsy
- Lumbar puncture with cytology in patients at risk for central nervous system (CNS) disease— DLBCL with elevated LDH level and more than one extranodal site and/or aggressive lymphoma in the BM. All Burkitt lymphoma and AIDS-related lymphoma (ARL) cases should be assessed.

Definitions:

- B symptoms: unexplained weight loss of more than 10% of body weight over the previous 6 months, fever, and "drenching" night sweats
- X: bulky disease (10 cm maximal dimension)
- E: extranodal disease
- Single E site is sufficiently limited in extent/location that it can be subjected to definitive treatment with radiation.

Diagnostic confirmation by tissue biopsy:

Sufficient material is critical to conduct the studies that ensure accurate diagnosis. Needle biopsies generally yield inadequate tissue for these studies and should be avoided for use in primary diagnosis. Important studies for diagnostic confirmation often include assessment of clonality, immunophenotyping, cytogenetic analysis, and molecular studies. Oncogene rearrangement and/or overexpression of oncoproteins can be diagnostically useful:

- t(8;14) or MYC in Burkitt lymphoma
- t(14;18) or bcl-2 in follicular lymphoma
- t(2;5) or anaplastic lymphoma kinase (ALK) in anaplastic large-cell lymphoma
- t(11;14) or bcl-1 in mantle cell lymphoma

TABLE 28.3. *Staging system in non-Hodgkin lymphomas*

Stage	Ann Arbor/AJCC and Cotswolds	St. Jude lymphoblastic NHL	Mycosis fungoides
I	Single node region or lymphoid structure or single extranodal site mediastinum or abdomen	Single tumor (extranodal) or single anatomic area (nodal), excluding	Confined to the skin
II	Two or more nodes on same side of diaphragm or single nodal site with extranodal extension	Single tumor (extranodal) with regional node involvement • Primary gastrointestinal tract tumor (usually ileocecal) ± mesenteric nodes	Clinically positive nodes
III	Nodal regions or lymphoid structure on both sides of the diaphragm	Node regions or lymphoid structures on both sides of the diaphragm • All primary intrathoracic tumor (i.e., mediastinal, pleural, and thymic) • All extensible primary intraabdominal disease; unresectable • All primary paraspinal or epidural tumors regardless of other sites	Histologically proven nodes
IV	Bone marrow or liver or extranodal site(s) beyond those designated as "E"	Any of the above with initial CNS or BM involvement	Visceral disease

- Trisomy 3 or trisomy 18 (marginal zone lymphoma)
- Some tumors (e.g., T-cell–rich B-cell lymphoma or lymphomatoid granulomatosis) have an excess of reactive T cells that may obscure the minority of diagnostic malignant B cells if inadequate tissue is obtained.

The Ann Arbor/American Joint Commission for Cancer (AJCC) and Cotswolds staging systems are applicable to all histologies except lymphoblastic and mycosis fungoides (MF) (see Table 28.3).

Restaging for Response Evaluation

- On completion of therapy, staging studies should be repeated. Restaging is also recommended after the first four cycles (all tests with abnormal results should be repeated). Disease progression or inadequate response implies extremely poor prognosis. If residual masses are present after systemic chemotherapy, a PET scan may help distinguish active disease from residual scar. If residual masses are unclear on imaging, evaluation biopsy may be required.
- Response to therapy may be slower in indolent lymphomas than in aggressive and highly aggressive lymphomas. Restaging can be performed less frequently in these cases.

Prognostic Features

- The disease-related prognostic features include histologic type and tumor histogenesis. Indolent lymphomas are rarely curable, but often have a prolonged natural history. DLBCL is potentially curative, with outcome depending on histogenesis: a better prognosis is associated with a germinal center B cell (GCB) gene expression pattern, and a worse prognosis is associated with a non-GCB gene expression pattern.

- Adverse clinical characteristics such as tumor bulk, advanced stage, many extranodal sites, and high tumor proliferation (MIB-1 and LDH) may be overcome with infusional regimens such as dose-adjusted EPOCH (doxorubicin, etoposide, vincristine, cyclophosphamide, and prednisone). *Bcl-2* expression has been associated with CHOP (cyclophosphamide, doxorubicin, vincristine, and prednisone) failure but may be partially overcome with rituximab.
- Prognostic assessment and modeling: The International Prognostic Index (IPI) was initially developed for aggressive NHL, but it has been applied to other NHL subtypes also.
- One point is assigned for each of the following:
  - Individuals older than 60 years
  - Eastern Cooperative Oncology Group (ECOG) performance status more than one
  - LDH level greater than normal
  - More than one extranodal site
  - Ann Arbor stage III or IV disease
  - Age-adjusted International Index for patients younger than 60 years.

CLASSIFICATION OF NON-HODGKIN LYMPHOMAS

The World Health Organization (WHO) classification is the currently accepted system and incorporates immunophenotypic, molecular, and clinical elements to distinguish NHL subtypes (see Tables 28.4 and 28.5). NHLs are broadly classified as B-cell lymphomas or T-cell lymphomas depending on the lymphocyte lineage giving rise to the tumor.

- B lymphocytes give rise to B-cell NHL; this accounts for 88% of NHLs.
- T lymphocytes give rise to T-cell NHL; this accounts for 12% of NHLs.

TABLE 28.4. *B-cell immunophenotype*

Histology	SIg	CIg	CD 5	10	11	15	23	30	34	43	45
CLL/SLL[a]	±	±	+	−	±		+			+	
Lymphoplasmacytoid lymphoma[a]	+	+	−	−	±		−				±
FCC grade I/II/IIIa[a,b]	+	−	−	±			±			−	
Marginal zone[a,c]	+	+	−	−	±		−			±	
Mantle cell lymphoma[a,d]	+	−	+	±	−		−			+	
Diffuse large B-Cell[a]	±	±	±	±			−				±
Primary mediastinal large B-cell[a,e]	−	−	±	±			−	−	±		±
Precursor B lymphoblastic Lymphoma /leukemia[a,f]	−	±			±				±		
Burkitt lymphoma[a]	+	−			+		−				

CLL, chronic lymphocytic leukemia; SLL, small lymphocytic lymphoma; FCC, follicular center cell.
[a]Positive B-cell–associated antigens: CD19, CD20, CD22, and CD79.
[b]SIg$^+$: IgM±, IgD > IgG > IgA.
[c]SIg M > IgG >IgA and IgD$^-$; CIg$^+$ in 40%.
[d]SIgM$^+$ usually IgD$^+$, $\kappa > \lambda$ and CD11c$^-$.
[e]IgM > IgG >IgA and IgD$^-$; CIg$^+$ in 40%.
[f]TdT$^+$, HLA – Dr$^+$ and CD20$^{-/+}$.

TABLE 28.5. *T-cell immunophenotype*

Histology	CD 1a	2	3	4	5	7	8	25	56	TdT
T-CLL /T-PLL[a]		+	+	+	+	+	+	−		
Mycosis fungoides		+	+	+	+	−/+	−	−		
Peripheral T-cell lymphoma unspecified[b]		±	±	+	±	−/+	±			
Angioimmunoblastic lymphoma		+	+	+	+					
Enteropathy T cell[c]			+	−		+	±			
Adult T-cell lymphoma/leukemia		+	+	+	+	−	−	+		
Systemic ALCL[d]			−/+					±		
Hepatosplenic γ/δ			+	−			−		+	
Precursor T-lymphoblastic lymphoma/leukemia	±	±	+	+	±	+	+			+

CLL, chronic lymphocytic leukemia; PLL, prolymphocytic leukemia; ALCL, anaplastic large-cell lymphoma.

[a]T-CLL: 60% are CD4+ and 21% CD4+8+; rare cases are CD4−8+ and CD25−.
[b]Peripheral T-cell are most commonly CD4 > CD8. It can be CD 4−8−; CD45RA may be + and CD45RA −.
[c]Intestinal T cell is CD103+.
[d]ALCL are CD30+, CD45±, EMA+ and CD15+.

- Expression (or lack thereof) of cell surface antigens and immunoglobulin proteins depends on the type of lymphocyte and its stage of differentiation. Thus, analysis of these proteins in tumor cells is diagnostically useful and may help determine tumor histogenesis.

There is an increasing appreciation of the relation between tumor histogenesis and clinical behavior, such as previously discussed with DLBCL. Patients with chronic lymphocytic leukemia/lymphoma (CLL) can be grouped according to whether the variable region of the Ig genes (IgV_H) shows sequence homology to germline IgV_H genes, or on the basis of evidence of somatic mutations. Prognosis is poorer in patients with unmutated IgV_H genes (pregerminal center histogenic origin) than in patients with somatic mutations (germinal center B-cell histogenic origin).

The World Health Organization (WHO) recognizes three major categories of lymphoid neoplasms:

1. B-cell neoplasms
2. T- and NK-cell neoplasms
3. Hodgkin lymphoma.

Both lymphomas and lymphoid leukemias are included in the WHO classification. Solid and leukemic phases are present in many lymphoid neoplasms. The WHO classification stratifies these neoplasms primarily according to lineage. A cell of origin is postulated for each neoplasm, and for many neoplasms, this cell of origin represents the stage of differentiation of the tumor cells in the tissues and may or may not reflect the stage of differentiation during which the initial transforming events occur, because it is not possible to know these events in many cases.

Each histologic entity is grouped according to general clinical behavior as indolent, aggressive, or highly aggressive lymphomas for the sake of the reader. For further information about the WHO classification of tumors, see http://www.iarc.fr/who-bluebooks/.

Indolent Lymphomas

B Cell

- **B-chronic lymphocytic leukemia/Small lymphocytic lymphoma (SLL):** These diseases affect older patients (median age in the seventh decade) and involve the BM, peripheral blood (PB), lymph node (LN), liver, and spleen. SLL represents the nonleukemic equivalent of CLL. These diseases are incurable and have median survivals of approximately 10 years. They can transform to more aggressive prolymphocytic leukemia (PLL) or large B-cell NHL (Richter syndrome), which have median survivals of less than 1 year.
- **Lymphoplasmacytoid lymphoma/Waldenström macroglobulinemia:** This lymphoma affects primarily older patients (median age in the seventh decade). The sites of involvement include BM, LN, and spleen; rarely, PB or extranodal sites are involved. Paraproteinemia with IgM and hyperviscosity symptoms may occur. When disseminated, this entity is incurable and has a median survival of approximately 8 to 10 years.
- **Follicular center cell (FCC) grades I, II, and IIIa:** The median age occurrence of this lymphoma is in the sixth decade. It is the second most common subtype of NHL, comprising approximately 35% of lymphomas. FCC lymphomas are graded on the basis of the proportion of small and large cells. Grade I contains predominantly centrocytes (small B cells) and zero to five centroblasts (large B cells); grade II contains mixed centrocytes and 6 to 15 centroblasts; and grade IIIa contains centrocytes and more than 15 centroblasts per high power field (HPF). It commonly shows LN and BM involvement, splenomegaly, extranodal involvement, and a clinical leukemic phase. Advanced-stage disease is incurable in most patients and has a median survival of 8 to 10 years. Histologic transformation of this disease to an aggressive large B-cell lymphoma occurs in most patients, although it may not manifest clinically.
- **Marginal zone:** There are two major clinical presentations of MZ: extranodal and nodal types. Extranodal types are associated with autoimmune diseases like Sjögren syndrome, Hashimoto thyroiditis, or *H. pylori* gastritis. Recent evidence indicates that proliferation may be antigen driven in some mucosa-associated lymphoid tissue (MALT) lymphomas such as *H. pylori* gastritis, and eradication of the antigen may result in tumor regression. Median age of occurrence of MZ lymphomas is in the seventh decade. These tumors are usually indolent but incurable and have a median survival of 10 years. Nodal types may represent the nodal dissemination of extranodal types of MZ. However, isolated nodal types occur, and are less indolent than the extranodal types.

T Cell

- **T-chronic lymphocytic leukemia/T-prolymphocytic leukemia:** T-CLL/T-PLL comprise 1% of CLLs but up to 20% of PLLs. Patients often have high white blood cell (WBC) counts (e.g., >100,000 per mm^3) and may have cutaneous or mucosal infiltrates. T cells are more aggressive than their B-cell counterparts and have a median survival of 8 years.
- **Mycosis fungoïdes:** MF is a cutaneous T-cell lymphoma that often has multiple cutaneous plaques, nodules, and/or generalized erythroderma. Nodal involvement and leukemic phases (Sézary syndrome) are late occurrences. Large-cell lymphoma may develop as a terminal event. The disease may be relatively indolent over prolonged periods and may have a median survival of 10.2 years, but in the group with poor prognosis (patients older than 65 years and stage IVB), the median survival is 1.1 years.

Treatment Principles

Patients with early-stage FCC and MZ lymphomas may be potentially cured with radiation treatment. In stage I FCC lymphoma, radiation treatment (e.g., 30 to 50 Gy) has a disease-free survival of 54% to 88% at 10 years, although recent evidence suggests that radiation does not increase overall survival (OS) (see Fig. 28.1). In advanced-stage patients, the Stanford group showed no difference in survival between watching until medical symptoms required treatment (called "watch and wait") and early intervention. On the basis of this approach, therapy is often not begun until symptoms or impending organ compromise occurs or until the lymphoma transforms to an aggressive subtype.

Selection of treatment is based on the clinical situation. Generally, radiation may be used to palliate local disease, whereas cytotoxic or monoclonal antibody therapies may be used in disseminated disease. The choice of agents depends on the cell type (B versus T cell), histology, and treatment history (see Table 28.6). Standard chemotherapy is not usually curative.

Some of the treatment possibilities are oral chlorambucil, CVP (cyclophosphamide, vincristine, and prednisone), fludarabine, or rituximab (monoclonal anti-CD20 antibody). Rituximab, as a single agent in previously untreated follicular lymphoma, yields up to 75% response rates. Maintenance rituximab may prolong remission. At 3 years of median follow-up, the duration of remission is 23 months for maintenance rituximab versus 12 months for rituximab as a single agent, thereby favoring the rituximab maintenance group receiving 375 mg per m² every 2 months for four doses after induction. As a single agent in previously treated follicular lymphoma, rituximab can yield responses in 50% to 60% of cases, with median response duration ranging from 6 to 16 months. Rituximab combinations, like rituximab with CHOP, induce complete responses in up to 95% of previously untreated follicular lymphomas, with the median response duration not being achieved until 50 months of follow-up. Rituximab combined with fludarabine yields results similar to the combination of CHOP and rituximab.

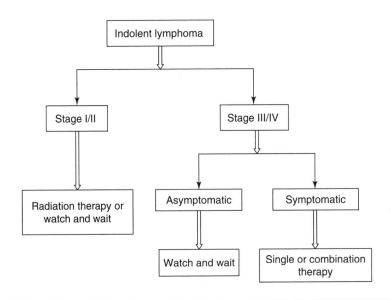

FIG. 28.1. Indolent non-Hodgkin lymphoma (NHL) approach.

TABLE 28.6. *Indolent lymphoma treatment*

	Treatment description
Combination chemotherapy	
CVP	Cyclophosphamide 400 mg/m^2 PO daily for 5 d, d 1–5 (total dose/cycle = 2,000 mg/m^2)
	Vincristine 1.4 mg/m^2 i.v. on d 1 (maximum dose/cycle = 2 mg; total dose/cycle = 1.4 mg/m^2)
	Prednisone 100 mg/m^2 PO daily for 5 d, d 1–5 (total dose/cycle = 500 mg/m^2)
	• treatment is repeated every 21 d
Single agents	
Fludarabine	Fludarabine 25 mg/m^2/d i.v. for 5 d, d 1–5 (total dose/cycle = 125 mg/m^2)
	• treatment is repeated every 28 d
Rituximab	Rituximab 375 mg/m^2 i.v. weekly (total dose/wk = 375 mg/m^2)
Radiolabeled monoclonal antibody	Zevaline and Bexxar

- **Radioimmunotherapy for relapsed disease:** Yttrium 90-ibritumomab tiuxetan (Zevalan) is FDA approved and is well tolerated. A randomized trial indicated a marginally statistically significant higher ORR and CR, but not response duration, for Zevalan than for rituximab alone in relapsed or refractory low-grade, follicular, or transformed B-cell NHL. Tositumomab and Iodine I 131 tositumomab (Bexxar) are also U.S. Food and Drug Administration (FDA)–approved for the treatment of CD20-positive, follicular lymphoma that is refractory to rituximab and that relapses following chemotherapy.
- **CLL/SLL:** Fludarabine and rituximab, given concurrently or sequentially, increase response rates. Alemtuzumab is approved for fludarabine-refractory disease, with response rates of approximately 30%.
- **Lymphoplasmacytoid lymphoma/Waldenström macroglobulinemia:** Initial therapy with rituximab has produced overall response rates of 30% to 60%. Other conventional therapies include alkylating agents (especially chlorambucil) with or without corticosteroids. Treatment with CHOP is sometimes used. Purine analogs such as fludarabine are also active. Response rates to first-line therapy range from 38% to 85%. Response rates to fludarabine in previously treated patients range from 30% to 50%.
- In MF, a variety of active treatments are available for good-prognosis disease, but the extent to which outcomes are related to therapy or to the natural history of the disease is often not well documented. Reported treatments include low-dose oral methotrexate, topical bexarotene gel, topical gel formulation combining methotrexate and laurocapram, and topical nitrogen mustard. Combined modality therapy, including subcutaneous interferon-α and oral isotretinoin followed by total-skin electron beam therapy and long-term maintenance therapy with topical nitrogen mustard and interferon-α, has been reported as being useful. Extracorporeal photopheresis with or without other modalities has been reported.

Aggressive Non-Hodgkin Lymphomas

B Cell

- **Mantle cell lymphoma:** This lymphoma occurs primarily in older patients (median age in the seventh decade), with a high male-to-female ratio. It often involves the spleen, BM, LN, and extranodal sites, particularly the gastrointestinal tract (lymphomatous polyposis) in up to 90% of cases. Unlike other aggressive lymphomas, it is incurable and has a short median survival of 3 to 5 years. The blastic variant is more aggressive than the other forms, with a propensity for CNS involvement and shorter survival.

- **FCC grade IIIb:** Histologically, FCC grade IIIb lymphoma presents with sheets of centroblasts and no centrocytes. This entity is rare and is biologically similar to *de novo* DLBCL. It should be treated like DLBCL and appears to have a similar rate of cure.

- **DLBCL:** This lymphoma constitutes up to 30% of adult lymphomas. As in other lymphomas, the median age is in the sixth decade. Patients frequently exhibit a rapidly enlarging mass or an acute onset of symptoms. Extranodal involvement is seen in 40% of cases. DLBC can be cured with combination chemotherapy and should be treated promptly and aggressively. The OS and progression-free survival (PFS) are approximately 50% and 32%, respectively, at 5 years.

- **Primary mediastinal (thymic) large cell lymphoma:** This recently recognized subtype of DLBCL is believed to arise in thymic tissue and commonly forms a large anterior mediastinal mass. It occurs most commonly in young women in their third or fourth decade and may involve extranodal sites such as the kidney, lung, and liver. The OS and PFS are similar to other large B-cell lymphomas.

- **HIV-associated B-cell lymphomas:** The incidence of lymphoma is 60 times higher than that expected among HIV-infected individuals. The median age of occurrence is in the fourth decade, compared with the sixth decade in patients with non–HIV-related lymphomas. Most patients have advanced-stage disease and often have extranodal involvement, including the gastrointestinal tract, BM, and CNS. CNS may be the only site involved, as in primary CNS lymphoma, or the lymphoma may form a part of systemic disease. Histologically, these lymphomas are aggressive B cells and are divided between the large B-cell (>70%) and Burkitt subtypes of lymphoma.

T Cell

- **Peripheral T-cell lymphomas (PTLs):** These lymphomas are less common, comprising less than 15% of lymphomas in the developed countries, but have a higher incidence in other parts of the world. They are divided into specified and unspecified types. The unspecified PTLs are so named because they do not fit the requirements for the specified types and do not share a common biology or clinical behavior. Patients typically have generalized disease and may have pruritus and eosinophilia. PTLs frequently involve LN, skin (subcutis), liver, and spleen. In general, PTLs have an aggressive clinical course, although some may be relatively indolent. T-cell lymphomas have a lower rate of cure and higher rate of relapse than B-cell lymphomas, with an OS and failure-free survival (FFS) of 25% and 18%, respectively, at 5 years.

- **Intestinal T-cell lymphoma:** Adult patients often have a history of gluten-sensitive enteropathy, or uncommonly, there may be no evidence of an underlying enteropathy. The geographic distribution of intestinal T-cell lymphomas is similar to that of intestinal enteropathies and hence is rare in western countries. Patients may have abdominal pain and jejunal perforation.

- **Angiocentric lymphoma:** These lymphomas are seen most commonly in Asia, where they usually occur in the nasopharyngeal area with symptoms of obstruction and pain. Nasal angiocentric lymphoma, the most common type, is caused by T/natural killer cells that express Epstein–Barr antigens. Treatment for localized disease primarily involves radiation, and the role of chemotherapy is unclear. At relapse, and less commonly at presentation, the disease may disseminate to extranodal sites such as the lungs and skin.

- **Angioimmunoblastic T-cell lymphoma (AILT):** This subtype of lymphoma was commonly known as angioimmunoblastic lymphadenopathy with dysproteinemia (AILD). It occurs in older patients who often have fever, rash, diffuse adenopathy, and polyclonal hypergammaglobulinemia. It was previously considered to be a reactive process but studies have demonstrated clonal T-cell rearrangements in most cases. The course is quite aggressive but very responsive to steroids and chemotherapy. Patients may develop opportunistic infections and secondary EBV lymphomas, and most patients die from the disease.

- **Adult T-cell Lymphoma/Leukemia (ATLL):** This lymphoma occurs mostly in HTLV-1–endemic regions such as Japan and the Caribbean basin. It is an aggressive T-cell lymphoma caused by HTLV-1 infection. The clinical presentation includes high WBC count, hypercalcemia, hepatosplenomegaly, and lytic bone lesions. Clinically, ATLL has been classified into four distinct clinical presentations called smoldering, chronic, lymphomatous, and acute, with clinical behaviors that range from indolent to highly aggressive.

- **Anaplastic large-cell lymphoma:** There are two clinical entities of this lymphoma, systemic and primary cutaneous. The systemic form occurs in both children and adults and usually expresses ALK kinase, because of t(2;5). It has either a T-cell or null phenotype. True anaplastic large-cell lymphomas (ALCL) of B-cell phenotype are very rare and are biologically unrelated to T-cell ALCL. Systemic ALCL may involve lymph nodes or extranodal sites, including the skin, and 50% of the patients may have constitutional symptoms and advanced stages at presentation. It is highly responsive to chemotherapy and is curable, with an OS and FFS of 75% and 60%, respectively, at 7 years. The primary cutaneous form occurs mostly in adults and has isolated skin nodules. The clinical behavior is indolent, and the skin lesions may regress spontaneously. Systemic disease is uncommon and has a late occurrence. This entity appears to be incurable, and some cases appear to be within the spectrum of lymphomatoid papulosis type A.

Treatment Principles

Many subtypes of aggressive lymphomas are potentially curable with appropriate therapy. However, histologic subtype and prognostic factors influence their curative potentials. Among the various histologies, the aggressive B-cell lymphomas have a better PFS than T-cell lymphomas, with the exception of systemic anaplastic lymphoma, which is among the most curable subtypes. It is important to recognize that some T-cell subtypes, such as ATLL and primary cutaneous anaplastic lymphoma, have no curative potential and should be approached in a palliative mode. Other T-cell subtypes such as angioimmunoblastic lymphomas and PTL have low curative potential with conventional-dose treatment and should be considered for trials targeting high-risk patients. Prognostic factors are helpful in identifying patients at various risk levels for curative purposes. The International NHL Prognostic Factor Project evaluated 3,273 patients from 16 institutions to develop a validated prognostic model. The model, known as the IPI, identified five adverse prognostic factors, which, based on the number of factors, could stratify patients into low-, low-intermediate–, high-intermediate–, and high-risk groups (see Table 28.7). This model can be used to identify patients at high risk for failure who should be considered for more aggressive

TABLE 28.7. *International prognostic index for aggressive diffuse large B-cell lymphomas*

Risk category (International Prognostic Index)	Score	Patients in risk group (%)	Complete responses (%)	5-year disease-free survival (%)	5-year survival (%)
Low	0 or 1	35	87	70	73
Low-intermediate	2	27	67	50	51
High-intermediate	3	22	55	49	43
High	4 or 5	16	44	40	26

TABLE 28.8. *Standard therapy for aggressive non-Hodgkin lymphoma*

Combination chemotherapy	Treatment description	Reference
CHOP-R	Cyclophosphamide 750 mg/m^2 i.v. d 1 (total dose/cycle = 750 mg/m^2) Doxorubicin 50 mg/m^2 i.v. d 1 (total dose/cycle = 50 mg/m^2) Vincristine 1.4 mg/m^2 i.v. d 1 (maximum dose/cycle = 2 mg; total dose/cycle = 1.4 mg/m^2) Prednisone 50 mg/m^2/d PO for 5 d, d 1–5 (total dose/cycle = 250 mg/m^2) Rituximab 375 mg/m^2 i.v. d 1 Treatment is repeated every 21 d	8

therapy, preferably in a clinical trial. A molecular model of outcome has been developed recently on the basis of cDNA microarrays and is independent of the IPI. Early and appropriate treatment will improve outcome in patients with curable lymphomas. Doxorubicin-containing combination chemotherapy should be used in patients with advanced-stage disease, the standard being cyclophosphamide, hydroxydaunomycin, vincristine (Oncovin), prednisone, and rituximab (CHOP-R). Recent evidence, however, suggests that dose-adjusted EPOCH-R, an infusional regimen with pharmacodynamic dosing, may be more effective than CHOP-R. These regimens will be compared in a phase III randomized study. Patients should be restaged after four and six cycles of treatment. Patients showing complete response (CR) or with stable minimal residual disease (i.e., unconfirmed CR) after four cycles usually receive two to four more cycles. However, patients with persistent disease after six cycles should receive salvage treatment. CHOP-R (see Table 28.8) was shown to produce 76% CRs in patients in all risk groups, with a 2-year event-free survival (EFS) and OS of 57% and 70%, respectively. The greatest benefit of rituximab appears to be in tumors with *bcl-2* overexpression. Patients with early-stage disease (i.e., stage I and nonbulky stage II) may receive full-course CHOP-R or, alternatively, may receive limited chemotherapy followed by involved radiation therapy. With this approach, the 5-year estimates of OS and PFS are 82% and 77%, respectively.

Salvage therapy: Patients with potentially curable lymphomas who are refractory or who have relapsed after standard treatment may still be cured with salvage approaches. High-dose therapy with autologous transplantation has been shown to be superior to conventional-dose salvage therapy with high-dose Ara-C and dexamethasone (DHAP) and is now a standard of care. The curative potential of transplantation, however, is influenced by multiple factors including disease responsiveness (i.e., sensitive versus resistant relapse), number of earlier regimens, and presence of bulky (>10 cm) disease. Depending on the study, the long-term survival of patients after autologous transplantation ranges from 20% to 50% depending on prognostic factors and length of follow-up. Patients at high risk for salvage failure should be considered for experimental approaches such as allogeneic transplantation. Patients who are not candidates for transplantation or those who have relapsed thereafter may be effectively palliated with single-agent or combination chemotherapy or radiation.

Chemotherapy regimens for NHL are listed in Table 28.9. The approach of aggressive NHL treatment is shown in Fig. 28.2.

Highly Aggressive NHL

B Cell

- **Precursor B lymphoblastic lymphoma/leukemia** is mostly a disease found in children and presents as leukemia in 80% and as lymphoma in 20% of cases. Involvement of nodes, skin,

TABLE 28.9. *Alternative or salvage regimens for aggressive non-Hodgkin lymphoma*

Combination chemotherapy	Treatment description	Reference
EPOCH-R (dose adjusted)[a]	Rituximab 375 mg/m² i.v. d 1 of each cycle prior to beginning infusions	9, 10
	Etoposide 50 mg/m²/d by continuous i.v. infusion for 4 d, d 1–4 (total dose/cycle = 250 mg/m²)	
	Doxorubicin 10 mg/m²/d by continuous i.v. infusion for 4 d, d 1–4 (total dose/cycle = 40 mg/m²)	
	Vincristine 4 mg/m²/d by continuous i.v. infusion for 4 d, d 1–4 [total dose/cycle = 1.6 mg/m² (no cap)]	
	Prednisone 60 mg/m²/dose PO every 12 h for 5 d, d 1–5 (total dose/cycle = 600 mg/m²)	
	Cyclophosphamide 750 mg/m² i.v. d 5 (total dose/cycle = 750 mg/m²)	
	Filgrastim 5 µg/kg/d s.c. starting d 6; continues until ANC >5,000 cells/mm³	
	• treatment is dose adjusted on the basis of neutrophil nadirs and repeated every 21 d	
CHOEP	CHOP with etoposide 100 mg/m² i.v. d 1, 2, and 3	11
R-ICE	Rituximab 375 mg/m² i.v. 48 h prior to cycle 1 and on d 1 of cycles one to three	12
	Etoposide 100 mg/m² i.v. d 3, 4, and 5	
	Carboplatin AUC 5: dose = 5 × (25 + creatinine clearance) capped at 800 mg i.v. on d 4	
	Ifosfamide 5,000 mg/m² mixed with an equal amount of Mesna continuous i.v. for 24 h on d 4	
DHAP	Cisplatin 100 mg/m² by continuous i.v. infusion for 24 h on d 1 (total dose/cycle = 100 mg/m²)	13
	Cytarabine 2,000 mg/m²/d i.v. over 3 h every 12 h for 2 doses on d 2 (total dose/cycle = 4,000 mg/m²)	
	Dexamethasone 40 mg/d PO or i.v. for 4 d, d 1–4 (total dose/cycle = 160 mg/m²)	
	• treatment is repeated every 21–28 d	
ESHAP	Etoposide 40 mg/m²/d over 1 h i.v. for 4 d, d 1–4 (total dose/cycle = 160 mg/m²)	14
	Methylprednisolone 250–500 mg/d i.v. for 5 d, d 1–5 (total dose/cycle = 1,250–2,500 mg)	
	Cytarabine 2,000 mg/m² i.v. over 2 h on d 5 (total dose/cycle = 2,000 mg/m²)	
	Cisplatin 25 mg/m²/d by continuous i.v. infusion for 4 d, d 1–4 (total dose/cycle = 100 mg/m²)	
	• treatment is repeated every 21–28 d	
ACVBP	Doxorubicin 75 mg/m² i.v. d 1	15
	Cyclophosphamide 1,200 mg/m²/dose i.v. d 1	
	Vindesine 2 mg/m² i.v. d 1 and 5	
	Bleomycin 10 mg i.v. d 1 and 5	
	Prednisone 60 mg/m²/d PO d 1–5	

[a]Etoposide, cyclophosphamide, and doxorubicin dosages may be increased by 20% from the previous cycle's dosage if there is no evidence of absolute neutropenia (ANC >500/mm³) or thrombocytopenia (platelet count >25,000/mm³).

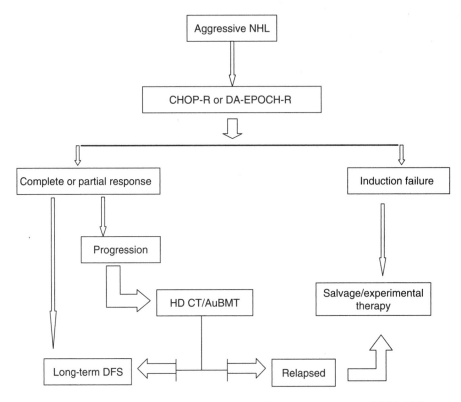

FIG. 28.2. Algorithm for the treatment of aggressive non-Hodgkin lymphoma (NHL). NHL, non-Hodgkin lymphoma; CHOP-R , cyclophosphamide, hydroxydaunomycin, vincristine (Oncovin), prednisone, and rituximab; DA-EPOCH-R, dose-adjusted doxorubicin, etoposide, vincristine, cyclophosphamide, prednisone, and rituximab; HD CT, high dose chemotherapy; AuBMT, autologous bone marrow transplantation; DFS, disease-free survival.

bone and/or BM may be seen. Poor prognostic factors include translocations of t(1;19), t(9;22), and 11q13 abnormalities, and tumors that lack expression of CD10, CD34, and CD24. Patients with more than 50 chromosomes have a better prognosis. The EFS at 5 years is 85% and 64% for localized and advanced disease, respectively.

- **Burkitt lymphoma** occurs primarily in children, although occasional cases, which are often called Burkitt-like lymphoma, are seen in adults. Burkitt and Burkitt-like lymphomas are believed to be similar diseases, with the latter showing some "atypical" pathologic features. The disease was initially identified in equatorial Africa, where it was found to be associated with EBV and translocation of the c-*myc* oncogene, and is regarded as the endemic form of lymphoma. In the western countries, a sporadic "nonendemic" form, which is infrequently associated with EBV, occurs commonly, and Burkitt lymphoma often involves mesenteric LN and the distal ileum and cecum. Burkitt lymphoma is highly curable with aggressive chemotherapy, with PFS being more than 90% (see Tables 28.10 and 28.11).

TABLE 28.10. *Adults and children with Burkitt and Burkitt-like non-Hodgkin lymphoma have similar outcomes when treated with cyclophosphamide, vincristine, doxorubicin, high-dose methotrexate/ifosfamide, etoposide, and high-dose cytarabine (CODOX-M/IVAC) regimen*

Number	CR (%)	EFS at 2 yr (%)
Children: 21	90	85
Adults: 20	100	100
Total: 41	95	92

Adapted from Magrath I, Adde M, Shad A, et al. Adults and children with small noncleaved cell lymphoma have a similar excellent outcome when treated with the same chemotherapy regimen. *J Clin Oncol* 1996;14(3):925–934, with permission.

TABLE 28.11. *Estimate of 1-year event-free survival for subgroups of high-risk patients treated with cyclophosphamide, vincristine, doxorubicin, high-dose methotrexate/ifosfamide, etoposide, and high-dose cytarabine (CODOX-M/IVAC) regimen*

Variable	n	1-yr EFS (%)	(95% CI)	Log-rank P value
International Prognostic Index score				
0–1	6	83.3	(53.5–99.0)	—
2	19	63.2	(41.5–84.9)	—
3	14	57.1	(31.2–83.1)	0.8852

From Mead GM, Sydes MR, Walewski J, et al. An international evaluation of CODOX-M and CODOX-M alternating with IVAC in adult Burkitt's lymphoma: results of United Kingdom Lymphoma Group LY06 study. *Ann Oncol* 2002;13:1264–1274, with permission.

T Cell

Precursor T-lymphoblastic lymphomas/leukemias are most common in young adult men in their third decade of life. In children, these cancers constitute 40% of all lymphomas and 15% of lymphoblastic leukemias. Patients often have a rapidly enlarging mediastinal mass, with or without peripheral LN involvement. The distinction between lymphoma and leukemia is based on the percentage involvement of the BM, with 25% to 30% defining the disease as a leukemia. The EFS at 5 years is 85% and 64% for localized and advanced disease, respectively.

Treatment Principles

The most highly aggressive lymphomas are curable by chemotherapy and should be treated expeditiously and with appropriate therapy. A number of aggressive regimens have shown equal results and are outlined in Tables 28.12, 28.13, and 28.14. The aggressive treatment of adults with Burkitt lymphoma has achieved results similar to those obtained in children and justifies the higher toxicity associated with these regimens. However, older patients often tolerate these aggressive regimens poorly.

TABLE 28.12. Hyper CVAD alternating with high-dose methotrexate and Ara-C

Cycle	Day	Drug	Dose	Route	Time
Odd number cycles 1, 3, 5, and 7	1–3	Cyclophosphamide	300 mg/m^2 (total dose 1,800 mg/m^2)	i.v.	Each dose given over 2 h every 12 h for six doses
	1–3	Mesna	600 mg/m^2	Continuous i.v.	Infused over 24 h daily for 3 d. Start 1 h before cyclophosphamide and continue for 12 h after last dose.
	4	Doxorubicin	50 mg/m^2	i.v.	Over 2 h
	4 and 11	Vincristine	2 mg	i.v.	DI–4 and 11–14
	4–11 and	Dexamethasone	40 mg/d	PO or i.v.	Daily, starting 24 h after the last dose of doxorubicin, until granulocytes are
	11–14	G-CSF	10 µg/kg	s.c.	>30,000/lL or until d 21 (whichever comes first).
Even number cycles 2, 4, 6, and 8	1	Methotrexate	1 g/m^2	Continuous i.v. i.v. or PO	Infused over 24 h
		Leucovorin	50 mg i.v. or PO is given		12 h after the completion of methotrexate, followed by 15 mg i.v. or PO every 6 h for eight doses. The methotrexate level is checked at 24 h and 48 h after the completion of the methotrexate infusion. If the level is >1 µM at 24 h or >0.1 µM at 48 h, the leucovorin dose is increased to 50 mg i.v. every 6 h until the level is <0.1 µM.
	2–3	Ara-C,	3 g/m^2	i.v.	Given over 2 h every 12 h for four doses
		G-CSF	5 µg/kg,	s.c.	Begin after chemotherapy completion until the ANC is >30,000/lL or until d 21 (whichever comes first). Then it is held for 1 d and the next cycle is started.

CNS prophylaxis: Methotrexate 12 mg intrathecal on d 2 and Ara-C 100 mg intrathecal on d 8 of each cycle for 16 intrathecal treatments in high-risk patients; four intrathecal treatments in low-risk patients.

TABLE 28.13. *Cyclophosphamide, vincristine, doxorubicin, high-dose methotrexate (CODOX-M) regimen*

Day	Drug	Dose	Route	Time
1	Cyclophosphamide	800 mg/m^2	i.v.	
	Vincristine	1.5 mg/m^2 (max 2 mg)	i.v.	
	Doxorubicin	40 mg/m^2	i.v.	
	Cytarabine	70 mg	Intrathecal	
2–5	Cyclophosphamide	200 mg/m^2	i.v.	Daily
3	Cytarabine	70 mg	Intrathecal	
8	Vincristine	1.5 mg/m^2 (max 2 mg)	i.v.	
10	Methotrexate	1,200 mg/^{2}	i.v.	Over 1 h
		240 mg/m^2	i.v.	Each h over 23 h
11	Leucovorin	192 mg/m^2	i.v.	At h 36
		12 mg/m^2	i.v.	Every 6 h until MTX level <5 × 10^{-8} M
13	G-CSF	5 μg/kg	s.c.	Daily until AGC > 10^9/L
15	Methotrexate	12 mg	Intrathecal	
16	Leucovorin	15 mg	PO	24 h after intrathecal methotrexate

MTX, methotrexate; G-CSF, granulocyte colony stimulating factor; AGC, absolute granulocyte count; ANC, absolute neutrophil count.

Next cycle should be started on the day the unsupported ANC is >1.0 × 10^9/L, and unsupported platelet >75 × 10^9/L.

TABLE 28.14. *Ifosfamide, etoposide, and high-dose cytarabine (IVAC) regimen*

Day	Drug	Dose	Route	Time
1–5	Etoposide	60 mg/m^2	i.v.	Daily over 1 h
	Ifosfamide	1,500 mg/m^2	i.v.	Daily over 1 h
	Mesna	360 mg/m^2 (mixed with ifosfamide) followed by 360 mg/m^2	i.v.	3 hourly (seven doses/24 h period)
1 and 2	Cytarabine	2 g/m^2	i.v.	Over 3 h, 12 hourly (total of four doses)
5	Methotrexate	12 mg	Intrathecal	
6	Leucovorin	15 mg	PO	24 h after intrathecal MTX
7	G-CSF	5 μg/kg	s.c.	Daily until AGC > 1.0 × 10^9/L

MTX, methotrexate; G-CSF, granulocyte colony-stimulating factor; AGC, absolute granulocyte count.

Next cycle should start (CODOX-M) on the day the unsupported ANC is >1.0 × 10^9/L, and unsupported platelet is >75 ×10^9/L.

SUGGESTED READINGS

Armitage JO, Vose JM, Bierman PJ. Salvage therapy for patients with non-Hodgkin's lymphoma. *J Natl Cancer Inst* 1990;10:39–43.

Bagley CM Jr, Devita VT Jr, Berard CW, et al. Advanced lymphosarcoma: intensive cyclical combination chemotherapy with cyclophosphamide, vincristine, and prednisone. *Ann Intern Med* 1972;76:227–234.

Cabanillas F, Hagemister F, McLaughlin P, et al. Results of MIME salvage regimen for recurrent or refractory lymphoma. *J Clin Oncol* 1987;5:407–412.

Chabner BA, Longo D. *Cancer chemotherapy and biotherapy principles and practice*, 2nd ed. Philadelphia, PA: Lippincott–Raven Publishers, 1996:1–16.

Chao NJ, Rosenberg SA, Horning SJ. CEPP(B): an effective and well-tolerated regimen in poor-risk, aggressive non-Hodgkin's lymphoma. *Blood* 1990;76:1293–1298.

Coiffier B, Lepage E, Briere J, et al. CHOP chemotherapy plus rituximab compared with CHOP alone in elderly patients with diffuse large-B-cell lymphoma. *N Engl J Med* 2002;346:235–242.

Czuczman MS, Grillo-Lopez AJ, White CA, et al. Treatment of patients with low-grade B-cell lymphoma with the combination of chimeric anti-CD20 monoclonal antibody and CHOP chemotherapy. *J Clin Oncol* 1999;17:268.

Dana B, Dahlberg S, Miller T, et al. m-BACOD treatment for intermediate-and high-grade malignant lymphomas: a Southwest Oncology Group phase II trial. *J Clin Oncol* 1990;8:1155–1162.

Danhauser L, Plunkett W, Keating M, et al. 9-beta-D-arabinofuranosyl-2-fluoroadenine 5'-monophosphate pharmacokinetics in plasma and tumor cells of patients with relapsed leukemia and lymphoma. *Cancer Chemother Pharmacol* 1986;18:145–152.

Goldstein L, Galaski H, Fojo A, et al. Expression of a multidrug resistance gene in human cancers. *J Natl Cancer Inst* 1989;81:116–120.

Gutierrez M, Chabner BA, Pearson D, et al. Role of a doxorubicin-containing regimen in relapsed and resistant lymphomas: an 8-year follow-up of study of EPOCH. *J Clin Oncol* 2000;18:3633–3642.

Hersh MR, Kuhn JG, Phillips JL, et al. Pharmacokinetic study of fludarabine phosphate (NSC 312887). *Cancer Chemother Pharmacol* 1986;17:277–280.

Hohenstein M, Augustine S, Rutar F, et al. Establishing an institutional model for the administration of tositumomab and iodine I 131 tositumomab. *Semin Oncol* 2003;30:39–49.

Hutton JJ, Von Hoff DD, Kuhn J, et al. Phase I clinical investigation of 9-beta-D-arabinofuranosyl-2-fluoroadenine 5'-monophosphate (NSC 312887), a new purine antimetabolite. *Cancer Res* 1984;44:4183–4186.

Kaiser U, Uebelacker I, Abel U, et al. Randomized study to evaluate the use of high-dose therapy as part of primary treatment for "aggressive" lymphoma. *J Clin Oncol* 2002;20(22):4413–4419.

Kewalramani T, Zelenetz AD, Nimer SD, et al. Rituximab and ICE (RICE) as second-line therapy prior to autologous stem cell transplantation for relapsed or primary refractory diffuse large-B-cell lymphoma. *Blood* 2004;103:3684–3688.

Kitada S, Andersen J, Reed JC, et al. Expression of apoptosis-regulating proteins in chronic lymphocytic leukemia: correlations with in vitro and in vivo chemoresponses. *Blood* 1998;91:3379–3389.

Klimo P, Connors J. MACOP-B chemotherapy for the treatment of diffuse large cell lymphoma. *Ann Intern Med* 1985;102:596–602.

Legha SS, Benjamin RS, MacKay B, et al. Reduction of doxorubicin cardiotoxicity by prolonged continuous intravenous infusion. *Ann Intern Med* 1982;96:133–139.

Magrath I, Adde M, Shad A, et al. Adults and children with small noncleaved cell lymphoma have a similar excellent outcome when treated with the same chemotherapy regiment. *J Clin Oncol* 1996;14:925–934.

McKelvey EM, Gottlieb JA, Wilson HE, et al. Hydroxyldaunomycin (Adriamycin) combination chemotherapy in malignant lymphoma. *Cancer* 1976;38:1484–1493.

McLaughlin P, Grillo-Lopez AJ, Link BK, et al. Rituximab chimeric anti-CD20 monoclonal antibody therapy for relapsed indolent lymphoma: half of patients respond to a four-dose treatment program. *J Clin Oncol* 1998;16:2825–2833.

Mead GM, Sydes MR, Walewski J, et al. An international evaluation of CODOX-M and CODOX-M alternating with IVAC in adult Burkitt's lymphoma: results of United Kingdom Lymphoma Group LY06 study. *Ann Oncol* 2002;13:1264–1274.

Non-Hodgkin's Lymphoma Classification Project. A clinical evaluation of the international lymphoma study group classification of non-Hodgkin's lymphoma. N Engl J Med 1993;329:987.

Reed JC. Dysregulation of apoptosis in cancer. *Cancer J Sci Am* 1999;4:S8–S13.

Rosenwald A, Wright G, Chan WC, et al. The use of molecular profiling to predict survival after chemotherapy for diffuse large-B-cell lymphoma. *N Engl J Med* 2002;346:1937–1947.

Thomas DA, Cortes J, O'Brien S, et al. Hyper-CVAD program in Burkitt's-type adult acute lymphoblastic leukemia. *J Clin Oncol* 1999;17:2461–2470.

Velasquez WS, Cabanillas F, Salvador P, et al. Effective salvage therapy for lymphoma with cisplatin in combination with high-dose Ara-C and dexamethasone (DHAP). *Blood* 1988;71:117–122.

Velasquez WS, McLaughlin P, Tucker S, et al. ESHAP—an effective chemotherapy regimen in refractory and relapsing lymphoma: a 4-year follow-up study. *J Clin Oncol* 1994;12:1169–1176.

Vose JM, Link BK, Grossbard ML, et al. Phase II study of rituximab in combination with CHOP chemotherapy in patients with previously untreated, aggressive non-Hodgkin's lymphoma. *J Clin Oncol* 2001;19:389–397.

Wagner HN Jr, Wiseman GA, Marcus CS, et al. Administration guidelines for radioimmunotherapy of non-Hodgkin's lymphoma with 90Y-labeled anti-CD20 monoclonal antibody. *J Nucl Med* 2002;43:267–272.

Weick J, Dahlberg S, Fisher R, et al. Combination chemotherapy of intermediate-grade and high-grade non-Hodgkin's lymphoma with MACOP-B: a Southwest Oncology Group study. *J Clin Oncol* 1991; 9:748–753.

Wilson WH, Grossbard ML, Pittaluga S, et al. Dose-adjusted EPOCH chemotherapy for untreated large B-cell lymphomas: a pharmacodynamic approach with high efficacy. *Blood* 2002;99:2685–2693.

29

Hodgkin Lymphoma

Gisa Schun[*], Jame Abraham[†], and Marcel P. Devetten[‡]

[*]Section of Hematology/Oncology, West Virginia University, Morgantown, West Virginia; [†]Section of Hematology/Oncology, Mary Babb Randolph Cancer Center, West Virginia University, Morgantown, West Virginia; and [‡]Department of Medicine, University of Nebraska Medical Center, Omaha, Nebraska

EPIDEMIOLOGY

Hodgkin lymphoma (HL) is among the most common malignancies of young adults. It constitutes approximately 1% of all malignancies and 18% of all lymphomas, and, in the United States, 3 of every 100,000 people develop this condition. In Europe and North America, there is a bimodal age distribution, with an increasing frequency between the second and third decades, and a second peak in the seventh decade.

ETIOLOGY AND RISK FACTORS

- The etiology of HL is unclear and may be multifactorial.
- Same-sex siblings of patients with HL have a ten times higher risk of developing HL than siblings of a different sex. This association may be caused by genetic factors and/or environmental factors.
- Approximately 40% to 50% of the cases of "classic" HL have clonal integration of Epstein–Barr virus (EBV) in the Reed–Sternberg (RS) cells.
- Smoking has recently been linked to HL.

PATHOLOGY

HL is a neoplastic disorder of the lymphoid system, usually arising from B lymphocytes. Typically, a small number of scattered giant neoplastic cells (RS cells) are surrounded by an inflammatory background.

Reed–Sternberg Cells or Variants

- The RS cell is a lymphoid cell, and in most of the cases studied, it is a clonal B cell.
- Cytologically, the RS cell is a multinucleated giant cell with large eosinophilic inclusion-like nucleoli, with a thick, well-defined nuclear membrane and pale-staining chromatin.
- The classic RS cell has two mirror-image nuclei, which are often described as "owl's eyes."
- A background of lymphocytes, eosinophils, and histiocytes is usually present (see Fig. 29.1).

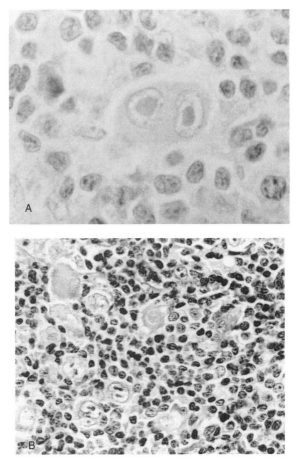

FIG. 29.1. A: Diagnostic Reed–Sternberg cell, seen in classic types of Hodgkin lymphomas (mixed cellularity, nodular sclerosis, lymphocyte depletion). **B:** Variants of Reed–Sternberg cells seen in nodular lymphocyte-predominant Hodgkin lymphomas: popcorn cells or L and H cells (lymphocytic or histiocytic predominance). Reed–Sternberg cells of the classic type generally are not seen in a nodular lymphocyte-predominant Hodgkin lymphoma.

Histopathologic Classification

In 1994, the International Lymphoma Study Group introduced a classification incorporating immunologic and molecular data as part of a Revised European–American Lymphoma classification (REAL) for HL, which replaced the older Rye classification. The REAL classification was incorporated in the classification of the World Health Organization (WHO) in 2001 (see Table 29.1).

The REAL/WHO classification recognizes two distinct diseases with distinguishing histopathologic features and immunophenotypes:

1. Classic Hodgkin Lymphoma (CHL)
2. Lymphocyte-predominant Hodgkin Lymphoma (LPHL).

Features and immunophenotypes of classic HL and LPHL are described in Table 29.2.

TABLE 29.1. *Classification systems*

REAL Classification, 1994	Rye Classification, 1965
Lymphocyte predominance Classic Hodgkin lymphoma	Lymphocyte predominance, nodular
	Lymphocyte predominance, diffuse (most cases)
Lymphocyte-rich classic HL	Lymphocyte predominance, nodular (some cases)
Nodular sclerosis (NSHL)	Nodular sclerosis (NSHL)
Mixed cellularity (MCHL)	Mixed cellularity (MCHL)
Lymphocyte depletion	Lymphocyte depletion

REAL, Revised European–American Lymphoma.

TABLE 29.2. *Features and immunophenotypes of Hodgkin lymphomas*

Cells/Antigen	Classic HL	Lymphocyte-predominant HL
Diagnostic RS cells	Always present	Rare to absent
Lymphocytes (background)	T > B cells	B > T cells
CD30 (Ki-1)	Usually positive	Often positive
CD15 (Leu M1)	Usually positive	Negative
CD45 (LCA)	Usually negative	Positive
CD20 (L26)	Usually negative	Positive
EBV	40%–50% positive	Usually negative

HL, Hodgkin lymphoma.

CLINICAL FEATURES

- More than 80% of patients present with cervical lymph node enlargement, and more than 50% have mediastinal adenopathy.
- Lymph nodes are usually nontender, firm, and rubbery.
- Constitutional symptoms ("B" symptoms):
- Unexplained fever (temperature, >38°C)
  - Drenching night sweats
  - Unexplained weight loss (>10% of body weight, more than 6 months before the diagnosis)
  - Other symptoms are important to note but are not considered "B" symptoms: fatigue, weakness, anorexia, alcohol-induced nodal pain, and pruritus.

Staging [Ann Arbor/American Joint Committee for Cancer (AJCC) and Cotswold] is outlined in Table 29.3.

Pretreatment Evaluation

1. Excisional biopsy of an enlarged lymph node: evaluation of the specimen by a hematopathologist, including immunophenotyping. Generally, needle biopsies are insufficient for a proper diagnosis.
2. History with attention to B symptoms.
3. Complete physical examination and documentation of measurable disease.
4. Laboratory tests include:
   - Complete blood count (CBC), erythrocyte sedimentation rate (ESR)
   - Biochemical tests of liver function, renal function, and serum uric acid, lactate dehydrogenase (LDH), serum albumin.

TABLE 29.3. *Staging*

Stage I	Involvement of single lymph node region or lymphoid structure (spleen, thymus, Waldeyer ring), or involvement of a single extralymphatic site (IE)
Stage II	Involvement of two or more lymph node regions on the same side of the diaphragm (II), which may be accompanied by localized contiguous involvement of an extralymphatic organ or site (IIE). The number of anatomic sites may be indicated by numeric subscript
Stage III	Involvement of lymph node regions on both sides of the diaphragm (III), which may also be accompanied by localized involvement of an associated extralymphatic organ or site (IIIE), by involvement of the spleen (IIIS), or both (IIIE+S)
Stage IV	Disseminated involvement of one or more extralymphatic organs, with or without associated lymph node involvement, or isolated extralymphatic organ involvement with distant (nonregional) nodal involvement
	Each stage is divided into A and B categories: B for those with defined systemic symptoms, and A for those without
X	A mass >10 cm or a mediastinal mass larger than one third of the thoracic diameter
E	Involvement of a single extranodal site contiguous to a known nodal site
CS	Clinical staging
PS	Pathologic staging

5. Radiologic studies:
   - Chest radiograph and computerized tomography (CT) scan of the chest, abdomen, and pelvis are used for evaluation. CT scan of the neck is useful, particularly if the neck or upper chest is involved.
   - Baseline gallium scans or positron emission tomography (PET) scans can be useful. PET scan is increasingly favored for staging because of evidence of higher sensitivity and accuracy, particularly in the spleen.
   - Bone scan or radiographs are used if bone pain or tenderness is present.
6. Bone marrow biopsy of at least one posterior iliac crest for those with abnormal CBC or clinical stage IIB, III, or IV.

Staging laparotomy and splenectomy were done routinely in the past for patients with early stage disease above the diaphragm and for whom definitive radiation treatment was considered. Now, with newer radiologic testing such as PET scans, it is rarely used.

Unfavorable Prognostic Features

The most important unfavorable prognostic features are advanced stage, B symptoms, and presence of bulky disease.

1. Advanced stage (IIIB and IV)
2. Presence of B symptoms (i.e., fever, weight loss, and drenching night sweats)
3. Bulky disease defined as >10-cm diameter, particularly in the mediastinum (more than one third of chest diameter)
4. Extranodal involvement (liver, spleen, and bone marrow)
5. Patients older than 40 years
6. Increased ESR (B symptoms + ESR >30, or no B symptoms and ESR >70)
7. Histology
   Unfavorable: mixed cellularity and lymphocyte depletion
   Favorable: lymphocyte-predominant and nodular sclerosis
8. Low serum albumin.

MANAGEMENT OF NEWLY DIAGNOSED HODGKIN LYMPHOMA

HL is treated with a curative intent. In view of the high cure rates, studies have increasingly addressed long-term toxicities to define best treatment strategies. Treatment selection is therefore not only influenced by stage and unfavorable prognostic factors but also by toxicity.

Risk Stratification and Prognosis

Two major risk groups are distinguished, early and advanced disease:

1. Stages I and II without B symptoms or bulky disease are considered "favorable early stage" and are at low risk for recurrence. Cure rate is greater than 90%.
2. Stage IIB and stages I to IIB with bulk are variably considered "early" or "advanced" by different study groups. Most U.S. groups treat them as "unfavorable early disease." Cure rate is greater than 80%.
3. Stages III and IV are considered "advanced stage" and are at significant risk for recurrence. Cure rate is about 60% to 70%.

Other criteria might be included to subdivide the two major risk groups further to avoid under- or overtreatment of patients with early stage disease.

For example, the Canada Clinical Trials Group and the Eastern Cooperative Oncology Group (ECOG) separate early stage Hodgkin Disease HD into:

Low risk: includes nodular lymphocyte-predominant Hodgkin disease (NLPHD) and nodular sclerosing histology, affects individuals younger than 40 years, ESR is less than 50, and three or less disease-site regions are involved.

High risk: includes all other diseases in stages I to II, excluding bulky disease >10 cm.

Radiation Treatment

Radiation is the most effective single therapeutic modality for HL. In general, the management of HL with radiation therapy consists of treating regions of known disease ("involved field"). An "extended field" treats unaffected adjacent nodal groups in addition to the involved regions (see Table 29.4).

Radiation covering extended fields is used to three major fields, known as the mantle, paraaortic, and pelvic or inverted-Y fields (see Fig. 29.2).

The usual dose of radiation is 25 to 30 Gy to uninvolved areas and 35 to 44 Gy to the involved field. Radiation doses can be lower when used in conjunction with chemotherapy

- Radiation therapy alone is reserved for early stages of HL without unfavorable prognostic features.
- In patients with advanced disease, radiation contributes to disease-free survival shown for bulky disease and nodular sclerosis histology, but whether it prolongs overall survival is not evident. Adding long-term toxicity with radiation remains a concern because of the high cure rate even in advanced disease.
- When choosing modalities, one should consider the higher risk of young women (younger than 27 years old) for breast cancer and the higher risk of lung cancer in smokers as late toxicity from radiation to the chest.
- Patients who relapse after treatment with radiation therapy alone are frequently salvaged successfully with combination chemotherapy.

TABLE 29.4. *Radiation guidelines*

Tumoricidal dose	40–45 By at the rate of 10 Gy/wk
Clinically negative nodal regions	35 Gy
Consolidation (after chemotherapy)	15–20 Gy

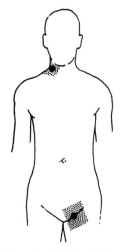

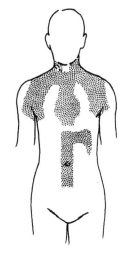

A Involved field irradiation

B Subtotal nodal irradiation
including mantle and spade fields

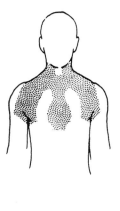

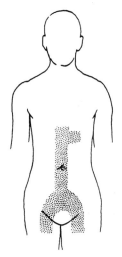

C Mantle field irradiation   D Inverted-Y field irradiation

FIG. 29.2. Radiation therapy fields used in treating Hodgkin disease (**A, B, C,** and **D**). When the fields shown in **C** and **D** are combined, this is commonly called total nodal irradiation (TNI). (From Haskell CM. *Cancer Treatment.* 4th ed. Philadelphia: WB Saunders, 1995:965, with permission.)

Chemotherapy

The first "curative regimen" was mechlorethamine, Oncovin, procarbazine, prednisone (MOPP), which resulted in a 70% complete remission in patients with stage III and stage IV cancer. Subsequently, many regimens have been developed, including MOPP variants, doxorubicin (Adriamycin), bleomycin, vinblastine, and dacarbazine (ABVD) and its variants, and hybrids of MOPP/ABVD.

Choosing between MOPP, ABVD, and MOPP/ABVD

In a randomized study, the Cancer and Leukemia Group B (CALGB) showed ABVD and MOPP/ABVD to be superior to MOPP alone in terms of remission, freedom from progression, and survival. At 10 years, the risk of developing treatment-related leukemia with the MOPP regimen is 2% to 3%, whereas it is 0.7% with ABVD. Infertility rates are much lower with ABVD than with MOPP (see Table 29.5).

A recent randomized intergroup trial demonstrated that MOPP/ABV is associated with a greater incidence of acute toxicity, myelodysplasia (MDS), and leukemia than ABVD is, with no difference in failure-free survival or overall survival at 5 years. ABVD should be considered the standard regimen for treatment of advanced HD (see Table 29.6).

Combined Modality Treatment

A meta-analysis of 23 trials of patients with early stage HD showed that the 10-year rate of freedom from relapse was higher with combined modality therapy than with radiation, but survival rates were not significantly different.

Primary Treatment Options

1. Favorable early disease
   a. Two to four cycles ABVD with involved field radiation to follow
   b. Extended field radiation alone.
2. Unfavorable early disease
   a. Four to six cycles ABVD with involved or extended field radiation. One European randomized trial showed no difference in freedom from treatment failure or overall survival when extended field radiation was replaced by involved field radiation (30 Gy to field, 10 Gy to bulk).
3. Advanced disease
   a. ABVD for six to eight cycles is the current standard. Treatment is usually continued two cycles after resolution of disease by imaging studies.
   b. Addition of involved field radiation is usually considered, particularly for bulky disease. Recent evidence from a randomized trial suggests there may be no need to add radiation, if a complete response can be achieved with combination chemotherapy.
   c. Stanford V is an effective regimen with shorter treatment duration (3 months) and is currently undergoing randomized comparison with ABVD-based treatment in intergroup trial E2496.

TABLE 29.5. *Cancer and Leukemia Group B study comparing combination treatments*

Regimen	Complete response rate (%)	Survival rate (%)
MOPP	67	64
ABVD	82	72
MOPP/ABVD	83	73

MOPP, mechlorethamine, Oncovin, procarbazine, and prednisone; ABVD, doxorubicin (Adriamycin), bleomycin, vinblastine, and dacarbazine.

TABLE 29.6. *Commonly used treatment regimens*

ABVD

Doxorubicin, 25 mg/m^2/dose i.v. push for two doses, d 1 and 15 (total dose/cycle, 50 mg/m^2)
Bleomycin, 10 units/m^2/dose i.v. push for two doses, d 1 and 15 (total dose/cycle, 20 units/m^2)
Vinblastine, 6 mg/m^2/dose i.v. push for two doses, d 1 and 15 (total dose/cycle, 12 mg/m^2)
Dacarbazine, 375 mg/m^2/dose i.v. infusion for two doses, d 1 and 15 (total dose/cycle, 750 mg/m^2)
Treatment cycle repeats every 28 d

MOPP

Mechlorethamine, 6 mg/m^2/dose i.v. push for two doses, d 1 and 8 (total dose/cycle, 12 mg/m^2)
Vincristine, 1.4 mg/m^2/dose i.v. push for two doses, d 1 and 8 (total dose/cycle, 2.8 mg/m^2)
Procarbazine, 100 mg/m^2/d PO for 14 doses, d 1–14 (total dose/cycle, 1,400 mg/m^2)
Prednisone, 40 mg/m^2/d PO for 14 doses, d 1–14 (cycles 1 and 14 only) (total dose/cycle, 560 mg/m^2)
Treatment cycle repeats every 28 d

Alternating MOPP/ABVD

Alternate MOPP and ABVD cycles by 28 d

MOPP/ABV hybrid

Mechlorethamine, 6 mg/m^2 i.v. push d 1 (total dose/cycle, 6 mg/m^2)
Vincristine, 1.4 mg/m^2 i.v. push d 1 (total dose/cycle, 1.4 mg/m^2; maximal dose, 2 mg)
Procarbazine, 100 mg/m^2/d PO for 7 doses, d 1–7 (total dose/cycle, 700 mg/m^2)
Prednisone, 40 mg/m^2/d PO for 14 doses, d 1–14 (total dose/cycle, 560 mg/m^2)
Doxorubicin, 25 mg/m^2 i.v. push d 8 (total dose/cycle, 25 mg/m^2)
Hydrocortisone, 100 mg i.v. d 8, before bleomycin (total dose/cycle, 100 mg)
Bleomycin, 10 units/m^2 i.v. push d 8 (total dose/cycle, 10 units/m^2)
Vinblastine, 6 mg/m^2 i.v. push d 8 (total dose/cycle, 6 mg/m^2)
Treatment cycle repeats every 28 d

Stanford V

Mustard, 6 mg/m^2 i.v. wk 1, 5, 9
Vincristine, 1.4 mg/m^2 i.v. wk 2, 4, 6, 8, 10, 12 (maximal dose, 2 mg)
Prednisone, 40 mg/m^2/d PO every other d wk 1–9, taper
Doxorubicin, 25 mg/m^2 i.v. wk, 1, 3, 5, 7, 9, 11
Bleomycin, 5 units/m^2 i.v. wk 2, 4, 6, 8, 10, 12
Vinblastine, 6 mg/m^2 i.v. wk, 1, 3, 5, 7, 9, 11
VP-16 60 mg/m^2 i.v. × 2 wk 3, 7, 11

1. The maximum dose of vincristine is 2 mg
2. All drugs are administered on d 1, except for VP-16, which is given on d 1 and 2
3. Taper prednisone by 10 mg of the total dose q.o.d. (every other day) on wk 10 and 11
4. Reduce the dose of vinblastine to 4 mg/m^2 if on wk 9 and 11 for patients over the age of 50 yr old
5. Reduce the dose of vincristine to 1 mg on wk 10 and 12 for patients over the age of 50 yr
6. If mustard is not available, a substitution with 650 mg/m^2 of cyclophosphamide can be made on wk 1, 5, 9
7. Patients will receive total of 12 wk of treatment.

---

4. Lymphocyte-predominant Hodgkin lymphoma: This subtype has the propensity to cause multiple relapses even up to 15 years.
   a. Early stages of LPHL without risk factors are treated with radiation alone.
   b. Advanced stages are rare at diagnosis and carry a poor prognosis. They are treated like nodular sclerosing histology.
   c. Phase II trials show single-agent activity of rituximab for the usually CD20-positive LPHL. It is possibly effective in the chemotherapy-refractory setting, although the effect is of short duration. The use of rituximab has to be considered investigational and affected patients should be referred for trials because of the rarity of the disease.

High-dose Therapy and Autologous Stem Cell Transplantation

High-dose therapy with autologous transplant has no defined role for consolidation in the treatment programs for newly diagnosed unfavorable-risk HL that respond to standard chemotherapy. One randomized trial from the United Kingdom demonstrated no advantage in patients with highly unfavorable prognosis in achieving complete response with the European regimen PVACE-BOP.

Evaluation of Treatment Response with Positron Emission Tomography

PET is a new tool in managing patients with lymphomas. A negative PET scan at completion of therapy indicates a favorable prognosis. Persistently positive PET scans at the end of chemotherapy seem to have a high sensitivity for predicting subsequent relapse and need close follow-up; however, some of those patients may remain in prolonged remission. More prospective studies are needed to define the usefulness and limitations of PET scans more precisely.

TREATMENT OF RELAPSED HODGKIN LYMPHOMA

In general, relapsed HL is still curable.

Relapses usually occur within 2 to 3 years after primary therapy. There are currently no clear parameters to predict the 15% to 20% of patients who will progress during treatment or relapse early. Patients with relapse within 1 year of primary treatment or with a second relapse have a survival of less than 20% at 5 years. For successful choice of management, one should consider the following:

1. Sites of relapse (i.e., prior radiated area, single or multiple nodes, extranodal, bulky).
2. Details of previous treatment.
   If the relapse is due to inadequate initial treatment, retreatment with chemotherapy or radiation is considered.
   Relapse after primary radiation is best managed with chemotherapy.
3. Achievement and duration of first remission:
   Early relapse (<1 year) or persistent disease after primary therapy with adequate numbers of cycles of combination chemotherapy should be treated with salvage chemotherapy followed by autologous stem cell transplantation with curative intent.
   Late relapse (particularly with favorable features: no B symptoms, long disease-free interval, no bulk, disease confined to lymph nodes, best only one site) has a chance for cure with salvage chemotherapy (and radiation if applicable). But consolidation with autologous stem cell transplantation should always be considered. Chemosensitive relapse treated with transplantation has the best prognosis.
4. Primary refractory HL is associated with a poor overall survival. However, some (15% to 20%) patients experience prolonged disease-free survival (DFS) after high-dose chemotherapy with autologous stem cell transplantation.

SALVAGE CHEMOTHERAPY REGIMENS

Non–Anthracycline-Containing Regimens

1. ESHAP (etoposide, methylprednisolone, high-dose cytarabine, and cisplatin)
2. ICE (ifosfamide, carboplatin, and etoposide)
3. EIP (etoposide, ifosfamide, and cisplatin)
4. DHAP (dexamethasone, high-dose cytarabine, and cisplatin)
5. MINE [mitoguazone (500 mg per m^2 on days 1 and 5), ifosfamide (1,500 mg/m^2 per day from day 1 to day 5), vinorelbine (15 mg per m^2 on days 1 and 5), and etoposide (150 mg/m^2/day from day 1 to day 3) for two 28-day cycles]

Anthracycline-Containing Regimens

EVA (etoposide, vincristine, and doxorubicin)
ASHAP (doxorubicin, cisplatin, high-dose cytarabine, and methylprednisolone)

Prognostic Factors in Relapse (Stanford Study)

1. 10-year DFS worsens with disease stage at the time of initial radiation:
   - Stage IA, 88%.
   - Stages IIA and IIIA, 58%.
   - Stage IV or B symptoms, 34%.
2. 10-year DFS depends on histology
   - LPHL and Nodular Sclerosis Hodgkin Lymphoma (NSHL), 67%.
   - Mixed Cellular Hodgkin Lymphoma (MCHL) and LPHL, 44%

Palliative Treatments

1. Investigational treatment
2. Radiation treatment
3. Sequential single-agent chemotherapy
   Gemcitabine emerges as new active agent in refractory HL
4. Steroids

COMPLICATIONS OF THERAPY

Radiation Therapy

Early Complications

- Mantle field radiation: mouth dryness, pharyngitis, cough, and dermatitis
- Subdiaphragmatic radiation: anorexia, nausea, and diarrhea
- Myelosuppression

Late Complications of Radiation for Hodgkin Lymphoma

- Hypothyroidism
- Pericarditis and pneumonitis
- Lhermitte sign: Six to 12 weeks after the treatment, 15% of the patients receiving mantle radiation may experience electric shock sensation radiating down the back of the legs when their head is flexed. This sensation may be caused by the transient demyelinization of the spinal cord, and it usually resolves spontaneously.
- Coronary artery disease (CAD): Increased risk in patients who receive cardiac radiation. Patients should be monitored and evaluated for other risk factors for CAD.

Secondary Neoplasm

Secondary neoplasms arise 20 years after radiation treatment in 75% of cases in the radiation field at a rate of 20% to 25%. Studies raise the possibility that splenic field radiation and splenectomy increase the risk of treatment-related cancer.

- Lung cancer:
  • Twofold to eightfold increase in lung cancer is observed more than 5 years after the radiation treatment and persists through the second decade.
  • The increase in lung cancer occurs mostly in smokers, who should be encouraged to stop smoking.
- Breast cancer:
  • The increase in breast cancer is inversely proportional to the age at radiation treatment. The relative risk (RR) is 136 if the patient is younger than 15 years. RR is 19 for age group 15 to 24 years and is 7 for age group 24 to 29 years.
  • Women irradiated before age 30 years are at high risk.
  • Average interval between radiation and diagnosis of breast cancer is 15 years.
  • Breast examination should be part of follow-up for women at risk.
  • Routine mammography should begin about 8 years after completion of the radiation.
- Thyroid cancer
- Stomach and esophageal cancer
- Sarcomas

Chemotherapy

Early Complications

• Nausea and vomiting
• Alopecia
• Myelosuppression
• Infection
• Pneumonitis (bleomycin)

Late Complications

Long-term follow-up for chemotherapy has not been documented beyond 15 years and is therefore not yet comparable with long-term data for radiation toxicity.

• Sterility
  – High risk with MOPP-based regimens
  – ABVD has a very low risk for permanent amenorrhea in women younger than 25 years. Male fertility returns to normal in most patients.
• Neuropathy (primarily with vincristine)
• Cardiomyopathy (doxorubicin)
• Pulmonary fibrosis (bleomycin)
• Secondary leukemia (MOPP ± radiation).

SUGGESTED READINGS

Aisenberg AC. Problems in Hodgkin's disease management. *Blood* 1999;93:761–779.

Aleman BM, Raemaekers JM, Tirelli U, et al. Involved-field radiotherapy for advanced Hodgkin's lymphoma. *N Engl J Med* 2003;3482396–2406.

Canellos GP, Anderson JR, Propert KJ, et al. Chemotherapy of advanced Hodgkin's disease with MOPP, ABVD, or MOPP alternating with ABVD. *N Engl J Med* 1992;327:1478–1484.

Cardep, Hagenbeek A, Hayat M, et al. Clinical staging versus laparotomy and combined modality with MOPP versus ABVD in early-stage Hodgkin's disease: the H6 twin randomized trials from the European Organization for Research and Treatment of Cancer Lymphoma Cooperative Group. *J Clin Oncol* 1993;11:2258–2272.

Connors JM. An update on the Vancouver experience in the management of advanced Hodgkin's disease treated with the MOPP/ABV hybrid program. *Semin Hematol* 1988;25:34–40.

Connors JM, Klimo P. MOPP/ABV hybrid chemotherapy for advanced Hodgkin's disease. *Semin Hematol* 1987;24:35–40.

Connors JM, Klimo P, Adams G, et al. Treatment of advanced Hodgkin's disease with chemotherapy: comparison of MOPP/ABV hybrid regimen with alternating courses of MOPP and ABVD: a report from the National Cancer Institute of Canada clinical trials group [published erratum appears in *J Clin Oncol* 1997;15:2762]. *J Clin Oncol* 1997;15:1638–1645.

Duggan DB, Petroni GR, Johnson JL, et al. Randomized comparison of ABVD and MOPP/ABV hybrid for the treatment of advanced Hodgkin's disease: report of an intergroup trial. *J Clin Oncol* 2003;21607–614.

Fabian CJ, Mansfield CM, Dahlberg S, et al. Low-dose involved field radiation after chemotherapy in advanced Hodgkin disease. A Southwest Oncology Group randomized study. *Ann Intern Med* 1994;120:903–912.

Federico M, Bellei M, Brice P, et al. High-dose therapy and autologous stem-cell transplantation versus conventional therapy for patients with advanced Hodgkin's lymphoma responding to front-line therapy. *J Clin Oncol* 2003;21:2320–2325.

Harris NL. Hodgkin's disease: classification and differential diagnosis. *Mod Pathol* 1999;12:159–176.

Horning SJ, Hoppe RT, Breslin S, et al. Stanford V and radiotherapy for locally extensive and advanced Hodgkin's disease: mature results of a prospective clinical trial. *J Clin Oncol* 2002;20:607–609.

Klimo P, Connors JM. MOPP/ABV hybrid program: combination chemotherapy based on early introduction of seven effective drugs for advanced Hodgkin's disease. *J Clin Oncol* 1985;3:1174–1182.

Lister TA, Crowther D, Suteliffe SB, et al. Report of a committee convened to discuss the evaluation and staging of patients with Hodgkin's disease: Cotswolds meeting. *J Clin Oncol* 1989;7:1630–1636.

Mauch PM. Controversies in the management of early stage Hodgkin's disease. *Blood* 1994;83:318–329.

Proctor SJ, Mackie M, Dawson A, et al. A population-based study of intensive multi-agent chemotherapy with or without autotransplant for the highest risk Hodgkin's disease patients identified by the Scotland and Newcastle Lymphoma Group (SNLG) prognostic index. A Scotland and Newcastle Lymphoma Group study (SNLG HD III). *Eur J Cancer* 2002;38(6):795–806.

Schmitz N, Pfistner B, Sextro M, et al. Aggressive conventional chemotherapy compared with high-dose chemotherapy with autologous haemopoietic stem-cell transplantation for relapsed chemosensitive Hodgkin's disease: a randomised trial. *Lancet* 2002;359(9323):2065–2071.

Specht L, Gray RG, Clarke MJ et al. International Hodgkin's Disease Collaborative Group. Influence of more extensive radiotherapy and adjuvant chemotherapy on long-term outcome of early-stage Hodgkin's disease: a meta-analysis of 23 randomized trials involving 3,888 patients. *J Clin Oncol* 1998;16:830–843.

Swerdlow AJ, Douglas AJ, Hudson GV, et al. Risk of second primary cancers after Hodgkin's disease by type of treatment: analysis of 2846 patients in the British National Lymphoma Investigation. *BMJ* 1992;304:1137–1143.

van Leeuwen FE, Klokman WJ, Hagenbeek A, et al. Second cancer risk following Hodgkin's disease: a 20-year follow-up study. *J Clin Oncol* 1994;12:312–325.

Diehl V, Stein H, Hummel M, et al. Hodgkin's lymphoma: biology and treatment strategies for primary, refractory, and relapsed disease. Proceedings of the American Society of Hematology, Education Program Book, 2003.

Viviani S, Bonnadonna G, Santoro A, et al. Alternating versus hybrid MOPP and ABVD combinations in advanced Hodgkin's disease: ten year results. *J Clin Oncol* 1996;14:1421–1430.

30

Hematopoietic Stem Cell Transplantation

Michael Craig*, Jame Abraham†, and Richard W. Childs‡

*Section of Hematology/Oncology, Department of Medicine, West Virginia University, Morgantown, West Virginia; †Mary Babb Randolph Cancer Center, West Virginia University, Morgantown, West Virginia; and ‡National Heart, Lung, and Blood Institute, National Institutes of Health, Bethesda, Maryland

Hematopoietic stem cell transplantation (HSCT) remains an effective treatment option for many patients with a wide range of malignant and nonmalignant conditions. In addition to autologous and matched related donor allogeneic transplantations, many patients may be offered unrelated donor, nonmyeloablative, or cord blood transplantation. An estimated 40,000 to 50,000 transplantations were performed worldwide in 2002. Although transplantation may be associated with significant morbidity and mortality, recent advances in supportive care, human leukocyte antigen (HLA) typing, and treatments for graft versus host disease (GVHD) have led to improved outcomes for patients undergoing the procedure. An overview of autologous and allogeneic transplantation is provided in this chapter, along with a discussion of the complications and their management.

HEMATOPOIETIC STEM CELLS

Hematopoietic stem cells (HSCs) are immature precursor cells residing within the marrow space that are capable of giving rise to most of the cellular elements within the blood, including lymphoid, erythroid, and myeloid lines. These cells are defined by their ability to rescue lethally irradiated animals from marrow aplasia. In humans, most HSCs express the CD34 antigen and lack lineage-specific markers, although a population of CD34⁻ stem cells has also been described. The number of CD34⁺ cells that are present in the graft has an impact on transplant outcome; in the allogeneic setting, fewer CD34⁺ cells are associated with a higher risk of transplant-related mortality and delays in the time to hematopoietic recovery in contrast to more CD34⁺ cells where transplant-related mortality and the risk of disease relapse is decreased. HSCs can be obtained from peripheral blood, bone marrow, or umbilical cord blood (discussed in subsequent text).

Peripheral Blood Stem Cell Collection

- Growth factors [granulocyte colony stimulating factor (G-CSF) or granulocyte-macrophage colony stimulating factor (GM-CSF)] are used to "mobilize" or increase the number of HSCs and progenitor cells in the peripheral blood.
- Cells are collected by apheresis procedure on day 5 or 6.
- In the autologous transplant setting, chemotherapy may be given (providing an additional antineoplastic effect) before growth factors, with apheresis being performed during hematopoietic recovery.

- Fewer complications and morbidity are experienced by the donor.
- Peripheral blood stem cell (PBSC) grafts result in more rapid engraftment than marrow grafts.
- The minimum goal of PBSC collection is 2×10^6 CD34$^+$ cells per kg (range 2.0 to 8.0).
- More T cells (CD3$^+$) are collected in the allogeneic setting.

Bone Marrow Harvest

- Traditional source of HSCs; used less often than peripheral blood grafts.
- Bone marrow is harvested from posterior iliac crests under general anesthesia.
- A harvest of 15 mL per kg of aspirated marrow is generally considered safe to the donor.
- The goal cell dose is 2.0×10^8 mononuclear cells per kg of recipient weight.
- Complications to the donor may include pain, neuropathy, and anemia.
- Severe complications occur in less than 0.5% of procedures.

CURRENT INDICATIONS FOR TRANSPLANTATION

Many malignant and nonmalignant disorders have been treated successfully with HSCT [the National Marrow Donor Program (NMDP) currently lists more than 70 diseases]. Most transplantations are performed for malignant conditions, including acute myeloid and lymphocytic leukemias, chronic myelogenous leukemia (CML), multiple myeloma, non-Hodgkin lymphoma, and Hodgkin lymphoma. Stem cell disorders (e.g., aplastic anemia and paroxysmal nocturnal hemoglobinuria), inherited immune-system defects (e.g., severe combined immunodeficiency and Wiskott-Aldrich syndrome), erythrocyte disorders (e.g., sickle cell anemia and β-thalassemia), and congenital metabolic diseases have been cured by allogeneic HSCT.

PRETRANSPLANTATION EVALUATION

Prior to treatment, a thorough discussion highlighting the transplantation procedure itself as well as risks and benefits associated with the procedure should take place between the physician and the patient.

1. Human leukocyte antigen testing (HLA typing) of the patient and a search for a HLA-matched donor (beginning with siblings) is required if an allogeneic transplant is being considered.
2. Medical history and evaluation
   - Review of original diagnosis and previous treatments, including radiation
   - Concomitant medical problems
   - Current medications and allergies
   - Determination of current disease status (i.e., in remission, relapse, minimal residual disease, etc.)
   - Restaging and confirmation of metastatic spread
   - Transfusion history and complications, as well as ABO typing
   - Psychosocial evaluation and delineation of a caregiver.
3. Physical examination
   - Thorough physical examination
   - Evaluation of oral cavity and dentition
   - Neurologic evaluation if disease could involve the central nervous system
   - Karnofsky performance status (preferred value >70%).
4. Organ function analysis
   - Renal function: creatinine clearance >60 mL per minute
   - Hepatic function: alanine aminotransferase (AST) and aspartate aminotransferase (ALT) less than twice the upper level of normal and bilirubin <2

- Cardiac evaluation [electrocardiogram (ECG) and echocardiography (ECHO) or multiple-gated acquisition imaging (MUGA) with ejection fraction >40%]
- Chest x-ray and pulmonary function testing including diffusing capacity of lung for carbon monoxide (DLCO) and forced vital capacity (FVC).

5. Infectious disease evaluation
   - Serology for cytomegalovirus (CMV), human immunodeficiency virus (HIV), and hepatitis
   - Serology for herpes simplex virus (HSV), Epstein–Barr virus (EBV), and varicella
   - Assess for prior history of invasive fungal (aspergillus) infection.

6. Consideration of referral to reproductive center for sperm banking or *in vitro* fertilization.

AUTOLOGOUS STEM CELL TRANSPLANTATION

High-dose chemotherapy (HDCT) without stem cell rescue may result in prolonged cytopenias. Autologous stem cells are collected and are reinfused into the patient after the completion of HDCT to reconstitute the hematopoietic system.

- Autologous transplantation is most effective in chemotherapy-sensitive tumors or as a consolidation therapy for patients in remission.
- HDCT may also overcome intrinsic tumor resistance to chemotherapy.
- Most grafts use PBSCs collected by apheresis.
- The product is frozen viably in dimethyl sulfoxide (DMSO) and thawed just prior to infusion.
- Reactions during transfusion are rare and may include bronchospasm, flushing, or hypotension secondary to DMSO.
- Pancytopenia typically persists for 10 to 20 days and is shortened using PBSC and growth factors.
- Antimicrobials and blood products are typically given to support the patient in the first few weeks following transplantation.
- Infectious complications may occur as a consequence of the patient being profoundly immunosuppressed.
- New protocols are currently exploring tandem autologous transplants (two stem cell rescues after HDCT) and autologous followed by nonmyeloablative allogeneic transplantation.
- Late toxicities include the development of myelodysplasia, especially in regimens with total body irradiation (TBI).

ALLOGENEIC STEM CELL TRANSPLANTATION

Introduction

Allogeneic stem cell transplantation has progressed from a treatment of last resort to first-line therapy for some patients. Extensive planning and coordination of care is required for all transplantation candidates, usually involving a network of physicians and support staff. The NMDP is an invaluable resource for physicians and their patients for the purpose of transplantation. The NMDP Web site is www.marrow.org. All physicians may perform a free initial search for an HLA-matched unrelated donor in the NMDP, which maintains a registry of more than 5 million potential donors.

Graft versus Malignancy

The main therapeutic benefit of allogeneic transplant depends on the potential of the donor's immune system to recognize and eradicate the malignant or abnormal stem cell clone [the so called graft-versus-leukemia (GVL) or graft-versus-tumor (GVT) effect]. This immune effect is evidenced by the lower relapse rate of hematologic malignancies in patients who undergo allogeneic transplantation than in those who undergo autologous transplantation, as well as by an increased relapse rate in patients receiving a transplant from a syngeneic (identical twin) donor or an allograft that has undergone T-cell depletion. In addition, patients who develop GVHD have a lower risk of relapse than those who do not, and those who relapse after transplantation may be induced into a second remission with a donor lymphocyte infusion (DLI). CML, low-grade lymphoma, and acute myelogenous leukemia (AML) are most susceptible to the GVT effect, whereas acute lymphoblastic leukemia and high-grade lymphomas are relatively resistant to GVT. GVL is predominantly mediated by donor-derived T cells, although new evidence supports a potential contribution from nonspecific cytokines (both host and/or donor derived) and donor-derived natural killer (NK) cells in some settings.

Sources of Donor Hematopoietic Progenitor Cells

Matched Related Donor

- The probability of HLA-identity between siblings is 25%.
- In the United States, approximately 30% of patients will have an HLA-matched sibling.
- The risk of GVHD increases as the HLA disparity between the patient and donor increases; therefore, most transplant centers prefer a 6/6 or 5/6 HLA match.

Syngeneic Donor

- Rarely, an identical twin can serve as the donor.
- Because GVHD does not occur, posttransplantation immunosuppression is not required (although the risk of disease relapse is higher in this setting).

Matched Unrelated Donor

- Search through the NMDP for appropriate HLA match.
- Time from identifying a preliminary donor to collecting the allograft is typically 3 to 4 months.
- Seventy percent of whites will have an HLA-matched donor.
- It is more difficult to find matched donors for certain minority groups.
- Thirty percent of searches through the NMDP result in a transplant.
- The risk of GVHD and graft failure increases with increasing HLA mismatches.

Umbilical Cord Transplantation

- Umbilical cords are obtained from umbilical vessels at delivery and are cryopreserved; a registry records the HLA type of the donor.
- Lymphocytes from cord grafts are immunologically immature, which appears to decrease the risk of GVHD that is associated with using an HLA-mismatched graft.
- Low stem cell numbers in the graft lead to increased risk of graft failure and a prolonged interval to hematopoietic recovery.

Haploidentical Donor

- Parent or sibling may serve as donor, with HLA match restricted to three loci.
- Large numbers of CD34$^+$ cells increase the chances of engraftment.
- T-cell depletion of the allograft is required to reduce the risk of lethal GVHD.
- The process requires prolonged immunosuppression, which increases the risk of infection.

Donor Evaluation

Careful donor selection and evaluation is an integral part of the pretransplantation workup. The donor must be healthy and able to withstand the apheresis procedure or a bone marrow harvest.

1. Donor HLA typing
2. ABO typing
3. History-relevant information of the donor
   - Any previous malignancy within 5 years except nonmelanoma skin cancer (absolute exclusion criteria)
   - Cardiac or coronary artery disease
   - Complications to anesthesia
   - History of lung disease
   - Back or spine disorders
   - Medications
4. Infection exposure
   - HIV, human T-lymphotropic virus (HTLV), hepatitis, CMV, HSV, and EBV.
5. Pregnancy.

Human Leukocyte Antigen Typing

The HLA system is a series of cell surface proteins, which play an important role in immune function. The system is intimately involved in cell-to-cell interactions and recognition. The genes encoding the HLA system are located on chromosome 6 and are codominantly expressed. A striking feature of the HLA system is its enormous diversity. HLA class I molecules include HLA-A, HLA-B, and HLA-C loci. HLA class II molecules are made up of more than 15 antigens, with HLA-DR having the greatest impact on transplantation outcome. Further complexity of the HLA system was revealed with the advent of molecular-based HLA typing, showing that HLA antigens previously identified by serologic testing were actually diverse when classified by DNA analysis. Current recommendations include matching of the donor and recipient at the allele level for HLA-A, HLA-B, and HLA-DRB1 loci.

Stages of Transplant

Conditioning ("The Preparative Regimen")

- The goals of the conditioning regimen include immunosuppression of the recipient to prevent graft rejection and to eradicate residual disease or abnormal cell populations.
- Conditioning strategies can be categorized as myeloablative (conventional conditioning) or nonmyeloablative (see section on nonmyeloablative transplants) strategies. Several myeloablative conditioning regimens are currently being used, with the most common regimens incorporating high-dose cyclophosphamide combined with either TBI or busulfan. The choice of a particular conditioning regimen is guided by factors such as the sensitivity of the malignancy to drugs in the regimen, the toxicities inherent to individual conditioning agents, and the age and performance status of the patient.
- Initial side effects of the transplantation procedure that are related to the preparative regimen include mucositis, nausea, diarrhea, alopecia, pancytopenia, and seizures (with busulfan).
- Late effects of transplant conditioning include lung toxicity, growth retardation, and second malignancy.

Transplantation Phase

- The transplantation phase usually starts 24 hours after completing the preparative regimen.
- Infusion of donor product is usually well tolerated by the recipient.
- The day of transplantation is traditionally referred to as "Day 0."

Engraftment

- Engraftment is defined as time to develop a sustained absolute granulocyte count of >500 cells per μL.
- Platelet recovery usually lags behind granulocyte recovery.
- Duration of conditioning-induced cytopenias depends on the CD34$^+$ cell count in the graft, use of growth factors, and agents used for GVHD prophylaxis.

Supportive Care Phase

- Hematologic support is provided with blood products.
- Infection prophylaxis and treatment form a part of this phase.
- GVHD and other transplantation-related complications occur in this phase.

Infections

Infection remains a major cause of morbidity for patients undergoing HSC transplantation. Figure 30.1 displays an overview of potential pathogens. Indwelling catheters are a common source of infections, and sepsis may occur during the neutropenia phase of the transplantation. Current approaches to minimize the risk of life-threatening infections include the use of prophylactic antimicrobial, antifungal, and antiviral agents, as well as aggressive screening for common transplantation-associated infections.

Neutropenic Fever

See Chapter 36 for overview of management of neutropenic fever.

Cytomegalovirus Infection

- Cytomegalovirus infection is a major cause of morbidity and mortality, especially pneumonia.
- In addition to pneumonia, symptoms may include fever, hepatitis, enteritis, and marrow suppression.
- CMV infection most commonly occurs as a result of the reactivation of a prior infection in the patient or because of the transfer of an infection from the donor (rare).
- The infection usually occurs after engraftment and may coincide with GVHD or with the use of immunosuppressive agents used to treat GVHD. The window of risk for viral reactivation is greatest from the day of engraftment to 100 days after transplantation.
- Screening for viral reactivation is performed weekly after transplantation by measuring the CMV antigen levels or by polymerase chain reaction (PCR).
- Initial treatment is with intravenous ganciclovir ± intravenous immunoglobulin treatment.
- Foscarnet is an alternative treatment (especially in patients with cytopenias).

Invasive Fungal Infection

- Invasive fungal infection is another cause of significant morbidity, with presentation of pneumonia, sinusitis, cellulitis, or blood infection.
- Common agents are *Aspergillus*, *Fusarium*, *Zygomycetes*, as well as *Candida* species.
- Expanded selection of antifungal agents may improve outcome.
- *Candida* fungal prophylaxis with fluconazole is used by many centers.

Hematologic Support

- Hematologic support is provided by replacement of blood and platelet products as needed.
- All blood products should be irradiated prior to infusion.
- Leukocyte reduction filters are indicated to reduce CMV transmission and to reduce febrile reactions.

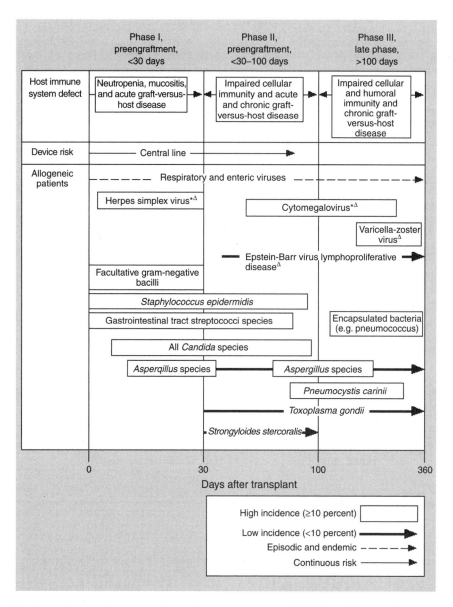

FIG. 30.1. Phases of opportunistic infections among allogenic HSCT recipients. *without standard prophylaxis; △primarily among persons who are seropositive before transplant. (From Centers for Disease Control and Prevention. Guidelines for preventing opportunistic infections among hematopoietic stem cell transplant recipients: recommendations of CDC, the Infectious Disease Society of America, and the American Society of Blood and Marrow Transplantation. *MMWR Morb Mortal Wkly Rep* 200;49(No. RR-10):[1–60], with permission.)

Venoocclusive Disease

Hepatic venoocclusive disease (VOD) is characterized by jaundice, tender hepatomegaly, and unexplained weight gain or ascites. VOD remains extremely difficult to treat, with the risk for this complication increasing with the use of busulfan-containing preparative regimens. Treatment typically involves supportive care measures focused on maintaining renal function, the coagulation system, and fluid balance. Monitoring busulfan drug levels with appropriate dose adjusting appears to decrease the incidence of this complication. Defibrotide, an investigational agent, has recently been used with success to treat severe VOD.

Pulmonary Toxicity

- Bacterial, viral, or fungal organisms may cause pneumonia.
- Diffuse alveolar hemorrhage (usually conditioning related) may respond to high-dose steroids.
- Interstitial pneumonitis with fever, diffuse infiltrates, and hypoxia may occur in 10% to 20% of patients; although commonly idiopathic, CMV needs to be excluded as the cause in all the cases.
- The need for ventilator support is associated with poor outcome.

Graft Versus Host Disease

GVHD remains a main toxic effect associated with allogeneic transplantation. This clinical condition results when donor-derived T cells recognize and react against normal recipient tissues. Acute GVHD occurs most commonly within the first 100 days of the transplantation, whereas chronic GVHD occurs most commonly more than 100 days after transplantation. Up to 50% of matched sibling allogeneic transplants are complicated by acute GVHD. Current approaches to lessen the risk include the use of prophylactic pharmacologic agents and T-cell depletion of the graft. The clinical presentation of GVHD may be variable but the most commonly affected organs are skin, liver, and the gastrointestinal system. The staging system for GVHD is presented in Table 30.1. Risk factors for acute GVHD are shown in Table 30.2.

TABLE 30.1. *Staging system for graft versus host disease (GVHD)*

Level of injury	Skin	Liver (bilirubin)	Gut
1	Maculopapular rash <25% of body surface	2–3 mg/dL	500–1,000 mL liquid stool/d
2	Maculopapular rash 25%–50% of body surface	3–6 mg/dL	1,000–1,500 mL liquid stool/d
3	Generalized erythroderma	6–16 mg/dL	>1,500 mL liquid stool/d
4	Generalized erythroderma with bullae or desquamation	>15 mg/dL	Severe abdominal pain with or without ileus

| Clinical grade | Level of injury | | |
	Skin	Liver	GI tract
I	1 or 2	None	none
II	1–3	1	1
III	2 or 3	2 or 3	2 or 3
IV	2–4	2–4	2–4

GI, gastrointestinal.

TABLE 30.2. *Risk factors for acute graft versus host disease (GVHD)*

Level of HLA mismatch
Infection (e.g., CMV, varicella, etc.)
Use of unrelated donors
Older patients
Donor with a prior history of pregnancy
Sex-mismatched transplant (female allografts into male recipients)
Intensive conditioning regimens

HLA, human leukocyte antigen; CMV, cytomegalovirus.

Prevention of Acute Graft Versus Host Disease

- T-cell depletion of the allograft or combinations of cyclosporine, methotrexate, tacrolimus, prednisone, or mycophenolate mofetil prevent acute GVHD.
- A common regimen for sibling donor transplants is cyclosporine, PO or i.v., and methotrexate i.v. on days 1, 3, 6, and 11.
- Cyclosporine dose 5 mg/kg/day, divided in two doses; the goal is to maintain blood levels of cyclosporine at 150 to 300 ng per mL.
- Tacrolimus dose 0.05 to 0.1 mg/kg/day, divided in two doses; the goal is to maintain levels at 5 to 15 ng per mL.
- Many medications may interact with immunosuppressant drugs.
- Donor T-cell depletion prior to transplant decreases risk of GVHD but may increase the risk of relapse.
- T-cell depletion may be accomplished by various methods, such as $CD34^+$ selection of the graft or the use monoclonal antibodies directed against T-cell antigens.

Treatment of Acute Graft versus Host Disease

- Initially, methylprednisolone should be given at a dose of 1 to 2 mg/kg/day.
- For those patients who do not respond or for those who have a partial response, additional agents can be added with variable success (see Table 30.3); clinical trials should be considered.

Chronic Graft versus Host Disease

- Chronic GVHD typically occurs after 100 days from transplantation.
- Prior history of acute GVHD and the use of PBSC allografts are risk factors.

TABLE 30.3. *Treatments that may be useful for acute graft versus host disease (GVHD) treatment*

Methylprednisolone
Cyclosporine/tacrolimus
Azathioprine
Daclizumab
Infliximab
Muromonab-CD3 (OKT3)
Photopheresis
Antithymocyte globulin

- Chronic GVHD presents with variable organ involvement and symptoms, including clinical presentations that may resemble autoimmune disorders (i.e., lichenoid skin changes, sicca syndrome, scleroderma-like skin changes, chronic hepatitis, and bronchiolitis obliterans).
- Chronic GVHD is often accompanied by cytopenias and immunodeficiency.
- Treatment involves prolonged courses of steroids and other immunosuppressive agents as well as prophylactic antibiotics (e.g., penicillin). Some trials have shown a benefit from thalidomide, mycophenolate mofetil, photopheresis, and Psoralen-UV-A (PUVA) (for chronic skin GVHD).

Relapse after Transplant

Relapse of malignant disease after allogeneic transplant is an ominous event. Most relapses occur within 2 years of transplantation. Immunosuppression is typically withdrawn to enhance a GVT effect, and in some cases, a DLI is given (lymphocytes from the original stem cell donor). This frequently results in GVHD, which may also be associated with a GVT response. The most favorable responses to DLI have been seen in patients with CML, especially those in the molecular or chronic phase of relapse.

Nonmyeloablative Transplantation

Nonmyeloablative transplantation (NST) relies principally on the graft versus malignancy effect. Instead of intense myeloablative preparative regimens, this technique incorporates immunosuppression to allow for engraftment of donor cells. The most common preparative regimen consists of fludarabine combined with an alkylating agent or low-dose TBI. Nonmyeloablative transplants may be performed in older adults (i.e., older than 60 years) because regimen-related toxicities are less in this case. A mixture of donor and recipient hematopoietic cells is present just after transplant (called *mixed chimerism*). As immune suppression is removed, the surviving recipient cells are gradually eradicated by the donor immune system, ultimately resulting in full donor engraftment. GVT effects have been observed to occur in CML, AML, chronic lymphocytic leukemia (CLL), lymphoma, multiple myeloma, as well as in select metastatic solid tumors.

A number of small studies have recently reported that GVT effects may be observed in patients with cytokine-refractory metastatic renal cell carcinoma. Disease regression is usually delayed, occurring 4 to 6 months after transplantation following the withdrawal of immunosuppression and occurring frequently in association with either acute or chronic GVHD. Clinical trials investigating GVT effects in renal cell carcinoma and a variety of other metastatic solid tumors are ongoing.

CONCLUSION

HSC transplantation has dramatically improved over the last several decades into an effective therapeutic treatment for a variety of malignant and nonmalignant conditions. The number of patients who benefit from this procedure will likely increase as future transplantation strategies continue to evolve that limit complications while maximizing beneficial donor immune-mediated graft-versus-malignancy effects.

SUGGESTED READINGS

American Society of Blood and Marrow Transplantation. Web site www.asbmt.org 2004.

Barrett AJ, Rezvani K, Solomon S, et al. New developments in allotransplant immunology. In: Broudy V, Prchal J, Tricot G, eds. *Hematology 2003: the American Society of Hematology education program book.* Washington, DC: American Society of Hematology, 2003:350–371. http://www.hematology.org.

Bensinger W, Martin P, Storer B, et al. Transplantation of bone marrow as compared to peripheral-blood cells from HLA-identical relatives in patients with hematological cancers. *N Engl J Med* 2001; 344:175–181.

Centers for Disease Control and Prevention. Guidelines for preventing opportunistic infections among hematopoietic stem cell transplant recipients: recommendations of the CDC, the Infectious Disease Society of America, and the American Society of Blood and Marrow Transplantation. *MMWR Morb Mortal Wkly Rep* 2000;49(No. RR-10):1–125.

Champlin R, Khouri I, Kornblau S, et al. Allogeneic hematopoietic stem cell transplantation as adoptive immunotherapy: induction of graft-versus-malignancy as primary therapy. *Hematol Oncol Clin North Am* 1999;13:1041–1057.

Childs R, Chernoff A, Contentin N, et al. Regression of metastatic renal-cell carcinoma after nonmyeloablative allogeneic peripheral-blood stem-cell transplantation. *N Engl J Med* 2000;343:750–758.

Hurley C, Lowe L, Logan B, et al. National Marrow Donor Program HLA-matching guidelines for unrelated marrow transplants. *Biol Blood Marrow Transplant* 2003;9:610–615.

International Bone Marrow Transplant Registry. Web site www.ibmtr.org 2004.

National Marrow Donor Program. Web site www.marrow.org 2004.

SECTION 10

Other Malignancies

31

Acquired Immunodeficiency Syndrome–Related Malignancies

Pallavi P. Kumar and Richard F. Little

*HIV and AIDS Malignancy Branch, Center for Cancer Research,
National Cancer Institute, National Institutes of Health, Bethesda, Maryland*

Individuals with human immunodeficiency virus (HIV) infection are at increased risk for developing neoplastic disease. The clinical behavior of specific malignancies is often markedly altered in the setting of HIV infection as compared to the HIV-negative counterpart.

- Three neoplasms are considered as acquired immunodeficiency syndrome (AIDS)–defining conditions when they occur in HIV-infected patients:
  1. Kaposi sarcoma (KS)
  2. Aggressive B-cell non-Hodgkin lymphoma, both peripheral and primary central nervous system (CNS) lymphomas
  3. Cervical cancer.
- A number of other cancers that are not considered AIDS-defining occur with increasing frequency in HIV-infected patients, including Hodgkin disease (HD), multicentric Castleman disease, angiosarcoma, multiple myeloma, brain cancer, lung cancer, and seminoma.
- Highly active antiretroviral therapy (HAART) for HIV infection has resulted in fewer AIDS complications, including malignancies.
  1. There is no cure for AIDS, but HAART increases longevity, thereby increasing the prevalence of people living with HIV and AIDS.
  2. Cancer prevalence in the HIV-infected population may be expected to increase over time.

KAPOSI SARCOMA

Epidemiology

- KS was first described in 1872 by Moritz Kaposi.
- KS is the most common HIV-associated tumor.
- There are four epidemiologic forms of KS:
  1. Classic KS
     a. This is found predominately in elderly men of the Mediterranean and Eastern Europe.
  2. Epidemic KS
     a. In Africa, especially in the Nile–Congo watershed, KS is the most commonly diagnosed tumor.
     b. KS can be aggressive in children, involving the lymph nodes, internal organs, and skin.
     c. The seroprevalence of Kaposi sarcoma–associated herpesvirus (KSHV) exceeds 60% in some parts of sub-Saharan Africa (see subsequent text).

3. AIDS-related KS
   a. AIDS-related KS heralded the emerging AIDS epidemic in 1981.
      i. This previously rare tumor was suddenly seen with an unexpectedly high prevalence in young gay men, a population previously unaffected by this disease.
      ii. Coinfection with HIV increases the risk of KS by more than 100,000 times, and the clinical course can be more aggressive than that of classical KS.
   b. In the developed world, the incidence of KS is highest among men who have sex with other men (MSM) and with their female sex partners. In the early stages of the epidemic, KS was the AIDS-defining diagnosis in nearly 50% of HIV-infected MSM.
   c. Currently, KS is the AIDS-defining diagnosis in less than 11% of HIV-infected MSM; the reasons for this include
      i. a change in the case definition of AIDS in 1992 that included less than 200 CD4 cells per mm^3
      ii. safer sex practices possibly leading to a decrease in KSHV transmission
      iii. induction of immune reconstitution by HAART, which can lower the risk of developing AIDS-related KS.
4. Immune suppression from other causes (e.g., iatrogenic immune suppression in solid organ transplantation) can also increase the risk of KS in individuals infected with KSHV.

Pathophysiology of Kaposi Sarcoma

- Kaposi sarcoma is an angioproliferative lesion caused by KSHV, also known as human herpesvirus 8 (HHV-8).
  - This novel gammaherpes virus was discovered in 1994.
  - It encodes for a number of viral mimics of human cytokines and other factors involved in KS pathogenesis.
    - Interleukin 6 (IL-6), macrophage inhibitory protein, and interferon regulatory factor upregulates vascular endothelial growth factor (VEGF) and its receptors.
    - KSHV-infected spindle-shaped cells are most likely of vascular endothelial origin.
    - KSHV-driven proangiogenic factors promote endothelial cell hyperproliferation and spindle-like morphogenesis.
    - KS endothelial/spindle cells respond to
      i. basic fibroblast growth factor (bFGF)
      ii. VEGF
  - Most cells are latently infected and express latency-associated nuclear antigen (LANA). LANA promotes cell survival by interacting with the tumor suppressor protein p53. LANA interacts with p53 and inhibits its ability to promote apoptosis, thereby contributing to viral persistence and oncogenesis in KS. Some cells show lytic infection.
  - Transmission routes have not been established.
    - The possibilities include mother to infant, child to child, and sexual transmission.
    - Saliva contains high concentrations of KSHV.
    - KSHV appears to be transmitted inefficiently by transfusion of blood products.
  - It is an angioproliferative neoplastic disease.
  - The vascularity of the lesion gives it a purplish appearance.
  - The lesions can be flat or nodular.
  - Lymphadenopathy and edema may be present in the absence of cutaneous involvement.
  - KS arises simultaneously in multiple nonmetastatic sites.
  - Skin involvement is typical, but virtually any internal organ except the brain can be affected.

Diagnosis

KS is diagnosed using the following techniques:

- A 4- to 6-mm skin punch biopsy: Extensive surgical excision is not required and may not be clinically useful.
- Differential diagnosis: Bacillary angiomatosis, melanoma, granulomatous conditions, or prominent vascularity in the lymph nodes.
- HIV serology should be obtained whenever KS is suspected.

Clinical Presentation

- Variable clinical course
  - Indolent waxing and waning of cutaneous involvement.
  - Relentless progression with ulceration, severe tumor-associated edema, pain, and disfigurement.
- Patients with minimal KS may require no treatment unless the psychological impact, which can be severe, warrants therapy.
- Extensive pulmonary involvement may be associated with a particularly poor prognosis (median survival less than 7 months in the pre-HAART era).
  - Substantial morbidity and death can ensue from involvement of other viscera (e.g., gastrointestinal tract).

Kaposi Sarcoma Staging

- The TIS staging system (see Table 31.1), devised by the AIDS Clinical Trials Group Oncology Committee, is commonly used.
  1. T refers to tumor extent
  2. I refers to immune status
  3. S refers to other AIDS-related systemic illness.
- The TIS system stages patients, overall, as being either at good risk, designated by the subscript 0, or at poor risk, designated by the subscript 1, the summary taking the form $T_{0 \text{ or } 1} I_{0 \text{ or } 1} S_{0 \text{ or } 1}$.
- In the HAART era, two different risk categories have been identified
  1. Good risk (T_0S_0, T_1S_0, T_0S_1)
  2. Poor risk (T_1S_1).
     The immune status of the two risk categories appears not to be predictive. This most likely depends on the effectiveness of HAART; the original TIS may be more applicable for patients with multidrug-resistant HIV infection.
- The staging of KS includes (a) enumeration and bidirectional measurement of cutaneous and oral lesions; (b) baseline chest x-ray: if this is abnormal, computerized tomography (CT) scan of the chest should be performed; (c) CD4 cell count; (d) endoscopy if symptoms referable to the gastrointestinal (GI) tract are present.
  1. Lesions should be characterized as
     a. flat or nodular
     b. lesions with or without tumor-associated edema.
  2. If there are more than 50 cutaneous lesions, representative areas containing at least 20 lesions are designated for individual lesion assessment for response to therapy.
  3. Abnormalities on chest CT may indicate pulmonary involvement by KS. Bronchoscopic evaluation can establish the diagnosis of pulmonary KS if lesions are visualized

TABLE 31.1. *Revised Acquired Immunodeficiency Syndrome Clinical Trial Group (ACTG) staging classification for Kaposi sarcoma[a]*

	Good risk (0) (all of the following)	Poor risk (1) (any of the following)
Tumor (T)	Confined to skin and/or lymph nodes and/or nonnodular oral disease confined to the palate	Tumor-associated edema or ulceration Extensive oral KS Nonnodal viscera
Immune system (I) (May not be predictive in those responding to HAART[b])	CD4 count $\geq$150/mm^3	CD4 count <150/mm^3
Systemic illness (S)	No history of opportunistic infection or thrush. No "B" symptoms (unexplained fever, night sweats, >10% involuntary weight loss, or diarrhea) persisting for more than 2 wk. Performance status <70 (Karnofsky)	History of opportunistic infections and/or thrush; "B" symptoms present. Performance status <70. Other HIV-related opportunistic illness

KS, Kaposi sarcoma; HAART, highly active antiretroviral therapy; HIV, human immunodeficiency virus.

The revised CD4 cutoff of 150 cells/mm^3 is lower than the original proposal of 200 cells/mm^3. Example of staging: A patient with only nodular oral KS, CD4 count of 175 cells/mm^3, and a history of PCP would be $T_1 S_0 I_1$. In the HAART era, two prognostic categories are considered good risk ($T_0 S_0$, $T_1 S_0$, $T_0 S_1$) and one category is considered poor risk ($T_1 S_1$).

[a]Adapted from Krown SE, Testa MA, et al., AIDS Clinical Trials Group Oncology Committee. AIDS-related Kaposi's sarcoma: prospective validation of the AIDS Clinical Trials Group staging classification. *J Clin Oncol* 1997;15(9):3085–3092.

[b]Adapted from Nasti G, Talamini R, et al., AIDS-related Kaposi's Sarcoma: evaluation of potential new prognostic factors and assessment of the AIDS Clinical Trial Group Staging System in the Haart Era—the Italian Cooperative Group on AIDS and Tumors and the Italian Cohort of Patients Naive from Antiretrovirals. *J Clin Oncol* 2003;21(15):2876–2882.

in the airways. Endobronchial or open lung biopsy should be avoided, because of risk of hemorrhage.

Prognostic Factors

- Response to KS therapy may be related to a variety of factors:
  - Tumor extent
  - Performance status
  - Presence of a HAART-sensitive HIV (this may predict a better prognosis)
  - Extent of HIV replication: A better control of HIV may result in a more indolent course of KS. In addition, the HIV viral load predicts the rate of progressive immunosuppression.

Management of Kaposi Sarcoma

- The goal of treatment is palliation.
  - KS is not yet curable.
  - It frequently reappears or progresses when therapy is suspended.
    - Complete response does not imply cure.
  - Well-controlled HIV infection (e.g., low HIV viral loads and high CD4 cell counts) may decrease the need for chronic KS-specific therapy.

- HAART is fundamental to the oncologic therapy of AIDS-KS.
  - For patients with minimal, slowly progressing KS, HAART alone may be the only therapeutic maneuver required.
    - Successful therapeutic effect is most likely if the increase in the CD4 cell count above the pretreatment baseline value is 150 cells per mm^3 or more and if HIV level is suppressed to undetectable levels.
    - Improvements are often noticeable within 3 to 4 weeks.
    - Responses may not be noticeable for several months or even longer.
  - Additional antitumor therapy will most likely be required if
    - HAART does not result in immunologic and virologic response
    - patients have been previously treated for HIV or KS
    - aggressive or widely disseminated tumor is present.

Additional Therapeutic Considerations
Local Therapy

Local therapy is reserved for minimal disease that is restricted to the skin or the oral cavity. It is limited by inadequate cosmetic outcome in some cases.

- Surgical excision
  1. Acceptable cosmetic results are seen in very limited circumstances.
  2. It is not to be used as definitive therapy in any case.
  3. Its use is not appropriate in many cases.
- Cryotherapy
  1. It is useful for small lesions.
  2. Permanent destruction of melanocytes may yield unacceptable cosmetic outcome, particularly in dark-skinned individuals.
- Photodynamic therapy
  1. Many lesions can be treated during a single session.
  2. Moderate pain and photosensitivity is experienced for a number of weeks following the treatment.
- Intralesional injection
  1. Vinblastine (0.1 mL of 0.1 mg per mL) or 3% sodium tetradodecyl sulfate injection (0.1 to 0.3 mL).
  2. This injection causes nonspecific necrosis or sclerosis of mucocutaneous tissue.
  3. Reasonable cosmetic outcome is exhibited for small lesions.
- Topical 9-*cis*-retinoic acid (Panretin gel)
  1. Topical 9-*cis*-retinoic acid is approved by the U.S. Food and Drug Administration (FDA).
  2. Approximately 45% of lesions show responses.
  3. Inflammation and lightening of the skin yields inadequate cosmesis in some cases.
- Radiotherapy
  Radiotherapy may be useful as adjunctive therapy in severe disease.
  1. The painful areas involved may respond rapidly; therefore, radiation therapy is useful when the potentially slower responses to systemic therapy may compromise the therapeutic outcome. For example, oral lesions causing poor nutritional intake may best be treated with radiotherapy in some patients. Severe mucositis and xerostomia may result from radiotherapy. Tolerance to radiation may be decreased among AIDS-KS patients, particularly on the mucosal surfaces.
  2. Radiotherapy is also useful for cosmetic purposes. For example, when the eyelid or conjunctiva is involved, other local therapies are not practical.
  3. Reappearance of KS in the area of previous irradiation is common.
  4. Residual or late-occurring radiation-induced hyperpigmentation or telangiectasias can be severe and may compromise the cosmetic outcome.

5. Palliation of visceral disease, including pulmonary involvement, may be reasonably well tolerated in some circumstances, when chemotherapy is not an option.
- Carbon dioxide laser therapy
  1. Carbon dioxide laser therapy may result in immediate improvement; for example, treatment of tumor involving the oropharynx and larynx can result in improved oral intake, with less toxicity than is sometimes seen with radiation to the oral cavity.

Systemic Therapy

- *Immunotherapy:* Interferon-α
  1. Immune therapy with interferon-α is most successful if the CD4 cell count is more than 200 per mm^3 in conjunction with antiretroviral therapy.
  2. Toxicity includes flu-like symptoms, depression, and decreased white cell count.
  3. Dose escalation to 5×10^6 to 10×10^6 U per day or intramuscular or subcutaneous therapy three times weekly is the schedule that is given. Other dosing schedules may also be effective.
- *Cytotoxic Chemotherapy*
  1. Monotherapy has replaced combination therapy as the standard of care.
     a. Liposomal anthracyclines or paclitaxel (see Table 31.2)
     b. Advantages of monotherapy over combination therapy include
        i. Better palliation
        ii. Reduced toxicity
        iii. Simplicity of administration with concurrent complicated antiretroviral regimens.
  2. Liposomal daunorubicin (DaunoXome): The FDA has approved liposomal daunorubicin as first-line therapy for KS.
  3. The FDA approved second-line therapy for KS.
     a. Liposomal doxorubicin (Doxil)
     b. Paclitaxel (Taxol): Often reserved for particularly severe disease on the basis of high response rates seen in phase II trials, but is perhaps more toxic than liposomal anthracyclines.

TABLE 31.2. *Commonly used standard therapies in Kaposi sarcoma*

	Doses	Response rates
Standard KS therapy		
Liposomal anthracyclines		
Doxorubicin	20 mg/m^2 intravenously over 30 min q2–3wk	59%
Daunorubicin	40–60 mg/m^2 intravenously over 60 min q2wk	25%
Paclitaxel	135 mg/m^2 intravenously over 3 h every 3 wk or 100 mg/m^2 intravenously over 3 h every 2 wk	59%–71%
Alternative therapies		
Doxorubicin/bleomycin/vinca alkaloids (ABV)	ABV q2–4wk Doxorubicin 10–40 mg/m^2 Bleomycin 15 U Vincristine 1 mg (or vinblastine 6 mg/m^2)	24%–88% (higher response rates with higher doxorubicin doses, but greater toxicity)
Vincristine/vinblastine	Vincristine 1 mg alternating with vinblastine 2–4 mg q wk	45%
Bleomycin/vinca alkaloids	Bleomycin 10 U and vincristine 1 mg or vinblastine 2–4 mg weekly	23%

From Yarchoan R. Therapy for Kaposi's sarcoma: recent advances and experimental approaches. *J Acquir Immune Defic Syndr* 1999;21(Suppl 1):S66-73, with permission.

4. Combination chemotherapy was the previous standard of care. Regimens include doxorubicin, bleomycin, and vinca alkaloid (either vincristine or vinblastine) (ABV).
   a. Response rates range from 28% to 84%, depending on the dose of doxorubicin.
   b. The higher doses tend to be associated with unacceptable toxicity, with pronounced myelosuppression.
   c. Toxic regimens are unsuited for the chronic dosing needed for many patients with this disease.

Experimental Therapies

- Because KS requires long-term treatment, there is strong interest in pathogenesis-based therapies, which may have less associated toxicity.
- The use of antiangiogenic therapies and antiviral therapies are being investigated.
  1. Thalidomide: Two phase II trials suggest activity in a subset of KS patients.
  2. Interleukin 12: Interleukin 12 has antiangiogenic and immunomodulatory properties.
  3. COL-3: COL-3 exhibits antiangiogenic and antimetastasic effects.
  4. Bevacizumab: Bevacizumab is a monoclonal antibody that blocks VEGF binding to its receptors.

ACQUIRED IMMUNODEFICIENCY SYNDROME–RELATED LYMPHOMAS

Epidemiology

- In 1985, the Centers for Disease Control and Prevention (CDC) included the aggressive and high-grade B-cell type of non-Hodgkin lymphoma (NHL) as an AIDS-defining condition.
- AIDS-related lymphoma (ARL) is the second most frequently occurring AIDS-associated malignancy.
  - It is the AIDS-defining diagnosis in approximately 3% of HIV-infected patients.
  - Estimated incidence of up to 10% per year, with a prevalence of 4.5% to 25%, has been documented in certain patient populations.
  - The risk of developing NHL in the HIV-infected population increases by nearly 100 times the risk in the non–HIV-infected population.
  - The true incidence is not known because lymphoma is not a reportable condition among patients already defined as having a prior AIDS-indicating condition, such as less than 200 CD4 cells per mm^3.
  - Risk of ARL is independent of the HIV-risk group.
- HAART has affected the incidence of ARL.
  - The incidence of ARL decreased by up to 50% compared to the pre-HAART period.
  - The greatest decrease in incidence is in the immunoblastic diffuse large B-cell lymphomas (DLBCL): AIDS-related primary CNS lymphoma (AIDS-PCNSL).
  - The incident cases of Burkitt lymphoma have not changed. These tend to occur when the CD4 cell count remains relatively well preserved.
  - Median overall ARL survival has increased in the HAART era.
    - It is approximately 21 months compared to 4 to 18 months in the pre-HAART era.
    - This increase in survival is most likely related to a relative shift to tumor types with better prognosis.

Classification of Acquired Immunodeficiency Syndrome–Related Lymphomas

- The World Health Organization (WHO) recognizes the predominant ARLs as
- Burkitt lymphoma
- DLBCL: includes AIDS-PCNSLs, which, in almost all cases, are of immunoblastic histology and are associated with Epstein–Barr virus (EBV).

- Primary effusion lymphoma (PEL); also termed body-cavity lymphoma.
- Plasmablastic lymphoma of the oral cavity.
- The non–AIDS-defining conditions (seen in the setting of HIV but not AIDS-defining) include
  - Hodgkin disease
  - Multicentric Castleman disease (MCD)

Acquired Immunodeficiency Syndrome–Related Lymphoma Pathology

- Distinct clinical, histogenetic, and pathobiologic features correlate with the different ARL subtypes (Table 31.3).
- Tumor histogenesis correlates with immunologic status (e.g., CD4 cell count).
- The relative upward shift in CD4 cell count among patients with access to HAART has changed the epidemiology and biology of ARL. This change in bioepidemiology may be the most biologically plausible explanation for the increased survival in patients with ARL in the HAART era.

Peripheral Acquired Immunodeficiency Syndrome–Related Lymphoma

Presentation

- Peripheral ARL frequently presents as advanced stage 3 or 4 disease.
- The lymphoma frequently behaves aggressively, with unusual patterns of organ involvement.
- Most patients will present with
  - rapidly growing mass lesion
  - systemic "B" symptoms (i.e., unexplained fever, drenching night sweats, or unexplained weight loss in excess of 10% of the normal body weight).
- Extranodal involvement is common.
  - bone marrow; 25% to 40%
  - gastrointestinal tract; 26%
  - CNS; 17% to 32%.
- PEL
  - shows 100% association with KSHV.
  - presents as lymphomatous effusions of the pleural spaces but can occasionally present initially as nodal disease.
- Plasmablastic lymphomas of the oral cavity
  - is localized in the oral cavity or jaw
  - is often associated with EBV.

Staging

- Standard staging—using the Ann Arbor Staging Classification for NHL (as is done in non–HIV-infected patients)
- History and physical examination
- Clinical laboratory assessment of organ function
- CD4 cell count
- Bilateral bone marrow biopsies
- CT scan of the chest, abdomen, and pelvis
- CNS assessment for all patients
  - Radiologic imaging
    - CT scan of the brain with contrast is adequate to assess for larger parenchymal brain lesions.
    - Magnetic resonance imaging (MRI) with gadolinium has the potential advantage of revealing smaller lesions and providing evidence of leptomeningeal involvement by the lymphoma.

TABLE 31.3. Genetic and clinical features of peripheral AIDS-related lymphomas

Histogenetic origin	Histology	Viral associations		Immunophenotype and pathobiologic markers					CD4 cells	Relative proportionate incidence in HAART compared to pre-HAART era	Prospects for chemosensitivity
		EBV (%)	KSHV (%)	CD20 (%)	BCL-2 (%)	BCL-6 (%)	p53 (%)	c-MYC (%)			
Germinal center	Burkitt	<50	0	~100	0	100	60	100	May be relatively well preserved	Increased	Favorable
	DLBCL centroblastic	<30	0	~100	0	>75	rare	0–50			
	Primary brain DLBCL (immunoblastic)	100	0	variable	90	<50	0	0	<50/mm³	Markedly decreased	Responds to radiation
Postgerminal center	DLBCL immunoblastic	>80	0	variable	30	0	0	0–20	Usually low	Decreased	Poor
	Primary effusion lymphoma	>90	100	<20	0	0	0	0			
	Plasmablastic (oral cavity associated)	>70	0	Rare	0	0	Rare	0			

HAART, highly active antiretroviral therapy; EBV, Epstein–Barr virus; KSHV, Kaposi sarcoma-associated herpes virus; DLBCL, diffuse large B-cell lymphomas.

Adapted from Yarchoan R, Little R. Cancer: AIDS-related malignancies. In: Devita VT, Hellman S, Rosenberg A, eds. *Cancer principles and practice of Oncology.* Philadelphia, PA: Lippincott Williams & Wilkins, 2005:2247–2263, with permission.

- – CNS evaluation is not indicated for patients with human immunodeficiency virus–Hodgkin disease (HIV-HD) because the CNS is not commonly involved.
- • Cytologic evaluation of the cerebrospinal fluid to assess for potential CNS involvement.

Prognosis

- • The CD4 cell count is the primary prognostic indicator.
- • The international prognostic index is not widely validated in ARL.
  - • Other factors associated with poor outcome are
    - – patients older than 35 to 40 years
    - – high concentration of lactate dehydrogenase (LDH)
    - – presence of extranodal sites
    - – intravenous drug use
    - – preexisting AIDS diagnosis.
- • HAART era
  - • Median overall survival is nearly 2 years; it may be less in cases of resistant HIV and lower CD4 cell counts (e.g., may behave as pre-HAART).
- • Pre-HAART era
  - • If CD4 cell count is less than 100 cells per mm^3, a median survival of about 4 months was observed.
  - • If CD4 cell count is 100 or cells per mm^3 or greater, a median survival of 11 to 18 months was observed.

Treatment

- • Optimal therapy has not been defined (see Table 31.4).
- • Comparison of ARL clinical trial results should consider the effect of
  - • CD4 cells
  - • the different times the trials were conducted (HAART versus pre-HAART).
- • Many experts advocate routine CNS prophylaxis in ARL.
  - • There is a predilection for leptomeningeal involvement (15% to 20% of cases).
  - • Prophylaxis with intrathecal methotrexate or Ara-C should be considered standard practice for treatment of ARL.
- • Prophylaxis for opportunistic infections
  - • All patients should receive prophylaxis for *Pneumocystis carinii* pneumonia (PCP) regardless of the CD4 count.
  - • Prophylaxis should be considered for patients at risk for *Mycobacterium avium* complex (MAC) (CD4 cell count <50 to 100 per mm^3).
  - • The CD4 cell count should be periodically monitored during chemotherapy because cytotoxic chemotherapy in itself can cause a profound drop in CD4 cell count.
- • Standard-dose chemotherapy has supplanted low-dose approaches in the HAART era.
  - • For patients with advanced AIDS and drug-resistant HIV, less aggressive therapy may be useful.
  - • Randomized study of standard versus low-dose m-BACOD (methotrexate, bleomycin, doxorubicin, cyclophosphamide, vincristine, and dexamethasone) was completed in 1997 (pre-HAART).
    - – Equivalent results were observed in both groups.
    - – Complete responses ranging from 41% to 52% were obtained.
    - – There was lower incidence of febrile neutropenia in the low-dose group; this finding formed the basis for its recommended use in ARL.

TABLE 31.4. Selected regimens and outcomes for peripheral AIDS-related non-Hodgkin lymphoma

Course of therapy	Number of evaluable patients	Median CD4 cells/mm^3 at baseline	Complete response rate (%)	Median overall/disease-free survival (mo)	Author
m-BACOD low dose	175	100	41	8 mo/8 mo	Kaplan et al. (randomized)
Standard dose CHOP HAART Low dose	40	122 138	52 30	Not reached; follow-up time not of sufficient duration to assess long-term disease-free survival	Ratner et al.
Standard dose Infusional CDE + rituximab + HAART	23 29	122 132	48 86	Not reached; follow-up time not of sufficient duration to assess long-term disease-free survival	Tirelli et al.
CHOP-rituximab	95	133	58	Median complete response duration has not been reached	Kaplan et al. (randomized)
CHOP Dose-adjusted EPOCH	47 39	198	50 74	60%/92% at 53 mo	Little et al.

m-BACOD, methotrexate, bleomycin, doxorubicin, cyclophosphamide, vincristine, and dexamethasone; CHOP, cyclophosphamide, doxorubicin, vincristine, and prednisone; HAART, highly active antiretroviral therapy; CDE, cyclophosphamide, doxorubicin, and etoposide; EPOCH, etoposide, vincristine, doxorubicin, prednisone, and cyclophosphamide.

- Recent trials are generally phase II trials.
  - Low-dose cyclophosphamide, doxorubicin, vincristine, and prednisone (CHOP) (COHOT 1) and standard-dose CHOP (COHOT 2)
    - All patients received HAART (i.e., stavudine, lamivudine, and indinavir).
    - The trials showed a trend for superior results with standard-dose CHOP.
    - The follow-up time has been too short for assessment of long-term disease-free survival (see list on considerations for role of HAART during chemotherapy in ARL).
  - A large phase II trial of infusional cyclophosphamide, doxorubicin, and etoposide (CDE)
    - 182 patients
    - complete response rate of 46%
    - median overall survival of 8.2 months.
- Dose-adjusted EPOCH (etoposide, vincristine, doxorubicin, prednisone, cyclophosphamide) (see Table 31.5)
  - The study had a long follow-up time of 53 months.
  - There were 39 patients in the study.
  - ARL outcomes were the same as those of similar tumors in non-AIDS NHL.
  - Complete remission was seen in 74% of patients (87% for those with CD4 counts >100 per mm^3).
  - The disease-free and overall survivals were 92% and 60%.
- Rituximab in ARL
  - On the basis of current available data, rituximab should not, at present, be considered as the standard of care in ARL.
  - Rituximab has been of considerable interest in ARL because it confers substantial therapeutic benefit in certain HIV-unrelated NHL types.
  - Preliminary results of a phase II study of CDE with HAART and rituximab are as follows:
    - Complete response rate of 85% has been observed.
    - Follow-up time is too brief to fully assess this approach.

TABLE 31.5. *Dose-adjusted EPOCH for acquired immunodeficiency syndrome–related lymphoma*

Drug	Dose			Route	Time
Etoposide	50 mg/m^2/d			CIV	d 1–4 (total dose/cycle = 250 mg/m^2)
Doxorubicin	10 mg/m^2/d			CIV	d 1–4 (total dose/cycle = 40 mg/m^2)
Vincristine	0.4 mg/m^2/d			CIV	d 1–4 (total dose/cycle = 1.6 mg/m^2 (no cap))
Prednisone	60 mg/m^2			PO	daily, d 1–5
Cyclophosphamide	Cycle one dependent on CD4 cell count				
	CD4/mm^3	<100	187 mg/m^2	i.v.	On d 5
		≥100	375 mg/m^2	i.v.	On d 5
	Cycles two and beyond dependent on ANC nadir				
	ANC nadir	<500	Decrease dose by 187 mg/m^2		
		≥500	Increase dose by 187 mg/m^2 (maximum dose is 750 mg/m^2)		
Filgrastim	300 µg/d s.c., starting d 6; continues until ANC >5,000 cells/mm^3				
	Treatment is repeated every 21 d				

CIV, continuous intravenous; ANC, absolute neutrophil count.
HAART is suspended until completion of all EPOCH cycles.
PCP Prophylaxis for all patients and continues until CD4 >200 cells/mm^3.
Mycobacterium avium complex (MAC) prophylaxis for all patients with CD4 <100 cells/mm^3.

- A randomized trial conducted by investigators of the National Cancer Institute (NCI)–sponsored AIDS Malignancies Consortium assessed the role of rituximab in ARL, with CHOP combined with HAART.
    - The differences in complete responses were not statistically significant—the complete response with rituximab was 58% and that without rituximab was 50%.
    - There were more treatment-related deaths in the rituximab group ($p = 0.02$)—15% in the group randomized to receive rituximab and 2% in the group with no rituximab.
- In HIV-unrelated aggressive DLBCL, rituximab may confer the greatest additional benefit when added to standard chemotherapy for the subset of tumors expressing BCL2. Most ARL do not express BCL-2. Further research is needed in this regard.
- Considerations for the role of HAART during chemotherapy in ARL:
- Most studies have demonstrated the feasibility of administering HAART along with the chemotherapy regimens. This is a complicated issue, and no study has shown a benefit specifically attributable to such an approach.
- Complicated pharmacokinetic interactions have been documented in pharmacokinetic studies that assess condition HAART and chemotherapy:
    - CHOP given with stavudine, lamivudine, and indinavir decreases cyclophosphamide clearance by approximately 50% as compared to historic control patients treated with CHOP alone. No obvious excess toxicity ensues.
    - A study of infusional CDE showed that cycles administered with didanosine tended to be associated with lower plasma etoposide levels than the cycles administered with CDE alone.
- No controlled trials that assess toxicity have been performed.
- Some retrospective studies have suggested that increased toxicity may be a concern when chemotherapy and HAART are coadministered.
- Other retrospective studies suggest that HAART leads to improved tolerance to chemotherapy:
    - A higher response rate and better tolerance to more dose-intensive chemotherapy have been observed in patients with long-term HIV suppression on HAART than in those patients who fail HAART or are HAART naïve.
    - These results suggest that HAART does not undermine the efficacy of combination chemotherapy and is consistent with other prospective feasibility studies.
- The dose-adjusted EPOCH (DA-EPOCH) study indicates that such a combination therapy is not needed for superior results.
- Considerations for omission of HAART during chemotherapy include the following:
    - Actually chemotherapy causes substantially more lymphocyte depletion than HIV does.
    - HAART is unlikely to protect against chemotherapy-induced lymphocyte depletion.
    - In HIV not-infected individuals lymphocyte depletion occurs during chemotherapy, with recovery over 12 to 18 months after completion of therapy.
    - Similar dynamics in HIV sensitive to HAART.
    - Temporary suspension of HAART until completion of ARL therapy is consistent with Guidelines for the Use of Antiretroviral Agents in HIV-1-Infected Adults and Adolescents as developed by the Panel on Clinical Practices for Treatment of HIV Infection convened by the Department of Health and Human Services (DHHS) and the Henry J. Kaiser Family Foundation and published in http://aidsinfo.nih.gov/guidelines.
- Because of potential interactions and toxicity, if HAART is to be combined with chemotherapy, care should always be taken to refer to appropriate drug information manuals when considering the therapeutic plan.

Acquired Immunodeficiency Syndrome–Primary Central Nervous System Lymphoma

Presentation

- AIDS-PCNSL accounts for 19% of ARL in pre-HAART era.
    - In patients with non–AIDS-NHL, PCNSL accounts for approximately 1% of NHL.

- Since the introduction of HAART, there has been a three-fold decrease in the incidence of PCNSL.
- PCNSL is the second most common mass lesion found in patients with AIDS and the most common brain tumor in this population.
- AIDS-PCNSL occurs almost exclusively when the CD4 cell count is <50 per mm^3.
- The presenting signs and symptoms include:
  - may be asymptomatic
  - altered mental status
  - lateralizing signs
  - subtle personality changes, decreased alertness, or headache
  - seizures, seen in approximately 10% of cases.

Diagnosis

- A definitive histopathologic diagnosis requires biopsy.
  - There is often some reluctance to do this procedure.
- There have been major advances in the diagnosis of AIDS-PCNSL:
  - EBV is nearly ubiquitous in AIDS-PCNSL
  - Nuclear medicine studies can distinguish malignant lesions from infectious lesions.
    - Thallium-201 single–photon emission computerized tomography (SPECT)
    - Fluorodeoxyglucose positron emission tomography (FDG-PET)
  - Combined assessment of EBV in the cerebrospinal fluid by polymerase chain reaction (PCR) and imaging with either SPECT or positron emission tomography (PET) is diagnostic of PCNSL
    - If both EBV PCR and nuclear imaging are positive, the positive predictive value for PCNSL is 100% in this setting. In this case,
      - i. initiation of antitumor therapy is justified
      - ii. biopsy confirmation may be omitted.
    - If both tests are negative, the lesion is highly unlikely to be lymphoma.
    - Discordance of the test results requires biopsy to establish the diagnosis.
- In many medical centers, it has become standard practice to treat AIDS patients presenting with focal brain lesions and antitoxoplasma antibodies empirically with antitoxoplasmosis therapy, reserving biopsy for those patients who are seronegative for antitoxoplasma antibodies or who fail to respond to treatment. However, delay in diagnosis can adversely affect survival in AIDS-PCNSL.
- If biopsy is to be performed, corticosteroids should be withheld until a diagnosis is made, unless the patient is in immediate danger of herniation, because corticosteroids can obscure the pathologic diagnosis owing to brisk tumor response.

Staging

- The staging of PCNSL includes evaluation for potential peripheral lymphoma because its occurrence, by definition, indicates the central lesions to be of metastatic origin.
- Because ocular involvement is frequent, ophthalmologic examination with a slit lamp should be included in the evaluation, and its finding should be interpreted as part of the CNS involvement.

Prognosis and Treatment

- Median overall survivals are reported to be from 2 to 5 months.
- Prognosis may be improved with adequate immune reconstitution. HAART initiation/optimization on diagnosis of AIDS-PCNSL may help decrease the risk of recurrence and opportunistic infection if adequate immune reconstitution can be achieved. The outcome may be favorably affected in this setting.

- The treatment modalities (with the exception of high-dose chemotherapy) used for immuno-competent patients are also applied to patients with AIDS-PCNL, but with greater toxicity and poorer results.
  - PCNSL is highly responsive to whole-brain irradiation. The generally recommended dose of whole-brain radiotherapy is 40 Gy. There is a high rate of recurrent lymphoma and opportunistic infection, leading to poor outcome.
  - Relapse can not only occur at a site remote from the primary site but can also occur within the radiation port.
  - Combining chemotherapy with radiotherapy has not benefited most patients, and the negative effects of this combination on immune reconstitution should be considered while assessing its role in a given patient.
  - Surgery has no therapeutic role in PCNSL because microscopic tumor infiltration into brain parenchyma extends from the site of primary involvement.

Human Immunodeficiency Virus–Associated Hodgkin Disease

- HIV-HD is not an AIDS-defining condition.
- The most common histologic subtypes are
  - mixed cellularity
  - lymphocyte depleted
  - nodular sclerosing Hodgkin disease, the most common histologic subtype in HIV-negative (primary-HD) patients.
- EBV accounts for
  - 78% to 100% of cases in patients with HIV-HD
  - 15% to 48% of patients with non–HIV-related HD.
- Compared to patients with non–HIV-related HD, those with HIV-HD have the following characteristics:
  - younger age
  - higher stage disease
  - less frequent mediastinal involvement
  - more frequent involvement of extranodal sites of disease
  - more frequent occurrence of "B" symptoms.
- Prognosis is generally poorer for patients with HIV-HD than for those with primary HD, although patients often present with relatively well-preserved CD4 cell counts (median CD4 cell count is more than 275 per mm^3 in some series).

Treatment of Human Immunodeficiency Virus–Hodgkin Disease

- Many physicians advocate the use of systemic chemotherapy for all stages.
  - The commonly presented disease features are associated with a poor prognosis
    – male gender
    – a large number of sites being involved
    – mixed cellularity or lymphocyte-depleted histology.
  - Treatment includes
    – radiotherapy and/or chemotherapy
    – doxorubicin, bleomycin, vinblastine, and dacarbazine (ABVD)
    – epirubicin, bleomycin, vinblastine, and prednisone (EBVP).
  - Complete response rates range from 50% to more than 80%.
  - Relapse of HD and progression of AIDS are common, contributing to poor overall survival.
  - Survival improvements may be seen in the HAART era.
  - Most patients are not diagnosed with AIDS when they develop HIV-HD.
- Because the CNS is rarely involved, CNS prophylaxis is not commonly utilized.

Kaposi Sarcoma–Associated Herpesvirus–Associated Multicentric Castleman Disease

- KSHV-MCD is a rare lymphoproliferative disorder.
  - KSHV is associated with MCD in approximately 50% of non–HIV-infected patients.
- It has a short median survival:
  - Approximately 2 years
  - In many cases, delay in diagnosis may lead to bias in the statistical calculations.
- The syndrome is possibly related to the high levels of IL-6 produced by the tumors. Other factors include:
  - fevers
  - cytopenias
  - multiorgan dysfunction.
- Treatment—there is no defined standard of care. Most of the information has been obtained from case reports.
  - Single agent and combination chemotherapy
  - Interferon-α
  - Splenectomy
  - Rituximab
  - Antiviral therapy
  - Published reports of monoclonal antibody to IL-6 being useful in KSHV-MCD support the role of IL-6 in the pathogenesis of the disease.

ANOGENITAL CANCERS IN HUMAN IMMUNODEFICIENCY VIRUS INFECTION

Overview

- Cervical cancer is an AIDS-defining condition.
- Anal cancer is not an AIDS-defining condition.
  - It is relatively prevalent in
    - HIV-infected women
    - homosexual and bisexual men with HIV infection.
- Anogenital cancers in HIV infections are associated with human papilloma virus (HPV).

Screening

- The CDC recommends cytologic screening as part of initial evaluation when HIV-seropositivity is diagnosed.
  - If the initial PAP smear is normal, at least one additional evaluation should be repeated within 6 months. If the results of the repeat test are normal, then reevaluation should be done at least annually.
  - If the initial or follow-up Papanicolaou smear shows severe inflammation with reactive squamous cellular changes, another Papanicolaou smear should be collected within 3 months.
  - If the initial or follow-up Papanicolaou smear shows squamous intraepithelial lesions (SILs) or atypical squamous cells of undetermined significance, the patient should be referred for a colposcopic examination of the lower genital tract and, if indicated, should undergo colposcopically directed biopsies.
- HIV infection is not an indication for colposcopy among women with normal Papanicolaou smears.
- HPV-associated cytologic abnormalities are common in the anal mucosa of both HIV-infected women and homosexual men. Some experts have suggested that routine periodic cytologic examination of the anal mucosa should also be considered in high-risk individuals.

Cervical Cancer

Epidemiology

- SIL, vulvovaginal condyloma acumináta, and anal intraepithelial neoplasia are seen approximately five times more in HIV-infected women than in women who are not infected with HIV.
- The prevalence of cervical intraepithelial neoplasia has been reported to range from 11% to 29% overall for HIV-infected women.
- Among sexually active women, HIV-infected women have a substantially higher rate of persistent HPV infections of the types most strongly associated with intraepithelial lesions and invasive cervical cancer, for example, HPV-16 or HPV-18–associated viral types.
- HPV infection is associated with the development of SIL, and increased prevalence of HPV infection among HIV-infected women may explain the increased incidence of SIL in this population.
- Women with a CD4 cell count <500 per mm^3 appear to be at greater risk for poor outcome.
- The incidence of invasive cervical cancer appears unchanged since the advent of HAART.
  - It is unclear whether this is due to the reduced usage of these medications among the women at highest risk for both HIV and HPV or whether this is related to some other factor.

Therapy

- Standard therapy for preinvasive cervical neoplasia includes
  - cryotherapy
  - laser therapy
  - cone biopsy
  - loop excision.
- Recurrence of preinvasive cervical neoplasia among HIV-infected women (even among those with high CD4 cell count) is twice that found in HIV-seronegative women.
  - The lower the CD4 count, the higher the risk for recurrence.
  - Preliminary data suggest that early preinvasive lesions can regress with effective antiretroviral therapy.
  - HAART may reduce recurrence and progression following standard excisional therapy.
- Invasive cervical cancer should be approached with the same principles of oncologic management that guide the treatment of cervical cancer in HIV-negative patients.
  - Patients with well-controlled HIV infection and relative immune preservation can be expected to have outcomes similar to that of HIV-negative women.
  - Patients with advanced HIV disease may be less tolerant of the myelosuppressive effects of radiation therapy and combination chemotherapy.
  - Following surgery, recurrence is common.
  - When antineoplastic therapy is administered concomitantly with antiretroviral therapy, the potential for overlapping toxicity of the various agents should be considered in the therapeutic plan.

Anal Cancer

- HPV infection of the anal canal, and anal cancer and the immediate precursor lesions, high-grade anal intraepithelial neoplasia, are common among HIV-infected women and among MSM, especially those with HIV or immunosuppression.
- The prevalence of cytologically abnormal anal epithelium has been reported to be as high as 39% and the incidence of high-grade anal intraepithelial lesions has been reported to be as high as 15% among HIV-seropositive men.
- Anal SILs do not appear to regress in patients receiving HAART, except perhaps in some patients with high CD4 cell count.

- In invasive anal cancer, the standard combined chemotherapy and radiation appears to effectively control disease in most patients.
  - Patients with CD4 cell counts of 200 per mm^3 or greater appear to have better disease control, with acceptable morbidity.
  - Patients with CD4 cell counts of $<$200 per mm^3 appear more likely to experience treatment-related toxicity including cytopenias, intractable diarrhea, moist desquamation requiring hospitalization, or a colostomy either for a therapy-related complication or for salvage.
  - In the non–HIV-infected population, the considerations for using therapies that may be associated with less toxicity include the use of infusional cisplatin and 5-flourouracil with concomitant radiotherapy, although this has not been formally assessed in the HIV-infected population.

SUGGESTED READINGS

Antinori A, Cingolani A, et al. Better response to chemotherapy and prolonged survival in AIDS-related lymphomas responding to highly active antiretroviral therapy.*AIDS* 2001;15(12):1483–1491.

Antinori A, De Rossi G, et al. Value of combined approach with thallium-201 single-photon emission computed tomography and Epstein-Barr virus DNA polymerase chain reaction in CSF for the diagnosis of AIDS-related primary CNS lymphoma. *J Clin Oncol* 1999;17(2):554–560.

Antman K, Chang Y. Kaposi's sarcoma. *N Engl J Med* 2000;342(14):1027–1038.

Besson C, Goubar A, et al. Changes in AIDS-related lymphoma since the era of highly active antiretroviral therapy. *Blood* 2001;98(8):2339–2344.

Biggar RJ, Rabkin CS. The epidemiology of AIDS-related neoplasms. *Hematol Oncol Clin North Am* 1996;10(5):997–1010.

Boshoff C, Weiss R. AIDS-related malignancies. *Nat Rev Cancer* 2002;2(5):373–382.

Carbone A, Gloghini A, et al. Expression profile of MUM1/IRF4, BCL-6, and CD138/syndecan-1 defines novel histogenetic subsets of human immunodeficiency virus-related lymphomas. *Blood* 2001;97(3):744–751.

Chin-Hong PV, Palefsky JM. Natural history and clinical management of anal human papillomavirus disease in men and women infected with human immunodeficiency virus. *Clin Infect Dis* 2002;35(9): 1127–1134.

Eltom MA, Jemal A., et al. Trends in Kaposi's sarcoma and Non-Hodgkin's lymphoma incidence in the United States from 1973 through 1998. *J Natl Cancer Inst Cancer Spectrum* 2002;94(16):1204–1210.

Grulich AE, Li Y, et al. Rates of non-AIDS-defining cancers in people with HIV infection before and after AIDS diagnosis. *AIDS* 2002;16(8):1155–1161.

Grulich AE, Wan X, et al. Risk of cancer in people with AIDS. *AIDS* 1999;13(7):839–843.

Kaplan, L. No benefit from rituximab in a randomized phase III trial of CHOP with or without rituximab for patients with HIV-associated non-Hodgkin's lymphoma: AIDS malignancies consortium study 010. 7th International Conference on Malignancies in AIDS and Other Immunodeficiencies, Bethesda, MD, 2003.

Kaplan LD, Straus DJ, et al., National Institute of Allergy and Infectious Diseases AIDS Clinical Trials Group. Low-dose compared with standard-dose m-BACOD chemotherapy for non-Hodgkin's lymphoma associated with human immunodeficiency virus infection. *N Engl J Med* 1997;336(23):1641–1648.

Knowles DM. Molecular pathology of acquired immunodeficiency syndrome-related non-Hodgkin's lymphoma. *Semin Diagn Pathol* 1997;14(1):67–82.

Krown SE, Testa MA et al., AIDS Clinical Trials Group Oncology Committee. AIDS-related Kaposi's sarcoma: prospective validation of the AIDS Clinical Trials Group staging classification. *J Clin Oncol* 1997;15(9):3085–3092.

Kumar PP, Little RF, et al. Update on Kaposi's sarcoma: a gammaherpesvirus-induced malignancy. *Curr Infect Dis Rep* 2003;5(1):85–92.

Little RF, Pittaluga S, et al. Highly effective treatment of acquired immunodeficiency syndrome-related lymphoma with dose-adjusted EPOCH: impact of antiretroviral therapy suspension and tumor biology. Blood 2003;101(12):4653–4659.

Mbulaiteye SM, Parkin DM, et al. Epidemiology of AIDS-related malignancies: an international perspective. *Hematol Oncol Clin North Am* 2003;17(3):673–96, v.

Nasti G, Talamini R, et al. AIDS-related Kaposi's Sarcoma: evaluation of potential new prognostic factors and assessment of the AIDS Clinical Trial Group Staging System in the Haart Era—the Italian Cooperative Group on AIDS and Tumors and the Italian Cohort of Patients Naive From Antiretrovirals. *J Clin Oncol* 2003;21(15):2876–2882.

Ratner L, Lee J, et al. Chemotherapy for human immunodeficiency virus-associated non-Hodgkin's lymphoma in combination with highly active antiretroviral therapy. *J Clin Oncol* 2001;19(8):2171–2178.

Tirelli U, Errante D, et al. Hodgkin's disease and human immunodeficiency virus infection: clinico-pathologic and virologic features of 114 patients from the Italian Cooperative Group on AIDS and Tumors. *J Clin Oncol* 1995;13(7):1758–1767.

Tirelli U, Spina M, et al. Infusional CDE with rituximab for the treatment of human immunodeficiency virus-associated non-Hodgkin's lymphoma: preliminary results of a phase I/II study. *Recent Results Cancer Res* 2002;159:149–153.

Von Roenn JH, Cianfrocca M. Treatment of Kaposi's sarcoma. *Cancer Treat Res* 2001;104:127–148.

Yarchoan R. Therapy for Kaposi's sarcoma: recent advances and experimental approaches. *J Acquir Immune Defic Syndr* 1999;21(Suppl. 1):S66–S73.

Yarchoan R, Little R. Cancer : AIDS–Related Malignancies. In: DeVita VT, Hellman S, Rosenberg SA, eds. *Cancer principles and practice of oncology*. Philadelphia, PA: Lippincott Williams & Wilkins, 2005:2247–2263.

32

Carcinoma of Unknown Primary

Hung T. Khong

Departments of Medicine and Pharmacology, USA Cancer Research Institute, University of South Alabama, Mobile, Alabama

DEFINITION

Carcinoma of unknown primary (CUP) is defined as the detection of one or more metastatic tumors for which routine evaluation, including history and physical examination, routine blood work, urinalysis, chest x-ray (CXR), and histologic evaluation, fails to identify the primary site.

EPIDEMIOLOGY

- Incidence: 3% of all diagnosed oncologic cases are CUP.
- Gender: male-to-female ratio is approximately 1:1.
- Age: highest incidence is in the sixth decade of life.

CLINICAL FEATURES AND PROGNOSIS

Clinical Features

- At presentation, most patients (97%) complain of symptoms at metastatic site(s). Common presenting sites and common metastatic sites are listed in Tables 32.1 and 32.2.
- Nonspecific constitutional symptoms also are common: anorexia, weight loss, and fatigue.
- At diagnosis, more than 50% of patients (59%) have multiple sites (more than two) of metastatic involvement.

Prognosis

- In general, the median survival time of patients with CUP is 3 to 4 months; however, some recent studies have reported a median survival duration of 5 to 12 months.
- Most patients (55% to 85%) die within 1 year; 5% to 10% survive at 5 years (see Fig. 32.1).

Poor Prognostic Factors

- Male gender
- Adenocarcinoma histology
- Increasing number of involved organ sites
- Hepatic involvement
- Supraclavicular lymphadenopathy.

TABLE 32.1. *Common presenting sites*

Site	%	Range (%)
Lymph node	26	14–37
Lung	17	16–19
Bone	15	13–30
Liver	11	4–19
Brain	8	7–10
Pleura	7	2–12
Skin	5	0–22
Peritoneum	4	1–6

In each patient, the metastatic site that was apparent or symptomatic first was the only one counted. Data were collected from three series involving a total of 611 patients.

From Le Chevalier T, Cvitkovic E, Caille P, et al. Early metastatic cancer of unknown primary origin at presentation. A clinical study of 302 consecutive autopsied patients. *Arch Intern Med* 1988;148(9):2035–2039; Kirsten F, Chi CH, Leary JA, Ng AB, Hedley DW, Tattersall MH. Metastatic adeno or undifferentiated carcinoma from an unknown primary site-natural history and guidelines for identification of treatable subsets. *Q J Med* 1987;62(238):143–161; and Lyman GH, Preisler HD. Carcinoma of unknown primary: natural history and response to therapy. *J Med* 1978;9(6):445–459, with permission.

TABLE 32.2. *Common metastatic sites*

Site	%	Range (%)
Lymph nodes	41	20–42
Liver	34	33–43
Bone	29	29
Lung	27	26–31
Pleura	11	11–12
Peritoneum	9	—
Brain	6	6
Adrenal gland	6	4–6
Skin	4	—
Bone marrow	3	—

All principal metastatic sites in each patient were counted. Data were collected from two series involving a total of 1,051 patients. Data reported from subspecialty practices were excluded.

From Shildt RA, Kennedy PS, Chen TT, Athens JW, O'Bryan RM, Balcerzak SP. Management of patients with metastatic adenocarcinoma of unknown origin: a Southwest Oncology Group study. *Cancer Treat Rep* 1983;67(1):77–79 and Hess KR, Abbruzzese MC. Lenzi R, Raber MN, Abbruzzese JL. Classification and regression tree analysis of 1000 consecutive patients with unknown primary carcinoma. *Clin Cancer Res* 1999;5(11): 3403–3410, with permission.

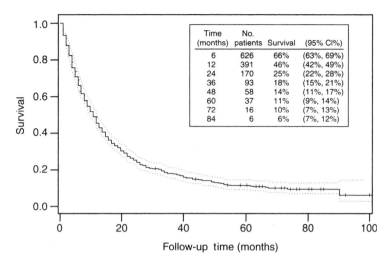

FIG. 32.1. Kaplan–Meier survival curve of 1,000 consecutive patients with cancer of unknown primary (CUP). Median survival is 11 months (95% confidence interval [CI], 10 to 12 months).

Advantageous Prognostic Factors

• Nonsupraclavicular lymphadenopathy
• Neuroendocrine histology
• A recent study of 1,000 patients (from M.D. Anderson) revealed several prognostic subgroups. Some subgroups are shown in Table 32.3.

DIAGNOSIS

• The recommended initial evaluation is listed in Table 32.4.
• Generous tissue samples should be obtained at the first biopsy.
• Accurate pathologic evaluation is critical.
• Light microscopic examination: four major histologic subtypes can be identified by the initial light microscopic examination (see Fig. 32.2).
• Immunoperoxidase staining (IPS) should be performed in all CUP cases of poorly differentiated carcinomas (PDCs). Table 32.5 lists some immunoperoxidase stains that are most useful.

TABLE 32.3. *Median survival in some prognostic subgroups*

Median survival time (mo)			
40	24	5	5
<3 metastatic organ sites; nonadenocarcinoma; no involvement of liver, bone, adrenal, or pleura	Liver mets and nonneuroendocrine histology	Liver mets; neuroendocrine histology; age >61.5 yr	Adrenal mets

Mets, metastasis.
The median survival for all patients in this study was 11 mo.

TABLE 32.4. *Initial evaluation*

Complete H & P (attention to breast and pelvic examination in women; prostate and testicular examination in men; and head/neck and rectal examination in all patients)
CBC
Chemistry profiles
Urinalysis
Stool testing for occult blood
CXR

H & P, history and physical; CBC, complete blood count; CXR, chest x-ray.

TABLE 32.5. *Immunoperoxidase staining in the differential diagnosis of carcinoma of unknown primary site*

Tumor type	Immunoperoxidase stains				
	Cytokeratin	Leukocyte common antigen	S100 protein, HMB 45	Neuron-specific enolase, chromogranin	Vimentin desmin
Carcinoma	+	−	−	±	−
Lymphoma	−	+	−	−	−
Melanoma	−	−	+	±	−
Sarcoma	−	−	−	−	+
Neuroendocrine	+	−	−	+	−

HMB, β-hydroxy β-methylbutyrate monohydrate.

- Electron microscopy should be considered if the tumor cannot be identified by IPS.
- Most common primary sites are listed in Table 32.6.

WELL-DIFFERENTIATED OR MODERATELY DIFFERENTIATED ADENOCARCINOMA OF UNKNOWN PRIMARY

Clinical Features

- Typically elderly patients
- Metastatic tumors at multiple sites
- Poor performance status (PS) at diagnosis
- Common metastatic sites: lymph nodes, liver, lung, and bone
- Most common primary sites identified: the lung and pancreas (45%) (Table 32.6)
- Poor prognosis (median survival of 3 to 4 months)
- Primary site is rarely found (<15% before death); an exhaustive search is not indicated.

Further Workup

Additional studies that should be performed include prostate-specific antigen (PSA) serum level and/or IPS for men and mammography, serum CA 15-3, serum CA 125, and estrogen receptor/progesterone receptor (ER/PR) (IPS) for women. Computerized tomography (CT) scan of the abdomen can identify a primary site in approximately 30% of cases. In patients with CUP who have metastatic adenocarcinoma to the axillary lymph nodes and a negative mammogram, breast magnetic resonance imaging (MRI) detected a primary breast cancer in 9 (75%) of 12 patients in one study and in 19 (86%) of 22 patients in another study.

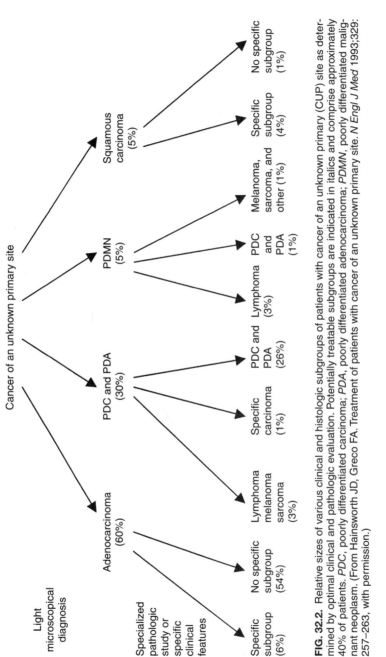

FIG. 32.2. Relative sizes of various clinical and histologic subgroups of patients with cancer of an unknown primary (CUP) site as determined by optimal clinical and pathologic evaluation. Potentially treatable subgroups are indicated in italics and comprise approximately 40% of patients. *PDC,* poorly differentiated carcinoma; *PDA,* poorly differentiated adenocarcinoma; *PDMN,* poorly differentiated malignant neoplasm. (From Hainsworth JD, Greco FA. Treatment of patients with cancer of an unknown primary site. *N Engl J Med* 1993;329:257–263, with permission.)

TABLE 32.6. *Primary sites (diagnosed during life or at autopsy)*

Primary sites	%
Lung	23.7
Pancreas	21.1
Ovary	6.4
Kidney	5.5
Colorectal	5.3
Gastric	4.6
Liver	4.3
Prostate	4.1
Breast	3.4
Adrenal	2.2
Thyroid	2.2
Urinary tract/bladder	1.9
Esophagus	1.5
Lymphoma	1.5
Gall bladder/biliary tree	1.2
Testicular germ cell	1
Mesothelioma	0.5
Uterus	0.3
Others	9.3
Total	100

Data were collected from nine series involving a total of 1,453 patients with CUP. A diagnosis was made either during life or at autopsy in 582 patients. Head/neck primary and data from subspecialty practices have been excluded in the calculation (to avoid artifactual representation of certain cancers such as the high rates of pancreatic primary reported by clinics specializing in gastrointestinal malignancy).

Treatment

- Most cases (90%) of well-differentiated or moderately differentiated adenocarcinoma of unknown primary show low response rates (RRs) and few complete responses with systemic chemotherapy.
- Patients in this group have a poor prognosis.
- The empiric chemotherapy for CUP has been discussed in Table 32.7.
- The various subsets of patients with different types of CUPs who can be treated are discussed in the following sections.

Peritoneal Carcinomatosis in Women

Characteristics:

- Typical of ovarian cancer
- Occasionally associated with cancers from the gastrointestinal (GI) tract or breast
- Serum CA125 level is often elevated.

Treatment:

- Treatment is the same as for stage III ovarian cancer (laparotomy with surgical cytoreduction, followed by taxane or platinum-based combination chemotherapy) (see Chapter 17). It should be noted that about 20% of patients have complete remission (CR) and 16% have prolonged disease-free survival.

TABLE 32.7. *Empiric chemotherapy for carcinoma of unknown primary*

Drug regimen	Treatment description	Cycle
EP[a] Cisplatin Etoposide	60–100 mg/m^2 i.v. on d 1 80–100 mg/m^2 i.v. on d 1–3	21 d
FAM[b] Fluorouracil Doxorubicin Mitomycin	600 mg/m^2 i.v., d 1, 8, 29, 36 30 mg/m^2 i.v., d 1, 29 10 mg/m^2 i.v., d 1	8 wk
Paclitaxel[c] Carboplatin Etoposide	200 mg/m^2 i.v. over 1 h, d 1 followed by dose calculated by Calvert formula to AUC 6 i.v., after paclitaxel 50 mg PO qd, alternating with 100 mg PO qd, d 1–10	21 d

In this study, there was an overall response rate (RR) of 47%, with 13% complete responses, and a median survival of 13.4 mo. Activity was seen in both well-differentiated adenocarcinoma (45% RR) and poorly differentiated carcinoma (48% RR). *AUC,* area under the curve.

[a]Adapted from Goldberg RM, Smith FP, Ueno W, et al. 5-Fluorouracil, adriamycin, and mitomycin in the treatment of adenocarcinoma of unknown primary. *J Clin Oncol* 1986;4(3):395–399.

[b]From Greco FA, Hainsworth JD. Cancer of unknown primary site. In: DeVita VT Jr, Hellman S, Rosenberg SA, eds. *Cancer: principles and practice of oncology.* 5th ed. Philadelphia: Lippincott-Raven Publishers, 1997:2423–2443, with permission.

[c]From Shepherd FA. Treatment of advanced non-small cell lung cancer. *Semin Oncol* 1994; 21:7–18, with permission.

Women with Axillary Lymph Node Metastases

Characteristics:

- Suggests breast cancer.
- ER/PR should be checked
- Occult breast primary is found in 55% to 75% of cases.

Treatment:

- Axillary node metastases should be treated in the same manner as stage II breast cancer.
- Modified radical mastectomy has been recommended.
- Alternatively, radiation therapy (XRT) to the breast can be performed after axillary node dissection.
- Adjuvant systemic chemotherapy should also be considered (see Chapter 17).
- Patients with metastatic sites in addition to axillary nodes should be treated for metastatic breast cancer (see Chapter 12).

Men with Elevated Prostate-specific Antigen or Osteoblastic Bone Metastasis

- If the PSA serum level or tumor staining is positive, a regimen of hormonal therapy similar to that used for metastatic prostate cancer (Chapter 14) should be started.
- If osteoblastic bone metastases are present, empiric hormonal therapy should be started regardless of the PSA levels.

Patients with a Single Metastatic Site

- Surgical excision and/or XRT is performed.

POORLY DIFFERENTIATED CARCINOMA/ADENOCARCINOMA OF UNKNOWN PRIMARY

Introduction

- Poorly differentiated carcinoma and poorly differentiated adenocarcinoma (PDA) account for 30% of CUP (PDC accounts for two thirds of CUP and PDA accounts for one third of CUP).

- Patients with PDC and PDA show poor response to fluorouracil-based chemotherapy and exhibit a short survival.
- Some patients have neoplasms that are highly responsive to platinating agent–based combination chemotherapeutic treatments. Some long-term survivors and cures have been described for both PDC and PDA.

Clinical Features

- Younger median age (about 40 years)
- Rapid progression of symptoms
- Evidence of rapid tumor growth
- Most common sites of metastatic involvement (50% of cases): lymph nodes, mediastinum, and retroperitoneum.

Pathologic Evaluation

- IPS is useful in the pathologic evaluation of PDC and PDA.
- Electron microscopic evaluation should be performed if tumor cannot be identified by IPS.
- Genetic analysis may be useful [e.g., i(12p), del(12p), or multiple copies of (12p) are diagnostic of germ cell tumor].

Further Workup

- Additional workup should include CT scan of chest and abdomen, and serum β-human chorionic gonadotropin (β-HCG) and α-fetoprotein (AFP).

Treatment

1. Extragonadal germ cell cancer syndrome
   - This syndrome is commonly found in young men.
   - These are predominantly midline tumors (mediastinum or retroperitoneum).
   - The syndrome is characterized by elevated levels of β-HCG, AFP, or both.
   - Genetic analysis may be diagnostic (e.g., abnormalities in chromosome 12).
   - This syndrome should be treated in the same manner as a germ cell tumor (Chapter 16).
2. Poorly differentiated neuroendocrine carcinoma
   - These carcinomas are high-grade tumors.
   - It is characterized by multiple metastatic sites.
   - The carcinomas are highly responsive to cisplatin-based chemotherapy.
   - The overall RR for combination chemotherapy was 71% (33 of 46 patients), with a complete response (CR) in 28% (13 of 46 patients); 17% of patients (8 of 46 patients) showed durable disease-free survival.
   - Patients in this group should be treated with a regimen of combination chemotherapy including a platinating agent and etoposide (Table 32.7). It should be noted that other patients with PDC or PDA should receive an empiric therapy of platinating agent–based chemotherapy (Table 32.7). (In a prospective study of 220 patients, the overall RR was 62%, with a complete RR of 26%. Thirteen percent of patients were considered cured.)

POORLY DIFFERENTIATED MALIGNANT NEOPLASMS OF UNKNOWN PRIMARY

- Poorly differentiated malignant neoplasms of unknown primary are found in 5% of all patients with CUP.
- Specialized pathologic study found 35% to 65% of the malignant neoplasms to be lymphomas; carcinomas accounted for most of the remaining cases. Less than 15% of the neoplasms are melanoma and sarcoma.

SQUAMOUS CELL CARCINOMA OF UNKNOWN PRIMARY

Cervical Node Involvement

High Cervical Node(s)

- Workup and treatment of squamous cell carcinoma of unknown primary in the high cervical nodes is the same as that for primary head and neck cancer (see Chapter 1).
- High long-term survival rates (30% to 70%) have been reported after local treatment.
- The role of chemotherapy is undetermined.

Low Cervical or Supraclavicular Node(s)

- Histology can be either squamous, adenocarcinoma, or poorly differentiated tumors.
- Poorer prognosis (particularly for adenocarcinoma histology) is because lung and GI tract are frequent primary sites.
- If no other sites of disease are found, a few patients (10% to 15%) will have a long-term disease-free survival with aggressive local therapy (surgery and/or XRT).
- The role of chemotherapy is undetermined.

Inguinal Lymph Node(s)

- A primary site in the genital or anorectal areas is often identified in most patients.
- Curative therapy is available for some of these patients.
- If no primary is found, surgical node dissection (with or without XRT) can offer long-term survival.

SUGGESTED READINGS

Abbruzzese JL, Abbruzzese MC, Hess KR, et al. Unknown primary carcinoma: natural history and prognostic factors in 657 consecutive patients. *J Clin Oncol* 1994;12:1272–1280.

Bataini JP, Rodriguez J, Jaulerry C, et al. Treatment of metastatic neck nodes secondary to an occult epidermoid carcinoma of the head and neck. *Laryngoscopy* 1987;97:1080–1089.

Ellerbroek N, Holmes F, Singletary E, et al. Treatment of patients with isolated axillary nodal metastases from an occult primary carcinoma consistent with breast origin. *Cancer* 1990;66:1481–1491.

Eltabbakh GH, Piver MS. Extraovarian primary peritoneal carcinoma. *Oncology* 1998;12:813–819.

Goldberg RM, Smith FP, Ueno W, et al. 5-Fluorouracil, adriamycin, and mitomycin in the treatment of adenocarcinoma of unknown primary. *J Clin Oncol* 1986;4(3):395–399.

Greco FA, Hainsworth JD. Cancer of unknown primary site. In: DeVita VT Jr, Hellman S, Rosenberg SA, eds. *Cancer: principles and practice of oncology*, 5th ed. Philadelphia, PA: Lippincott–Raven Publishers, 1997:2423–2443.

Greco FA, Oldham RK, Fer MF. The extragonadal germ cell cancer syndrome. *Semin Oncol* 1982;9:448–455.

Hainsworth JD, Johnson DH, Greco FA. Cisplatin-based combination chemotherapy in the treatment of poorly differentiated carcinoma and poorly differentiated adenocarcinoma of unknown primary site: results of a 12-year experience. *J Clin Oncol* 1992;10:912–922.

Hess KR, Abbruzzese MC, Lenzi R, et al. Classification and regression tree analysis of 1000 consecutive patients with unknown primary carcinoma. *Clin Cancer Res* 1999;5(11):3403–3410.

Kirsten F, Chi CH, Leary JA, et al. Metastatic adeno or undifferentiated carcinoma from an unknown primary site-natural history and guidelines for identification of treatable subsets. *Q J Med* 1987;62(238):143–161.

Le Chevalier T, Cvitkov́ic E, Caille P, et al. Early metastatic cancer of unknown primary origin at presentation. A clinical study of 302 consecutive autopsied patients. *Arch Intern Med* 1988;148(9):2035–2039.

Lyman GH, Preisler HD. Carcinoma of unknown primary: natural history and response to therapy. *J Med* 1978;9(6):445–459.

Morris EA, Schwartz LH, Dershaw DD, et al. MR imaging of the breast in patients with occult primary breast carcinoma. *Radiology* 1997;205(2):437–440.

Orel SG, Weinstein SP, Schnall MD, et al. Breast MR imaging in patients with axillary node metastases and unknown primary malignancy. *Radiology* 1999;212(2):543–549.

Shepherd FA. Treatment of advanced non-small cell lung cancer. *Semin Oncol* 1994;21:7–18.

Shildt RA, Kennedy PS, Chen TT, et al. Management of patients with metastatic adenocarcinoma of unknown origin: a Southwest Oncology Group study. *Cancer Treat Rep* 1983;67(1):77–79.

Sporn JR, Greenberg BR. Empirical chemotherapy in patients with carcinoma of unknown primary. *Am J Med* 1990;88:49–55.

http://www.nci.nih.gov/cancer/topics/pdq/treatment/unknownprimary/HealthProfessional, 2004.

33

Central Nervous System Tumors

Patrick J. Mansky[*], J. Paul Duic[†], and Howard A. Fine[††]

[*]*National Center for Complementary and Alternative Medicine, National Institutes of Health, Bethesda, Maryland;* [†]*Department of Emergency Medicine, Johns Hopkins University, Baltimore, Maryland and* [††]*Neuro-Oncology Branch, National Cancer Institute and National Institute of Neurologic Disorders, National Institutes of Health, Bethesda, Maryland*

Primary brain tumors represent a diverse spectrum of diseases that uniformly pose a unique problem to the practitioner because of their intracranial location. Brain tumors represent the second most common neurologic cause of death after stroke, but only the tenth most common cause of death from cancer. Nevertheless, they are a major cause of mortality from cancer in young adults and children. Most adult brain tumors occur in the cerebral hemispheres, but two thirds of all pediatric brain tumors are infratentorial.

During autopsy, metastatic brain tumors can be found in 25% to 40% of patients with systemic cancer. Early detection and accuracy of diagnosis have markedly improved because of advances in computerized tomography (CT) and magnetic resonance imaging (MRI). Despite the improvements, the prognosis for most forms of malignant brain tumors remains extremely poor. The mainstays of therapy remain surgery and radiation, whereas chemotherapy is beneficial only in a select group of tumors.

EPIDEMIOLOGY

According to the Surveillance, Epidemiology, and End Results (SEER) registry for 1973 through 1987, the range of incidence of brain tumors is 2 to 19 cases per 100,000 persons per year, depending on age at diagnosis.

- Peak age: 0 to 4 years, 3.1 per 100,000 persons
- Plateau: 65 to 79 years, 17.9 to 18.7 per 100,000 persons
- 17,000 to 20,000 new cases per year
- Primary brain tumors comprise 2% of newly diagnosed malignancies per year in the United States.

Distribution

The most common central nervous system (CNS) tumors are derived from glial precursors. The distribution of tumor frequency by age is demonstrated in Table 33.1.

Mortality

There are an estimated 13,000 deaths from primary brain tumors per year. CNS tumors are the most prevalent solid tumors in childhood. In children younger than 15 years, brain tumors

433

TABLE 33.1. *Distribution of tumor frequency by age*

Histology	0–9	10–19	20–29	30–39	40–49	50–59	60–74
Astrocytoma	60%	59%	76%	81%	86%	87%	91%
Low-grade	10%	7%	5%	5%	3%	2%	2%
Anaplastic	47%	43%	51%	55%	48%	39%	40%
GBM	1%	7%	14%	18%	33%	44%	51%
Mixed glioma	3%	4%	5%	6%	6%	4%	2%
Oligodendroglioma	1%	4%	5%	6%	6%	4%	2%
Ependymoma	9%	3%	4%	2%	1%	1%	1%
Medulloblastoma	21%	10%	6%	2%	1%	0%	0%
Embryonal/teratoid	1%	1%	0%	0%	0%	0%	0%
Meningioma	0%	0%	1%	2%	1%	2%	2%

Age (yr) spans the numeric columns.

GBM, glioblastoma multiforme.
From DeVita VT Jr, Hellman S, Rosenberg SA, eds. *Cancer: principles and practice of oncology*, 6th ed. Philadelphia: Lippincott-Raven, 2001, with permission.

are the most frequent cancer-related causes of death. In the age group 15 to 59 years, CNS tumors are the third leading cause of cancer-related deaths. However, 80% of all primary brain tumor–related deaths occur in patients older than 59 years.

CLINICAL DIAGNOSIS

Common symptoms (by decreasing frequency):

- Headache
- Seizure
- Cognitive/personality changes
- Focal weakness
- Nausea/vomiting
- Speech abnormalities
- Altered consciousness

Common signs (by decreasing frequency):

- Hemiparesis
- Cranial nerve palsies
- Papilledema
- Cognitive dysfunction
- Sensory deficits
- Hemianesthesia
- Hemianopia
- Dysphasia

DIFFERENTIAL DIAGNOSIS

Tumors of the cerebrum may be differentiated by location according to age at onset of symptoms (see Table 33.2 and Fig. 33.1).

Acute Complications of Intracranial Tumors

Because the skull's rigid nature does not allow for processes associated with intracranial expansion, brain lesions routinely result in structural displacement and life-threatening consequences. Following the path of least resistance, tentorial or foramen magnum herniation may ensue. Neurologic findings are described in Tables 33.3 and 33.4.

TABLE 33.2. *Differential diagnosis*

Location	Adult	Child
Supratentorial	Metastatic disease	Astrocytoma
	Glioblastoma	Glioblastoma
	Astrocytoma	Oligodendroglioma
	Meningioma	Sarcoma
	Oligodendroglioma	Neuroblastoma
	Mixed glioma	Mixed glioma
Infratentorial	Metastatic disease	Astrocytoma
	Astrocytoma	Medulloblastoma
	Glioblastoma	Ependymoma
	Ependymoma	Brainstem glioma
	Brainstem glioma	
Sellar/parasellar	Pituitary tumor	Craniopharyngioma
	Meningioma	Optic glioma
		Epidermoid
Base of skull	Neurinoma	
	Meningioma	
	Chordoma	
	Carcinoma	
	Dermoid/epidermoid	

TABLE 33.3. *Neurologic findings*

Tentorial/temporal lobe herniation
Pupillary dilation
Ptosis
Ipsilateral hemiplegia
Contralateral hemiplegia
Homonymous hemianopia
Midbrain syndrome
Coma with rising blood pressure/bradycardia

TABLE 33.4. *Neurologic findings*

Cerebellar/foramen magnum herniation
Head tilt
Stiff neck
Neck paresthesias
Tonic tensor spasms of limbs and body
Coma
Respiratory arrest

PRIMARY BRAIN TUMORS VERSUS BRAIN METASTASES

Primary Brain Tumors

Gliomas

Four major types of gliomas have been recognized on the basis of their presumed normal glial cell of origin:

1. Astrocytoma
2. Oligodendrocytoma

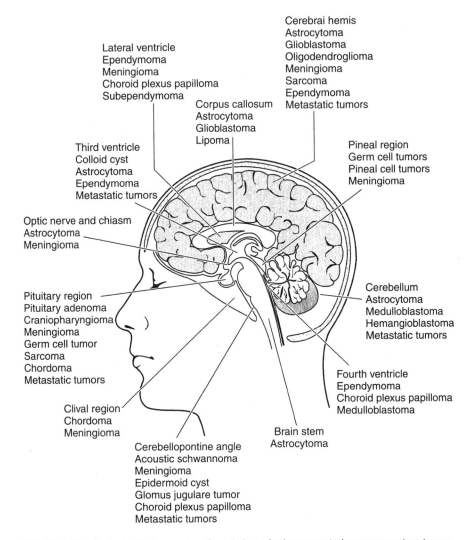

FIG. 33.1. Topologic distribution and preferred sites of primary central nervous system tumors. (From Burger PC, Scheithauer BW, Vogel FS. *Surgical pathology of the nervous system and its coverings*, 3rd ed. New York: Churchill Livingstone, 1991, with permission.)

3. Oligoastrocytoma (mixed glioma)
4. Ependymoma

Grading

The pathologic classification of primary brain tumors has been a controversial and constantly changing area secondary to the lack of prognostic relevance for most classification systems. In addition, the considerable intraobserver variability between neuropathologists in assessing the specific histologic subtypes of a given tumor, secondary to the subjective criteria of each pathologic classification schema, has made the classification of brain tumors even more confusing. A pathologic grading system recently proposed by the World Health Organization (WHO) has been generally accepted by most neuropathologists and incorporates the following features for determining the grade (level of aggressiveness) of each histologic subtype of tumor:

- Cellular atypia
- Mitotic activity
- Degree of cellularity
- Vascular proliferation
- Degree of necrosis

A general classification of primary brain tumors can be found in the subsequent text:

Grade 1

- Pilocytic astrocytoma
- Giant cell astrocytoma
- Ganglioglioma
- Dysembryoplastic neuroepithelial tumors

Grade 2

- Well-differentiated low-grade astrocytomas
- Oligodendrogliomas
- Ependymomas

Grade 3

- Anaplastic astrocytomas (AAs)
- Anaplastic oligodendrogliomas
- Anaplastic ependymal tumors

Grade 4

- Glioblastoma multiforme (GBM)
- Embryonal tumors

Epidemiology

Gliomas comprise 45% of all intracranial tumors, with peak age in the seventh decade. Table 33.5 shows the prevalence of the pathologic subtypes of gliomas in relation to other more common primary brain tumors.

Molecular Genetics of Gliomas

Genetic alterations form a continuum of progressive anaplasia in gliomas (see Table 33.6). Whereas secondary or progressive gliomas often harbor mutations of p53 and overexpression

TABLE 33.5. *Epidemiology*

Type	%
Glioblastoma	55.0
Astrocytoma	20.5
Ependymoma	6.0
Medulloblastoma	6.0
Oligodendroglioma	5.0
Choroid plexus papilloma	2.0
Colloid cyst	2.0

TABLE 33.6. *Molecular genetics of gliomas*

Genetic alteration	Anaplasia	Glioma variant

TP53 mutation
  PDGF overexpression
  Loss of chromosome 17p and 22q
	Low-grade	Low-grade astrocytoma

CDKN2/p16 deletion
  RB mutation
  CDK4 amplification
  Loss of chromosome 9p, 19q, 11p
	Anaplastic astrocytoma	

MDM2 amplification/overexpression
  EGFR amplification rearrangements
  PTEN mutation
  Loss of chromosome 10
	High-grade GBM	

GBM, glioblastoma multiforme; EGFR, epidermal growth factor receptor.

of the platelet-derived growth factor (PDGF) receptor, they seldom show amplification of epidermal growth factor receptor (EGFR). By contrast, primary or *de novo* GBM usually lack p53 mutations and contain an amplified EGFR. To date, none of the molecular parameters has demonstrated any significant association with patient survival in GBM.

Glioblastoma Multiforme

- GBM is the most common adult primary brain tumor, accounting for 10% to 15% of intracranial tumors.
- The age of peak incidence is 45 to 55 years; overall incidence is two to three per 100,000 population; sex distribution, male-to-female ratio is 3:2.
- Median survival is 6 months.

Localization

- GBM occurs equally everywhere in the brain and is proportional to the volume of brain tissue in that particular anatomic location.
- It is more likely to be bihemispheric than other types of tumors are.

Development

Development of GBM is *de novo* ("primary") or is a progression from a lower grade precursor lesion ("secondary").

Genetics

- p53 mutations
- EGFR amplification
- Loss of heterozygosity (LOH) on chromosome 10; phosphatase and tensin homolog (PTEN) deletions
- LOH on chromosome 17p
- Significant aneuploidy

Imaging Characteristics on Magnetic Resonance Imaging

- Heterogeneous hypointense or isointense mass on CT scan or on Tesla 1 (T1, relaxation time 1) MRI.
- Heterogeneously contrast-enhancing mass

- Hypervascular appearance
- Calcifications are rare

Differential Diagnosis

- Brain metastasis
- Cerebral abscess
- Demyelinating/inflammatory process (i.e., multiple sclerosis)
- Radiation necrosis
- Single photon emission computerized tomography (SPECT) and MR cerebral perfusion imaging may be used to distinguish radiation necrosis (hypovascular) from tumor recurrence (hypervascular)

MR spectroscopy is being increasingly used to help distinguish tumor from other processes that are visualized on MRI.

Gliosarcoma is a variant, with a mesenchymal component and a greater tendency for dural invasion.

GBMs are characteristically infiltrative within brain parenchyma but rarely show extracerebral metastasis.

Therapy

Current treatment recommendations for malignant gliomas (i.e., high-grade astrocytomas and GBM) include surgical resection, adjuvant radiotherapy, and, in select patients, the addition of chemotherapy. Secondary to the infiltrative growth characteristics of malignant gliomas, tumors recur even after gross total primary resection.

An analysis of several Radiation Therapy Oncology Group (RTOG) trials created the survival categories according to patient characteristics, as shown in Table 33.7.

Radiation therapy has demonstrated a clear survival benefit in several randomized clinical trials, increasing the median survival from 20 to 36 weeks. Irradiation usually includes the contrast-enhanced tumor volume or peritumoral edema with a margin of 2 to 3 cm. A total dose of 60 Gy is delivered in 30 to 33 fractions. Palliative treatment courses provide radiation to 30 Gy in 10 fractions over 2 weeks.

The role of chemotherapy in the treatment of malignant gliomas was established by the Brain Tumor Study Group (BTSG) in several phase III trials, introducing nitrosoureas as effective agents. Carmustine (BCNU), at a dose of 80 mg per m^2 given daily for 3 days, repeated every 6 weeks, increased median survival from 38 to 51 weeks in patients with GBM. There is no real rationale for administering the BCNU over 3 days, and, more commonly, it is now given as a single intravenous (i.v.) infusion of 200 mg per m^2 every 6 weeks.

TABLE 33.7. *Survival categories by patient characteristics*

Patient characteristics	Tumor	Median survival (mo)
Age <50 yr, normal mental status Age >50 yr, KPS >70, symptoms >3 mo	Anaplastic astrocytoma	40–60
Age <50 yr, abnormal mental status Age >50 yr, symptoms <3 mo	Anaplastic astrocytoma	11–18
Age >50 yr	Glioblastoma	11–18
Age <50 yr, KPS >70		
Age >50 yr, KPS <70 or abnormal mental status	Glioblastoma	5–9

KPS, Karnofsky performance status.

Recent data from a randomized European Organization for Research and Treatment of Cancer (EORTC) trial have established a new standard of care for patients with newly diagnosed glioblastoma. In this trial, temozolomide was given at a dose of 75 mg/m^2/day every day throughout the 6 weeks of standard external-beam radiotherapy (60 Gy in 30 fractions). Temozolomide was then administered postradiotherapy at a dosage of 200 mg/m^2/day for 5 days every 28 days for six cycles. Patients who received this regimen had a statistically significant increase in prolongation of survival compared to patients who received radiotherapy alone (median survival increased by approximately 2.5 months; 2-year survival increased from 9% with radiation alone to 28% with combined treatment).

The role of multiagent chemotherapy versus single-agent therapy with BCNU remains controversial. The most commonly used regimen is PCV (see Table 33.8), which has demonstrated durable responses of more than 50% in anaplastic oligodendrogliomas. Anaplastic astrocytomas, mixed gliomas, and recurrent oligodendrogliomas also have shown favorable responses to this regimen. Temozolomide is also active in these glial tumors; however, currently, there is no basis for comparing the activity of PCV and temozolomide (although the PCV regimen tends to be associated with a higher incidence of side effects).

Given the overall poor prognosis for patients with high-grade gliomas, new treatment strategies are needed. Possibly the most promising of such strategies is the use of new inhibitors of signal transduction pathways such as inhibitors of the EGFR, platelet-derived growth factor receptor (PDGFR), ras, and mTOR pathways. Other treatment strategies currently under investigation include therapeutic gene transfer and antiangiogenic and immunotherapeutic approaches.

Astrocytoma

Astrocytomas comprise 25% to 30% of all hemispheric gliomas.

Low-grade Diffuse Astrocytoma

- Grade II
- Accounts for approximately 5% of primary brain tumors
- Mean age, 34 years
- Distribution: mostly cerebral hemispheres but also in the brainstem
- Imaging characteristics on MRI:
  - Little edema/mass effect
  - Difficulty in distinguishing the astrocytoma from nonmalignant infarct/cerebritis/demyelination
  - Rare calcifications
  - Large area of white/gray matter changes
  - Differential diagnosis: infarct or cerebritis

TABLE 33.8. *PCV regimen: Procarbazine, lomustine (CCNU), vincristine*

Procarbazine, 60 mg/m^2/d PO for 14 d, on cycle d 8–21 (d 8–21; total dose/cycle, 840 mg/m^2)
Lomustine (CCNU), 110 mg/m^2 PO d 1 (d 1; total dose/cycle, 110 mg/m^2)
Vincristine, 1.4 mg/m^2/dose i.v. on d 8 and 29 (d 8 and 29; total dose/cycle, 2.8 mg/m^2)
  Cycle duration is 6 wk; may be extended to 8 wk for hematologic recovery

From Levin VA, Silver P, Hannigan J, et al. Superiority of post-radiotherapy adjuvant chemotherapy with CCNU, procarbazine, and vincristine (PCV) over BCNU for anaplastic astrocytoma: NCOG 6G61 final report. *Int J Radiat Oncol Biol Phys* 1990;18:321–324, with permission.

Median survival for patients after surgery of 19% to 32% at 5 years and 10% at 10 years is surpassed by that for the patients treated with surgery and postoperative irradiation, which is 36% to 55% after 5 years and 26% to 43% after 10 years.

Therapy

Historically, radiation therapy has been the standard treatment. The timing and dose of radiation therapy have been questioned. Recent studies of several hundred patients with low-grade gliomas from the EORTC have demonstrated no survival benefit for 60 Gy of radiation compared to 54 Gy. Thus, 54 Gy of radiation is currently considered standard. In another EORTC trial, patients with low-grade gliomas were randomized between immediate radiation at the time of diagnosis versus delayed radiation until radiographic and/or clinical progression. Although median time to tumor progression was longer for the immediate radiotherapy group, there was no difference in overall survival.

Recent data demonstrated that temozolomide can induce significant (albeit slow) preradiation tumor regressions in low-grade astrocytomas, although it does not appear that such responses are generally prolonged.

Low-grade supratentorial astrocytomas of children respond for prolonged periods to carboplatin and vincristine, although pilocytic tumors (see subsequent text) tend to be more responsive than diffuse astrocytomas.

Pilocytic astrocytomas are a special subset of low-grade astrocytomas and represent the most common childhood astrocytic tumor. This is virtually the only type of astrocytoma for which cure is possible with complete surgical resection.

Prolonged stabilization and tumor regression can be seen both with radiotherapy and chemotherapy, with the carboplatin and vincristine regimen being the most commonly used.

High-grade Diffuse Astrocytoma

- Grade III
- Accounts for approximately 5% of primary brain tumors; mean age, 41 years
- Macroscopically indistinguishable from low-grade astrocytomas
- Survival: 2 to 5 years

Therapy

Early trials established the role of postoperative radiation therapy at a dose of approximately 60 Gy, increasing median survival time from 14 to 36 weeks. The introduction of postoperative chemotherapy with nitrosourea-based regimens such as PCV significantly increased survival, particularly in anaplastic astrocytoma, with 50% of patients being alive at 157 weeks. Two large retrospective studies from the University of California, San Francisco (UCSF) and the RTOG, however, suggest that the outcomes are just as good for patients treated with postradiation single-agent nitrosourea [i.e., BCNU and lomustine (CCNU)] as for those treated with PCV. There are currently no prospective data on the use of temozolomide in the postradiation setting for anaplastic gliomas. Nevertheless, on the basis of the proven activity of nitrosoureas in the postradiation setting in anaplastic gliomas and the proven activity of temozolomide in recurrent anaplastic gliomas, it is reasonable to extrapolate that temozolomide will prove to be active in the postradiation setting for anaplastic gliomas.

Brainstem Gliomas

Brainstem gliomas occur predominantly in children as a group of diffuse astrocytomas of all grades.

The clinical course is often malignant, regardless of grade, with a typical presentation of cranial nerve VI and VII palsies.

Management

- Surgery: Brainstem gliomas are rarely resectable unless there is a very large exophytic component. Even then, the intrinsic component is never completely resectable. Infiltrating pontine gliomas are one of the few (if not the only) brain tumors for which treatment based purely on radiographic criteria, and without a tissue diagnosis, is considered appropriate.
- Radiation therapy: A dose of 60 Gy of radiation is delivered in standard fractionation. Earlier data pointing to an advantage for hyperfractionation have not held up.
- Chemotherapy: Regimens including CCNU, PCV, 5-fluorouracil, and hydroxyurea have been tested without clear survival benefits.

Oligodendrogliomas and Oligoastrocytomas (Mixed Gliomas)

- Diffuse cerebral tumors; often appear with prominent areas of calcification on CT scan
- Accounts for 5% to 10% of all gliomas
- May have better prognosis than astrocytomas
- Chemosensitive, particularly anaplastic oligodendroglioma; most promising regimen includes PCV and temozolomide
- Like astrocytomas, low-grade gliomas may progress to higher grade gliomas

Treatment

- Low-grade oligodendrogliomas are best treated by surgical resection if most of the radiographically visible tumor can be safely removed.
- Radiation therapy has been the historic treatment of choice for low-grade progressive and anaplastic oligodendrogliomas. Increasingly so, chemotherapy with PCV or temozolomide is being used either in the postradiation adjuvant setting or as neoadjuvant therapy in order to delay the potential long-term neurotoxicity of radiation therapy; particularly in the settings of large diffuse tumors that would require large-field radiation.

EPENDYMOMA

Ependymomas comprise a spectrum of tumors ranging from aggressive childhood intraventricular tumors to low-grade adult spinal cord lesions. Typical locations are on the ventricular surface and the filum terminale.

Epidemiology

- Ependymomas account for 2% to 7.8% of all CNS neoplasms.
- 75% of ependymomas are of low grade.
- 50% occur before the age of 5 years.
- Intracranial tumors: 60% infratentorial, 40% supratentorial (with 50% intraventricular).
- Overall incidence of spinal seeding, approximately 7% to 15.7% for high-grade infratentorial lesions, is increased in patients with uncontrolled primary lesions.

Imaging

CT scanning and MRI are highly suggestive of the presence of ependymomas (i.e., calcified mass on the fourth ventricle) but are not diagnostic.

Management

Surgery

Survival benefit is noted only for complete resections that are confirmed by neuroimaging.

Radiotherapy

- When complete surgical resection is achieved, no adjuvant therapy is recommended for low-grade ependymomas.
- Radiation therapy is usually warranted for low-grade ependymomas that show radiographic signs of tumor progression and for which complete surgical resection is no longer possible. Radiation is also warranted for anaplastic ependymomas.
- The entire posterior fossa is treated in case of infratentorial ependymomas, whereas local fields are treated in case of supratentorial ependymomas.
- Craniospinal irradiation is warranted for evidence of seeding by cerebrospinal fluid (CSF) cytologic or radiographic studies, or for anaplastic ependymoma.

Chemotherapy

Multiple chemotherapeutic regimens have been tested in recurrent and anaplastic ependymomas. Generally, response rates have been very low, with few responses being maintained. The role of chemotherapy in this disease remains investigational.

Prognosis

- Low-grade tumors: 5-year survival, 60% to 80%
- Anaplastic ependymoma: 5-year survival, 10% to 47%
- With surgery alone: long-term survival, 17% to 27%
- Surgery plus radiation: long-term survival, 40% to 87%
- Age is dominant prognostic factor; infants do poorly.

CHOROID PLEXUS TUMORS

These tumors occur mostly in ventricles; in adults, the occurrence is predominantly in the fourth ventricle. The spectrum of tumors ranges from aggressive supratentorial childhood tumors to benign cerebellopontine angle tumors of adulthood. An association with Li–Fraumeni syndrome and von Hippel–Lindau syndrome has been described.

Diagnosis

- Signs of increased intracranial pressure (ICP)
- Focal findings of the fourth ventricle: ataxia and nystagmus
- Anaplastic histologic changes warrant CSF examination for increased risk of disseminated disease.

Management

Surgery

Complete resection is the goal of surgery.

Radiation Therapy/Chemotherapy

Given the rarity of these tumors, there are few prospective studies to evaluate any uniform approach. Radiation therapy, in conjunction with chemotherapy, has been used with some benefit for choroid plexus carcinoma and anaplastic tumors. Combinations of doxorubicin, cyclophosphamide, vincristine, and nitrosoureas have been used, as well as intraventricular methotrexate and cytarabine. Studies to evaluate these approaches have not been undertaken.

MEDULLOBLASTOMA

Medulloblastoma is a malignant, "small, blue, round cell tumor" of the CNS.

Epidemiology

- Medulloblastoma forms 25% of all pediatric tumors, and is found predominantly in the posterior fossa in children.
- It is uncommon in adults.
- 30% to 50% of medulloblastomas have isochromosome 17q.
- It is associated with Gorlin syndrome and Turcot syndrome.

Clinical Presentation

The most common presenting symptoms include signs of increased ICP, and cerebellar and bulbar signs. Five percent to 25% of patients have CSF dissemination at diagnosis, with less than 10% of patients exhibiting systemic metastasis, commonly to the bone; 40% of patients have brainstem infiltration.

Risk Stratification

- Average risk: With incidence of localized disease at diagnosis, total or near-total resection achieved
- High risk: Perceived with disseminated disease and/or partial resection

Imaging

Typically, contrast-enhancing posterior fossa midline lesion, most frequently arising from cerebellar vermis, is visualized on CT scan or MRI.

Staging

- A modified Chang staging system (see Table 33.9), where the presence of disseminated disease is the most important factor, is currently used. The other important prognostic factors are age (worse in children younger than 3 years) and extent of resection (controversial).
- Evaluation is performed according to size, local extension, and presence of metastasis.
- CSF and spinal axis should be evaluated for metastasis with lumbar puncture and contrast-enhanced MRI scan.

Management

- Surgery: goal is complete resection.
- Radiation therapy: involves postoperative 35-Gy radiation to whole brain, with 15- to 20-Gy boost to posterior fossa. Average-risk patients may be cured with radiation alone.
- In children with nondisseminated disease, there is emerging evidence that 23.4-Gy radiation to the craniospinal axis, supplemented by 31-Gy local irradiation, in conjunction with vincristine, 1.5 mg per m² for eight doses, followed by adjuvant CCNU, 75 mg/m² PO, and cisplatin, 75 mg per m² i.v. every 6 weeks, along with vincristine once every week for three consecutive weeks out of every cycle of 6 weeks duration, showed equivalent overall survival to that for

TABLE 33.9. *Chang staging system*

Stage	Description
T1	Tumor <3 cm in diameter, limited to midline position in the vermis, the roof of the fourth ventricle, and less frequently to the cerebellar hemisphere
T2	Tumor >3 cm, further invading one adjacent structure or partially filling the fourth ventricle
T3a	Tumor invading two adjacent structures or completely filling the fourth ventricle, with extension into aqueduct of Sylvius, foramen of Magendie, or foramen of Luschka, producing marked hydrocephalus
T3b	Tumor arising from the floor of the fourth ventricle or brainstem and filling the fourth ventricle
T4	Tumor further spreading through the aqueduct of Sylvius to involve the third ventricle or midbrain, or extending to the upper spinal cord
M0	No evidence of gross subarachnoid or hematogenous metastasis
M1	Microscopic tumor cells found in cerebrospinal fluid
M2	Gross nodule seedings demonstrated in cerebellar–cerebral subarachnoid space or in the third or lateral ventricles
M3	Gross nodule seedings in the spinal subarachnoid space
M4	Extraneuraxial metastasis

the regimen that included 36-Gy craniospinal radiation, with less long-term cognitive seque-lae. Progression-free survival at 5 years was 79%.
- The most commonly used chemotherapeutic regimen is adjuvant CCNU, 75 mg per m^2 PO; cisplatin, 75 mg per m^2 i.v. every 6 weeks; vincristine, 1.5 mg per m^2 weekly during radiation for eight doses, and then once weekly for 3 weeks during adjuvant chemotherapy cycles.
- Small nonrandomized trials with select patients suggest that a small (<20%) percentage of patients who relapse after primary treatment can be successfully re-treated and remain disease free for more than 5 years with high-dose chemotherapy and stem cell support.

Prognosis

Progression-free survival after chemotherapy and radiation are as follows:

- High-risk patients: 40% to 60%
- Average- risk patients: 65% to 91%.

MENINGIOMAS

Epidemiology

Meningiomas are common, composing up to 39% of primary CNS tumors (usually benign).

Genetics

- Monosomy 22, with frequent mutation of *NF2* gene on 22q
- Malignant meningiomas frequently show loss of 1p, 10, and 14q
- Predisposition: female sex, ionizing irradiation, *NF2*, and breast carcinoma

Clinical Presentation

- Most common areas of presentation are parasagittal region, cerebral convexity, and sphenoidal ridge.
- Signs and symptoms include seizures, hemiparesis, visual field loss, and other focal findings.

Management

Surgery

- Treatment goal is complete resection.
- Recurrence rate after complete resection is 7% at 5 years and 20% at 10 years (higher for incompletely resected meningiomas).

Radiotherapy

- Adjuvant irradiation should be considered only for meningiomas that have been subtotally resected. Radiation probably reduces recurrence after subtotal resection.
- Malignant meningiomas: Irradiation probably increases survival and should be considered in the postoperative adjuvant setting even after complete surgical resection.
- Dosing: benign meningiomas, 54 Gy in 1.8- to 2.0-Gy fractions; malignant meningiomas, dose should be increased to 60 Gy.

Chemotherapy

- There are no known effective drugs for meningiomas.
- Despite harboring estrogen and/or progesterone receptors, meningiomas have generally not been responsive to hormonal therapy with agents such as tamoxifen. Although a small phase II trial suggested that the antiprogestin, RU-486, had antimeningioma activity, a subsequent large randomized trial by the Southwestern Oncology Group (SWOG) of RU-486 versus placebo for locally unresectable meningiomas showed no benefit for the drug compared to the placebo.

PRIMARY BRAIN LYMPHOMA

Intracerebral lymphoma most frequently presents as parenchymal lymphoma; however, other anatomic sites such as the eye, meninges, or ependymal nodules may be found.

Primary CNS lymphoma is a rare tumor, accounting for less than 2% of all primary brain tumors. Over the last few decades, there has been a dramatic increase in the prevalence of this tumor in immunocompetent patients, currently exceeding the incidence of non-Hodgkin lymphoma (NHL).

Risk Factors

- Acquired immunodeficiency syndrome (AIDS)
- Immunosuppression for organ transplantation
- Autoimmune disease
- Congenital immunodeficiencies such as Wiscott–Aldrich syndrome

Clinical Presentation

- The clinical presentation of primary brain lymphoma includes symptoms of intracranial mass, with headaches and signs of increased ICP.
- The frontal lobe is the most commonly involved site, often with multiple lesions; personality changes and decreased level of alertness are common.
- Multifocal disease; 42% leptomeningeal seeding at diagnosis

Clinical Diagnosis

A tissue diagnosis is of paramount importance.

Staging studies should include

- MRI of brain with gadolinium
- lumbar puncture
- ophthalmologic evaluation
- complete physical examination and blood work (including liver function tests)
- chest radiograph
- abdominal CT scan (optional if no other signs of systemic disease).

Management

Approximately 40% to 70% of tumors are highly steroid sensitive; therefore, steroids should be withheld, if at all possible, until a tissue diagnosis has been established. A ring-enhancing lesion that "disappears" after starting steroids is strongly suggestive of a CNS lymphoma, although other infectious (i.e., toxoplasmosis) and inflammatory/demyelinating diseases (i.e., multiple sclerosis) must be considered.

Surgery

Surgery has no role in therapy, but is used for confirmation of diagnosis.

Radiotherapy

Radiotherapy yields 80% to 90% radiographic complete response (CR), and is commonly dosed at 40 to 60 Gy to the entire brain and meninges ("C2" radiation); median survival is 12 to 18 months.

Chemotherapy

- Recent studies suggest that preradiation chemotherapy with high-dose methotrexate significantly increases median survival and the number of long-term survivors.
- Role of radiotherapy for patients who have CR to chemotherapy remains unknown.
- The likelihood of long-term treatment-induced neurocognitive toxicity is probably enhanced considerably in patients who receive combined-modality treatment.
- The two most widely utilized regimens for treating primary CNS lymphoma are the NABTT (New Approaches to Brain Tumor Therapy) high-dose methotrexate regimen and the MSKCC (Memorial Sloan-Kettering Cancer Center) regimen, both of which are detailed in Table 33.10.

TABLE 33.10. *Chemotherapy*

NABTT Regimen: HD MTX 8 g/m^2 q2wk, with leucovorin rescue to maximal response; Delay XRT until tumor progression; 22 patients treated; Overall response rate 74%; Median progression-free survival 12.8 mo; Median overall survival 22.8+ mo; No reported cases of delayed severe neurologic toxicity

MSKCC Regimen: Five cycles of methotrexate 2.5 g/m^2, vincristine 1.4 mg/m^2 with maximum dose at 2.8 mg (2m^2), procarbazine 100 mg/m^2/day for 7 days (cycle 1,3,5), and intra-ventricular methotrexate 12 mg followed by whole-brain XRT to 45 Gy; 102 patients; 94% response to preradiation chemotherapy; Median progression-free survival 24.0 mo; Overall survival 3.9 mo; 15% of patients experienced severe delayed neurologic toxicity (1)

HD MTX, high-dose methotrexate; XRT, radiation therapy.
From DeAngelis LM, Seiferheld W, Schold Sc et al. Combination chemotherapy and radiotherapy for primary central nervous system lymphoma: Radiation Therapy Oncology Group Study 93–10. *J Clin Oncol* 2002;20(24):4643–4648.

GERM CELL TUMORS

Epidemiology

CNS germ cell tumors (GCTs) are typically located in the pineal region. The most common histologic type is germinoma, comprising 30% to 50% of all pineal tumors. Overall, however, this group of tumors represents a rare subgroup of less than 1% of all intracranial tumors.

Diagnosis

Because the pineal region involves an area close to the center of the brain, symptoms are generally related to increased ICP and ocular pathway cranial nerve palsies.

- Obstructive hydrocephalus: headache, nausea, vomiting, and lethargy
- Cranial nerve palsies: diplopia and upward-gaze paralysis
- Elevations in serum tumor marker levels: α-fetoprotein (AFP), β-human chorionic gonadotropin (β-HCG), and placental alkaline phosphatase (PLAP)

Management

Surgery

- Microsurgical infratentorial supracerebellar or supratentorial approach under the occipital lobe is used to establish diagnosis and to attempt resection in radioresistant tumors.

Radiation Therapy

Germinomas are exquisitely radiosensitive.

- Localized germinomas are treated with 24-Gy radiation to the ventricular system, and with 26 Gy to tumor.
- Disseminated germinomas are treated with 20- to 35-Gy radiation to craniospinal axis in addition to systemic chemotherapy.
- Nongerminomatous GCTs are irradiated after chemotherapy. Localized tumors: 24 Gy to ventricular system, 54- to 60-Gy boost to tumor. Disseminated tumors: craniospinal irradiation with 54 to 60 Gy to tumor, 45 Gy to ventricles, and 35 Gy to spinal cord.

Chemotherapy

- Chemotherapy is used primarily for nonseminomatous GCTs; the overall contribution of chemotherapy remains unclear.
- Commonly used regimens include cisplatin/etoposide/bleomycin (PEB), carboplatin/etoposide/vinblastine in doses used for extragonadal GCTs.
- Teratoma: treatment is primarily surgical, possibly with radiation.

Prognosis

Germinomas: 5-year survival is greater than 80% with radiation only. The prognosis is significantly poorer for nonseminomatous, mixed GCTs.

- High survival is seen in mature teratomas.

BRAIN METASTASES

Epidemiology

Brain metastases represent the most prevalent intracranial malignancy. With an estimated incidence of 80,000 to 170,000 cases per year in the United States, compared to 17,000 to

20,000 newly diagnosed primary brain tumors, the importance of diagnosis and management of this disease is well understood (see Table 33.11 and 33.12).

Ten percent to 30% of adults and 6% to 10% of children with cancer develop symptomatic brain metastases, with lung and breast cancers being the most common primary cancers in adults. Sarcomas, neuroblastomas, and GCTs appear to be most common in pediatric metastatic brain disease (Tables 33.13 to 33.14).

Differential Diagnosis

• Primary brain tumors
• Abscess
• Demyelination

TABLE 33.11. *Frequency of brain metastases*

Primary tumor	Frequency (%)
Lung cancer	50
Breast cancer	15–20
Unknown primary	15–19
Melanoma	10
Colon cancer	5

TABLE 33.12. *Distribution by location*

Location	Frequency (%)
Hemispheres	80
Cerebellum	15
Brainstem	5

TABLE 33.13. *Diagnosis: clinical signs*

Sign	Frequency (%)
Hemiparesis	44
Mental status changes	35
Gait ataxia	13
Hemisensory loss	9
Papilledema	9

TABLE 33.14. *Diagnosis: clinical symptoms*

Symptom	Frequency (%)
Headache	42
Mental changes	31
Focal deficit	27
Seizure	20
Gait ataxia	17
Speech disturbance	10
Sensory problems	6

- Cerebral infarction
- Cerebral hemorrhage
- Progressive multifocal leukoencephalopathy
- Radiation necrosis

The false-positive rate for single brain metastasis may be as high as 30%. Nonmetastatic brain lesions are equally divided between primary brain tumors and infections. Meningioma must be considered in patients with primary breast cancer with a dural-based brain lesion because the prevalence of this primary brain tumor increases in breast cancer.

Imaging

Contrast-enhanced MRI is the diagnostic imaging modality of choice. Features of MRI that favor the diagnosis of brain metastasis include

- multiple lesions
- location at gray–white matter junction
- high ratio of vasogenic edema to tumor size.

If imaging modalities and clinical history do not provide sufficient information to render a diagnosis, a biopsy of the lesion is indicated.

Brain Metastasis with Unknown Primary

A chest radiograph should be obtained in any patient with a new brain mass because 60% of patients with brain metastasis of unknown primary have a lung mass from a pulmonary malignancy or pulmonary metastasis of a primary in a different location. A CT scan of the chest considerably increases the likelihood of finding a lung mass if the chest radiograph is nondiagnostic.

To determine the extent of metastatic disease, CT scans of the abdomen and pelvis and a bone scan should be performed.

Management

Symptomatic Therapy

Reduction of symptomatic edema: Dexamethasone, 10 mg loading dose, followed by 4 mg four times a day.

- Symptomatic improvement should be expected within 24 to 72 hours.
- Imaging studies may not show a decrease of cerebral edema for up to 1 week.
- Steroid should be tapered after completion of irradiation or earlier if cerebral edema is minimal.

Seizure Management

Because infratentorial metastases carry a very low risk for seizures, anticonvulsant therapy is usually not indicated. The role of prophylactic anticonvulsant therapy remains controversial in patients with supratentorial brain metastasis without prior seizures who have not had surgery. Generally after seizure activity has occurred or after a patient has undergone craniotomy, phenytoin therapy is initiated. Close monitoring is advised because dexamethasone and phenytoin mutually increase the clearance of phenytoin, and the number of reports suggesting a correlation between Stevens–Johnson syndrome and palliative whole-brain irradiation in patients taking phenytoin is increasing. Secondary to the fact that phenytoin (like most other older antiepileptic drugs) induces hepatic cytochrome P450 isoenzymes, thereby considerably altering the metabolism and pharmacology of many other drugs such as chemotherapeutic agents, some physicians are moving toward initiating seizure prophylaxis with newer agents that do not induce hepatic enzymes, such as Keppra, despite the fact that most of these agents (including Keppra) are not approved by the U.S. Food and Drug Administration (FDA) for monotherapy.

Surgery

Factors influencing the decision favoring surgical resection include

- extent of systemic disease
- neurologic status of patient
- number of cerebral metastases
- interval between diagnosis of primary cancer and occurrence of brain metastasis
- primary cancer
- location of tumor.

Single brain metastasis: Several controlled studies suggest a benefit of surgery combined with whole-brain irradiation for patients with single brain metastasis and stable extracranial disease.

Multiple brain metastases: For patients with multiple brain metastases, the role of surgery is generally limited to

- large, symptomatic, or life-threatening lesions
- tissue diagnosis in unknown primary
- differentiation of metastasis from primary brain tumor like meningioma.

The value of resection of multiple brain metastases with therapeutic intent has not been established.

Radiation Therapy

- Radiation therapy is considered the primary therapy for patients with brain metastasis.
- Whole-brain irradiation increases median survival to 3 to 6 months.
- Overall response rate is 64% to 85%.
- Cranial nerve deficit improvement is seen in 40% of patients.

Fractionation Schedule

- From 30 to 50 Gy in 1.5- to 4-Gy fractions
- Most common schedule: 30 Gy in 10 fractions over 2 weeks
- Patients with good prognosis: more prolonged fractionation such as 40 Gy in 2-Gy fractions may reduce long-term morbidity.

Postoperative Radiation Therapy

- A 62% reduction in treatment failure is observed with postoperative radiation therapy.
- There is a 30% reduction in risk of death from neurologic causes.
- There is no improvement of overall survival or duration of functional independence.
- Dosing: 50.4 Gy in 28 fractions.

Late Toxicities

- Dementia occurs in 11% of patients receiving a total dose of radiation > 30 Gy
- Recommended dosing: 40 to 45 Gy in 1- to 2-Gy fractions.

Reirradiation

- Radiosurgery is recommended for patients with solitary or fewer than three metastases.
- Whole or partial brain irradiation is for patients who are not eligible for radiosurgery/chemotherapy.
- Clinical response is from 42% to 75%.
- Median survival is from 3.5 to 5 months.
- Dosing schedules vary without established consensus.

Radiosurgery

Indications

- Young patient
- Good performance status
- Limited extracranial disease
- One to two small lesions
- Recurrent brain metastasis after whole-brain irradiation.

Adverse Prognostic Factors

- Poor performance status
- Progressive systemic disease
- Infratentorial location
- Large tumor size
- Multiple lesions.

Interstitial Brachytherapy

- There is, at present, no real indication for interstitial brachytherapy.

Chemotherapy

In select malignancies, brain metastases may show responses to systemic treatment of the underlying cancer.

Breast Cancer

Regimens including cyclophosphamide/5-fluorouracil/cisplatin (CFP), cyclophosphamide/methotrexate/5-fluorouracil (CMF), and doxorubicin (Adriamycin)/cyclophosphamide (AC) have been used, and are generally directed at the systemic cancer. Responses are noted in 50% to 70% of cases. There appears to be a survival advantage in patients who respond.

Small Cell Lung Cancer

Regimens including etoposide and platinating agents have been used. Overall response rates for primary brain metastasis approach 76%. Response rates decrease to 43% on CNS relapse.

Prognostic Factors

- Karnofsky Performance Status more than 70
- Age less than 65 years
- Controlled primary disease
- No extracranial metastasis

TABLE 33.15. Prognosis (median survival in months)

Untreated brain metastasis	1 mo
Addition of steroids	2 mo
With whole-brain irradiation	3–6 mo
Single metastasis, limited extracranial disease, surgery and whole-brain radiation	10–16 mo

- Median survival ranges from 2.3 to 7.1 months depending on the presence of good prognostic indicators (Table 33.15).

REFERENCES

1. DeAngelis LM, Seiferheld W, Schold SC, et al. Combination chemotherapy and radiotherapy for primary central nervous system lymphoma: Radiation Therapy Oncology Group Study 93-10. *J Clin Oncol* 2002;20:4643–4648.

SUGGESTED READINGS

Ahmed Rasheed BK, Wiltshire RN, Bigner SH, et al. Molecular pathogenesis of malignant gliomas. *Curr Opin Oncol* 1999;11:162–167.

Avgeropoulos NG, Batchelor TT. New treatment strategies for malignant gliomas. *Oncologist* 1999; 4:209–224.

Batchelor T, Carson K, O'Neil A, et al. Treatment of primary CNS lymphoma with methotrexate and deferred radiotherapy: a report of NABTT 96-07. *J Clin Oncol* 2003;21:1044–1049.

Black PM. Meningiomas. *Neurosurgery* 1993;31:643–657.

Davey P. Brain metastases. *Curr Probl Cancer* 1999;23:59–98.

DeVita VT Jr, Hellman S, Rosenberg SA. *Cancer: principles and practice of oncology*, 6th ed. Philadelphia: Lippincott–Raven Publishers, 2001.

Haskell CM, ed. *Cancer treatment*, 4th ed. Philadelphia: WB Saunders, 1995.

Hoffman HJ. Brain stem gliomas. *Clin Neurosurg* 1997;44:549–558.

Kyritsis AP, Yung WKA, Bruner JB, et al. The treatment of anaplastic oligodendrogliomas and mixed gliomas. *Neurosurgery* 1993;32:365–370.

Levin VA, Silver P, Hannigan J, et al. Superiority of post-radiotherapy adjuvant chemotherapy with CCNU, procarbazine, and vincristine (PCV) over BCNU for anaplastic astrocytoma: NCOG 6G61 final report. *Int J Radiat Oncol Biol Phys* 1990;18:321–324.

Maldjian JA, Patel RS. Cerebral neoplasms in adults. *Semin Roentgenol* 1999;34:102–122.

Newton HB, Turowski RC, Stroup TJ. Clinical presentation, diagnosis, and pharmacotherapy of patients with primary brain tumors. *Ann Pharmacother* 1999;33:816–832.

Packer RJ. Brain tumors in children. *Arch Neurol* 1999;56:421–425.

Packer RJ, Goldwein J, Nicholson HS, et al. Treatment of children with medulloblastomas with reduced-dose craniospinal radiation therapy and adjuvant chemotherapy: a Children's Cancer Group study. *J Clin Oncol* 1999;17:2127–2136.

Pech IV, Peterson K, Cairncross JG. Chemotherapy for brain tumors. *Oncology* 1998;12:537–547.

Perez CA, Brady LW, eds. *Principles and practice of radiation oncology*, 3rd ed. Philadelphia: Lippincott–Raven Publishers, 1998.

Pizzo PA, Poplack DG, eds. *Principles and practice of pediatric oncology*, 3rd ed. Philadelphia: Lippincott–Raven Publishers, 1997.

Sanford RA, Gajjar A. Ependymomas. *Clin Neurosurg* 1997;44:559–570.

Schiffer D. Classification and biology of astrocytic gliomas. *Forum* 1998;8:244–255.

Schild SE, Haddock MG, Scheithauer BW, et al. Nongerminomatous germ cell tumors of the brain. *Int J Radiat Oncol Biol Phys* 1996;36:557–563.

Shaw EG, Daumas-Duport C, Scheithauer BW, et al. Radiation therapy in the management of low-grade supratentorial astrocytomas. *J Neurosurg* 1989;70:853–861.

Tomlinson FH, Kurtin PJ, Suman VJ, et al. Primary intracerebral malignant lymphoma: a clinicopathologic study of 89 patients. *J Neurosurg* 1995;82:558–566.

Wen PY, Loeffler JS. Management of brain metastases. *Oncology* 1999;13:941–961.

34

Endocrine Tumors

Michael E. Menefee* and Tito Fojo†

*Medical Oncology Clinical Research Unit, National Cancer Institute, National Institutes of Health, Bethesda, Maryland, and †Cancer Therapeutics Branch, National Cancer Institute, National Institutes of Health, Bethesda, Maryland

Endocrine tumors are relatively uncommon. These tumors may cause morbidity and mortality not only by local and distant spread of tumor cells but also through mediators produced by the tumor cells that may have systemic effects. The tumors are often difficult to diagnose and treat effectively.

This chapter discusses

1. thyroid cancer
2. cancer of the parathyroid gland
3. adrenocortical cancer
4. pheochromocytoma
5. pancreatic endocrine tumors
6. carcinoid tumors
7. multiple endocrine neoplasia (MEN).

The epidemiology of endocrine tumors is outlined in Table 34.1.

THYROID CARCINOMA

Thyroid carcinoma is not a common type of cancer. However, it is the most common endocrine malignancy and remains a diagnostic as well as therapeutic challenge to the clinician.

Epidemiology

- Thyroid carcinoma accounts for more than 90% of all endocrine tumors.
- There are approximately 20,000 new cases per year.
- The occurrence of thyroid carcinoma is greater in women than in men (2–3:1).
- Risk factors include:
  - irradiation to the head and neck during childhood
  - family history.

Etiology

- Rearrangements of the tyrosine kinase domains of the *RET* and *TRK* genes with the amino terminal sequence of an unlinked gene are found in some papillary carcinomas.
- *RET* rearrangements are found in 3% to 33% of the papillary carcinomas that are not associated with irradiation and in 60% to 80% of those that occur after radiation.

455

TABLE 34.1. *Incidence and proportion of all endocrine cancers and relative proportions of different primary thyroid cancer subtypes*

	Number	Total (%)
All endocrine cancers		
Thyroid	18,100	91
Endocrine pancreas	800	4
Adrenal	550	2.8
Thymus	425	2.1
Pineal gland	128	0.6
Pituitary gland	77	0.4
Parathyroid	48	0.2
Carotid body, paraganglia	33	0.16
Primary thyroid cancers		
Well differentiated		87–90
Papillary		75
Follicular		10
Hürthle cell		2–4
Anaplastic		1–2
Medullary thyroid cancer		5–9
Sporadic		6
Familial		3
Lymphoma		1–3
Sarcoma and others		<1

From DeVita VT, Hellman JS, Rosenberg SA. *Cancer: principles and practices of oncology*, 6th ed. Philadelphia: Lippincott-Raven, with permission.

Clinical Manifestations

- Most patients with thyroid carcinoma present with an asymptomatic thyroid nodule
- Hoarseness is caused by invasion of the recurrent laryngeal nerve or by direct compression of the larynx
- Cervical lymphadenopathy
- Dysphagia
- Horner syndrome.

Subtypes

Papillary Thyroid Carcinoma

- Papillary thyroid carcinoma is the most common subtype of thyroid carcinomas (60% to 75%).
- The carcinoma is well differentiated.
- Papillary thyroid carcinoma tends to be unilateral, although it may be multifocal within a lobe.
- The carcinoma metastasizes via lymphatic invasion; vascular invasion is uncommon.
- The prognosis is related to stage and age of the patient. Patients with early-stage disease have a prolonged survival. Ten-year survival in patients with distant metastases ranges from 30% to 50%.
- Variants include tall-cell, columnar, and diffuse sclerosis.

Follicular Thyroid Carcinoma

- Follicular thyroid carcinomas are well differentiated.
- The carcinoma affects a slightly older patient population than does papillary thyroid carcinoma.
- The carcinoma metastasizes at a late stage to the lungs and bones via a vascular route and may occur late.
- Lymph node involvement is rare.
- Prognosis is good, but is slightly less favorable than that of papillary thyroid carcinoma.

Medullary Thyroid Carcinoma

- Medullary thyroid carcinoma is a neuroendocrine tumor of the parafollicular (C) cells.
- It represents 3% to 5% of all thyroid carcinomas.
- The carcinoma may be a part of the MEN type 2 (MEN-2) syndrome; however, most cases are sporadic.
- Sporadic tumors tend to be solitary, whereas familial tumors tend to be bilateral and multifocal.
- The tumors secrete calcitonin.
- Approximately 50% of patients with this carcinoma present with regional lymphadenopathy.
- Distant metastases typically occur late in the disease and usually involve the lungs, liver, bones, and the adrenal glands.

Anaplastic Thyroid Carcinoma

- Anaplastic thyroid carcinoma accounts for 2% to 5% of all thyroid cancers; up to 50% of patients will have either antecedent or concurrent history of a well-differentiated thyroid carcinoma.
- It is a high-grade tumor, often with lymphovascular invasion and regional or distant spread at diagnosis.

Other

- Hürthle cell carcinoma
- Radiation-induced carcinoma—25- to 30-year latency period between exposure and the development of cancer
- Lymphoma
- Metastatic tumors

Staging

- The TNM definitions and the staging for thyroid carcinoma are discussed in Tables 34.2 and 34.3.

Evaluation of a Thyroid Nodule

- Fine needle aspiration biopsy (FNAB) is a more cost-effective technique than ultrasonography.
- Ultrasonographic evaluation is warranted in patients with a history of neck irradiation.
- The evaluation of palpable thyroid nodules is discussed in Fig. 34.1 and Table 34.4.

Prognostic Factors of Well-differentiated Thyroid Carcinoma

- Overall survival rate at 10 years for middle-aged adults is about 80% to 95%.
- Five percent to 20% of patients will have local or regional recurrences.
- Ten percent to 15% of patients will have distant metastatic disease.
- The prognostic indicators for recurrent disease and death are age at the time of diagnosis, histologic subtype, and extent of the tumor.

Treatment of Well-differentiated Thyroid Carcinoma

Surgery

- If the lesion is <1.5 cm, lobectomy is appropriate.
- Lobectomy: contralateral lobe is not dissected, but is examined only for abnormalities.

TABLE 34.2. *TNM definitions for thyroid carcinoma*

Primary tumor

TX	Primary tumor cannot be assessed
T0	No evidence of primary tumor
T1	Tumor 2 cm or less in greatest dimension, limited to the thyroid
T2	Tumor more than 2 cm but not more than 4 cm in greatest dimension, limited to the thyroid
T3	Tumor more than 4 cm in greatest dimension, limited to the thyroid, or any tumor with minimal extrathyroid extension
T4a	Tumor of any size extending beyond the thyroid capsule to invade subcutaneous soft tissues, larynx, trachea, esophagus, or recurrent laryngeal nerve
T4b	Tumor invades prevertebral fascia or encases carotid artery or mediastinal vessels.

All anaplastic carcinomas are considered T4 tumors

T4a	Intrathyroidal anaplastic carcinoma—surgically resectable
T4b	Extrathyroidal anaplastic carcinoma—surgically unresectable

Regional lymph nodes

NX	Regional lymph nodes cannot be accessed
N0	No regional lymph node metastasis
N1	Regional lymph node metastasis
N1a	Metastasis to level IV lymph nodes
N1b	Metastasis to unilateral, bilateral, or contralateral cervical or superior mediastinal lymph nodes

Distant metastasis

MX	Distant metastasis cannot be accessed
M0	No distant metastasis
M1	Distant metastasis

From *American Joint Committee on Cancer Staging Manual*, 6th ed. New York: Springer, with permission.

TABLE 34.3. *Staging of thyroid cancer*

	Well differentiated		Medullary	Anaplastic
Stage	Age >45 yr	Age <45 yr		
1	Any T, any N, M_0	T_1	T_1	—
2	M1	T_{2-3}	T_{2-4}	—
3	—	T_4 or N_1	N_1	—
4	—	M_1	M_1	Any

- Subtotal thyroidectomy: leaves 2 to 4 g of the thyroid tissue in the upper part of the contralateral thyroid. It also preserves the recurrent laryngeal nerve and the blood supply to the upper parathyroid glands.
- Near-total thyroidectomy: leaves a much smaller portion of the thyroid tissue near the ligament of Berry. It also preserves the recurrent laryngeal nerve, but not the blood supply to the parathyroid glands.
- Total thyroidectomy: removes all thyroid tissue. It can cause permanent hypocalcemia. Replacement calcium and vitamin D supplementation should therefore be considered.
- The choice of surgery is a controversial topic.

Iodine-131

- Iodine-131 is used in papillary or follicular thyroid carcinoma for the following reasons:
  - Ablation of the normal, residual thyroid tissue after thyroid surgery, thereby increasing the sensitivity of subsequent iodine-131 total body scanning (TBS), and measurement of serum thyroglobulin for the presence of recurrent disease.

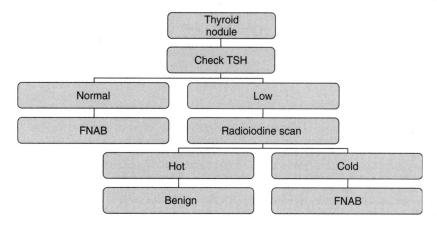

FIG. 34.1. Evaluation of a palpable thyroid nodule.

TABLE 34.4. *Analysis of thyroid fine needle aspiration (FNA) results*

FNAB diagnosis	Biopsies (%)	Malignant[a] (%)	Next step
Benign	60–70	1–2	Follow-up
Malignant	5–10	98	Surgery
Suspicious	20	20–30	Surgery (in most cases)
Inadequate	5–10	5–10	Consider repeat FNA with ultra-sound guidance

FNAB, Fine needle aspiration and biopsy.
[a]Percentage found to be malignant at surgery.

- Treatment of microscopic occult thyroid cancer in the neck or in the metastatic sites.
- Radioiodine treatment decreases cancer-related death, tumor recurrence, and development of distant metastases.
- The dose of iodine-131 varies from 30 to 150 mCi or higher.
- Table 34.5 discusses the indications for iodine-131 treatment after surgery.
- Fig. 34.2 provides the recommended follow-up of patients after total thyroid ablation.

Complications of Iodine-131 Treatment

- Sialadenitis
- Nausea
- Marrow suppression
- Testicular dysfunction
- Leukemia

Chemotherapy

Chemotherapy has only a limited role in thyroid carcinoma. Doxorubicin is considered the most active agent; other single agents like UP-16, carboplatin, and cisplatin have low response rates.

TABLE 34.5. *Indications for ablative treatment with iodine-131 after surgery in patients with thyroid cancer*

No indication

• Low risk of cancer-specific mortality and low risk of relapse

Indication

• Distant metastases
• Incomplete excision of tumor
• Complete excision of tumor but high risk of mortality associated with thyroid carcinoma
• Complete excision of tumor but high risk of relapse because of age (younger than 16 yr or older than 45 yr), histologic subtype (i.e., tall cell, columnar cell, or diffuse sclerosing papillary variants; widely invasive or poorly differentiated follicular subtypes; Hürthle cell carcinomas), or extent of tumor (i.e., large tumor mass, extension beyond the thyroid capsule, or lymph node metastases)
• Elevated serum thyroglobulin concentration >3 mo after surgery

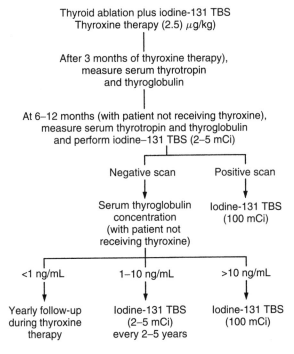

FIG. 34.2. Recommended follow-up of patients after total thyroid ablation based on serum thyroglobulin [assessment and iodine-131 total body scanning (TBS)]. (From Schlumberger MJ. Papillary and follicular thyroid carcinoma. *N Engl J Med* 1998;338:297–308, with permission.)

External Radiation

External-beam radiation therapy has only a limited role in thyroid carcinoma. Indications include incomplete surgical resection and tumors that do not take up iodine-131.

Thyroxine Treatment

- The growth of the thyroid tumor cells is controlled by thyrotropin, and the recurrence and survival rates are improved by inhibition of thyrotropin secretion with thyroxine.
- Levothyroxine should be given to all patients with thyroid carcinoma regardless of the extent of the surgery and other treatments.
- In patients without evidence of thyroid carcinoma, the level of the thyroid-stimulating hormone (TSH) should be maintained below the normal range (0.5 to 5 mU per mL).
- In patients with thyroid carcinoma, the level of the TSH should be maintained below 0.1 mU per mL.

Follow-up of Patients with Well-differentiated Thyroid Carcinoma

The goals after initial therapy are to maintain a euthyroid state and to detect recurrent or persistent disease.

- Clinical examination for recurrent nodes in thyroid bed
- Ultrasonography in patients with clinical findings suggestive of the disease and in those who are at high risk
- Serum thyroglobulin

Thyroglobulin

- Thyroglobulin (Tg) is an important tumor marker in the follow-up of thyroid cancer (Fig. 34.2).
- Tg should be undetectable after thyroidectomy and radioablation.
- If there are detectable Tg levels after suppressive therapy, it is indicative of persistent or recurrent thyroid cancer.
- Thyroxine can suppress Tg secretion and mask recurrent disease.
- Combined rTSH-stimulated radioiodine and Tg testing is as sensitive as thyroid hormone withdrawal in detecting recurrent thyroid cancer and causes less morbidity.
- Tg may be more sensitive than whole-body scan in detecting cancer.

Treatment of Medullary Thyroid Carcinoma

- Chemotherapy and external-beam radiation are ineffective in treating medullary thyroid carcinoma.
- Total thyroidectomy with central nodal dissection is the treatment of choice.

Treatment of Anaplastic Thyroid Carcinoma

- The options available for the treatment of anaplastic thyroid carcinoma are limited, and prognosis is extremely poor.
- Surgery: Patients should be considered for aggressive local resection.
- Radiation treatment: Radiation therapy after surgery should be considered, although response rates are low.
- Chemotherapy: Paclitaxel is the single most effective agent.

PARATHYROID CARCINOMA

Parathyroid carcinoma is an extremely rare cause of hyperparathyroidism. It is different from other endocrine tumors, which usually are hypofunctional. Clinically, it is important to distinguish this disease from other benign disorders of the parathyroid gland that result in hyperparathyroidism (see Table 34.6).

Epidemiology

- Parathyroid carcinoma accounts for less than 1% of all cases of hyperparathyroidism.
- Its incidence is approximately 0.015 per 100,000 population.
- It is equally prevalent in men and women.
- It occurs in the fifth or sixth decade of life.

Natural History

- The recurrence rates of parathyroid carcinoma approach 50%.
- The 10-year survival rate is 49%.
- The morbidity and mortality are usually related to the hypercalcemia rather than to the complications of metastases.

Etiology

- Unknown
- Familial tumor, renal failure, prior neck irradiation.

Pathology

- Thick fibrous bands, a large number of mitotic figures, and trabecular pattern are characteristic of parathyroid carcinoma.
- There is invasion of the glandular capsule and vascular tissue.

Staging

- There is no American Joint Committee for Cancer (AJCC) staging for parathyroid carcinoma because of the low incidence of the disease.

Clinical Manifestations

- Symptoms of moderate to severe hypercalcemia, with calcium levels usually more than 14 mg per dL
- Palpable neck mass; if >3 cm, suggestive of carcinoma

TABLE 34.6. *Benign versus malignant*

	Benign	Malignant
Weight	<200 g	>500 g
Mitoses	Few	Many
Ploidy	Diploid	Aneuploid
Necrosis	Some	More
Metastases	Never	Frequent
Neuropeptide Y	Yes	±

- Elevated parathyroid hormone levels
- Vocal cord paralysis in more advanced disease
- Sites of metastases: lungs, cervical lymph nodes, and liver.

Diagnostic Evaluation

- Differential includes parathyroid adenoma and hyperplasia, with carcinoma being suggested by a large neck mass and markedly elevated calcium levels.
- Most cases are diagnosed at surgery; however, some cases are not diagnosed until after the initial resection has been completed or until the time of local recurrence or metastases.
- Fine needle aspiration (FNA) is inappropriate for diagnosis.

Treatment

- Surgical
  - Primary modality consists of an *en bloc* resection of the tumor and involved structures, as well as of the ipsilateral lobe of thyroid.
  - Recurrent tumor and oligometastases should be resected as well.
- Medical
  - Chemotherapy is of limited value.
  - Agents with activity include DTIC (dacarbazine); 5-fluorouracil; cyclophosphamide.
  - Management of hypercalcemia is essential while treating parathyroid carcinoma.
- Radiation
  - Tumors are generally radioinsensitive.
  - Radiation only has a palliative benefit.

ADRENAL CORTICAL CARCINOMA

Epidemiology

- Adrenal cortical carcinoma is rare; it accounts for 0.05% to 0.2% of all cancers.
- It shows a bimodal age distribution, with the first peak in children younger than 5 years and with a second peak in adults in their fourth to fifth decade.

Natural History

- The 5-year survival rate is 23%.
- The 10-year survival rate is 10%.
- The prognosis is better in children.
- The common sites of distant spread are liver, lungs, lymph nodes, and bone.

Etiology

- The etiology of adrenal cortical carcinoma is not known.

Pathology

- Differentiation between adenomas and carcinomas can represent a histologic challenge. However, carcinomas will tend to display mitotic activity, aneuploidy, and venous invasion.
- Carcinomas may also secrete abnormal amounts of androgens and 11-deoxysteroids.

Staging

MacFarlane classification of various stages of adrenal cortical carcinoma is given in Fig. 34.3.

Stage I – Tumor <5 cm without regional extension

Stage II – Tumor >5 cm without regional extension

Stage III – Regional extension ± lymphnode

Stage IV – Distant metastases (e.g., liver, lung, and bone)

FIG. 34.3. MacFarlane classification. (From DeVita VT, Hellman JS, Rosenberg SA. *Cancer: principles and practices of oncology*, 6th ed. Philadelphia: Lippincott-Raven, with permission.)

Clinical Manifestations

- Endocrine dysfunction:
  - Features of hypercortisolism
  - Virilization/feminization
  - Mineralocorticoid excess.
- Approximately 50% of patients present with evidence of hormonal excess.
- Symptoms arising from local mass effect or distant metastases are evident.

Diagnostic Evaluation

- Adrenal incidentalomas are being detected more often, with improved quality and with more frequent utilization of imaging studies. See Fig. 34.4.
- Biochemical evaluation is performed if clinically warranted (i.e., urinary steroids, suppression tests).

Treatment

- *En bloc* resection is appropriate for all stages initially, and further surgical resection should be attempted for local recurrence and for metastatic disease whenever feasible.
- Radiofrequency ablation may be implemented for local control or metastases in patients with unresectable disease.
- Mitotane has induced hormonal response rates in up to 75% of patients with functional tumors, without any change in overall survival.
- Other active agents include doxorubicin, etoposide, and cisplatin.

PHEOCHROMOCYTOMA

Epidemiology

- Pheochromocytoma is found in less than 0.2% of all patients with hypertension.
- Classically, approximately 10% of pheochromocytomas are malignant; however, the true number may be higher.
- Approximately 10% of pheochromocytomas are bilateral; it tends to occur more frequently in the familial syndromes.
- Approximately 10% of the disease is extraadrenal; malignancy is more likely to be found in extraadrenal tumors.
- Approximately 10% of the disease is associated with a familial genetic syndrome [e.g., MEN-2 or von Hippel–Lindau (VHL)].

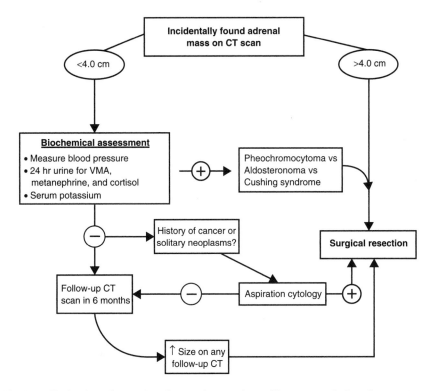

FIG. 34.4. Evaluation of an adrenal mass in a patient with suspected pheochromocytoma. (From DeVita VT, Hellman JS, Rosenberg SA. *Cancer: principles and practices of oncology*, 6th ed. Philadelphia: Lippincott-Raven, with permission.)

Natural History

- Pheochromocytomas generally are indolent tumors.
- It metastasizes most commonly to the lungs, brain, and bone.
- Morbidity and mortality is related to the secretory products of the tumor.

Etiology

- The etiology of pheochromocytoma is not known.

Pathology

- Pheochromocytomas arise from chromaffin cells, most of which nest in the adrenal medulla.
- Both malignant and benign tumors have the capability of vascular invasion and extension into the cortex.
- The only absolute criterion for malignancy is the presence of secondary tumors in sites where chromaffin cells do not usually exist.

Clinical Manifestations

- The clinical features of pheochromocytomas are summarized in Table 34.7.

TABLE 34.7. *Clinical features*

Mild labile hypertension to hypertensive crisis; sustained hypertension is also common
Myocardial infarction
Cerebral infarction
Classic pattern of paroxysmal hypertension occurs in 30%–50% of cases
Spells of paroxysmal headache
Pallor or flushing
Tremor
Apprehension
Palpitation
Orthostasis
Mild weight loss
Diaphoresis

Diagnostic Evaluation

- Metabolic assessment:
  - Twenty-four-hour urinary catecholamines, vanillylmandelic acid (VMA), and metanephrine (most specific)
  - Clonidine suppression test is recommended for intermediate catecholamine levels. Catecholamine levels will not be suppressed in patients with pheochromocytoma.
- Radiologic assessment:
  - Both computerized tomography (CT) scan and magnetic resonance imaging (MRI) are equally sensitive.
  - Labeled metaiodobenzylguanidine (^{131}I-MIBG) is structurally similar to norepinephrine and is taken up and concentrated in adrenergic tissue. It is highly sensitive and specific, particularly for malignant tumors and the familial syndromes.
  - Bone scan is superior to ^{131}I-MIBG in detecting bone metastases.
- Diagnostic evaluation helps to differentiate between benign and malignant tumors (Table 34.7).

Treatment

Surgical

- Surgery is the mainstay of treatment and should be considered for primary, recurrent, and metastatic disease.
- Appropriate preoperative evaluation and $\alpha \pm \beta$-blockade are required to minimize risk of a hypertensive crisis.
- The laparoscopic approach is acceptable if no obvious tumor invasion or metastases are visualized during imaging studies (see Fig. 34.5).

Medical

Chemotherapy

- Cyclophosphamide, vincristine, and dacarbazine (CVD)
- Biochemical response of 79%
- Fifty-seven percent reduction in measurable disease
- Median duration of response is greater than 20 months
- Small study (14 patients).

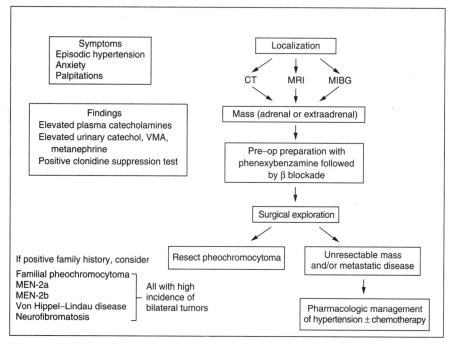

FIG. 34.5. Diagnosis and treatment of pheochromocytoma. (From Abeloff MD, et al. *Clinical oncology*, 3rd ed. Philadelphia: Elsevier Churchill Livingstone, with permission.)

Radiation

• Radiation has a limited role; it may be used for bone metastases and soft-tissue metastases.

NEUROENDOCRINE TUMORS

Neuroendocrine tumors are rare tumors that are distinguished from many other solid tumors by their ability to produce biologically active molecules that can produce systemic syndromes. The two primary subgroups of neuroendocrine tumors are carcinoid tumors and pancreatic endocrine tumors.

Carcinoid Tumors

Epidemiology

• The incidence of carcinoid tumors in the United States is 1 to 2 cases per 100,000 individuals.

Natural History

• Abdominal and rectal carcinoids tend to present with tumors of small size (<2 cm) and are amenable to surgical resection, with 5-year survival rates of approximately 95%.
• Small-bowel carcinoids present at a more advanced stage, but if resectable, the 20-year survival rates for these carcinoids are still approximately 80%. If unresectable, median survival is approximately 5 years.

Pathology

- It is difficult to differentiate between malignant and benign carcinoid tumors on the basis of histology.
- Malignancy is determined only if there is lymph node invasion or distant metastatic disease.

Clinical Manifestations

- Carcinoid syndrome, a result of excess production and secretion of serotonin, may result in multiple symptoms including flushing, diarrhea, abdominal cramps, cough, bronchospasm, valvular heart disease, and pellagra in severe cases.
- Eighty-five percent of tumors originate from the gut (predominantly from the appendix).
- The lungs are the second most common site of involvement and represent approximately 2% of lung cancers.

Diagnosis

- Twenty-four-hour urine for 5-hydroxyindoleacetic acid
- CT scan or MRI of the abdomen
- Octreotide scan
  - This scan has higher sensitivity for detecting pancreatic tumors as well as metastatic disease.
  - It may predict which patients will respond to therapy with a somatostatin analog.

Treatment

Surgical

- Appendiceal tumors
  - For tumors <2 cm: appendectomy
  - For tumors >2 cm: right hemicolectomy with lymph node dissection
- Small intestine and rectal tumors
  - Segmental resection with mesenteric lymphadenectomy
- Hepatic disease
  - Debulking by surgery, cryotherapy, or radiofrequency ablation
  - Transplantation may be of benefit to patients without extrahepatic disease.

Medical

- Symptoms of hormonal excess are mitigated with somatostatin analogs, steroids, and other agents.
- Carcinoids tend to be resistant to most chemotherapeutic agents.
  - Active agents include 5-fluorouracil (5-FU), doxorubicin, interferon α-2a and α-2b, and these agents achieve response rates between 10% and 20%.
  - Combining chemotherapeutic agents offers minimal clinical and survival benefit while increasing toxicity.

Radiation

- Radiation therapy is reserved for palliation.

Pancreatic Endocrine Tumors

Gastrinoma (Zollinger–Ellison Syndrome)

Epidemiology

- Gastrinoma accounts for 60% to 80% of all pancreatic endocrine tumors.
- Gastrinoma occurs in 0.1% to 1% of patients with peptic ulcer disease.
- It is usually diagnosed between the third and sixth decades, but can occur at any age.
- Twenty percent of gastrinomas are familial and 20% develop MEN-1.
- Approximately one third of patients with gastrinoma have metastatic disease at diagnosis.
- Male-to-female ratio is 1.5 to 2.0:1.

Pathology

- Gastrinomas are well differentiated, with few mitoses.
- The malignant potential of gastrinomas is determined by the presence of distant metastases and not by histologic grade. Most tumors are malignant.
- Primary tumors predominate in the pancreatic head but may also develop in the small intestine or stomach.

Clinical Manifestations

- Excess production of gastrin results in increased secretion of gastric acid.
- Severe, often refractory, peptic ulcer disease is a characteristic feature.
- Secretory diarrhea is commonly seen.
- Abdominal pain is a common symptom.

Diagnosis

- A gastric acid pH <3.0 in the setting of hypergastrinemia (1,000 pg per mL) indicates gastrinoma.
- Gastrin level that increase by more than 200 pg per mL within 15 minutes of an intravenous infusion of secretin is suggestive of gastrinoma.
- Ultrasonography, CT scan, MRI, endoscopic ultrasonography (EUS), angiography, and octreotide scanning are the commonly used diagnostic procedures.

Treatment

Surgical

- Surgery is potentially curative, but is only an option in 20% of patients.
- With the advent of better, effective medical therapies, surgery seems to be having a limited role. Controversy exists about operating on patients with MEN-1.
- Resection of the primary tumor can reduce the rate of liver metastases.

Medical

- Proton pump inhibitors are the drugs of choice
- Somatostatin analogs (e.g., octreotide)
- Chemotherapeutic agents with activity include 5-FU, etoposide, doxorubicin, DTIC, streptozotocin, and α-interferon (α-IFN)
- Tumor embolization.

Radiation

- The role of radiation in the adjuvant setting remains undefined.
- It may be effective in palliation in patients with unresectable disease.

Insulinoma

Epidemiology

- Insulinoma occurs most commonly in the fifth decade of life.
- There is a slight female predominance in the occurrence of insulinoma.
- Approximately 10% of cases are malignant.
- Gastrinomas account for 20% to 40% of pancreatic endocrine tumors.

Pathology

- Malignancy is defined by the presence of metastases. Most tumors are benign.

Clinical Manifestations

- Whipple triad:
  - Hypoglycemia
  - Neuroglycopenic and/or adrenergic symptoms
  - Relief from symptoms and hypoglycemia when the latter is corrected.
- Most tumors are solitary.

Diagnosis

- An inappropriately high level of insulin during an episode of hypoglycemia establishes the presence of insulinoma.
- In patients who are asymptomatic at the time of diagnosis, a prolonged fasting period, with serum sampling for glucose, insulin, and C-peptide levels every 6 to 12 hours, helps diagnose insulinoma.

Treatment

Surgical

- Surgery is the treatment of choice; it may result in a complete cure.

Medical

- Dietary management with small, frequent meals
- Oral diazoxide inhibits pancreatic secretion of insulin and stimulates the release of catecholamine as well as glucose from the liver.
- Streptozotocin, 5-FU, and doxorubicin are shown to be active in patients with malignant disease.

VIPoma (Verner–Morrison Syndrome)

- Elevated serum vasoactive intestinal peptide establishes the presence of VIPoma.
- VIPoma manifests with watery diarrhea, hypokalemia, and achlorhydria.
- Surgery is the treatment of choice, with limited roles for chemotherapy and or radiation; somatostatin analogs treat diarrhea effectively.

TABLE 34.8. *Syndromes of multiple endocrine neoplasia*

MEN-1	MEN-2
Pituitary tumors	MEN-2a and -2b
Eosinophilic adenoma (acromegaly)	Medullary carcinoma of the thyroid
Prolactinoma	Pheochromocytoma
Nonfunctional tumors	MEN-2a
ACTH-secreting tumors	Hyperparathyroidism
Hyperparathyroidism	MEN-2b
Pancreatic tumors	Mucosal neuromas
Most common	Marfanoid habitus
Gastrinoma	Typical facies
Insulinoma	Bowel abnormalities
Pancreatic polypeptide-secreting tumor	
Uncommon	
Glucagonoma	
VIPoma	
GRFoma	

MEN-2a, -2b, multiple endocrine neoplasia types 2a, 2b; ACTH, adrenocorticotropic hormone. From Abeloff MD, et al. *Clinical oncology*, 3rd ed. Philadelphia: Elsevier Churchill Livingstone, with permission.

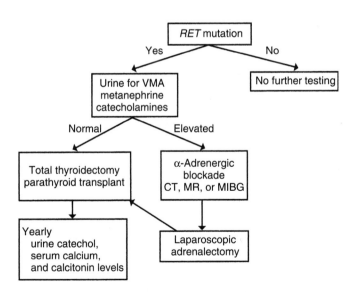

FIG. 34.6. Suggested diagram for treatment of individuals from kindreds of MEN-2a. (From Norton, JA. Adrenal tumors. In: DeVita VT Jr, Hellman S, Rosenberg SA, eds. *Cancer: principles and practice of oncology,* 5th ed. Philadelphia: Lippincott-Raven, 1997:1659–1677, with permission.)

Glucagonomas

- Glucagonomas are tumors that secrete excess glucagon. Serum levels of glucagons >500 pg per mL are diagnostic.
- Glucagonomas cause diabetes, weight loss, anemia, and increased risk for thromboembolism.
- Necrolytic migratory erythema is a common presenting symptom of glucagonomas.
- Surgery, somatostatin analogs, anticoagulants, and chemotherapy are therapeutic options for glucagonomas.
- Zinc supplementation and amino acid infusions may reduce the rash.

Somatostatin

- Tumors secrete excess somatostatin, resulting in inhibition of the secretion of insulin and pancreatic enzyme, and in the production of gastric acid.
- Surgery is the treatment of choice.
- Chemotherapy is the therapeutic option for unresectable disease.

MULTIPLE ENDOCRINE NEOPLASIA I AND II

MENs are characterized by the occurrence of tumors involving two or more endocrine glands within one patient. MENs are uncommon, but because they are inherited as autosomal dominant traits, they have important implications for other family members. First-degree relatives have about a 50% risk of developing the disease (see Tables 34.7 and 34.8 and Fig. 34.6).

SUGGESTED READINGS

Bellantone R, Lombardi CP, Raffaelli M, et al. Is routine supplementation therapy (calcium and vitamin D) useful after total thyroidectomy? *Surgery* 2002;132(6):1109–1112.

Grant CS, Hay ID, Gough IR, et al. Local recurrence in papillary thyroid carcinoma: is extent of surgical resection important? *Surgery* 1998;104:954–962.

Hundahl SA, Fleming ID, Fremgen AM, et al. A national cancer database report on 53,856 cases of thyroid carcinoma treated in the U.S., 1985–1995. *Cancer* 1998;83:2638–2648.

Icard P, Chapuis Y, Andreassian B, et al. Adrenocortical carcinoma in surgically treated patients: a retrospective study on 156 cases by the French Association of Endocrine Surgery. *Surgery* 1992;112:972–979.

Ladenson PW. Recombinant thyrotropin for detection of recurrent thyroid cancer. *Trans Am Clin Climatol Assoc* 2002;113:21–30.

Lairmore TC, Ball DW, Baylin SB, et al. Management of pheochromocytomas in patients with multiple endocrine neoplasia type 2 syndromes. *Ann Surg* 1993;217:595–603.

Luton JP, Cerdas S, Billaud L, et al. Clinical features of adrenocortical carcinoma, prognostic factors, and the effect of mitotane therapy. *N Engl J Med* 1990;322:1195–1201.

Mazzaferri EL. Treating differentiated thyroid carcinoma: where do we draw the line? *Mayo Clin Proc* 1991;66:105–111.

Neumann HP, Berger DP, Sigmund G, et al. Pheochromocytomas, multiple endocrine neoplasia type 2, and von Hippel-Lindau disease. *N Engl J Med* 1993;329:1531–1538.

Norton JA. Adrenal tumors. In: DeVita VT Jr, Hellman S, Rosenberg SA, eds. *Cancer: principles and practice of oncology*, 5th ed. Philadelphia: Lippincott-Raven, 1997:1659–1677.

Sanders LE, Cady B. Differentiated thyroid cancer: reexamination of risk groups and outcome of treatment. Arch Surg 1998;133:419–425.

Schlumberger MJ. Papillary and follicular thyroid carcinoma. *N Engl J Med* 1998;338:297–308.

Sclafani LM, Woodruff JM, Brennan MF. Extraadrenal retroperitoneal paragangliomas: natural history and response to treatment. *Surgery* 1990;108:1124–1129.

SECTION 11

Supportive Care

35

Hematopoietic Growth Factors

Philip M. Arlen and James L. Gulley

Laboratory of Tumor Immunology and Biology, Center for Cancer Research, National Cancer Institute, National Institutes of Health, Bethesda, Maryland

Hematologic toxicity from chemotherapy is the most prevalent serious side effect encountered in medical oncology clinical practice. Reduction in all three cell lineages (i.e., white blood cells, red blood cells, and platelets) can lead to complications such as fever, which complicates neutropenia and requires patient hospitalization, and severe anemia or thrombocytopenia, which may necessitate transfusion.

All three cell lines arise from differentiation of totipotent hematopoietic stem cells; the fully differentiated cells are mature leukocytes, erythrocytes, or platelets (the breakdown product of megakaryoctes). Hematopoietic growth factors are the regulatory molecules for all three cell lines. Several hematopoietic growth factors have been identified, synthesized, and approved for use in clinical practice to mitigate hematologic toxicity caused by chemotherapy. Recommendations in this chapter come primarily from the evidence-based clinical practice guidelines of the American Society of Clinical Oncology (ASCO) (1–3).

In many clinical situations, hematopoietic growth factor is used both judiciously (4) and in a cost-effective manner (5,6). New agents continue to be sought, developed, and evaluated in clinical trials.

MYELOID GROWTH FACTORS: GRANULOCYTE COLONY-STIMULATING FACTOR AND GRANULOCYTE MACROPHAGE COLONY-STIMULATING FACTOR

Currently, two myeloid growth factors have been approved for clinical use by the U.S. Food and Drug Administration (FDA). They are filgrastim (granulocyte colony-stimulating factor [G-CSF; Neupogen and Neulasta (Pegfilgrastim)]; Amgen, Inc. and sargramostim (granulocyte macrophage colony-stimulating factor [GM-CSF, Leukine; Berlex Laboratories (Schering AG)]. Whereas G-CSF is specific for the production of neutrophils, GM-CSF stimulates the production of monocytes and eosinophils in addition to neutrophils. There is no firm clinical evidence to indicate that one agent produces a superior clinical benefit over the other. Although exogenous myeloid growth factor decreases the duration of absolute neutropenia, it does not affect the extent of the neutropenia. FDA-recommended doses of growth factors are listed in Table 35.1.

TABLE 35.1. *Summary of growth factor indications*

Drug/FDA-recommended dosing	Indications
Filgrastim • 5 µg/kg/d s.c.—initiated 24 h after completion of chemotherapy—continued daily until the postchemotherapy ANC is = 10×10^9 cells/L—may require as many as 10–14 daily injections. • For stem cell mobilization and transplant—10 µg/kg/d s.c. may be used.	Cancer pts receiving myelosuppressive chemotherapy. Pts with nonmyeloid malignancy following BMT Pts with severe chronic neutropenia following induction chemotherapy for AML mobilization of stem cells for transplant
Pegfilgrastim • Single 6-mg fixed dose, once per chemotherapy cycle	Cancer pts receiving myelosuppressive chemotherapy
Sargramostim • Dose for chemotherapy-induced neutropenia is 250 µg/m²/d s.c • Following autologous bone marrow transplant—250 µg/m²/d given by a 2-hour i.v. infusion	Following autologous BMT Delay or failure of BMT engraftment Following induction chemotherapy for AML in older pts Mobilization of stem cells for transplant
Epoetin α chemotherapy for nonmyeloid malignancies • current FDA-approved recommended dose—150 U/kg s.c. three times a wk—can be increased to 300 U/kg three times weekly if an adequate response (rise in hemoglobin = 1 g/dL) does not occur after 4 wk of therapy. • 40,000 units s.c. weekly—well tolerated and as effective as a three times a week dosing.	Chemotherapy induced anemia
Darbopoetin α • approved recommended starting dose is 2.25 µg/kg s.c.—dose should be adjusted to maintain a target hemoglobin level – for a < 1.0 g/dL increase in hemoglobin after 6 wk of therapy, dose should be increased up to 4.5 µg/kg – if hemoglobin increases by more than 1.0 g/dL in a 2-wk period or exceeds 12 g/dL, the dose should be reduced by 25% – if hemoglobin exceeds 13 g/dL, doses should be temporarily withheld until the hemoglobin falls to 12 g/dL	Same as epoetin α
Oprelvekin • dose in adult is 50 µg/kg s.c. once daily • therapy begins 6–24 h after chemotherapy is completed • continues until the postnadir platelet count is = 50,000 µL.	Pts undergoing myelosuppressive chemotherapy for nonmyeloid malignancies who are at high risk for developing severe thrombocytopenia

FDA, U.S. Food and Drug Administration; pts, patients; ANC, absolute neutrophil count; BMT, bone marrow transplant; AML, acute myelogenous leukemia.

INDICATIONS

Primary Prophylaxis

Myeloid growth factors were initially recommended as primary prophylaxis after a first cycle of chemotherapy for patients with a more than 40% probability of experiencing febrile neutropenia (FN). This was based upon the Lyman study that examined the cost of hospitalization and the point at which G-CSF became a cost-effective option in preventing FN (5). ASCO guidelines are currently being updated to reflect the threshold value of the probability of experiencing FN as being greater than 20% to 25%, the value at which it currently becomes cost effective to use growth factors to prevent hospitalization. This probability includes patients who are receiving high-dose chemotherapeutic regimens. The use of growth factors may be strongly considered in patients who are thought to be at higher risk for chemotherapy-induced infectious complications because of (a) preexisting neutropenia caused by disease, (b) extensive earlier chemotherapy, (c) previous irradiation to areas containing large amounts of bone marrow, (d) a history of FN during earlier myelosuppressive treatments that have been equally or less myelosuppressive, or (e) conditions that potentially increase the risk of a serious infection (e.g., poor performance status, decreased immune function, open wounds, and preexisting active tissue infections).

Secondary Prophylaxis

To date, there have been no published regimens demonstrating a benefit of either disease-free survival or overall survival to patients when CSF support is implemented as a secondary prophylaxis along with dose-intense chemotherapy. Therefore, in the absence of clinical data or other compelling reasons for maintaining the dose intensity of chemotherapy, CSF support should be administered following FN or severe or prolonged neutropenia after a previous chemotherapy cycle while implementing conventional chemotherapy doses.

Treatment of Neutropenic Patients

A number of clinical trials strongly support the recommendation that growth factors should not be used routinely for uncomplicated fever and neutropenia, which are defined as fever for at least 10 days; when there is no evidence of pneumonia, cellulitis, abscess, sinusitis, hypotension, multiorgan dysfunction, or invasive fungal infection; and in the absence of uncontrolled malignancies (7–14). Although a decrease in the period of neutropenia [absolute neutrophil count (ANC) <500 per µL] has been demonstrated with growth factors, no clinical benefit has been consistently noted. Growth factors, however, may be considered along with antibiotics in some patients with FN who are at a higher risk for infection-associated complications and in those who have prognostic factors that are predictive of a poor clinical outcome. These factors include absolute neutropenia, ANC < 100 per µL, uncontrolled primary disease, hypotension, multiorgan dysfunction (sepsis syndrome), and invasive fungal infection. It is important to note that the benefits of CSF in these circumstances have not been proven.

Transplantation and Peripheral Blood Stem Cell Mobilization

CSFs are used to mobilize peripheral blood stem cells (PBSCs) and after PBSC infusion. Using both G-CSF and GM-CSF can lead to rapid hematopoietic recovery, shorter hospitalization, and, possibly, reduced costs (15–17).

Leukemias and Myelodysplastic Syndrome

CSFs can be given after induction chemotherapy to patients with acute myelogenous leukemia (AML) if the benefits in reducing the length of hospitalization outweighs the costs of administering the growth factor (18,19). Patients who are 55 years or older are more likely to benefit from the use of growth factors. Despite concerns that myeloid growth factors might actually induce the growth of the underlying leukemia, clinical studies have not shown any detrimental effect from their use in this setting. Data on the use of growth factors in leukemic patients younger than 55 years are limited.

There are sufficient data to recommend the administration of G-CSF in patients with acute lyphoblastic leukemia (ALL) after the completion of the first few days of initial induction chemotherapy or after the first postremission course, thereby shortening the duration of neutropenia (ANC <1000 per μL) by approximately 1 week (20,21). However, data are not sufficient to recommend CSF in patients with refractory or relapsed ALL.

In myelodysplastic syndrome (MDS), there are no data about the safety of long-term use of myeloid growth factors; however, its intermittent use may be considered in patients with MDS who have severe disease-related neutropenia and recurrent infections.

ERYTHROCYTIC GROWTH FACTOR: EPOETIN

Indication: Anemia in Cancer Patients

Erythropoietin is specific for differentiation of erythrocytes (Table 35.1). Anemia is multifactorial in patients with cancer. Before initiating supportive treatment with agents such as erythropoietin stimulating proteins (ESP), the selection of patients is important to ensure the cost-effectiveness of the treatment. Patients who have anemia before commencing the antineoplastic treatment and those who experience a decrease in hemoglobin level by more than 2 g per dL after the first cycle of chemotherapy are at greatest risk for transfusion of anemia.

American Society of Hematology and American Society of Clinical Oncology Clinical Practice Guidelines

The recommendations for using erythropoietin in chemotherapy-induced anemia are summarized in Table 35.2 (22). Recently, the FDA approved the use of darbepoetin-α for the treatment of chemotherapy-induced anemia. It has a longer half-life than epoetin-α and requires less frequent dosing. The recommended dosage of epoetin-α and darbepoetin-α is listed in Table 35.1.

PLATELET GROWTH FACTOR: INTERLEUKIN-11

Thrombocytopenia can be a life-threatening consequence of antineoplastic treatments and requires monitoring of platelet counts, and platelet transfusions are required when it is necessary to prevent or mitigate hemorrhagic complications. Patients who are at high risk for bleeding or who experience delays in receiving planned chemotherapy include those with poor bone marrow reserve or a previous history of bleeding, those who receive regimens highly toxic to bone marrow, and those with a potential bleeding site (e.g., necrotic tumor) (23).

Although several thrombopoietic agents are in clinical development, oprelvekin (Neumega; Genetics Institute, Inc.) is the only thrombocytopoietic agent that has received FDA approval for clinical use. Oprelvekin is a product of recombinant DNA technology and is nearly homologous with native interleukin-11 (IL-11), lacking only an amino-terminal proline residue. Oprelvekin promotes the proliferation of hematopoietic stem cells, induces the maturation of megakaryocytes, and has clinically been shown to shorten the duration of thrombocytopenia and reduce the need for platelet transfusions in patients who develop

TABLE 35.2. *American Society of Hematology/American Society of Clinical Oncology (ASH/ASCO) practice guidelines for anemia in cancer patients*

ESP use in chemotherapy-associated anemia	
ESP is indicated	Hgb = 12 g/dL[a]
ESP is used on the basis of clinical circumstance	Hgb 10–12 g/dL[a]
Insufficient data to suggest ESP use	Hgb = 12 g/dL
ESP use in hematologic disease states	
ESP is indicated	Low-risk MDS
Insufficient data to suggest ESP use	Multiple myeloma, non-Hodgkin lymphoma, or chronic lymphocytic leukemia in absence of chemotherapy[b]

Response to ESP Treatment
Goal Hgb 10–12 g/dL
If no response is seen in 6–8 wk (= 1 g/dL rise)
  with appropriate dose escalation, discontinue ESP[a]
Monitoring during ESP Treatment
Periodic total iron, TIBC, transferrin, and ferritin,
  with iron replacement as indicated

ESP, erythropoietin stimulating proteins; Hgb, hemoglobin; MDS, myelodysplastic syndrome; TIBC, total iron-binding capacity.
[a]Blood transfusion is also a therapeutic option
[b]If anemia persists despite optimal treatment of underlying disease, ESP may be indicated.

platelet counts of $<20 \times 10^3$ per μL after prior antineoplastic treatments (24). Table 35.1 provides the recommended dose of IL-11.

Fortunately, iatrogenic thrombocytopenia that requires platelet transfusion or causes major bleeding is relatively uncommon, although its occurrence tends to increase with cumulative cycles of chemotherapy that are toxic to hematopoietic progenitor cells. At present, neither the ASCO nor the National Comprehensive Cancer Network (NCCN) has published formal guidelines for using thrombopoietic growth factors, although they are under development. The results of clinical trials and economic analyses with this class of agents will aid in determining their optimal clinical use.

REFERENCES

1. Ozer H, Armitage JO, Bennett CL et al. American Society of Clinical Oncology. Update of recommendations for the use of hematopoietic colony-stimulating factors: evidence-based, clinical practice guidelines. *J Clin Oncol* 2000;20(18):3558–3585.
2. Rizzo JD, Lichtin AE, Woolf SH, et al. Use of ESP in patients with cancer: evidence-based clinical practice guidelines of the American Society of Clinical Oncology and the American Society of Hematology. *J Clin Oncol* 2002;20(19):4083–4107.
3. Bennett CL, Smith TJ, Weeks JC, et al. Use of hematopoietic colony-stimulating factors: the American Society of Clinical Oncology survey. *J Clin Oncol* 1996;14:2511–2520.
4. Croockewit AJ, Bronchud MH, Aapro MS, et al. A European perspective on haematopoietic growth factors in haemato-oncology: report of an expert meeting of the EORTC. *Eur J Cancer* 1997;33:1732–1746.
5. Lyman GH, Kuderer M, Grene J, et al. The economics of febrile neutropenia: implications for the use of colony-stimulating factors. *Eur J Cancer* 1998;34:1857–1864.
6. Schulman KA, Dorsainvil D, Yabroff KR, et al. Prospective economic evaluation accompanying a trial of GM-CSF/IL-3 in patients undergoing autologous bone marrow transplantation for Hodgkin's and non-Hodgkin's lymphoma. *Bone Marrow Transplant* 1998;21:607–614.
7. Maher DW, Lieschki GJ, Green M, et al. Filgrastim in patients with chemotherapy-induced febrile neutropenia: a double-blind, placebo-controlled trial. *Ann Intern Med* 1994;121:492–501.

8. Mitchell PLR, Morland B, Stevens MCG, et al. Granulocyte colony-stimulating factor in established febrile neutropenia: a randomized study of pediatric patients. *J Clin Oncol* 1997;15:1163–1170.

9. Vellenga E, Uyl-de Groot CA, de Wit R, et al. Randomized placebo-controlled trial of granulocyte-macrophage colony-stimulating factor in patients with chemotherapy-related febrile neutropenia. *J Clin Oncol* 1996;14:619–627.

10. Anaissie E, Vartivarian S, Bodey GP, et al. Randomized comparison between antibiotics alone and antibiotics plus granulocyte-macrophage colony-simulating factor (*Escherichia coli*-derived) in cancer patients with fever and neutropenia. *Am J Med* 1996;100:17–23.

11. Mayordomo JI, Rivera F, Diaz-Puente MT, et al. Improving treatment of chemotherapy-induced neutropenic fever by administration of colony-stimulating factors. *J Natl Cancer Inst* 1995;87:803–808.

12. Ravaud A, Chevreau C, Cany L, et al. Granulocyte-macrophage colony-stimulating factor inpatients with neutropenic fever is potent after low-risk but not after high-risk neutropenic chemotherapy regimens: results of a randomized phase III trial. *J Clin Oncol* 1998;16:2930–2936.

13. Riikonen P, Saarinen UM, Makipernaa A, et al. Recombinant human granulocyte-macrophage colony-stimulating factor in the treatment of febrile neutropenia: a double-blind placebo-controlled study in children. *Pediatr Infect Dis J* 1994;13:197–202.

14. Biesma B, de Vries EG, Willemse PH, et al. Efficacy and tolerability of recombinant human granulocyte-macrophage colony-stimulating factor in patients with chemotherapy-related leukopenia and fever. *Eur J Cancer* 1990;26:932–936.

15. Ho AD, Young D, Maruyama M, et al. Pluripotent and lineage-committed CD34+ subsets in leukapheresis products mobilized by G-CSF, GM-CSF vs. a combination of both. *Exp Hematol* 1996;24:1460–1468.

16. Meisenberg B, Brehm T, Schmeckel A, et al. A combination of low-dose cyclophosphamide and colony-stimulating factors is more cost-effective than granulocyte-colony-stimulating factors alone in mobilizing peripheral blood stem and progenitor cells. *Transfusion* 1998;38:209–215.

17. Cesana C, Carlo-Stella C, Regazzi E, et al. CD34+ cells mobilized by cyclophosphamide and granulocyte colony stimulating factor (G-CSF) are functionally different from CD34+ cells mobilized by G-CSF. *Bone Marrow Transplant* 1998;21:561–568.

18. Bennett CL, Stinson TJ, Laver JH, et al. Cost analyses of adjunct colony stimulating factors for acute leukemia: can they improve clinical decision-making. *Leuk Lymphoma* 2000;37:65–70.

19. Bennett DL, Hynes D, Godwin J, et al. Economic analysis of granulocyte colony-stimulating factor as adjunct therapy for older patients with acute myelogenous leukemia (AML): estimates from a Southwest Oncology Group clinical trial. *Cancer Invest* 2001;19(6):603–610.

20. Pui C, Boyett JM, Hughes WT, et al. Human granulocyte colony-stimulating factor after induction chemotherapy in children with acute lymphoblastic leukemia. *N Engl J Med* 1997;336:1781–1787.

21. Laver J, Amylon M, Desai S, et al. Effects of r-met HuG-CSF in an intensive treatment for T-cell leukemia and advanced stage lymphoblastic lymphoma of childhood: a Pediatric Oncology Group pilot study. *J Clin Oncol* 1998;16:522–526.

22. Rizzo JD, Lichtin AE, Woolf SH, et al. American Society of Clinical Oncology. American Society of Hematology. Use of ESP in patients with cancer: evidence-based clinical practice guidelines of the American Society of Clinical Oncology and the American Society of Hematology. *J Clin Oncol* 2002;20(19):4083–4107.

23. Rubenstein EB, Elting L. Incorporating new modalities into practice guidelines: platelet growth factors. *Oncology* 1998;12:381–386.

24. Tepler I, Elias S, Smith JW II, et al. A randomized placebo-controlled trial of recombinant human IL-11 in cancer patients with severe thrombocytopenia due to chemotherapy. *Blood* 1996;87:3607–3614.

36

Infectious Complications in Oncology

Sarah M. Wynne* and Juan C. Gea-Banacloche†

Laboratory of Immunoregulation, National Institute of Allergy and Infectious Diseases, National Institutes of Health, Bethesda, Maryland; and †Experimental Transplantation and Immunology Branch, National Cancer Institute, National Institutes of Health, Bethesda, Maryland

FEVER IN NONNEUTROPENIC CANCER PATIENTS

Patients with cancer may have fever for many reasons other than infection, including the underlying malignancy, medications, blood products, and graft-versus-host disease. Infections, however, are a significant problem in patients, regardless of the type of malignancy and the stage of treatment. In addition to neutropenia, there are several other factors that contribute to increased susceptibility to infection.

- Local factors include breakdown of barriers (i.e., mucositis and surgery) that provide a portal of entry for bacteria, and obstruction (i.e., biliary obstruction, ureteral obstruction, and bronchial obstruction) that facilitates local infection (e.g., cholangitis, pyelonephritis, and postobstructive pneumonia).
- Intravascular devices, drainage tubes, or stents may become colonized by microorganisms and may lead to local infection, bacteremia, or fungemia.
- Splenectomy increases the susceptibility to infection caused by *Streptococcus pneumoniae* and other encapsulated bacteria.
- Deficiencies of humoral immunity (e.g., multiple myeloma and chronic lymphoid leukemia) lead to increased susceptibility to encapsulated organisms such as *S. pneumoniae* and *Haemophilus influenzae*.
- Defects in cell-mediated immunity (e.g., lymphoma, hairy cell leukemia, treatment with steroids, fludarabine and other drugs, and T-cell–depleted hematopoietic stem cell transplantation) increase the susceptibility to opportunistic infections from *Legionella pneumophila*, *Mycobacterium* species, *Cryptococcus neoformans*, *Pneumocystis jiroveci*, cytomegalovirus (CMV), varicella-zoster virus (VZV), and other pathogens.

Antibiotic Therapy in Nonneutropenic Cancer Patients

- Antibiotics should be administered empirically in cases of fever in patients with cancer who do not exhibit neutropenia only when a bacterial infection is considered likely.
- In the absence of localizing signs and symptoms, bacteremia should be considered, particularly in patients with intravascular devices. Many authorities recommend empiric antibiotics (e.g., levofloxacin and ceftriaxone) until bacteremia is ruled out.
- Clinically documented infections and sepsis should be treated with antibiotics as warranted by the clinical scenario.

- Whenever antibiotics are started, a plan with specific endpoints should be formulated to avoid unnecessary toxicity, superinfection, and development of resistance.

FEVER IN NEUTROPENIC CANCER PATIENTS

Neutropenia is the most important risk factor for developing bacterial infection in patients with cancer. The risk of developing infection increases with the rapidity of onset and with the degree and duration of neutropenia. Patients with febrile neutropenia require immediate evaluation and prompt initiation of empiric antibiotics (see Fig. 36.1). Empiric broad-spectrum antibiotics with activity against *Pseudomonas aeruginosa* must be initiated as soon as the clinical evaluation is completed.

Definitions

- Fever: an oral temperature higher than 38.3C or two oral temperatures >38°C measured 1 hour apart.
- Neutropenia: an absolute neutrophil count (ANC) <500 per mm^3, or an ANC between 500 per mm^3 and 1,000 per mm^3, with a predicted decline to <500 per mm^3 within 48 hours.

Etiology

- There is a microbiologically documented infection (most commonly bacteremia) in 10% to 20% of patients with fever and neutropenia.
- There is clinical evidence of infection in 20% to 30% of patients with fever and neutropenia.
- There is no microbiologically documented infection and no clinical evidence of infection other than fever in 50% to 70% of patients with fever and neutropenia.
- Gram-positive and gram-negative bacteria are isolated with similar rates of occurrence.
- Gram-negative bacteremia may be associated with faster clinical decompensation and death; therefore, empiric treatment is targeted to cover gram-negative pathogens, particularly *Pseudomonas* species.
- *Candida* and *Aspergillus* species are the most common causes of fungal infections in patients with neutropenia and become more prevalent as the duration of neutropenia increases.

Evaluation

- History and physical examination should be performed, with special attention to potential sites of infection: skin, mouth, perianal region, and catheter exit site.
- Routine complete blood count, chemistries, urinalysis, blood and urine cultures, and chest x-ray should be obtained.
- Any accessible sites of possible infection should be sampled for Gram stain and culture (i.e., catheter site, sputum, etc.).
- Antibiotics should be administered as soon as cultures have been obtained.

Empiric Antibiotic Therapy

Several options are available for the initial empiric therapy of neutropenic fever with no localizing signs or symptoms of infection. Either a single antibiotic regimen or a combination of antibiotics may be used.

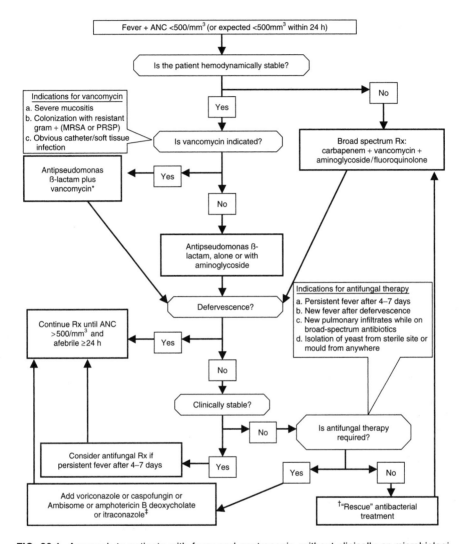

FIG. 36.1. Approach to patients with fever and neutropenia, without clinically or microbiologically documented infection. For specific infections, see text and Table 36.2. *Vancomycin should be discontinued after 48–72 hours if there is no bacteriological documentation of a pathogen requiring its use, except in soft-tissue or tunnel infections. †This "rescue" antibacterial regimen will vary between institutions depending on the local patterns of antibiotic resistance. Carbapenem + fluoroquinolone/aminoglycoside + vancomycin is typical. ‡For a detailed discussion of antifungal therapy options, see text. MRSA, methicillin (oxacillin)-resistant *Staphylococcus aureus*; PRSP, penicillin-resistant *Streptococcus pneumoniae*; ANC, absolute neutrophil count.

Monotherapy

Monotherapy with select broad-spectrum β-lactams with activity against *Pseudomonas* species is as effective as combination antibiotic regimens (β-lactam plus aminoglycoside) for empiric therapy for uncomplicated fever and neutropenia, and it has fewer toxicities.

Antibiotics recommended by the Infectious Diseases Society of America (IDSA) include (doses for adults with normal renal function)

- ceftazidime, 2 g i.v. every 8 hours
- cefepime, 2 g i.v. every 8 hours
- imipenem–cilastatin, 500 mg i.v. every 6 hours
- meropenem, 1 g i.v. every 8 hours.

Combination Therapy

Combination therapy should be used empirically to broaden the antibacterial spectrum in certain clinical circumstances.

Combination therapy should be used in the following cases:

- Severe sepsis or septic shock
- High prevalence of multi-drug resistant gram-negative bacilli.

Effective antibiotic combinations include one of the aforementioned β-lactams (i.e., ceftazidime, cefepime, imipenem, or meropenem) and an aminoglycoside. Ciprofloxacin may be used instead of an aminoglycoside if the prevalence of quinolone-resistant bacteria is low.

Role of Vancomycin

Vancomycin should *not* be part of the initial empiric regimen unless one or more of the following circumstances applies:

- Clinically suspected catheter-related infections (not the mere presence of an intravascular device)
- Known colonization with penicillin-resistant *S. pneumoniae* (PRSP) or methicillin-resistant *Staphylococcus aureus* (MRSA)
- Severe mucositis
- Severe sepsis or septic shock.

Adding vancomycin to the initial regimen because of persistent fever alone does not improve the outcome and is not recommended.

Oral Therapy

Oral therapy may be acceptable for initial empiric therapy in certain patients with febrile neutropenia who are at low risk for developing infection. A scoring system based on patient characteristics and clinical symptoms may be useful in selecting patients who are eligible for oral therapy (see Table 36.1). The patients with a score of greater than or equal to 21 of 26 possible points, indicating low risk, can be considered for oral therapy. The following drug regimen is recommended: Ciprofloxacin, 750 mg PO every 12 hours, plus amoxicillin/clavulanate, 125 mg, 875 mg (amoxicillin component) PO every 12 hours.

Most patients should be started on antibiotics as inpatients. Following discharge, these patients should see the physician daily and should be instructed to call or come to the clinic if new or worsening symptoms are noted or if persistent high fever is present.

TABLE 36.1. *Multinational Association for Supportive Care in Cancer (MASCC) index: A scoring system based on patient characteristics and symptoms used for selecting patients who are suitable candidates for oral therapy (score ≥21 of 26 possible points)*

Characteristic	Score
Burden of illness:	
– no or mild symptoms	5
– moderate symptoms	3
No hypotension	5
No chronic obstructive pulmonary disease	4
Solid tumor or no previous fungal infection	4
No dehydration	3
Outpatient status	3
Age <60 yr	2

From The Multinational Association for Supportive Care in Cancer risk index: a multinational scoring system for identifying low-risk febrile neutropenic cancer patients. *J Clin Oncol* 2000;18(16):3038–3051, with permission.

Modifications of the Initial Antibiotic Regimen

Modification of therapy is often necessary (30% to 50% of cases) during the course of treatment of fever and neutropenia. Specific clinical syndromes (see Table 36.2) or microbiologic isolates dictate specific modifications of therapy to the approach toward the management of the syndrome therapy.

Empiric Antifungal Therapy

Candida and *Aspergillus* infections are the most common fungal infections, and their occurrence increases with increased duration of neutropenia. An antifungal agent should be added empirically for patients with neutropenia who have persistent or recurrent fever after 4 to 7 days of broad-spectrum antibiotic therapy. Treatment options include the following:

- Amphotericin B deoxycholate, 0.6 to 1 mg/kg/day i.v.
- Liposomal amphotericin B (AmBisome), 3 to 5 mg/kg/day i.v.
- Voriconazole, 6 mg per kg i.v. every 12 hours for 24 hours, followed by 4 mg per kg i.v. every 12 hours
- Itraconazole, 200 mg i.v. every 12 hours for 48 hours, followed by a 200-mg daily dosage
- Fluconazole, 400 mg per day i.v. or PO
- Caspofungin, 70 mg i.v. loading dose, followed by 50 mg i.v. daily

The authors' recommendations:

- If the patient has not been receiving antifungal prophylaxis and if the patient has fever and neutropenia for more than 3 days, fluconazole 400 mg i.v. or PO daily should be added from day 4.
- If the patient has been receiving antifungal prophylaxis or is at high risk for an *Aspergillus* infection, he or she should be treated with voriconazole, caspofungin, liposomal amphotericin (5 mg/kg/day), or amphotericin B (1 mg/kg/day).

Duration of Antibiotic Therapy

- Documented bacterial infection: Antibiotics should be continued for the standard period for that bacterial infection or should be continued until neutropenia is resolved, whichever is longer.
- Uncomplicated fever and neutropenia of uncertain etiology: Antibiotics should be continued until the fever has resolved and until the ANC is >500 per mm^3 for 24 hours.
- Antifungal agents can also be discontinued when there is no documented fungal infection.

TABLE 36.2. *Specific infectious diseases syndromes in oncology patients and approach to diagnosis and management*

Clinical syndrome	Diagnostic considerations	Management

Intravascular catheter associated infections	• Infections can be local, involving the exit site or subcutaneous tunnel, or systemic, causing bacteremia
	• For local infections, check culture of exit-site discharge as well as blood cultures
		• For tunnel and systemic infections, empiric therapy should include vancomycin as well as gram-negative coverage (e.g., ceftazidime, cefepime, and ciprofloxacin)
		• Intravascular catheters should be removed in certain situations
		  – tunnel infections
		  – blood cultures remain positive for pathogens after 72 h of therapy
		  – specific pathogens: *Mycobacterium* spp, *Bacillus* spp., VRE, *S. aureus*, fungi
		  – case-by-case decision for *C. jeikeium* and gram-negative organisms

Skin/soft-tissue infections	• Prompt biopsy with histologic staining and culture for bacteria, mycobacteria, viruses, and fungi • Pathogens: *S. aureus*, *S. pyogenes*, gram-negative bacilli (e.g., *Pseudomonas*), VZV, HSV, *Candida* species • For vesicular lesions, scrape base for DFA for VZV and culture for HSV	• Ecthyma gangrenosum: include coverage of *Pseudomonas* (e.g., ceftazidime, cefepime, ciprofloxacin) • Infections with *S. pyogenes*: treat aggressively with penicillin G, clindamycin, IVIG, and surgical debridement • Perianal cellulitis: broad-spectrum coverage including anaerobes (e.g., imipenem) • VZV, HSV: acyclovir
Sinusitis	• Evaluate with CT scan and examine by otolaryngologist • Tissue should be biopsied if there is suspicion of fungal infection or if there is no response to antibiotic therapy after 72 h • Pathogens: *S. pneumoniae*, *H. influenzae*, *M. catarrhalis*, *S. aureus*, gram-negative bacilli (e.g., *Pseudomonas*), and fungi	• Nonneutropenic patient: levofloxacin or amoxicillin/clavulanate • Neutropenic: broad-spectrum coverage including *Pseudomonas* (e.g., imipenem), and consider antifungal coverage (e.g., amphotericin B)
Pulmonary infections	• CT scan and bronchoalveolar lavage should be performed early • Pneumonias in any patient with cancer are often caused by gram-negative bacilli and *S. aureus* as well as by community-acquired pneumonia pathogens: *S. pneumoniae*, *H. influenzae*, *Legionella* spp., *Chlamydia pneumoniae*	• For all patients, ensure adequate coverage of community-acquired pneumonia (e.g., newer-generation fluoroquinolone or azithromycin) • Neutropenic patients: include coverage of *S. pneumoniae* and *Pseudomonas* (e.g., newer-generation fluoroquinolone and ceftazidime); add antifungal coverage if pneumonia develops with treatment by antibiotics (e.g., amphotericin B and voriconazole)

continued on next page

TABLE 36.2. *Continued*

Clinical Syndrome	Diagnostic considerations	Management
	• Neutropenic patients are at risk for invasive fungal infections, particularly aspergillosis • Patients with cell-mediated defects are at risk for infections with PCP, viruses (i.e., CMV, VZV, and HSV), *Nocardia* spp., and *Legionella* • Mycobacteria should also be considered, particularly in patients with previous exposure	• Cell-mediated immunodeficiency: consider coverage of *Pneumocystis* with trimethoprim/sulfamethoxazole, CMV with ganciclovir and IVIG, and *Nocardia* with trimethoprim/sulfamethoxazole
Gastrointestinal tract infections	• Lesions associated with mucositis can be superinfected with HSV or *Candida* species • Esophagitis can be caused by *Candida* species, HSV, and CMV • Diarrhea is most commonly caused by *C. difficile* (send toxin assay) but can also be caused by *Salmonella, Shigella, Aeromonas, E. coli,* viruses, parasites, etc. • Enterocolitis in neutropenic patients is most commonly caused by a mix of organisms including *Clostridium* spp. and *Pseudomonas*	• Mucositis or esophagitis: acyclovir and fluconazole • C. difficile: metronidazole or vancomycin if refractory • Neutropenic enterocolitis: broad-spectrum antibiotics with activity against a *Pseudomonas* (e.g., imipenem)
Urinary-tract infections	• Pathogens: gram-negative bacilli, *Candida* species • Consider whether candiduria may represent disseminated candidiasis	• Remove catheter to clear colonization • Neutropenic patient: treat bacteriuria/candiduria regardless of symptoms • Nonneutropenic patient: reserve treatment for symptomatic episodes • Antibiotic treatment should be tailored to the organism
CNS infections	• Bacteria cause most cases of meningitis (e.g., *S. pneumoniae, Listeria,* and *N. meningitides*) • In patients with cell-mediated immunodeficiency, also consider *Listeria* or *Cryptococcus* • Encephalitis is most commonly caused by HSV but consider other viruses • Brain abscesses may be confused with tumor	• Bacterial meningitis: ceftriaxone, vancomycin, and ampicillin • Cryptococcal meningitis: amphotericin B with flucytosine • Encephalitis: acyclovir (consider ganciclovir)

VRE, vancomycin-resistant enterococci; VZV, varicella zoster virus; HSV, herpes simplex virus; DFA, direct fluorescent antibody; IVIG, intravenous immunoglobulin; CT, computerized tomography; CMV, cytomegalovirus.

SPECIFIC INFECTIOUS DISEASE SYNDROMES

If a patient presents with clinical signs and symptoms of a specific infection, with or without neutropenia, the workup and therapy are guided by the clinical suspicion for that infection (Table 36.2). After patients are started on empiric antibiotics for fever and neutropenia, they must be monitored closely for the development of signs or symptoms of infection, and antibiotic therapy must be modified accordingly.

Bacteremia/Fungemia

- A positive blood culture should prompt immediate initiation of therapy with appropriate antibiotics in a patient with neutropenia or in a patient who is not neutropenic and is febrile or unstable.
- If the isolated organism is commonly pathogenic, such as *S. aureus* or gram-negative bacilli, antibiotics should be started even if the patient is afebrile and clinically stable.
- If the isolate is a common contaminant, such as a coagulase-negative *Staphylococcus*, and if the patient is not neutropenic, is afebrile, and is clinically stable, it may be appropriate to repeat the cultures and observe before starting antibiotics.
- Whenever bacteremia is documented, blood cultures should be repeated to confirm the effectiveness of the therapy, and the source of the infection should be sought.

Gram-positive Bacteremia

Gram-positive Cocci

- Coagulase-negative *Staphylococcus* species is the most common cause of bacteremia. In the setting of neutropenia or clinical instability, vancomycin should be started.
- *S. aureus* bacteremia is associated with a high likelihood of metastatic complications if not treated adequately. Intravascular devices should be removed, and transesophageal echocardiogram should be performed to rule out endocarditis.
- Oxacillin and nafcillin are the drugs of choice for treating a *S. aureus* infection; vancomycin should be reserved for the treatment of patients who are allergic to penicillin or for methicillin-resistant *S. aureus* (MRSA) infection.
- Bacteremia with viridans group streptococci may cause overwhelming infection with sepsis and acute respiratory distress syndrome (ARDS) in a patient with neutropenia; vancomycin therapy should be used until susceptibility results are obtained.
- The risk factors for viridans group streptococci bacteremia include severe mucositis (particularly, following treatment with cytarabine), active oral infection, and prophylaxis with trimethoprim/sulfamethoxazole or a fluoroquinolone.
- Enterococci often cause bacteremia in debilitated patients who have been hospitalized for a long period and who have been receiving broad-spectrum antibiotics.
- Vancomycin-resistant enterococci (VRE) are an increasingly common cause of bacteremia and should be treated promptly with linezolid (600 mg q12h) or quinupristin–dalfopristin (7.5 mg per kg q8h).

Gram-positive Bacilli

- *Clostridium septicum* is associated with sepsis and metastatic myonecrosis during neutropenia. Treatment is with high-dose penicillin or a carbapenem.
- *Listeria monocytogenes* may cause bacteremia with or without encephalitis in patients with defects in cell-mediated immunity. Ampicillin plus gentamicin is the treatment of choice.
- Other gram-positive bacilli such as *Bacillus*, *Corynebacterium*, *Lactobacillus*, and *Propionibacterium* species are common contaminants of blood cultures, but, in the setting of neutropenia, these bacilli can cause true catheter-related infection.

Gram-negative Bacteremia

- Gram-negative bacteria in the blood should never be considered contaminants and should be treated immediately.
- Therapy should be initiated with two antimicrobials to ensure adequate coverage until susceptibility results are available.
- *Escherichia coli* and *Klebsiella* species are the most prevalent gram-negative pathogens in patients with neutropenia; however, the use of prophylactic antibiotics such as ciprofloxacin or trimethoprim/sulfamethoxazole may increase the prevalence of more resistant enteric organisms such as *Enterobacter*, *Citrobacter*, and *Serratia* species.
- The prevalence of strains of *Klebsiella* and *E. coli* that produce extended-spectrum β-lactamases (ESBLs) is increasing; carbepenems are the drugs of choice for these organisms.
- *P. aeruginosa* is among the most lethal agents of gram-negative bacteremia in the patient with neutropenia; combination therapy should be started to ensure that the patient is receiving at least one antimicrobial agent to which the isolate is susceptible.
- *Stenotrophomonas maltophilia* is an increasingly common cause of infection in patients who have been on broad-spectrum antibiotics or in those who have intravascular catheters; trimethoprim/sulfamethoxazole is the treatment of choice. For the allergic patient, ticar cillin–clavulanate or levofloxacin may be effective.
- *Acinetobacter baumannii* bacteremia is frequently associated with infected intravascular catheters in patients with cancer and is often resistant to multiple antibiotics, including imipenem–cilastatin. Ampicillin-sulbactam or colistin may be effective, but an infectious diseases specialist should be consulted.

Fungemia

- *Candida* species cause most cases of fungemia in patients with cancer. The prevalence of non-*albicans* candidemia is increasing.
- Non-albicans species are likely to be resistant to fluconazole and should be treated with caspofungin, amphotericin B, or a lipid formulation of amphotericin B.
- All patients with candidemia should undergo ophthalmologic evaluation with a funduscopic examination. In most cases, intravascular catheters should be removed.

Intravascular Catheter–Associated Infections

Definitions

- Exit-site infections are diagnosed clinically by the presence of erythema, induration, and tenderness within 2 cm of the catheter's exit site.
- A tunnel infection is characterized by erythema along the subcutaneous tract of a tunneled catheter that extends 2 cm beyond the exit site.
- Catheter-associated bloodstream infection is defined by positive blood cultures or by a positive catheter tip culture.

Management

- The following recommendations refer to management of implanted catheters of the Hickman-Broviac type and to long-term intravascular devices. The management of peripheral lines and non-permanenet lines includes a much lower threshold for removal of the catheter.
- If a local infection is suspected, a swab of the exit-site discharge should be sent for culture, in addition to blood cultures.
- Uncomplicated site infections (i.e., no signs of systemic infection or bacteremia) can be managed with local care and with oral antibiotics such as dicloxacillin.

- If the patient has fever in addition to an exit-site infection or if there is substantial cellulitis around the catheter site, vancomycin (i.v.) should be used empirically while awaiting culture results.
- Tunnel infections require intravenous antibiotics and removal of the catheter; empiric therapy should include vancomycin, as well as agents such as ceftazidime, cefepime, or ciprofloxacin for coverage of gram-negative bacilli. Therapy can then be modified if an organism is identified.
- Catheter-related bloodstream infections caused by coagulase-negative *Staphylococcus* or gram-negative bacilli should be treated with antibiotics for a total of 14 days. Initially, therapy should be delivered intravenously and continued as long as the patient remains neutropenic. Once cultures are found to be negative for the bacteria, therapy can be changed to oral antibiotics provided the patient is clinically stable and no longer neutropenic.
- The management of exit-site infections and tunnel infections is illustrated in Fig. 36.2.

Indications for Removal of Intravascular Catheters

Indwelling intravascular catheters should be removed in the following situations:

- Tunnel infections
- Blood cultures remain positive after 48 to 72 hours of therapy (regardless of the pathogen)
- Cultures are positive for
  - *S. aureus*
  - *Bacillus* species
  - Vancomycin-resistant enterococci
  - *Mycobacterium* species
  - *Candida* species

In case of catheter-related infections caused by *Corynebacterium jeikeium*, *Pseudomonas*, *Stenotrophomonas*, and other gram-negative pathogens, the decision of whether to remove the catheter should be made on a case-by-case basis.

Skin and Soft-tissue Infections

- Soft-tissue infections may represent local or disseminated infection.
- A biopsy for staining and culture for bacteria, mycobacteria, viruses, and fungi should be considered early in the evaluation of skin and soft-tissue infections.
- Ecthyma gangrenosum often presents in patients with neutropenia as a dark, necrotic lesion but can be variable in appearance. It is a typical manifestation of *P. aeruginosa* bacteremia and may also be caused by bacteremia from other gram-negative bacilli. Antibiotic therapy with coverage of *Pseudomonas* should be initiated and a surgeon should be consulted.
- VZV and herpes simplex virus (HSV) generally present as vesicular lesions. Scrapings from the base of vesicles should be sent for direct fluorescent antibody (DFA) testing to diagnose VZV and for shell-vial culture to diagnose HSV. Treatment of VZV in the immunocompromised host involves acyclovir 10 mg per kg i.v. every 8 hours and that for HSV involves acyclovir 5 mg per kg i.v. every 8 hours.
- Patients with cancer are at increased risk for streptococcal toxic shock syndrome and severe soft-tissue infections caused by *Streptococcus pyogenes*. The treatment is aggressive surgical debridement and antibiotic therapy with penicillin G and clindamycin, as well as intravenous immunoglobulin (IVIG).
- Perianal cellulitis may develop in patients with neutropenia. Antibiotic therapy should include gram-negative and anaerobic coverage (e.g., imipenem–cilastatin or meropenem as single agents or ceftazidime plus metronidazole). A computerized tomography (CT) scan should be obtained to rule out a perirectal abscess. Incision and drainage may also be required in the setting of abscess or unremitting infection, but, if possible, this should be delayed until neutropenia is resolved.

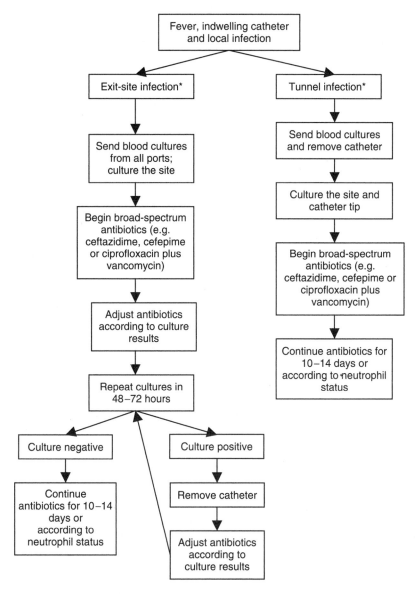

FIG. 36.2. Management of catheter-related infections. *Exit-site infection: erythema, induration, and tenderness within 2 cm of the catheter exit site; *tunnel infection: erythema, induration, and tenderness along the subcutaneous tract of a tunneled catheter that extends 2 cm beyond the exit site.

Sinusitis

- In the absence of an immunocompromised state, the common pathogens of acute sinusitis in patients who are not immunocompromised are *S. pneumoniae*, *H. influenzae*, and *Moraxella catarrhalis* as well as *S. aureus*. Acute sinusitis is treated with levofloxacin, 500 mg daily, or amoxicillin–clavulanate, 875 mg twice daily.
- In immunocompromised hosts, sinusitis can also be caused by aerobic gram-negative bacilli including *Pseudomonas*. Furthermore, patients with neutropenia are at high risk for fungal sinusitis.
- During neutropenia, sinusitis should be treated with broad-spectrum antibiotics including coverage of *Pseudomonas*. A sinus CT scan should be obtained and an otolaryngologist should be consulted. Biopsy should be obtained if there is any suspicion of fungal infection (e.g., bone erosion on CT scan, necrotic eschar of nasal turbinates) or if there is no response to antibiotic therapy within 72 hours.
- If fungal sinusitis is confirmed, it should be treated with surgical debridement, and antifungal treatment should be started at maximum dosing:
  - amphotericin B; 1 to 1.5 mg/kg/day
  - liposomal amphotericin B; 5 to 7.5 mg/kg/day
  - voriconazole may be substituted only after it is certain that the infection is not caused by *Zygomycetes* (i.e., *Mucor* or *Rhizopus*), which are not susceptible to voriconazole.

Pneumonia

Pulmonary infiltrates in the immunocompromised host can be from infectious or noninfectious causes. It is important to obtain an etiologic diagnosis, and the authors recommend early use of bronchoalveolar lavage (BAL) if a diagnostic sputum specimen cannot be obtained.

Pulmonary Infiltrates in the Neutropenic Patient

- Adequate coverage for community-acquired pneumonia should be added to the antibiotic regimen (e.g., newer-generation fluoroquinolone in addition to ceftazidime).
- CT scan and bronchoscopy for BAL should be performed early.
- If pulmonary infiltrates appear while the patient is treated with broad-spectrum antibiotic therapy, the likelihood of fungal pneumonia is high. Empiric antifungal coverage with voriconazole, liposomal amphotericin B, or amphotericin B should be started immediately.

Fungal Pneumonia

- *Aspergillus* species are the most common molds that cause disease in patients with cancer. Neutropenia is the most important risk factor followed by use of corticosteroids.
- Clinical presentation:
  - Persistent or recurrent fever
  - Development of pulmonary infiltrates while being treated with antibiotics
  - Chest pain, hemoptysis, or a pleural rub
- In the setting of allogeneic hematopoietic stem cell transplantation, most cases of *Aspergillus* pneumonia occur well into the engraftment period. The most important risk factors in this setting are graft-versus-host disease, use of corticosteroid, and CMV disease.
- The demonstration of fungal elements in tissue obtained by biopsy is necessary for a definitive diagnosis of fungal pneumonia. When a biopsy is not possible, positive respiratory cultures (i.e., sputum or BAL fluid) are highly predictive of invasive disease in a high-risk patient.
- Options for treatment of aspergillus pneumonia include:
  - voriconazole (6 mg per kg i.v. every 12 hours for 24 hours followed by 4 mg per kg i.v. every 12 hours)

- high-dose liposomal amphotericin B (5 to 7.5 mg/kg/day)
- amphotericin B (1 to 1.5 mg/kg/day)
- caspofungin (70 mg loading dose followed by 50 mg per day i.v.) has been approved for patients with invasive aspergillosis who are unresponsive to or intolerant of the above-mentioned antifungal agents.
- *Zygomycetes* such as *Rhizopus*, *Mucor*, and *Cunninghamella* species are less common causes of pulmonary infection in patients with neutropenia, and these species are resistant to voriconazole. Treatment should include early aggressive surgical debridement where feasible and high-dose amphotericin B.
- *Fusarium* species rarely cause pulmonary infection in patients with neutropenia. Voriconazole or high-dose amphotericin can be used for treatment. Response is usually contingent on neutrophil recovery.
- Dematiaceous fungi such as *Scedosporium*, *Alternaria*, *Bipolaris*, *Cladosporium*, and *Wangiella* species also rarely cause pneumonia in patients with neutropenia. Treatment is with itraconazole or voriconazole.

Pulmonary Infiltrates in Patients with Defects in Cell-mediated Immunity

- In addition to the common bacterial causes of pneumonia, patients with defects in cell-mediated immunity are at risk for infections with *P. jiroveci*, *Nocardia* species, and viruses, as well as with *Legionella*, mycobacteria, and fungi.
- Bronchoscopy for BAL should be performed.
- Empiric antibiotics should include a newer generation fluoroquinolone for coverage of bacterial pathogens such as *Legionella* and trimethoprim/sulfamethoxazole for coverage of *Pneumocystis*. Consideration should also be given to antifungal and antiviral agents depending on the clinical presentation.

Pneumocystis Pneumonia

- Patients with pneumonia from *P. jiroveci* usually present with rapid onset of dyspnea, nonproductive cough, hypoxemia, and fever.
- Radiologic studies generally show diffuse bilateral interstitial infiltrates but can show focal infiltrates.
- Treatment should be started on the basis of clinical suspicion: trimethoprim/sulfamethoxazole 5 mg per kg i.v. every 8 hours (prednisone should be added if the partial pressure of oxygen (P_{O_2}) is <70 mm Hg).

Nocardia

- Pneumonia from *Nocardia* species can cause a dense lobar infiltrate or multiple pulmonary nodules with or without cavitation.
- Diagnosis is made from material obtained at bronchoscopy, either by pathology or by culture.
- Treatment is with trimethoprim/sulfamethoxazole, with or without ceftriaxone. Depending on the species, imipenem–cilastatin with amikacin may also be used.

Viral Pneumonia

- Pneumonia caused by respiratory viruses [i.e., respiratory syncytial virus (RSV), influenza, parainfluenza, and adenovirus] is more common in patients with defects in cell-mediated immunity. Treatment with ribavirin (for RSV and parainfluenza) or with cidofovir (for adenovirus), may be considered, but these agents have not been shown to change outcome.

- CMV pneumonia is a considerable complication of allogeneic stem cell transplantation that typically develops between 40 and 100 days after transplantation. CMV pneumonia after day 100 is becoming more common and typically presents with fever, dyspnea, hypoxemia, and diffuse interstitial infiltrates.
- After allogeneic stem cell transplantation, the presence of CMV in the BAL culture is considered sufficient to establish the diagnosis of CMV pneumonia. In other settings, tissue biopsy is required.
- Treatment of CMV pneumonia is with ganciclovir (5 mg per kg i.v. every 12 hours) and with IVIG (500 mg per kg q48 h). Foscarnet (90 mg per kg q12 h) may be substituted.
- HSV, VZV, and human herpesvirus 6 (HHV-6) have also been associated with pneumonitis in the immunocompromised patient.

Gastrointestinal Infections

Mucositis

- The shallow painful ulcerations of the tongue and buccal mucosa caused by chemotherapy can become superinfected with HSV or with *Candida* species.
- If severe, HSV infection is treated with acyclovir 5 mg per kg i.v. every 8 hours for 7 days. If the infection is less severe, valacyclovir 1,000 mg PO every 12 hours or famciclovir 500 mg PO every 12 hours can be used.
- Candidiasis can be treated locally with clotrimazole troches 10 mg dissolved in the mouth 5 times daily or systemically with fluconazole 200 mg PO or i.v. once followed by 100 mg daily.

Esophagitis

- Odynophagia, dysphagia, and substernal chest discomfort can be a result of chemotherapy but may also be caused by herpes or candidal infections.
- Endoscopy with biopsy should be performed when possible.
- If endoscopy and biopsy are not possible, empiric therapy with fluconazole for *Candida* species and acyclovir for HSV is recommended.
- CMV can also cause esophagitis.

Diarrhea

- *Clostridium difficile* is the most common pathogen that causes diarrhea in cancer patients.
- Diagnosis is made by the presence of *C. difficile* antigen in the stool.
- Treatment is with metronidazole 500 mg PO three times a day or, in refractory cases, with vancomycin 125 mg to 250 mg PO four times a day. Metronidazole can be given intravenously in patients who are unable to tolerate oral therapy. Treatment is continued for 10 to 14 days.
- Bacteria such as *E. coli* and *Salmonella*, *Shigella*, *Aeromonas*, and *Campylobacter* species, as well as parasites and viruses are less common causes of diarrhea in patients with cancer. Stool should be sent for culture for bacterial pathogens and examined for ova and parasites. Specific therapy should be directed against the recovered pathogens.

Neutropenic Enterocolitis (Typhlitis)

- Typhlitis typically presents as abdominal pain, rebound tenderness, bloody diarrhea, and fever in the setting of neutropenia. The diagnosis should be considered in the case of abdominal pain during neutropenia.

- The diagnosis is frequently made on the basis of characteristic CT scan findings: a fluid-filled, dilated, and distended cecum, often with diffuse cecal wall edema and, possibly, with air in the bowel wall (pneumatosis intestinalis).
- Pathogens are typically mixed aerobic and anaerobic gram-negative bacilli (including *Pseudomonas*) and *Clostridium* species.
- Treatment is with broad-spectrum antibiotics including coverage of *Pseudomonas* (e.g., imipenem or meropenem or the combination of ceftazidime plus metronidazole plus vancomycin)
- Patients should be monitored closely for the development of complications that may require surgical intervention, such as bowel perforation, bowel necrosis, or abscess formation.

Hepatosplenic Candidiasis

- Hepatosplenic candidiasis presents typically as neutropenic fever without localizing signs or symptoms.
- When neutropenia resolves, the patient will continue to have fever, may develop right upper quadrant pain and hepatosplenomegaly, and will have significant elevations in alkaline phosphatase levels.
- CT scan, ultrasonography, or magnetic resonance imaging (MRI) will show hypoechoic and/or bulls-eye lesions in the liver and spleen.
- Treatment consists of a prolonged course of fluconazole 400 to 800 mg daily.

Urinary-tract Infections

- In the presence of neutropenia, bacteriuria should be treated even in the absence of symptoms.
- In a patient who does not have neutropenia, treatment should be reserved for symptomatic episodes.
- Candiduria may represent colonization in a patient with an indwelling urinary catheter, particularly in the setting of broad-spectrum antibiotics, and removal of the catheter is usually sufficient to clear it.
- Persistent candiduria can occasionally cause infections such as pyelonephritis or disseminated candidiasis in immunocompromised patients. In addition, candiduria can indicate disseminated candidiasis.
- Fluconazole 400 mg per day for 1 to 2 weeks is the treatment of choice for urinary tract infections. In the case of *non–albicans Candida*, another azole or amphotericin should be used. Caspofungin is minimally present in the urine, and there is no clinical experience in this setting.

Central Nervous System Infections

- Changes in mentation or level of consciousness, headache, or photophobia should be evaluated promptly with MRI and lumbar puncture.
- In addition to the usual bacterial causes of meningitis (i.e., *S. pneumoniae* and *Neisseria meningitides*), *Listeria* and *Cryptococcus* species should also be considered, particularly when a defect in cell-mediated immunity is present.
- For *Listeria* species, the treatment of choice is ampicillin 2 g i.v. every 4 hours in combination with gentamicin loading dose of 2 mg/kg i.v. followed by 1.7 mg/kg i.v. every 8 hours. Once daily dosing (5 mg/kg) is also possible, but there is less experience.
- For *Cryptococcus* species, treatment is with liposomal amphotericin B 3 mg/kg/day or with amphotericin B 0.5 to 0.7 mg/kg/day in combination with flucytosine 37.5 mg per kg q6h for 2 weeks. If the patient improves (i.e., is afebrile and cultures are negative for *Cryptococcus* species), the regimen can be changed to fluconazole 400 mg daily.

- Encephalitis in patients with cancer is most commonly caused by HSV and should be treated with acyclovir 10 mg per kg i.v. every 8 hours. VZV, CMV, and HHV-6 are other less common causes of encephalitis.
- Brain abscesses that develop during neutropenia are typically caused by fungi (most commonly *Aspergillus* and *Candida*). Bacterial abscesses may also be a local extension of infection (e.g., sinusitis and odontogenic infection) caused by mixed aerobic and anaerobic flora (e.g., streptococci, *Staphylococcus*, and *Bacteroides*). While the results from the biopsy and cultures are pending, empiric treatment with ceftazidime plus vancomycin plus metronidazole plus voriconazole is recommended.

PROPHYLAXIS

Antibacterial Prophylaxis

- Fluoroquinolones are the most commonly used antibiotics for prophylaxis against bacterial infections in patients with neutropenia and can considerably reduce the occurrence of gram-negative infections. However, they may *increase* the occurrence of gram-positive infections, and they do not appear to affect the outcome.
- Fluoroquinolone prophylaxis can result in the emergence of resistance among enteric gram-negative bacteria.
- The routine use of fluoroquinolone prophylaxis is not recommended for all patients with neutropenia but can be considered in high-risk patients such as those who are expected to have a long duration of neutropenia.

Antiviral Prophylaxis

Herpes Simplex Virus

- Prophylaxis against HSV should be considered in patients who are seropositive or who have a history of herpetic stomatitis and are undergoing allogeneic stem cell transplantation or highly immunosuppressive chemotherapy.
- Prophylaxis should be given, beginning with the conditioning chemotherapy before transplantation and continued for 100 days post-transplantation and until immunosuppressants are discontinued.
- The medications of choice are valacyclovir 500 mg PO daily or acyclovir 250 mg per m^2 i.v. every 12 hours.

Cytomegalovirus

- Ganciclovir, given prophylactically, can reduce the incidence of CMV disease, but its use is limited by myelosuppressive toxicity.
- Patients who have undergone allogeneic stem cell transplantation should be monitored for CMV replication by following CMV pp65 antigenemia.
- If patients are positive for CMV, they should be treated with ganciclovir 5 mg per kg i.v. every 12 hours for 7 days followed by 5 mg per kg i.v. daily until two CMV antigenemia results are negative for the virus 1 week apart.
- Alternative treatments include (a) foscarnet 90 mg per kg i.v. every 12 hours for 7 days followed by 90 mg per kg daily, (b) valganciclovir 900 mg i.v. every 12 hours for 7 days followed by 900 mg daily, or (c) cidofovir 5 mg per kg i.v. weekly for 2 weeks followed by 5 mg per kg i.v. every alternate week.

P. jiroveci Pneumonia Prophylaxis

- Prophylaxis against *Pneumocystis* species is generally administered to patients with lymphoma, to those who are within the 6-month post-stem cell transplantation period, and to those with a history of *Pneumocystis* pneumonia.
- The regimen of choice is trimethoprim (160 mg)/sulfamethoxazole (800 mg) PO 3 days a week.
- Alternative treatments include (a) inhaled pentamidine 300 mg every 4 weeks, (b) dapsone 100 mg daily [glucose-6-phosphate dehydrogenase (G6PDH) deficiency should be ruled out before using dapsone], or (c) atovaquone 1,500 mg daily.

Antifungal Prophylaxis

- Antifungal prophylaxis is aimed at reducing invasive *Candida* infections, particularly in patients undergoing allogeneic stem cell transplantation.
- Fluconazole 400 mg PO or i.v. daily is the regimen of choice.
- An alternative regimen is itraconazole 200 mg i.v. every 12 hours for 2 days followed by 200 mg i.v. daily for 12 days followed by 200 mg PO every 12 hours.
- Prophylaxis should be continued until 100 days post-transplantation and until immunosuppressants have been discontinued.
- Use of fluconazole has led to increased occurrence of fluconazole-resistant infections such as *Candida tropicalis*, *Candida parapsilosis*, and *Candida krusei*.
- It is not known if any intervention provides adequate prophylaxis for invasive fungal infections caused by *Aspergillus* or other molds. Currently there is not sufficient evidence upon which to base a specific recommendation.

SUGGESTED READINGS

Dykewicz CA. Summary of the guidelines for preventing opportunistic infections among hematopoietic stem cell transplant recipients. *Clin Infect Dis* 2001;33:139–144.

Hughes WT, Armstrong D, Bodey GP, et al. Guidelines for the use of antimicrobial agents in neutropenic patients with cancer. *Clin Infect Dis* 2002;34:730–751.

Klastersky J, Paesmans M, Rubenstein EB, et al. The multinational association for supportive care in cancer risk index: a multinational scoring system for identifying low-risk febrile neutropenic cancer patients. *J Clin Oncol* 2000;18:3038–3051.

Mermel LA, Farr BM, Sherertz RJ, et al. Guidelines for the management of intravascular catheter-related infections. *Clin Infect Dis* 2001;32:1249–1272.

NCCP. NCCP practice guidelines for fever and neutropenia. v.1.2004. Available at http://www.nccn.org/professionals/physician_gls/f_guidelines.asp

Picazo JJ. Management of the febrile neutropenic patient: a consensus conference. *Clin Infect Dis* 2004;39:S1–S6.

Pizzo PA. Fever in immunocompromised patients. *N Engl J Med* 1999;341:893–900.

Vidal L, Paul M, Ben dor I, et al. Oral versus intravenous antibiotic treatment for febrile neutropenia in cancer patients: a systematic review and meta-analysis of randomized trials. *J Antimicrob Chemother* 2004;54:29–37.

Walsh TJ, Pappas P, Winston DJ, et al. National Institute of Allergy and Infectious Diseases Mycoses Study Group. Voriconazole compared with liposomal amphotericin B for empirical antifungal therapy in patients with neutropenia and persistent fever. *N Engl J Med* 2002;346:225–234.

Walsh TJ, Teppler H, Donowitz GR, et al. Caspofungin versus liposomal amphotericin B for empirical antifungal therapy in patients with persistent fever and neutropenia. *N Engl J Med* 2004;351:1391–1402.

Wingard JR. Empirical antifungal therapy in treating febrile neutropenic patients. *Clin Infect Dis* 2004;39:S38–S43.

37

General Principles of
Cancer Pain Management

Jason R. Beckrow* and Richard A. Messmann†

*Department of Internal Medicine, Michigan State University, East Lansing,
Michigan; and †Department of Hematology/Oncology, Michigan State University,
East Lansing, Michigan

Inappropriate or inadequate pain management is a considerable problem that results in suffering and decreased quality of life for patients with cancer. Most patients with advanced cancer, and up to 60% of patients with any stage of cancer diagnosis, experience considerable pain. The problem is not trivial, and unrelieved pain is a risk factor for suicide in patients with cancer. This chapter is designed to help clinicians focus on the three major components of any comprehensive pain-management plan: (a) initial patient assessment followed by (b) analgesic therapy, and (c) reassessment. The chapter is not intended to be an exhaustive review of pain management, but it may act as a helpful guide to facilitate an understanding of pain assessment and control.

INITIAL PATIENT ASSESSMENT

The initial assessment of any patient with cancer who is in pain should include a comprehensive history, with documentation of the following:

- The primary cancer diagnosis and current extent of disease: This may help define the etiology of the painful stimuli (e.g., prostate cancer and bone pain).
- Any current or earlier treatment of pain: Is the patient opiate naïve? Earlier analgesic interventions and documentation of outcomes may affect dosing considerations. The type(s) of analgesics being used by the patient as well as the administration route (Is the delivery of the medication optimized?), dose (Is the dose sufficient for analgesia?), schedule (Is there appropriate regularly scheduled "around-the-clock" coverage? Is the dosing interval consistent with the duration of action of the prescribed drug?), and change in effectiveness of current regimen (Is there a tolerance developing to the current regimen?) should be identified.
- Location of pain: Identify the specific area, depth or site from which the pain originates.
- Date of onset: Is this an acute or a chronic problem?
- Quality of pain: Characterization may help elucidate the etiology of pain. Is the pain cramping, burning, aching, dull, or sharp?
- Character of pain: Is the pain waxing or waning? What are the aggravating and alleviating factors? Is it constant or intermittent?
- Intensity and severity of pain: A visual analog scale (VAS) and a numeric scale (see Fig. 37.1) should be used to quantify and document the intensity of pain. The patient's subjective interpretation of the level of pain should be believed. Chronic cancer pain may not be accompanied

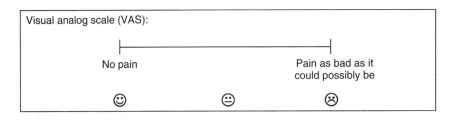

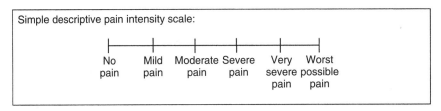

FIG. 37.1. Pain intensity scales: **(Top)** Visual analog scale (VAS). **(Bottom)** Simple descriptive pain intensity scale.

by sympathetic stimulation, which is normally manifested as tachypnea or tachycardia, despite severe pain.

- Psychosocial evaluation (any concomitant major stresses?): Psychological dependency on prescription or illicit drugs, and on alcohol, should be identified.
- Pertinent medical history should be documented. Physical examination: The physical examination should characterize the manifestations of pain, such as atrophy, muscle weakness, and trigger points. A thorough neurologic examination is essential, especially if neuropathic pain is suspected. Appropriate laboratory and imaging studies should be obtained.
- These baseline findings should be documented in the patient's chart to facilitate future management.

PHARMACOLOGIC THERAPY

The six principles of pharmacologic pain management modified from the World Health Organization (WHO) report are as follows:

1. **By the mouth:** The oral route is the preferred route whenever possible (for the sake of the patient's convenience and to avoid painful i.m. injections).
2. **By the clock:** Basal analgesic administration should be based on a fixed schedule— "around the clock" (ATC) and not on an "as needed" (p.r.n.) basis. A rationally designed, regularly scheduled ATC dosing avoids the peak-and-trough effect of prn dosing, in which high serum levels of the analgesic correlate with adverse effects such as nausea, pruritus, or somnolence, and low levels correspond to periods of suboptimal analgesia. Patients should not rely on prn analgesics to cover basal pain-control requirements. However, prn analgesics should always be ordered for breakthrough pain control.
3. **WHO three-step ladder** (see Fig. 37.2):
   Step 1: For mild pain, use nonopioid analgesics (see Table 37.1) with or without adjuvant therapy (see Table 37.2), at recommended dose and frequency.
   Step 2: For moderate pain, add a weak opioid analgesic (see Table 37.3) to the nonopioid analgesic, or, alternatively, use a narcotic analgesic combination (see Table 37.4) with or without adjuvant therapy.

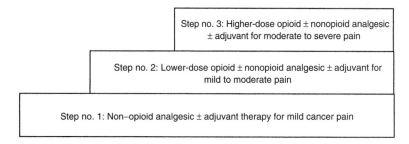

FIG. 37.2. Three-step World Health Organization (WHO) analgesic ladder. (From *Cancer pain relief*, 2nd ed. Geneva: World Health Organization, 1996, with permission.)

Step 3: For severe pain, substitute a strong opioid analgesic (Table 37.3) for the weak opioid analgesic, in addition to the nonopioid, with or without adjuvant therapy (Table 37.2).
- If a maximum dose of medication fails to adequately relieve pain, move up the ladder, and not laterally to a different drug in the same efficacy group.
- The initial point of entry into the WHO analgesic ladder should correspond to the patient's level of pain. For example, patients with mild pain may start at Step 1, whereas patients experiencing severe pain would start at Step 3 to attain prompt analgesia.

4. **Individualized treatment:** A comprehensive analgesic regimen requires therapeutic customization to the patient's needs, including careful dose titration and reassessment to eliminate cancer pain and the appropriate management of opioid-related side effects (see Table 37.5). Once the pain "type" is identified and characterized (e.g., bone, visceral, or neuropathic; see Table 37.6), initiate an appropriate regimen of analgesics by the appropriate route (see Table 37.7).
5. **Monitoring:** Monitoring is required to ensure that the benefits of treatment are maximized and the adverse effects are minimized.
6. **Use of adjuvant therapies (Table 37.2):** Examples of adjuvant therapies include antidepressants, benzodiazapines, steroids, anticonvulsants, and local anesthetics. Depression often accompanies chronic pain, and tricyclic antidepressants at low doses augment analgesia, whereas full-dose selective serotonin reuptake inhibitors (SSRIs) improve sleep and appetite and elevate mood. Use pain-management consultants (e.g., anesthesia pain-management service). Nonsteroidal antiinflammatory drugs (NSAIDs) are often most efficacious in controlling metastatic bone pain. Gabapentin is effective in controlling neuropathic pain.

GENERAL CONSIDERATIONS ABOUT PHARMACOTHERAPY

Use short-acting opioid analgesics [i.e., shorter acting i.v. or PO morphine sulfate versus long-acting morphine sulfate (MS Contin)] until the patient has attained adequate pain control. Short-acting analgesics may offer advantages over longer-acting formulations in the initial management of acute cancer pain, including (a) ease of dose adjustment and (b) rapid onset of analgesic effect. After attaining effective analgesia, the total daily-dose requirements can be determined, thereby facilitating conversion to long-acting formulations. Be aware that there is wide interpatient variability in the amount of analgesics required for pain control.

Consider using patient-controlled analgesia (PCA), which administers small intravenous or epidural doses of opioids on demand. This modality, often used for treatment of acute varying or postoperative cancer pain, affords a high degree of patient satisfaction and safety. Frequent

TABLE 37.1. Select nonopioid analgesics

Generic drug name	Usual dose and administration schedule	Maximum daily dose[a]	Comments
Aspirin	325–650 mg PO every 4–6 h	Usually ≤4,000 mg daily Therapeutic salicylate concentration range, 150–300 μg/mL	Analgesic, antiinflammatory, and antipyretic Irreversibly inhibits platelet aggregation; irritating to GI mucosa; may cause GI bleeding; may trigger allergic reactions inatopic patients
APAP	325–650 mg PO every 4–6 h, or 975–1,000 mg PO every 4–6 h	Limit total daily APAP dose to ≤4,000 mg	Analgesic and antipyretic; may be hepatotoxic high doses and in chronic alcohol users
Ibuprofen	200–400 mg PO every 4–6 h	Limit total daily Ibuprofen dose to ≤3,200 mg	See NSAIDs general statement[b]
Naproxen	Naproxen immediate release: 250–500 mg PO every 12 h Naproxen delayed release: 375–500 mg PO every 12 h Naproxen controlled release: 750–1,000 mg PO once daily	Limit total daily dose to ≤4,000 mg naproxen Limit total daily dose to ≤1,375 mg naproxen sodium	See NSAIDs general statement[b]
Ketorolac	Naproxen sodium: 275–550 mg PO every 12 h Parenterally Age <65 yr: 30 mg i.m./i.v. every 6 h For patients aged ≥65 yr, renal impairment, or with body weight <55 kg, the total daily dose should not exceed 60 mg. Age ≥65 yr, renal impairment, or with body weight <55 kg: 15 mg i.m./i.v. every 6 h	Limit total daily ketorolac dose to ≤40 mg PO, ≤120 mg i.v./i.m. Duration of use by all routes of administration should not exceed 5 consecutive days Doses and treatment duration greater than recommended and shorter dosing intervals increase the potential for adverse effects	See NSAIDs general statement[b]
Tramadol	50–100 mg PO every 4–6 h In renal impairment (GFR <30 mL/min), the recommended tramadol dosage is 50–100 mg PO every 12 h In patients with cirrhosis, the recommended dosage is tramadol, 50 mg PO every 12 h	Limit total daily tramadol dose to ≤400 mg For patients aged ≥75 yr, maximal daily tramadol dose should not exceed 300 mg In renal impairment (GFR, <30 mL/min) maximal daily tramadol dose should not exceed 200 mg	Potential adverse effects in drug accumulation and overdose include respiratory depression and seizure

GI, gastrointestinal; APAP, acetaminophen; NSAIDs, nonsteroidal antiinflammatory drugs; PO, orally; i.v., intravenously; i.m., intramuscularly; i.v., intravenously; GFR, glomerular filtration rate.

[a]In the absence of concomitant diseases and other contraindications.

[b]NSAIDs' analgesic, antiinflammatory, and antipyretic effects vary among compounds. Consider alternative NSAID if one agent is ineffective. Potency and duration of inhibitory effect on platelet aggregation varies among compounds but is reversible. NSAIDs are irritating to GI mucosa; these may cause GI erosion and bleeding. NSAIDs may produce dermatitis. NSAIDs decrease renal blood flow and may exacerbate renal insufficiency. NSAIDs may trigger allergic reactions in atopic patients.

TABLE 37.2. *Select adjuvant therapy*

Modality	Comments	Considerations
TCAs	Relieves neuropathic pain and posttherapeutic neuralgia Analgesic effects start at doses lower than those required for antidepressant effect	Use is associated with anticholinergic effects such as dry mouth, urinary retention, orthostatic hypotension, and conduction abnormalities
Benzodiazepines/ anxiolytics	Decrease anxiety, as a sedative or muscle relaxant	Prolonged use may affect REM sleep
Steroids	Decrease inflammatory component (i.e., nerve-root compression); may potentiate analgesia, provide euphoria, and increase appetite; particularly useful in managing neuropathic pain	Prolonged use associated with a variety of side effects including weight gain and adrenal insufficiency; increase risk of GI bleeding, especially when used with NSAIDs

TCAs, tricyclic antidepressants; REM, rapid eye movement; GI, gastrointestinal; NSAIDs, nonsteroidal antiinflammatory drugs.

evaluation to determine the analgesic effect and the need for dose modification suggests that PCA may be best used through formal consultation of an in-house anesthetist or multimodality "pain-management teams." Programmable PCA pumps often allow basal or maintenance rates of opioid infusion in addition to bolus dose amounts and "lockout" intervals. Maintenance PCA orders can be initiated after bolus opioid dosing achieves adequate analgesic effect.

Avoid using agents such as meperidine and pentazocine, as well as i.m. injections. Meperidine (Demerol) is metabolized to normeperidine, a metabolite with neuroexcitatory (seizure-producing) effects. The risk of toxicity is increased after prolonged administration (for more than 48 hours) and in patients with renal insufficiency. Pentazocine (Talwin) is not more potent than codeine, with a high incidence of hallucinations and agitation. Oral and subcutaneous routes of ingestion are as efficacious, without the pain and expense of i.m. injections.

ANESTHETIC AND NEUROABLATIVE MANAGEMENT

Referral to an anesthetist or a pain care team may be necessary to implement specific anesthetic blockade, neurolysis, and intrathecal or epidural analgesia. Local anesthetic neural blockade may achieve both diagnostic and therapeutic ends. Diagnostically, the nerve block may help predict the efficacy of neuroablation. Therapeutically, the intervention will provide pain relief and the pain-relieving effect may also outlast the drug effect. Neuroablation involves intentionally destroying the nervous structures implicated in the transmission of pain. Spinal administration of opioids produces analgesia without changes in motor or sensory function. Local anesthetics and/or steroids may be added in patients with refractory pain to enhance analgesia. Implantable intrathecal delivery systems are also available, with promising improvements in rapid and sustained pain relief.

PATIENT REASSESSMENT

Pain management is a dynamic process that requires frequent reassessment to determine the effectiveness of therapy and to facilitate dose adjustment. Disease progression often requires increasing doses of analgesics, whereas opioid tolerance is often manifested as decreased duration of analgesia.

The appropriate management of opioid-related side effects (Table 37.5), such as constipation or pruritus, is of paramount importance because the mismanagement of these side effects often acts as a barrier that precludes administration of adequate analgesia. Optimization of patient management requires that the clinician be proactive in managing opioid-related side effects and in assessing and reassessing pain related to cancer.

TABLE 37.3. *Select opioid analgesics*[a,b]

| Generic (proprietary) drug names | Equianalgesic doses[a,b] | | Duration of action | Comments |
	Parenteral	Oral		
Alfentanil (Alfenta)	0.4–0.8 mg (i.m.)	—	—	High potency; primarily used for anesthesia induction and maintenance
Codeine	120 mg	200 mg	4–6 h	Very low potency; high emetic potential; excellent antitussive activity at less-than-analgesic doses (~15 mg)
Fentanyl[c] [Sublimaze (injection); Duragesic (transdermal patches); Oralet (lozenges); Actiq (lozenge on a stick)]	0.1 mg[c]	—	1–2 h	Available formulations include injectable solution, patches for transdermal drug delivery, and lozenges for transmucosal delivery; *Caution:* transdermal patches deliver fentanyl continuously
Hydromorphone (Dilaudid)	1.5–2 mg	7.5 mg	3–5 h	Low emetic potential; solid and liquid oral formulations, rectal suppositories, and injectable formulations available
Levorphanol (Levo-Dromoran)	2 mg	4 mg	6–8 h	Very low emetic potential
Meperidine	100 mg	300 mg	2–4 h	Primary metabolite is a neuroexcitatory compound, normeperidine, which is eliminated more slowly than meperidine and may produce muscle tremors, fasciculations, or seizures in patients with renal insufficiency
Methadone[c] (Dolophine)	10 mg	10 mg	4–8 h[c]	Accumulates with repeated use
Morphine	10 mg	30–60 mg	4–6 h	Immediate-release and sustained-release oral formulations available
Oxycodone	—	20 mg	4–6 h	Immediate-release and sustained-release oral formulations available
Oxymorphone (Numorphan)	1–1.5 mg (injection) 5–10 mg (per rectum)	—	3–6 h	Injectable and rectal suppository formulations available
Propoxyphene (Darvon)	—	130 mg	3–6 h	Low potency; often used in combination with aspirin or acetaminophen
Sufentanil (Sufenta)	0.01–0.04 mg	—	—	High potency; primarily used for anesthesia induction and maintenance

i.m., intramuscularly.

[a]Equianalgesic doses are approximately equal to 10 mg parenterally administered morphine sulfate.

[b]Generally, elderly patients are much more sensitive to opioid pharmacologic effects.

[c]Duration of action increases with repeated or prolonged use.

504

TABLE 37.4. Select opioid analgesic combinations

Generic (proprietary) drug names	Drug content		Usual dose and Administration schedule	Notes
Acetaminophen (APAP) with codeine (Tylenol with codeine no. 2, no. 3, or no. 4; many others)	APAP w/codeine no. 2 APAP w/codeine no. 3 APAP w/codeine no. 4	APAP 300 mg 300 mg 300 mg	Codeine 15 mg 30 mg 60 mg	300–600 mg APAP + 15–60 mg codeine PO every 4–6 h	Limit patient's daily APAP use to ≤4,000 mg
Acetaminophen + hydrocodone	APAP and hydrocodone	APAP 500–750 mg	Hydrocodone 2.5–5 mg	5–10 mg Hydrocodone PO every 4–6 h	Limit patient's daily APAP use to ≤4,000 mg
Acetaminophen + propoxyphene (Darvocet-N 50, Darvocet-N 100, Wygesic)	Darvocet-N 50 Darvocet-N 100 Wygesic	APAP 325 mg 650 mg 650 mg	Propoxyphene 50 mg 100 mg 65 mg	50–100 mg Propoxyphene PO every 4–6 h	Limit patient's daily APAP use to ≤4,000 mg
Acetaminophen + oxycodone (Percocet, Roxicet, Tylox, Roxicet 5/500, Roxilox)	Percocet, Roxicet: Tylox, Roxicet 5/500, Roxilox:	APAP 325 mg 500 mg	Oxycodone 5 mg 5 mg	5–10 mg Oxycodone PO every 4–6 h	Limit patient's daily APAP use to ≤4,000 mg
Aspirin + oxycodone (Percodan)	Percodan	Aspirin 325 mg	Oxycodone ~5 mg	5–10 mg Oxycodone PO every 4–6 h	Gastrointestinal mucosal integrity and platelet aggregation may be adversely affected by aspirin

PO, orally.

505

TABLE 37.5. *Management of opioid-induced adverse effects*

Reaction	Comments	Therapeutic alternatives and suggestions
Constipation	Very common; requires aggressive vigilance and therapy; always order a bowel regimen for any patient on regularly scheduled opioids	Bowel regimen: Senna 2 tabs PO h.s. (up to maximum of 8 tabs/day) + 100 mg docusate sodium PO h.s. (titrate to effect) ± bisacodyl Obstipation: consider lactulose, milk of magnesia, etc., p.r.n. disimpaction
Nausea	Tolerance often develops in 3–5 d	Hydrate patient; relieve constipation; decrease opioid dose with increased frequency to avoid high serum peaks; consider antiemetics, anxiolytics, and anticholinergic agents such as prochlorperazine, metoclopramide, lorazepam, meclizine, or Transderm Scop —scopolamine patch
Pruritus	Morphine releases histamine; consider using fentanyl or oxymorphone	Consider using diphenhydramine, hydroxyzine, or cyproheptadine
Sedation	Patients may develop a varying degree of tolerance over several days	Decrease opioid dose with increased frequency to avoid high serum peaks; consider using stimulants like caffeine, 100–200 mg PO q3–4h, or methylphenidate, 5–10 mg PO at breakfast; repeat at lunch
Respiratory depression	Rarely a significant problem; patients develop rapid tolerance	May simply require physical stimulation; if severe/emergency use, 0.4 mg nalox one/10 mL NS as a 0.5 mL i.v. push q2 min, titrating to effect; use with caution; may precipitate acute pain, withdrawal, and/or seizures

PO, orally; h.s., at bedtime; p.r.n., as needed; NS, normal saline.

TABLE 37.6. *Treatment of cancer pain by etiology*

Type of pain	Characteristics	Suggested treatment options
Bone	Aching, dull	NSAIDs, opioids, strontium, pamidronate, plicamycin, samarium, lexidronam, calcitonin
Soft tissue infiltration/ nerve compression/ spinal cord compression		Corticosteroids (dexamethasone and prednisone), radiation therapy, neurolytic procedures
Neuropathic	Burning, tingling	Tricyclic antidepressants, opioids, anticonvulsants
Neuralgic	Lancinating (sharp, shooting)	Opioids, anticonvulsants (carbamazepine, clonazepam, phenytoin, gabapentin), antidepressants; herpetic neuralgia; sympathetic or epidural blocks
Somatic	Deep, dull	Chest wall pain: consider intrapleural analgesia, or intercostal nerve block
Visceral	Complaint depends on site of disease: If pleural or pericardial, worse with deep breathing, sharp; if organ-based, cramping, gnawing	Three-step ladder ± adjuvant therapy; versus mucositis, consider opioids, topical anesthetics, PCA, oral rinses

NSAIDs, nonsteroidal antiinflammatory drugs; PCA, patient-controlled analgesia.

TABLE 37.7. *Selected routes of analgesic administration*

Route	Advantages	Comments
Oral	Facilitates long-term administration. Tablet/capsule or liquid formulations	Preferred route whenever possible
Intramuscular	None	Painful administration, slower onset than i.v. route. Variable time to peak effect
Subcutaneous	Steady serum levels without peak/trough effect when used to administer continuous infusion of medication	As with i.v. and transdermal routes, subcutaneous route is ideal for certain infusional techniques
Intravenous	Rapid onset-to-peak effect and ease of titration	May require repeated i.v. boluses for titration to analgesic effect, followed by maintenance dosing
Sublingual	Circumvents first-pass hepatic metabolism; fast onset	Facilitates ease of use for liquid preparations (e.g., Roxanol)
Rectal	As an alternative to oral administration of drug	Not often considered
Transdermal	Convenient for nonfluctuating analgesic or basal requirements or for long-term administration	Slow onset (~48 h to steady-state levels). Difficult to titrate during changing analgesic requirements
Epidural or intrathecal	Can utilize opioid or local anesthetics or both in combination	Optimally requires "pain service" consult; respiratory depression if dermatome levels are too high
Injection techniques	Trigger-point injections and nerve blocks	Optimally requires "pain service" consult
Neurosurgery	Neuroablative techniques	Requires "pain service" or neurosurgical consult

SUGGESTED READINGS

Abraham J. *A physician's guide to pain and symptom management in cancer patients.* Baltimore, MD: The Johns Hopkins University Press, 2000.

Agency for Health Care Policy and Research. *Management of cancer pain guideline panel.* Rockville, MD: U.S. Department of Health and Human Services, Public Health Service Agency for Health Care Policy and Research, 1994.

American Association of Hospice and Palliative Medicine. *Hospice/palliative care training for physicians: pocket guide to hospice/palliative medicine.* Glenview, IL: American Academy of Hospice and Palliative Medicine, 2003.

American Pain Society. *Principles of analgesic use in the treatment of acute pain and cancer pain,* 3rd ed. Skokie, IL: American Pain Society, 1992.

Arbit E. *Management of cancer-related pain.* Mount Kisco, NY: Futura Publishing, 1993.

Brisman R. *Neurosurgical and medical management of pain: trigeminal neuralgia, chronic pain, and cancer pain.* Boston, MA: Kluwer Academic Publishers, 1989.

Brooks PM, Day RO. Nonsteroidal antiinflammatory drugs: differences and similarities [see comments]. N Engl J Med 1991;324:1716–1725 [published erratum appears in *N Engl J Med* 1991;325:747].

Cleeland CS, Gonin R, Hatfield AK, et al. Pain and its treatment in outpatients with metastatic cancer [see comments]. *N Engl J Med* 1994;330:592–596.

Djulbegovia B, Sullivan DM. *Decision making in oncology: evidence-based management.* New York: Churchill Livingstone, 1997.

Epps RP, Stewart SC. *American Medical Women's Association: guide to cancer and pain management.* New York: Dell Publishing, 1996.

Kaiko RF, Foley KM, Grabinski PY, et al. Central nervous system excitatory effects of meperidine in cancer patients. *Ann Neurol* 1983;13:180–185.

Kanner R. *Diagnosis and management of pain in patients with cancer.* Basel: Karger, 1988.

Magni G. The use of antidepressants in the treatment of chronic pain: a review of the current evidence. *Drugs* 1991;42:730–748.

McGuire DB, Yarbro CH. *Cancer pain management.* Orlando, FL: Grune & Stratton, 1987.

McGuire DB, Yarbro CH, Ferrell B. *Cancer pain management,* 2nd ed. Boston, MA: Jones & Bartlett, 1995.

Mellick LB, Mellick GA. Successful treatment of reflex sympathetic dystrophy with gabapentin [letter]. *Am J Emerg Med* 1995;13:96.

Parris WCV. *Cancer pain management: principles and practice.* Boston, MA: Butterworth-Heinemann, 1997.

Pazdur R, Coia LR, Hoskins WJ, et al. *Cancer management: a multidisciplinary approach,* 7th ed. New York: The Oncology Group, 2003.

Schug SA, Zech D, Dorr U. Cancer pain management according to WHO analgesic guidelines. *J Pain Symptom Manage* 1990;5:27–32.

Ventafridda V, Tamburini M, Caraceni A, et al. A validation study of the WHO method for cancer pain relief. *Cancer* 1987;59:850–856.

Waller A, Caroline NL. *Handbook of palliative care in cancer.* Boston: Butterworth-Heinemann, 1996.

Watson CP. Antidepressant drugs as adjuvant analgesics. *J Pain Symptom Manage* 1994;9:392–405.

38

Oncologic Emergencies and Paraneoplastic Syndromes

Muhammad K. Siddique* and Richard A. Messmann†

*Division of Hematology/Oncology, Department of Medicine, Michigan State University, East Lansing, Michigan, and †Great Lakes Cancer Institute, Lansing, Michigan

SPINAL CORD COMPRESSION

- Spinal cord compression (SCC) is a true oncologic emergency.
- Delay in evaluation and treatment can result in permanent bowel and bladder dysfunction or paralysis.
- Most cord compression cases involve tumor or collapsed bone fragments in the epidural space, a few cases are subdural, and intramedullary metastases are very rare.
- The thoracic spine is most often involved (60% to 70%), followed by the lumbosacral (20% to 30%) and cervical spine (10%) (1).

Etiology of Spinal Cord Compression

- Metastatic tumors from primary breast, lung, and prostate cancer; lymphoma; multiple myeloma; renal and gastrointestinal tumors (1).
- SCC, infrequently, is the first sign of cancer.

Clinical Signs and Symptoms of Spinal Cord Compression

- Back or radicular pain
- Muscle weakness
- Acute or slowly evolving changes in bowel or bladder function
- Sensory loss or autonomic dysfunction.

Any of these signs and symptoms should bring about the initiation of a prompt clinical evaluation for SCC (2,3).

A thorough physical and neurologic examination should be performed (4), including

- gentle percussion of the spinal column
- evaluation for motor or sensory weakness
- passive neck flexion
- straight-leg raising
- rectal examination (to evaluate the sphincter tone)
- pinprick testing from toe to head to establish whether a "sensory level" is present

A clinical suspicion of SCC should prompt the initiation of steroid therapy (see Treatment, in subsequent text) (5).

DIAGNOSTIC IMAGING

The choice of diagnostic imaging should be suggested by the results of the neurologic examination.

- Magnetic resonance imaging (MRI) with gadolinium contrast is the standard for diagnosis because of its high sensitivity and specificity for detecting SCC (2,4,5). The entire neuraxis is readily imaged such that the superior and inferior extent of the compression can be used to target radiotherapy.
  Some limitations include limited availability in some communities, inability of the patient to lie absolutely still and supine for 30 to 60 minutes of imaging, and issues that preclude MRI [e.g., history of metallic vertebral stabilization surgery, earlier pacemaker/automatic implantable cardioverter–defibrillator (AICD) placement, or presence of certain other implanted devices].
- Computerized tomography (CT) scan of the spinal region combined with myelogram (CT-myelogram) provides an excellent assessment of the epidural space and surrounding soft tissue and is useful in diagnosis and therapy planning.
  It is generally more available than MRI and is an acceptable imaging modality when MRI is not possible.
  Technical limitations include the need for lumbar puncture to administer radiocontrast, as well as a requirement that the ordering physician identifies the expected spinal region to be imaged. The procedure is impractical for the entire neuraxis and may require supplemental studies to exclude a more superior level of compression.
- Conventional radiographs are readily obtained and are inexpensive. Radiographs exploit the finding that almost all SCC begins as vertebral bone metastases that lead to subsequent fracture and cord compression by the bone and tumor. The value of conventional radiographs is limited to verifying a diagnostic impression of SCC, assessing surgical options, and evaluating spinal stability. Radiographs do not exclude the diagnosis of SCC even if they are "normal" and are insufficient to plan radiotherapy.

Diagnosis of Spinal Cord Compression

Symptomatic patients with *abnormal* neurologic examination:

- Receive steroid therapy at once, as detailed in subsequent text.
- Conventional radiographs detect abnormalities in most patients with SCC, which aids prompt confirmation of the diagnosis.
- MRI is then done to define the proximal and distal extent of the compression to facilitate the therapeutic plan.

Symptomatic patients with *normal* neurologic examination:

- Conventional radiographs of the spine should be followed by MRI if the conventional radiograph is abnormal (as for the patients with abnormal neurologic examination) or if clinical progression occurs or if the symptoms fail to resolve. It should be noted that a very small percentage of intradural tumor metastasis will be visible only in MRI.
- In addition, any abnormal findings should prompt initiation of steroid therapy. Myelography (often assisted by simultaneous CT scan) may be useful if an MRI is not available.

Treatment of Spinal Cord Compression

The goals of treatment for SCC include pain control, recovery of normal neurologic function, local tumor control, and avoidance of complications.

- Once SCC is suspected, administer steroids as follows:
  Begin treatment with a "loading" dose of dexamethasone, 10 mg by i.v. infusion.
  Six hours after the loading dose, and every 6 hours thereafter, administer dexamethasone, 4 mg by i.v. infusion (5,6).
  An alternative treatment strategy includes an initial bolus dose of dexamethasone, 100 mg by i.v. infusion, followed 6 hours later by dexamethasone, 4 mg by i.v. infusion every 6 hours; however, this regimen is associated with additional toxicities related to high-dose steroid administration (7) and no improvement has been seen compared to low-dose therapy with respect to pain, ambulation, and bladder function (8).
- Surgical and radiation oncology consultation(s) are required immediately after diagnosis, and further therapy is decided on the basis of the clinical signs and symptoms, availability of histologic diagnosis, spinal stability, and previous treatments. All symptomatic patients with SCC should be considered for decompression radical resection of metastatic tumor within 24 hours of onset of symptoms, regardless of spinal stability.
  In symptomatic patients with SCC caused by metastatic tumors other than lymphoma, initial debulking surgery followed by radiation results in a four times longer duration of maintained ambulation after treatment, and a three times higher chance of regaining ambulation for nonambulatory patients, than that with radiation alone. In addition, patients who receive combined-modality therapy achieve superior pain control and bladder continence. Patients treated with radiation therapy alone require more steroids and narcotics and are less likely to maintain continence (9).
  Patients with spinal instability even in the absence of clinical signs and symptoms should undergo surgery unless otherwise contraindicated.
  Additional surgical candidates include patients with relapsed compression at a site of earlier irradiation and patients with progression of deficits during radiation therapy.
- Radiotherapy is used to treat radiosensitive tumors in asymptomatic individuals and in those individuals who are symptomatic but are poor surgical candidates.
  Radiosensitive tumors include breast and prostate tumors, lymphoma, multiple myeloma, and neuroblastoma.
  Radiotherapy candidates may also include patients with multiple areas of compression.
  Standard radiation doses range from 2,500 to 4,000 cGy delivered in 10 to 20 fractions.
- Select patients with chemosensitive tumors may benefit from chemotherapy in addition to either radiation or surgical intervention (6,10).
- Chemotherapy may be an appropriate first-line therapy for patients with chemosensitive tumors (i.e., lymphoma, myeloma, germ cell tumors, and breast and prostate cancer) and in individuals who are not candidates for radiation or surgery. The reader is directed to a number of references for specific details (2,11–18).

SUPERIOR VENA CAVA SYNDROME

- Superior vena cava syndrome (SVCS) is a common occurrence in cancer patients and may occur as a manifestation of either primary or metastatic tumor, or as a thrombosis associated with central venous access devices.
- Superior vena caval obstruction can result in life-threatening cerebral edema (increased intracranial pressure) or laryngeal edema (airway compromise).

Etiology of Superior Vena Cava Syndrome

SVCS is most often caused by extrinsic compression of the SVC by a tumor (intrathoracic) in the setting of (1,4)

- lung cancer, especially right-sided bronchogenic carcinoma
- non-Hodgkin lymphoma, especially diffuse large cell or lymphoblastic lymphoma in the anterior mediastinum

- metastatic disease to the mediastinum, from primary
  - breast cancer
  - testicular cancer
  - gastrointestinal (GI) cancers
- primary tumors:
  - sarcomas (e.g., malignant fibrous histiocytoma)
  - melanomas.

Other causes include:

- central line thrombus and other iatrogenic causes
- fibrosing mediastinitis, either idiopathic or secondary to infections like histoplasmosis, tuberculosis, actinomycosis, aspergillosis, blastomycosis, or bancroftian filariasis
- retrosternal goiter.

Clinical Signs and Symptoms of Superior Vena Cava Syndrome

- Clinical evolution of SVCS may occur acutely or gradually.
- Physical examination findings may include neck or chest wall superficial venous distension, facial and periorbital edema, cyanosis, facial plethora, mental status changes, lethargy, or edema of the upper extremities.
- SVCS symptoms include dyspnea, orthopnea, facial swelling, complaint of head "fullness," cough, arm swelling, chest pain, dysphagia, hoarseness, and positional worsening of symptoms (5).

Diagnosis of Superior Vena Cava Syndrome

- A thorough physical examination may be sufficient to establish the diagnosis of SVCS (19).
- Noninvasive imaging that may facilitate the diagnosis of SVCS includes:
  - contrast-enhanced CT scan or MRI
  - chest radiograph that may show mediastinal widening.

Doppler ultrasonography examination of the jugular or subclavian vein may help differentiate thrombus from extrinsic obstruction.

Radiocontrast or other injections into veins of the affected extremity are not recommended because of the risk of extravasation and the delayed entry of the contrast into central circulation.

Treatment of Superior Vena Cava Syndrome

- Options for the treatment of SVCS depend on the underlying etiology and on the pace of symptom progression (19,20).
- Emergent radiation therapy is required when respiratory compromise (e.g., stridor) or central nervous system (CNS) symptoms are present.
- The endpoints of the nonemergent treatment are symptom relief and treatment of the malignant or infectious or other process causing the SVCS.
- If SVCS is a presenting symptom (i.e., no history of cancer), and if time allows (i.e., no respiratory distress or changing neurologic status), tissue should be obtained to establish a diagnosis before treatment (21).
- Diagnostic strategies may be limited by the patient's inability to lie supine (i.e., worsened SVCS symptoms). Most malignancies that cause SVCS can be identified without major thoracic surgical procedures by using thoracentesis, bronchoscopy, lymph node biopsy, and bone marrow biopsy, or by analyzing sputum cytology. Limited thoracotomy and mediastinoscopy may be required in some cases.
- Conservative treatment includes elevation of the head of the bed, supplemental oxygen, and bed rest.

- The emergent treatment of malignancy, or treatment once the histologic diagnosis is established, may include the following:
  - Adjunct medical therapy with steroids can be used, but the benefit is not well established (22). For severe respiratory symptoms, hydrocortisone, 100 to 500 mg i.v., may be administered initially, followed by lower doses of hydrocortisone every 6 to 8 hours.
  - Cautious use of loop diuretics may provide transient, symptomatic relief of edema. Overdiuresis may lead to dehydration and cardiovascular compromise.
  - Endovascular stent insertion provides relief of symptoms more rapidly and in higher proportion of patients than that with radiation or chemotherapy (4,5,22,23). The use of a stent is limited when intraluminal thrombosis is present.
  - Radiation therapy [especially for non–small cell lung cancer (NSCLC)].
  - Chemotherapy (for lymphoma or germ cell tumor).
  - Chemotherapy and radiation therapy is used for limited-disease small cell lung cancer.
  - Anticoagulant or thrombolytic therapy (for caval thrombosis and in catheter-associated thrombosis).
  - In cases of SVCS caused by catheter-associated thrombosis, removal of the catheter with a brief period of anticoagulant therapy remains an option. Alternatively, the catheter can be retained (if functional) and the patient can be treated indefinitely with therapeutic-dose warfarin.
  - Surgery (especially in the setting of refractory disease or nonmalignant causes).

HYPERCALCEMIA

Etiology of Hypercalcemia

Hypercalcemia most often occurs in the setting of the following cancers:

- Non–small cell lung cancer: squamous cell/bulky disease
- Breast: adenocarcinoma/during hormonal therapy
- Genitourinary tumors: renal, small cell ovarian cancer
- Multiple myeloma
- Head and neck tumors
- Lymphoma: older patients with Hodgkin lymphoma who have bulky disease, intermediate or high-grade non-Hodgkin lymphoma (NHL)/adult T-cell lymphoma
- Leukemias and unknown primary neoplasms (1,4)
- Patients with solid tumor metastasis to the bone comprise a large percentage of patients with cancer who have hypercalcemia (small cell lung and prostate cancers are seldom associated with hypercalcemia).

Clinical Signs and Symptoms of Hypercalcemia

The clinical signs and symptoms of hypercalcemia:

- May be general: dehydration, weakness, fatigue, and pruritus
- May involve many organ systems including CNS (i.e., hyporeflexia, mental status changes, seizure, coma, and proximal myopathy) and GI or genitourinary tract (GI: weight loss, nausea/vomiting, constipation, ileus, polyuria, polydipsia, azotemia, dyspepsia, and pancreatitis)
- May involve cardiac symptoms: bradycardia, short-QT interval, wide T wave, prolonged PR interval, arrhythmias, and arrest.

Diagnosis of Hypercalcemia

- It may be difficult to distinguish between hypercalcemia as a paraneoplastic syndrome and the hypercalcemia that results from metastatic disease to the bone.

- Hypercalcemia of malignancy: serum intact parathormone (iPTH) level is low or undetectable; serum parathormone-related peptide (PTH-RP) levels are elevated, whereas both 1,25-dihydroxyergocalciferol and inorganic phosphate levels are low or normal. Serum PTH-RP level has a high prevalence in malignancy-related hypercalcemia, which results from osteoclastic bone resorption and increased renal resorption of calcium.
- Osteolytic hypercalcemia is seen in the setting of multiple myeloma, NSCLC, and breast cancer.
- Calcitriol-mediated hypercalcemia is seen in relation to Hodgkin and non-Hodgkin lymphomas.
- In general terms, the degree of hypercalcemia can be characterized as follows: *Mild hypercalcemia* is characterized by a serum calcium level >10.5 mg/dL but <12 mg per dL, whereas in *moderate hypercalcemia*, serum calcium level ranges from 12 to 13.5 per dL, and *severe hypercalcemia* occurs at levels >13.5 mg per dL, although patients with chronic hypercalcemia may tolerate levels well in excess of 14 mg per dL without any apparent symptoms. The reader is cautioned, therefore, that the clinical manifestations and severity of hypercalcemia do not necessarily correlate with the absolute serum level of calcium but may be more directly related to the speed with which hypercalcemia develops (1).
- Albumin and certain serum proteins bind serum calcium and may distort "true" serum calcium levels; for example, in cases of myeloma, in which dramatic elevations in serum calcium levels simply reflect elevated concentrations of serum calcium–binding proteins as opposed to severe hypercalcemia. Approximation of the "corrected" serum calcium level can be calculated using one of several formulas that account for serum albumin levels, for example (15):

Formulae for corrected serum calcium concentration:

$$(mg/dL) = serum\ Ca_{(measured)} + 0.8 \times [4.0\ serum\ albumin\ concentration\ (g/dL)] \quad (1)$$
$$(mEq/L) = serum\ Ca_{(measured)} + 0.4 \times [4.0\ serum\ albumin\ concentration\ (g/dL)] \quad (2)$$
$$(mmol/L) = serum\ Ca_{(measured)} + 0.2 \times [4.0\ serum\ albumin\ concentration\ (g/dL)] \quad (3)$$

General Principles of Treatment of Hypercalcemia

- The most effective treatment of hypercalcemia requires effective therapy directed at the underlying malignancy (i.e., the source of the hypercalcemia). Unfortunately, hypercalcemia most often occurs in advanced states of disease and in patients who have progressed through available standard chemotherapy. In patients with solid tumor primary cancers, survival is often less than 6 months.
- Any symptomatic patient with hypercalcemia, regardless of absolute serum calcium level, should be treated for correction of the hypercalcemia (24–27).
- Symptomatic patients with severely elevated calcium levels often require profound fluid volume replacement, which makes outpatient therapy impractical and unsafe.
- Mild asymptomatic hypercalcemia with serum calcium concentration in range of 11 to 12 mg per dL should be treated, when there is associated hypercalciuria, because of the risk of nephrolithiasis and nephrocalcinosis.

Practical Management of Hypercalcemia

- Therapy for mild chronic hypercalcemia usually includes observation and oral rehydration. Corticosteroids can be considered in select patients. Corticosteroid administration inhibits osteoclastic bone resorption and is useful in patients with tumors responsive to this steroid effect. These tumors include lymphoma, leukemia, myeloma (prednisone, 40 to 100 mg per day), and breast cancers (prednisone, 15 to 30 mg per day) during hormonal therapy (4,28–30). The hypocalcemic effect of corticosteroid administration is inconsistent, however, in steroid-resistant tumor types, and caution is advised (4). Oral phosphate (1 to 3 g per day) can also be considered as long as serum phosphate concentrations do not exceed 4 mg per dL.

Oral phosphate usually lowers the serum calcium concentration by 0.5 to 1.0 mg per dL, but its use is frequently complicated by gastrointestinal symptoms.

- Acute therapy of patients with symptomatic or more severe hypercalcemia, (i.e., serum calcium concentration exceeding 12 mg per dL) requires hospitalization. Therapy should be initiated by increasing urinary calcium excretion through vigorous hydration and by decreasing bone resorption through osteoclast inhibition (see subsequent text).
- The fluid and hemodynamic status should be assessed by evaluating blood pressure, pulse, orthostatics, urine volume, and appropriate laboratory values of the patient (4,27). Patients with hypercalcemia are often severely dehydrated (i.e., they need many liters of fluid) and require immediate administration of isotonic saline (1 to 2 L over 1 hour followed by 300 to 400 mL per hour, unless the patient has heart failure or renal failure) to increase renal blood flow and calcium excretion. Small doses of furosemide may be used when the patient's volume status has first been restored.
- During treatment, patients require frequent monitoring of clinical status and metabolic laboratory testing because forced diuresis may be complicated by hypomagnesemia, hypokalemia, fluid overload, or subsequent pulmonary edema.
- Once rehydration is complete and urinary output is optimized, the need for bisphosphonate administration should be assessed. These pyrophosphate analogs interfere with osteoclast function, thereby inhibiting calcium release.
- Intravenous zoledronic acid (4 mg i.v., infused over at least 15 minutes) or pamidronate (60 or 90 mg i.v., infused over 2 to 4 hours) is commonly used in malignancy-induced hypercalcemia (31,32). Zoledronic acid has replaced pamidronate as the agent of choice. In a recent phase III trial, zoledronic acid was shown to normalize serum calcium level in 87% to 88% of patients as compared to 70% of patients who received pamidronate. The duration of response (32 to 43 days versus 18 days) was also in favor of zoledronic acid (33). Bisphosphonate administration is well tolerated by patients except for occasional i.v. site irritation and fever during infusion. Its onset of action is within 24 to 48 hours of administration; the maximal effect may not be achieved until 72 hours after treatment.
- An additional and perhaps more effective intervention for hypercalcemia includes the use of gallium nitrate (not the radioisotope), which also inhibits bone resorption (4).
- Intravenous administration (100–200 mg/m^2/day over 24 hours or up to 5 days) of gallium nitrate in rehydrated nonoliguric (target urine output: 1,500 to 2,000 mL per day) patients is highly effective (70% to 90%) in the treatment of hypercalcemia. Care should be taken to discontinue gallium nitrate once normocalcemia is achieved, but close metabolic monitoring should be maintained because maximal drug effect occurs days after cessation of administration. The concomitant use of nephrotoxic drugs should be avoided when using gallium nitrate.
- Patients with hypercalcemia who do not respond to pamidronate may benefit from subsequent gallium nitrate administration. Conversely, patients who do not respond to gallium nitrate may benefit from pamidronate (1,4).
- Calcitonin has a rapid onset of action (within 4 hours) and is often useful in severe and symptomatic hypercalcemia until the more slowly acting agents become effective (e.g., zoledronic acid, pamidronate, and gallium nitrate).
- Salmon calcitonin is initially given at 4 units per kg (body weight) s.c. or i.m. every 12 hours. If response is not satisfactory after 1 to 2 days, the dosage may be increased to 8 units per kg s.c. or i.m. every 12 hours. If response is still not adequate after a 1- to 2-day trial at the higher dose, the dosing interval should be decreased to 8 units per kg s.c. or i.m. every 6 hours. Although many patients initially will respond to calcitonin, tachyphylaxis often develops rapidly, which renders patients refractory to its hypocalcemic effect (26−32,34).
- Plicamycin (mithramycin) also has a rapid onset of hypocalcemic activity (< 12 hours), with a duration of response ranging from 3 to 7 days.
- The hypocalcemic effect of plicamycin is attributed to a direct cytotoxic effect on osteoclasts. Single doses of plicamycin, 0.025 mg per kg (body weight) in 150 to 250 mL of 0.9% sodium chloride injection or 5% dextrose injection by i.v. infusion over 30 to 60 minutes,

are usually well tolerated. The duration of the hypocalcemic response with plicamycin is typically 3 to 7 days; however, it is essential to note that a maximal hypocalcemic effect may not be achieved until 48 hours after treatment. Consequently, repeated doses should not be given more frequently than every 48 hours if hypocalcemia is to be avoided. Higher doses and shorter treatment intervals also increase the risk of plicamycin-induced hepatic and renal toxicities, hemorrhagic diathesis, and thrombocytopenia (4,34). Plicamycin is not commonly used in the United States because of its toxicities.

- Hemodialysis should be considered, in addition to the other treatments listed for hypercalcemia, in patients who have serum calcium level in the range of 18 to 20 mg per dL and/or in those who have neurologic symptoms but are hemodynamically stable.

TUMOR LYSIS SYNDROME

Etiology of Tumor Lysis Syndrome

- The administration of antitumor agents can lead to cell death, with subsequent release of intracellular contents.
- Tumor lysis syndrome (TLS) occurs when cellular disruption results in life-threatening lactic acidosis, with concomitant hyperuricemia, hyperkalemia, hyperphosphatemia, and hypocalcemia (4). The patient rapidly develops renal failure or has renal insufficiency at presentation.

Clinical Setting, Signs, and Symptoms of Tumor Lysis Syndrome

- TLS usually occurs in bulky disease treated with cytotoxic agents directed at rapidly proliferating tumors (1).
- TLS occurs most often during the treatment of leukemia or high-grade lymphomas but may also occur during the treatment of other solid tumors (35).
- Cardiac arrhythmias may result from the severe hyperkalemia or hypocalcemia that accompanies the TLS.
- Hypocalcemia can result in tetany, whereas hyperphosphatemia and hyperuricemia can result in acute renal failure.

Prevention and Treatment of Tumor Lysis Syndrome

- Preemptive measures include the pretreatment identification of individuals at risk, along with 24 to 48 hours of prehydration, use of pretherapeutic allopurinol, and vigilant metabolic monitoring (every 3- to 4-hour laboratory tests) after institution of therapy. These actions are the hallmarks of TLS prevention and management (35,36). Elevated levels of lactate dehydrogenase (LDH), uric acid, or creatinine at presentation identify a particularly high-risk patient.
- Corrective measures should be directed toward any metabolic abnormalities that occur in patients after starting cytotoxic therapy, and particular care should be given to the appropriate monitoring of responses [e.g., continuous or serial electrocardiograms (ECGs)] and to the provision of early interventions while correcting hyperkalemia, while admitting the patient to the intensive care unit (ICU) for severe hemodynamic instability, and during hemodialysis, when the patient is faced with worsening or severely compromised renal function (4).
- The correction of metabolic abnormalities during TLS is similar to the general management of ICU patient, with specific interventions for the following conditions.

Hyperphosphatemia

- In mild hyperphosphatemia, dietary phosphate is restricted to 0.6 to 0.9 g per day, and oral phosphate binder such as calcium carbonate is added.

- Severe hyperphosphatemia with symptomatic hypocalcemia can be life threatening. The hyperphosphatemia usually resolves within 6 to 12 hours if renal function is intact. Phosphate excretion can be increased by saline infusion, although this can further reduce the serum calcium concentration by dilution. Phosphate excretion can also be increased by administration of acetazolamide (15 mg per kg every 3 to 4 hours). Hemodialysis is often indicated in patients with symptomatic hypocalcemia, particularly if renal function is impaired.

Hypocalcemia

- The most appropriate treatment of hypocalcemia, in the absence of hypomagnesemia, is intravenous calcium, at a dose of 100 to 200 mg of elemental calcium (1 to 2 g of calcium gluconate) in 10 to 20 minutes. Such infusions do not raise the serum calcium concentration for more than 2 to 3 hours and, therefore, should be followed by a slow infusion of 10% calcium gluconate (90 mg of elemental calcium per 10 mL ampule) at the rate of 0.5 to 1.5 mg per kg i.v. per hour.
- Calcium chloride, 10% (272 mg of elemental calcium per 10 mL ampule) can also be used, with 5 to 10 mL given initially i.v. slowly over 10 minutes or diluted in 100 mL of 5% dextrose in water and infused over 20 minutes. This dosage should be repeated as often as every 20 minutes if the patient is symptomatic. Serum calcium levels should be monitored every 4 to 6 hours and hypomagnesemia be corrected as needed.
- Primary management of the hyperphosphatemia is critical to minimize metastatic deposition of insoluble calcium phosphate. Hemodialysis is almost always required by this time.

Hyperkalemia

- Confirm that the elevation in potassium level is genuine.
- If the patient is asymptomatic, with a plasma potassium concentration of 6.5 mEq per L and with an ECG that does not manifest signs of hyperkalemia, then withhold potassium and initiate the administration of cation exchange resins. If the patient is symptomatic, with peripheral neuromuscular weakness, electrocardiographic signs of hyperkalemia, or plasma potassium concentration above 7 mEq per L, consider calcium gluconate, 10% solution, 10 mL i.v. given over 2 to 5 minutes (dose can be repeated after 5 minutes if electrocardiographic changes persist), followed by glucose with insulin, sodium bicarbonate, or a nebulized β-agonist. Prepare for hemodialysis (37,38).
- Measures to reduce serum potassium level:
  1. Regular insulin, 10 U plus 50% glucose, 50 mL i.v. as a bolus (onset 15 to 60 minutes; duration 4 to 6 hours), followed by glucose infusion to prevent hypoglycemia. Insulin along with glucose lowers the potassium level by driving it into the cell.
  2. Adrenergic β2-agonist such as nebulized albuterol, 10 to 20 mg in 4 mL normal saline, inhaled over 10 minutes (onset 15 to 30 minutes; duration 2 to 4 hours) is effective in reducing serum potassium concentration. Adrenergic β2-agonists induce hypokalemia by stimulating the transport of potassium into skeletal muscle.
  3. Sodium bicarbonate, at the dose of is 45 mEq (1 ampule of a 7.5% sodium bicarbonate solution), is infused slowly over 5 minutes (onset 30 to 60 minutes; duration several hours); this dose can be repeated in 30 minutes if necessary. This also temporarily drives the potassium inside the cell.
  4. Kayexalate, orally or rectally, 15 to 50 g in 50 to 100 mL of 20% sorbitol solution, is repeated every 3 to 4 hours, as needed, for up to five times per day (onset, 1 to 3 hours, duration of several hours).
- Minimize administration of drugs that can cause or potentiate hyperkalemia [e.g., nonsteroidal antiinflammatory drugs (NSAIDs), β-blockers, angiotensin-converting enzyme (ACE) inhibitors, and potassium-sparing diuretics].

Hyperuricemia and Renal Failure

- Hyperuricemic acute renal failure following chemotherapy may be avoided by (a) prechemotherapeutic identification of patients at risk for developing TLS and (b) administration of allopurinol at doses of 600 to 900 mg every day, starting several days before chemotherapy, with tapering doses to maintain uric acid levels of <7 mg per dL.
- The therapy for hyperuricemic acute renal failure before chemotherapy consists of administering allopurinol (if it has not already been given) and attempting to wash out the obstructing uric acid crystals by a loop diuretic and by fluids. Sodium bicarbonate should not be given at this time because it is difficult to raise the urine pH in this setting. Hemodialysis to remove the excess circulating uric acid should be used in patients in whom a diuresis cannot be induced.
- Hyperuricemic acute renal failure following chemotherapy is usually refractory to conservative intervention (hydration, diuretics, etc.), and patients require hemodialysis for supportive therapy and renal recovery.

In an effort to improve the control of hyperuricemia in patients with leukemia or lymphoma, Pui et al. tested the recombinant urate oxidase (rasburicase) by i.v. administration of the uricolytic agent for five to seven consecutive days to children, adolescents, and young adults with newly diagnosed leukemia or lymphoma (39).

The recombinant enzyme produced a rapid and sharp decrease in plasma uric acid concentrations in all patients. Despite cytoreductive chemotherapy, plasma uric acid concentrations remained low throughout the treatment. The toxicity of the agent was negligible, and none of the patients required dialysis. The mean plasma half-lives of the agent were 16.0 ± 6.3 [standard deviation (SD)] hours and 21.1 ± 12.0 hours, respectively, in patients treated at doses of 0.15 and 0.20 mg per kg. Seventeen of the 121 assessable patients developed antibodies to the enzyme.

The authors concluded that rasburicase was safe and effective for the prophylaxis for or treatment of hyperuricemia in patients with leukemia or lymphoma.

REFERENCES

1. Abeloff MD. *Clinical oncology*, 2nd ed. New York: Churchill Livingstone, 1999.
2. Boogerd W, van der Sande JJ. Diagnosis and treatment of spinal cord compression in malignant disease. *Cancer Treat Rev* 1993;19:129–150.
3. Talcott JA, Stomper PC, Drislane FW, et al. Assessing suspected spinal cord compression: a multidisciplinary outcomes analysis of 342 episodes. *Support Care Cancer* 1999;7:31–38.
4. DeVita VT, Hellman S, Rosenberg SA. *Cancer: principles and practice of oncology*, 6th ed. Philadelphia: Lippincott–Raven Publishers, 2001.
5. Djulbegovic B, Sullivan DM. *Decision making in oncology: evidence-based management*. New York: Churchill Livingstone, 1997.
6. Loblaw DA, Laperriere NJ. Emergency treatment of malignant extradural spinal cord compression: an evidence-based guideline. *J Clin Oncol* 1998;16:1613–1624.
7. Heimdal K, Hirschberg H, Slettebo H, et al. High incidence of serious side effects of high-dose dexamethasone treatment in patients with epidural spinal cord compression. *J Neurooncol* 1992;12:141.
8. Vecht CJ, Haaxma-Reiche H, van Putten WL, et al. Initial bolus of conventional versus high-dose dexamethasone in metastatic spinal cord compression. *Neurology* 1989;39:1255–1257.
9. Regine WF, Tibbs PA, Young A, et al. Metastatic spinal cord compression: a randomized trial of direct decompressive surgical resection plus radiotherapy vs. Radiotherapy alone. *Int J Radiat Oncol Biol Phys* 2003;57(Suppl. 2):S125.
10. Byrne TN. Spinal cord compression from epidural metastases. *N Engl J Med* 1992;327:614–619.
11. Burch PA, Grossman SA. Treatment of epidural cord compressions from Hodgkin's disease with chemotherapy: a report of two cases and a review of the literature. *Am J Med* 1988;84:555–558.
12. Clarke PR, Saunders M. Steroid-induced remission in spinal canal reticulum cell sarcoma: report of two cases. *J Neurosurg* 1975;42:346–348.

13. Cooper K, Bajorin D, Shapiro W, et al. Decompression of epidural metastases from germ cell tumors with chemotherapy. *J Neurooncol* 1990;8:275–280.
14. Friedman HM, Sheetz S, Levine HL, et al. Combination chemotherapy and radiation therapy: the medical management of epidural spinal cord compression from testicular cancer. *Arch Intern Med* 1986;146:509–512.
15. Payne RB, Carver ME, Morgan DB. Interpretation of serum total calcium: effects of adjustment for albumin concentration on frequency of abnormal values and on detection of change in the individual. *J Clin Pathol* 1979;32:56–60.
16. Sanderson IR, Pritchard J, Marsh HT. Chemotherapy as the initial treatment of spinal cord compression due to disseminated neuroblastoma. *J Neurosurg* 1989;70:688–690.
17. Sinoff CL, Blumsohn A. Spinal cord compression in myelomatosis: response to chemotherapy alone. *Eur J Cancer Clin Oncol* 1989;25:197–200.
18. Sasagawa I, Gotoh H, Miyabayashi H, et al. Hormonal treatment of symptomatic spinal cord compression in advanced prostatic cancer. *Int Urol Nephrol* 1991;23:351–356.
19. Ostler PJ, Clarke DP, Watkinson AF, et al. Superior vena cava obstruction: a modern management strategy. *Clin Oncol* 1997;9:83–89.
20. Patel V, Igwebe T, Mast H, et al. Superior vena cava syndrome: current concepts of management. *N Engl J Med* 1995;92:245–248.
21. Schraufnagel DE, Hill R, Leech JA, et al. Superior vena caval obstruction. Is it a medical emergency? *Am J Med* 1981;70:1169.22.
22. Rowell NP, Gleeson FV. Steroids, radiotherapy, chemotherapy and stents for superior vena caval obstruction in carcinoma of the bronchus (Cochrane review). *Cochrane Database Syst Rev* 2001;4:CD001316.
23. Greenberg S, Kosinski R, Daniels J. Treatment of superior vena cava thrombosis with recombinant tissue type plasminogen activator. *Chest* 1991;99:1298–1301.
24. Chisholm MA, Mulloy AL, Taylor AT. Acute management of cancer-related hypercalcemia. *Ann Pharmacother* 1996;30:507–513.
25. Bilezikian JP. Management of acute hypercalcemia. *N Engl J Med* 1992;326:1196–1203.
26. Raisz LG, Trummel CL, Wener JA, et al. Effect of glucocorticoids on bone resorption in tissue culture. *Endocrinology* 1972;90:961–967.
27. Percival RC, Yates AJ, Gray RE, et al. Role of glucocorticoids in management of malignant hypercalcaemia. *Br Med J* 1984;289:287.
28. Kristensen B, Ejlertsen B, Holmegaard SN, et al. Prednisolone in the treatment of severe malignant hypercalcaemia in metastatic breast cancer: a randomized study. *J Intern Med* 1992;232:237–245.
29. Gucalp R, Theriault R, Gill I, et al. Treatment of cancer-associated hypercalcemia: double-blind comparison of rapid and slow intravenous infusion regimens of pamidronate disodium and saline alone. *Arch Intern Med* 1994;154:1935–1944.
30. Ralston SH, Gallacher SJ, Patel U, et al. Comparison of three intravenous bisphosphonates in cancer-associated hypercalcaemia. *Lancet* 1989;2:1180–1182.
31. Chan FK, Koberle LM, Thys-Jacobs S, et al. Differential diagnosis, causes, and management of hypercalcemia. *Curr Probl Surg* 1997;34:445–523.
32. Kiang DT, Loken MK, Kennedy BJ. Mechanism of the hypocalcemic effect of mithramycin. *J Clin Endocrinol Metab* 1979;48:341–344.
33. Major P, Lortholary A, Hon J, et al. Zoledronic acid is superior to pamidronate in the treatment of hypercalcemia of malignancy: a pooled analysis of two randomized, controlled clinical trials. *J Clin Oncol* 2001;19(2):558–567.
34. Green L, Donehower RC. Hepatic toxicity of low doses of mithramycin in hypercalcemia. *Cancer Treat Rep* 1984;68:1379–1381.
35. Jones DP, Mahmoud H, Chesney RW. Tumor lysis syndrome: pathogenesis and management. *Pediatr Nephrol* 1995;9:206–212.
36. Fleming DR, Doukas MA. Acute tumor lysis syndrome in hematologic malignances. *Leuk Lymphoma* 1992;8:315–318.
37. Tierney LM, McPhee SJ, Papadakis MA, eds. Fluid and electrolyte disorders. *Current medical diagnosis and treatment*, 38th ed. Stanford, CT: Appleton & Lange, 1999:847.
38. Cogan MG. *Fluid and electrolytes: physiology and pathophysiology*, 1st ed. Norwalk, CT: Appleton & Lange, 1991.
39. Pui C, Mahmoud H, Wiley J, et al. Recombinant urate oxidase for the prophylaxis or treatment of hyperuricemia in patients with leukemia or lymphoma. *J Clin Oncol,* 2001;19(3):697–704.

39

Psychopharmacologic Management in Oncology

Donald L. Rosenstein*, Maryland Pao*, and June Cai†

*National Institute of Mental Health, National Institutes of Health, Bethesda, Maryland;
and †Department of Pyschiatry and Human Behavior, Brown University Medical School,
Providence, Rhode Island

Psychiatric syndromes, predominantly depression and anxiety, occur commonly in patients with cancer, and, if misdiagnosed or poorly managed, can have a profoundly negative effect on optimal oncologic care. The comprehensive psychiatric care of patients with cancer includes psychosocial, behavioral, and psychoeducational interventions as well as pharmacologic and psychotherapeutic treatment. This chapter focuses on the psychopharmacologic management of the major psychiatric syndromes encountered in the oncology setting and concludes with specific recommendations for psychopharmacologic management in pediatric oncology.

CONSIDERATIONS BEFORE PRESCRIBING PSYCHOPHARMACOLOGIC AGENTS

1. Psychiatric symptoms are often manifestations of an underlying medical disorder or are complications of its treatment (see Table 39.1). For example, specific malignancies (e.g., lung, breast, gastrointestinal, renal, and prostate cancers) are prone to metastasize to the central nervous system (CNS). In addition, any advanced cancer can result in structural or metabolic CNS insults that precipitate psychiatric symptoms. For those patients whose psychiatric symptoms fail to respond to psychopharmacologic treatment, CNS involvement should be reconsidered, even in malignancies that do not commonly metastasize to the brain.
2. Medically ill patients are particularly susceptible to CNS adverse effects of medications. Specific examples of medications associated with mood, cognitive, and behavioral symptoms include the following: corticosteroids, interleukin-2, interferon-α, narcotics, and dopamine-blocking antiemetics. For patients who develop psychiatric symptoms after treatment with such agents, it is often more prudent to lower the dose or to discontinue the use of a currently prescribed medication than to introduce yet another agent (i.e., a psychotropic) that might exacerbate psychiatric symptoms.
3. Polypharmacy is often unavoidable in patients with cancer; however, most clinically significant interactions with psychotropic agents are predictable and can be avoided by choosing alternative agents or by making dose adjustments. The use of monoamine oxidase inhibitors (MAOIs) with either meperidine (Demerol) or selective serotonin reuptake inhibitors (SSRIs) is life threatening. Up-to-date drug interaction resources can be found at several internet websites (e.g., http://medicine.iupui.edu/flockhart/).

TABLE 39.1. *Medical conditions in oncologic and other disorders associated with anxiety and depression*

Neoplasms	Cardiovascular
Brain tumors	Ischemic heart disease
Insulinoma	Arrhythmias
Lymphoma	Congestive heart failure
Small cell carcinoma	
Pancreatic cancer	Metabolic
Leukemia	Electrolyte disturbances
	Uremia
Endocrinologic	Vitamin B_{12} or folate deficiency
Cushing syndrome	
Adrenal insufficiency	Other
Hypopituitarism	Substance abuse and withdrawal
Pheochromocytoma	Pain (uncontrolled)
Thyroid dysfunction	Hematologic (e.g., anemia)

4. Inadequate pain control frequently induces symptoms of anxiety, irritability, or depression. It is essential to have pain well-controlled so that the appropriate psychiatric diagnosis and treatment can proceed (see Chapter 37). One note of caution in this regard concerns the combined use of SSRIs and tricyclic antidepressants (TCAs), which are frequently used in the treatment of neuropathic pain. Some SSRIs (e.g., fluoxetine, paroxetine, and fluvoxamine) inhibit the metabolism of TCAs, which can in turn prolong the corrected QT interval (QTc) interval.

COMMON PSYCHIATRIC SYNDROMES IN THE ONCOLOGY SETTING

1. *Adjustment disorder:* This is a time-limited, maladaptive reaction to a specific stressor that typically involves symptoms of depression, anxiety, or behavioral changes and impairs psychosocial functioning. The diagnostic criteria include the onset of symptoms within 3 months of the stressor but the duration of symptoms is no more than 6 months. The differential diagnosis includes the following disorders:
   • Bereavement
   • Posttraumatic stress disorder
   • Other mood and anxiety disorders
   Management: The initial treatment approach consists of crisis intervention and brief psychotherapy. Time-limited symptom management with medications may be indicated. For example, anxiety, tearfulness, and insomnia are frequent reactions to the diagnosis of a new or recurrent malignancy. Short-term treatment of these symptoms with benzodiazepines (BZDs) (e.g., lorazepam and clonazepam) is appropriate, effective, and rarely associated with the development of abuse or dependence.
2. *Major depression:* Major depression and subsyndromal depressive disorders are common in patients with cancer. Prevalence rates vary between 5% and 50% depending on how depression is defined, whether study samples are drawn from outpatient clinics or hospital wards, and the type of cancer involved. Untreated depression has been correlated to poor compliance with medical care, increased pain and disability, and a greater likelihood to consider euthanasia and physician-assisted suicide.
   A major diagnostic task in the oncology setting is assorting symptoms attributable to depression from those symptoms that are caused by the cancer or its treatment. The patient with disseminated cancer who is undergoing chemotherapy is likely to experience fatigue, anorexia, weight loss, and insomnia, whether a clinical depression is

present or absent. Our practice is to institute empiric trials of antidepressants using a targeted symptom reduction approach. In borderline cases, a personal or family history of depression and symptoms of excessive guilt, poor self-esteem, anhedonia, and ruminative thinking strengthen the argument for a medication trial. Furthermore, because the number of well-tolerated, safe, and effective antidepressants has grown, we have lowered our threshold for treating subsyndromal depression in the oncology setting.

Particular attention should be paid to symptoms of hopelessness, helplessness, and suicidal ideation, accompanied by considerable increases in anxiety, because patients with cancer have an increased risk of suicide compared with the general population. The incidence of cancer at certain sites (e.g., head and neck, lung, gastrointestinal tract, urogenital tract, and breast) is associated with an even greater risk of suicide (see Table 39.2).

Differential diagnosis of major depression:
- Adjustment disorder
- Dysthymic disorder
- Delirium
- Dementia
- Substance abuse
- Bipolar disorder
- Bereavement
- Mood disorder caused by a medical disorder or medication (Table 39.1).

Management: Treatment modalities include pharmacotherapy (see Table 39.3), psychotherapy, and electroconvulsive therapy (ECT). Selection of an antidepressant should be based on a number of considerations such as prior treatment response, an optimal match between the patient's target symptoms and the side-effect profile of the antidepressant (e.g., using a sedating agent for the patient with anxiety and insomnia), and the potential for drug interactions. Mirtazapine (Remeron) has several properties that make it a particularly attractive antidepressant choice in patients with cancer: it is sedating, causes weight gain, has few significant drug interactions, and is a partial 5HT-3 receptor antagonist (i.e., has antiemtic properties).

3. *Anxiety disorders:* Many medical conditions seen in the oncology setting, such as heart failure, respiratory compromise, seizure disorders, pheochromocytoma, and chemotherapy-induced ovarian failure, may cause anxiety. Additional conditions that may cause both anxiety and depression are listed in Table 39.1. Similarly, anxiety is an adverse effect of numerous medications. In particular, dopamine-blocking antiemetics such as metoclopramide (Reglan), prochlorperazine (Compazine), and promethazine (Phenergan) frequently cause akathisia, an adverse effect characterized by subjective restlessness and increased motor activity, which is commonly misdiagnosed as anxiety.

The differential diagnosis of anxiety disorders in the oncology setting includes the following:
- Exacerbation of medical illness
- Agitated depression

TABLE 39.2. *Risk factors for suicide in patients with cancer*

Historical considerations	Clinical descriptors
Prior suicide attempts	Elderly men
Family history of suicide	Recent loss and poor social support
Prior psychiatric illness	Current depression, anxiety, substance abuse
History of substance abuse	Advanced cancer, pain, poor prognosis
Impulsive behavior	Delirium, psychosis, illogical thoughts

TABLE 39.3. *Commonly used antidepressants in patients with cancer*

Generic names (brand names)	Dose range (mg)	Important adverse effects and comments
SSRIs		
Fluoxetine (Prozac)[a,d]	5–60	Sexual dysfunction, diarrhea, weight changes, insomnia, agitation, anxiety, hyponatremia, night sweats
Sertraline (Zoloft)[a,d]	12.5–200	Sedation, weight gain, GI symptoms, sexual dysfunction, hyponatremia
Paroxetine (Paxil)[c,d]	10–60	Sexual dysfunction, sedation, akathisia, anticholinergic effects, hyponatremia, withdrawal syndrome
Citalopram (Celexa)[d]	10–60	Nausea, dry mouth, somnolence, ejaculation disorder, weak inhibition of CYP isoenzymes
Escitalopram (Lexapro)	5–40	Nausea, dry mouth, somnolence, ejaculation disorder, weak inhibition of CYP isoenzymes
Fluvoxamine (Luvox)[a]	25–300	Night sweats, sexual dysfunction, potent inhibitor of CYP1A2 and 3A3/4
Novel antidepressants		
Venlafaxine (Effexor)[c]	18.75–300	GI distress, sexual dysfunction, sedation, anticholinergic effects, hypertension at dose >225 mg
Mirtazapine (Remeron)[b]	7.5–45	Sedation, dry mouth, increased appetite and weight gain, constipation, asthenia, dizziness
Bupropion (Wellbutrin)[c]	37.5–450	GI distress, tremor, excitement, seizure at high dose or with brain tumors
Trazodone (Desyrel)	25–200	Sedation, anticholinergic effects, orthostatic hypotension, priapism, useful for anxiety and insomnia at low doses
CNS stimulants		
Methylphenidate (Ritalin)[a,c]	2.5–40	Insomnia, agitation, GI distress, headache, tics, rebound depression
Dextroamphetamine (Dexedrine)[a,c]	2.5–30	Insomnia, agitation, confusion, delusion, psychosis, tics, rebound depression
Tricyclic antidepressants		
Amitriptyline (Elavil)[a]	25–150	Dry mouth, sedation, weight gain, ECG changes, orthostatic hypotension, anticholinergic effects
Desipramine (Norpramin)	25–150	Dry mouth, tachycardia, ECG changes
Nortriptyline (Pamelor)	25–150	Tremor, confusion, anticholinergic effects

SSRI, selective serotonin reuptake inhibitor; GI, gastrointestinal; CYP, cytochrome P-450; CNS, central nervous system; ECG, electrocardiogram.

[a]FDA approval for use in children/adolescents.
[b]Orally disintegrating tablets or wafers available.
[c]Sustained release and extended release formulations available.
[d]Liquid formulation available.

TABLE 39.4. *Preferred BZDs in the oncology setting*

	Lorazepam (Ativan)[a]	Clonazepam (Klonopin)
Dose equivalency	1 mg	0.25 mg
Dose range	0.25–2 mg PO, sublingual, i.m. or i.v. routes, every 1–6 h (maximum daily dose, 8 mg)	0.25–1 mg PO route only, every 12 h
Advantages	Rapid onset of action	Less frequent dosing than with lorazepam

BZD, benzodiazepines; PO, orally; i.m., intramuscularly; i.v., intravenously.
[a]Liquid formulation available.

- Adverse effects of medications
- Substance or alcohol abuse or withdrawal
- Adjustment disorder
- Delirium.

Management of anxiety: In addition to behavioral therapy and psychotherapy, BZDs are the medications that are most frequently used for the short-term treatment of anxiety (see Table 39.4). For anxiety that persists beyond a few weeks, treatment with an antidepressant (Table 39.3) is indicated. If the patient has already been taking an SSRI, it is important to not discontinue an SSRI (with the exception of fluoxetine because of its long half-life) abruptly to avoid rebound anxiety from withdrawal. Low-dose atypical antipsychotics are often useful for severe and persistent anxiety or for conditions such as anxiety secondary to steroids and delirium (see Table 39.5).

The following issues associated with BZD use require attention:

- BZDs are the treatment of choice for delirium caused by alcohol or sedative–hypnotic withdrawal, but typically worsen other types of delirium.
- In patients with hepatic failure, lorazepam, temazepam, or oxazepam are the preferred BZDs.

TABLE 39.5. *Commonly used neuroleptics in the oncology setting*

	Initial dose (mg)	Administrative routes and schedules	Maximum daily dose (mg)	Important adverse effects
haloperidol[a,b] (Haldol)	0.25–1 PO, or i.v.	every 2–12 h s.c., i.m.,	20	Hypotension, EPS, elevated prolactin
chlorpromazine (Thorazine)	12.5–50 PO, i.m. or i.v.	every 4–12 h	300	Decreased seizure threshold, EPS, hypotension
risperidone[a,b] (Risperdal)	0.25–3 PO	every 12 h	6	Hypotension, sedation, elevated prolactin,
olanzapine (Zyprexa)	2.5–10 PO	every 12–24 h	20	Sedation, anticholinergic, insulin resistance
quetiapine (Seroquel)	25–50 PO	every 12–24 h	800	Sedation, increased QTc

EPS, extrapyramidal symptoms; PO, orally; s.c., subcutaneously; i.m., intramuscularly; i.v., intravenously.
[a]FDA approval for use in children/adolescents.
[b]Liquid formulation available.

- BZDs may result in "disinhibition," especially in delirium, substance abuse, organic disorders, and preexisting personality disorders.
- The abrupt discontinuation of BZDs with short half-lives [e.g., alprazolam (Xanax) and triazolam (Halcion)] can cause rebound anxiety and precipitate a withdrawal syndrome.

4. *Delirium:* Delirium is an acute confusional state characterized by a fluctuating course of cognitive impairment, perceptual disturbances, mood changes, delusions, and sleep–wake cycle disruption. Patients can have a hyperactive (agitated) or hypoactive (quiet) delirium. Virtually any psychiatric symptom can be a manifestation of delirium, among which anxiety and/or labile mood are common presentations often misdiagnosed as "depression." Patients who are elderly, who are on multiple medications, or who have underlying brain pathology are more prone to delirium. Delirium in terminally ill patients is common and often underdiagnosed. The differential diagnosis includes the following:

- Dementia
- Affective disorders with psychosis (mania or depression)
- Psychotic disorders
- Medication effects or substance or alcohol abuse or withdrawal.

Management: The first steps in the management of delirium are the identification and treatment of precipitating factors and the discontinuation of nonessential medications. Haloperidol (Haldol) continues to be the treatment of choice for delirium in most cases (Table 39.5). Newer atypical antipsychotics have fewer side effects and can be used as well, such as olanzapine (Zyprexa), quetiapine (seroquel) and risperidone (Risperdal). Delirium secondary to BZD, or sedative–hypnotic and alcohol withdrawal should be treated with BZDs.

ADDITIONAL CONSIDERATIONS FOR PSYCHOPHARMACOLOGIC MANAGEMENT IN PEDIATRIC ONCOLOGY

Cancer is the fourth leading cause of death, and the leading cause of nonacute death among children. Life-threatening illness in a child or an adolescent is traumatic and can be associated with anxiety and depression. Although many patients cope well with and adapt to the trauma, symptoms of depression such as fatigue, cognitive impairment, decreased social interaction and exploration, and anorexia may be part of a cytokine or immunologic response to cancer and its treatments. Psychotropic medications can dramatically improve the quality of life for children with cancer. These medications do not replace comprehensive, multimodal, multidisciplinary care, but are adjuncts to decrease discomfort and improve functioning of medically ill children.

Assessment and Diagnosis in Pediatric Oncology

A thorough psychiatric assessment is needed to make a correct diagnosis and to institute treatment. Typically, this assessment is based on multiple brief examinations of the child and information gathered from additional sources including family, staff, and teachers. A patient's biologic vulnerability to depression and anxiety may be inferred from (a) a family history of a mood or anxiety disorder, or other psychiatric disorder, and (b) previous psychiatric symptoms or psychiatric treatment.

Common complaints in medically ill children include:

- anxiety
- pain
- difficulty in sleeping
- fatigue
- feeling "bored."

Adult psychiatric syndromes of adjustment disorder, major depression, anxiety, and delirium apply to children as well, but anxiety, rather than depression, is the most frequent diagnosis. Important determining factors for pharmacologic intervention are severity and duration of psychiatric symptoms.

Psychopharmacologic Treatment of Pediatric Patients

In 1994, manufacturers and federally funded researchers were mandated to study medications such as antidepressants in children. Although there have been no well-controlled antidepressant trials in depressed medically ill children, and the dose of psychiatric medications for children with cancer has not been systematically studied, antidepressants have been useful for treating anxiety and depression. Body weight, Tanner staging, clinical status, and potential for medications to interact are weighed in deciding doses. See Tables 39.3 and 39.5 for psychotropics with U.S. Food and Drug Administration (FDA) approval for use in children and adolescents.

BZDs, such as lorazepam, used in low doses in conjunction with nonpharmacologic distraction techniques, may be appropriate for procedures that induce considerable anxiety in children. Clonazepam is longer acting and may be helpful with more pervasive and prolonged anxiety symptoms. BZDs can cause sedation, confusion, and behavioral disinhibition. Their use should be carefully monitored, especially in those patients with CNS dysfunction. BZD withdrawal precipitated by abrupt discontinuation occurs most frequently on transferring the patient from intensive care settings.

Antihistamines have been used to sedate anxious children. Diphenhydramine, hydroxyzine, and promethazine may be helpful for occasional insomnia. However, antihistamines are not helpful for persistent anxiety and their anticholinergic properties can precipitate or worsen delirium. Intravenous diphenhydramine may be sought because it can induce euphoria when given by i.v. push; very high doses can provoke seizures.

Fluoxetine is the only FDA-approved SSRI for depression in children older than 6 years. Fluoxetine and sertraline are approved for obsessive-compulsive disorder in children older than 6 years; fluvoxamine is approved for those who are 8 years and older. Fluoxetine, with its active metabolite norfluoxetine, and fluvoxamine are potent inhibitors of cytochrome P-450 (CYP) 3A3 and 3A4. They are contraindicated with macrolide antibiotics, azole antifungal agents, and several other medications. Amitriptyline is approved for depression in children who are 12 years or older. TCAs are useful for treating insomnia, weight loss, anxiety, and some pain syndromes.

Some antidepressants may contribute to suicidal thinking in children and adolescents. This possibility warrants careful monitoring of all children treated with antidepressants. Use of non-FDA approved psychopharmacologic agents in children with cancer may be considered in extreme or prolonged distress and poor functioning, but must be monitored closely. It is unusual for children with cancer to be suicidal in the absence of premorbid depression or inadequate pain management.

Children and adolescents who cannot tolerate antidepressants may benefit from stimulants for depression and apathy. Psychostimulants are generally well tolerated and have a rapid onset of action. Children with delirium, hallucinations, severe agitation, or aggression may be safely treated with low-dose antipsychotics such as haloperidol or atypical neuroleptics such as risperidone.

Although there is a dearth of research in pediatric cancer psychopharmacology, child psychiatry consultation may considerably improve the quality of life for children undergoing cancer treatment and dealing with cancer survival. Routine psychological screening of children with cancer and survivors can detect ongoing distress. Psychopharmacologic consultation may also help children with postradiation or postchemotherapy conditions related to attention, mood, and anxiety disorders.

SUMMARY

Psychiatric syndromes are frequently misdiagnosed and poorly treated in patients with cancer. Before initiating psychopharmacologic therapy, underlying medical disorders and adverse effects of medication must be addressed and potential drug interactions anticipated. Psychiatric symptoms should then be treated promptly and aggressively. Consultation from a psychiatrist is indicated in the following circumstances when the patient (a) has a complex psychiatric history and is taking multiple psychotropic medications; (b) exhibits depressive symptoms associated with extreme guilt, anxiety, and/or suicidal thoughts; (c) is confused, hallucinating, agitated, or violent; and (d) is noncompliant with treatment or rejects treatment and seeks physician-assisted suicide.

SUGGESTED READINGS

Academy of Psychosomatic Medicine. Psychiatric aspects of excellent end-of-life care: a position statement of the Academy of Psychosomatic Medicine. Available at: http://www.apm.org/eol-care.html. Accessed March 14, 2005.

American Psychiatric Association. *Diagnostic and statistical manual of mental disorders*, 4th ed. Washington, DC: American Psychiatric Association, 1994.

Cassem EH. Depressive disorders in the medically ill: an overview. *Psychosomatics* 1995;36:S2–S10.

Cleeland CS, Bennett GJ, Dantzer R, et al. Are the symptoms of cancer and cancer treatment due to a shared biologic mechanism? A cytokine-immunologic model of cancer symptoms. *Cancer* 2003;97:2919.

Coyle N, Adelhardt J, Foley KM, et al. Character of terminal illness in the advanced patient with cancer: pain and other symptoms during the last four weeks of life. *J Pain Symptom Manage* 1990;5:83.

Emanuel EJ, Fairclough DL, Daniels ER, et al. Euthanasia and physician-assisted suicide: attitudes and experiences of oncology patients, oncologists, and the public. *Lancet* 1996;347:1805.

Endicott J. Measurement of depression in patients with cancer. *Cancer* 1984;53:2243.

Fawzy I, Greenburg D. Oncology. *Textbook of consultation-liaison psychiatry*. Washington, DC: American Psychiatric Press, 2001.

Goldman LS, Wise TN, Brody DS. *Psychiatry for primary care physicians*. Washington, DC: American Psychiatric Press, 1997.

Holland J. *Psycho-oncology*. New York: Oxford University Press, 1998.

Lipsett DR, Payne EC, Cassem NH. On death and dying. Discussion. *J Geriatr Psychiatry* 1974;7:108.

Lynch ME. The assessment and prevalence of affective disorders in advanced cancer. *J Palliat Care* 1995;11:10.

McDaniel JS, Musselman DL, Porter MR, et al. Depression in patients with cancer: diagnosis, biology, and treatment. *Arch Gen Psychiatry* 1995;52:89.

Recklitis C, O'Leary T, Diller L. Utility of routine psychological screening in the childhood cancer survivor clinic. *J Clin Oncol* 2003;21:787.

Spiegel D, Sands S, Koopman C. Pain and depression in patients with cancer. *Cancer* 1994;74:2570.

Spiegel L. Pediatric psychopharmacology. *Psycho-oncology*. New York: Oxford University Press, 1998; Wise TN. The physician and his patient with cancer. *Prim Care* 1974;1:407.

40

Management of Emesis in Oncology

David R. Kohler

Pharmacy Department, National Institutes of Health,
Clinical Center, Bethesda, Maryland

TYPES OF TREATMENT-RELATED EMETIC SYMPTOMS

Radiation- and chemotherapy-associated emetic symptoms are categorized as acute, delayed, or anticipatory (see Fig. 40.1) (1).

Acute-phase symptoms correlate with serotonin (5-HT) release from enterochromaffin cells. Emetic signals are propagated at local $5\text{-}HT_3$ receptors and transmitted along afferent vagus nerve fibers, and a diffuse series of effector nuclei are activated in the medulla oblongata (the so-called "vomiting center"). This in turn integrates afferent emetic signals and subsequently activates and coordinates motor nuclei that produce the physiologic changes associated with vomiting.

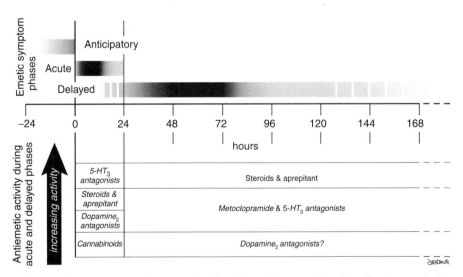

FIG. 40.1. Emetic symptom phases and antiemetic activity comparison. Top: The temporal relation between the start of emetogenic treatment [hour zero (0)] and emetic symptom phases. For each phase, shaded bars indicate generally the periods during which nausea and emesis occur; depth of shading correlates directly with the incidence of symptoms. Bottom: The most highly active drug categories are ranked by their relative effectiveness during the acute (0–24 hours) and delayed (after 24 hours) emetic phases.

TABLE 40.1. *Antineoplastic drugs implicated in causing delayed emesis*

Carboplatin $\geq$300 mg/m^2 ($\pm$ other cytotoxic agents)
Cisplatin $\geq$50 mg/m^2
Cyclophosphamide $\geq$600 mg/m^2
Cyclophosphamide $\pm$ other cytotoxic agents
Cyclophosphamide + anthracycline combinations
Doxorubicin $\geq$50 mg/m^2

Although an etiology for delayed symptoms remains elusive, such symptoms may be related to activation of neurokinin type 1 receptors (NK$_1$) for which substance P is the natural ligand. Delayed-phase symptoms have been associated with numerous chemotherapeutic regimens (see Table 40.1). Symptoms may occur as early as 16 to 18 hours after emetogenic treatment, with the period of most frequent incidence between 24 and 96 hours after treatment (2,3).

Delayed emesis may occur in patients who do not experience symptoms acutely, but its incidence characteristically decreases in patients who achieve complete control during the acute phase. Although the severity of emesis during the delayed phase is typically less than that which occurs during the acute phase, the severity of nausea is reportedly similar during both phases.

Repeated antineoplastic treatments that are characterized by poor emetic control give rise to anticipatory emetic symptoms, which are an aversive conditioned response. Consequently, complete control throughout antineoplastic treatment remains the best preventive strategy against developing symptoms. Although anxiolytic amnestic drugs are helpful in preventing the development of anticipatory symptoms, behavior-modification and cognitive-distraction techniques become the primary modalities of intervention after symptoms occur. After symptoms develop, the role of medical intervention during subsequent emetogenic treatment is limited to preventing reinforcement of conditioned stimulus, which may exacerbate anticipatory symptoms.

EMETIC (EMETOGENIC) POTENTIAL

The potential for producing emesis and the patterns in which symptoms manifest vary among antineoplastic medications and radiation therapy techniques.

Acute emetic symptoms:

- Generally, onset of emesis is within 1 to 3 hours after commencing chemotherapy administration (see Table 40.2).
  - Exceptions include mechlorethamine (nitrogen mustard), cyclophosphamide, and carboplatin.
- Most frequent incidence of emesis occurs during a 2- to 6-hour period after treatment.
- Emesis may persist or recur intermittently for 12 hours or longer after treatment.

Among antineoplastic drugs, the dose administered most often affects emetogenic potential and the duration for which symptoms occur. The number of emetogenic drugs administered in combination, administration schedule, treatment duration, and route of drug administration are also mitigating factors. Emetic potential is often a function of treatment duration; it may be decreased or eliminated by attenuating drug delivery over hours or days and is often increased by rapid administration, by repetitious emetogenic treatment, and by brief intervals between repeated doses.

For ionizing radiation, emetic potential correlates directly with the amount of radiation administered per dose and the dose rate. Large treatment volumes and fields including the upper abdomen, the upper hemithorax, and the whole body are prominent risk factors for

TABLE 40.2. *Time to onset after commencement of chemotherapy administration and duration of emesis*

Drug name	Time to onset (h)	Duration (h)
Aldesleukin	0–6	—
Altretamine	3–6	—
Asparaginase	1–3	—
Bleomycin	3–6	—
Carboplatin	6–8	>24
Carmustine	2–6	4–24
Chlorambucil	48–72	—
Cisplatin	1–6	24 to >48
Cyclophosphamide	6–18	6 to >24
Cytarabine	6–12	3–5
Dacarbazine	1–5	1–24
Dactinomycin	2–6	12–24
Daunorubicin	2–6	24
Doxorubicin	4–6	6 to >24
Etoposide	3–8	6–12
Fluorouracil	3–6	3–4
Hydroxyurea	6–12	—
Ifosfamide	1–6	6–12
Irinotecan	2–6	6–12
Lomustine	2–6	4–12
Mechlorethamine	0.5–2	1–24
Melphalan	6–12	—
Mercaptopurine	4–8	—
Methotrexate	4–12	3–12
Mitomycin	1–6	3–12
Mitotane	Long latency	Persistent
Paclitaxel	3–8	3–8
Pentostatin	Long latency	Persistent, >24
Plicamycin	4–6	12–24
Procarbazine	24–27	Variable
Streptozocin	1–4	12–24
Teniposide	3–8	6–12
Thioguanine	4–8	—
Thiotepa	6–12	Variable
Vinblastine	4–8	—
Vincristine	4–8	—
Vinorelbine	4–8	—

From Borison HL, McCarthy LE. Neuropharmacology of chemotherapy-induced emesis. *Drugs* 1983;25(suppl 1):8–17 and Aapro M. Methodological issues in antiemetic studies. *Invest New Drugs* 1993;11:243–253, with permission (4,5).

severe emesis. Generally, emetic risk is increased when radiation and chemotherapy are administered concomitantly.

PATIENT RISK FACTORS THAT AFFECT EMETIC CONTROL

It is generally more difficult to prevent and control emesis in

- women than in men, particularly among women with a history of persistent or severe emetic symptoms during pregnancy
- children and young adults than in older patients

- patients with a history of incomplete antiemetic control during earlier treatments, whether (a) acutely, (b) during the delayed phase, or (c) during both periods.
  - Patients in the category (c) are at greatest risk for poor antiemetic control during subsequent treatments (6).

Decreased performance status and a predisposition to motion sickness have also been associated with poor emetic control. In contrast, patients who have chronically consumed alcoholic beverages (generally, >100 g ethanol per day for several years) are more likely to have complete emetic control than "nondrinkers," even if the former are not using alcohol now.

For a minority of patients who receive treatment-appropriate antiemetic prophylaxis, effective emetic control is beyond the scope of evidence-based guidelines and requires a rational empiric approach. Unfortunately, empiric interventions predispose patients to a risk of overtreatment that may adversely affect their safety and unjustifiably increase treatment costs. In comparison, undertreatment is equally unsatisfactory because it places patients at risk for emesis and debilitating morbidity that may adversely affect their safety, comfort, and quality of life, and it complicates their care.

PRIMARY ANTIEMETIC PROPHYLAXIS

To prevent emetic symptoms during each emetogenic treatment, treatment-appropriate antiemetic prophylaxis should precede treatment and proceed on a fixed schedule. Unscheduled medications require patients to recognize prodromes or develop symptoms before an antiemetic is administered. It is essential that patients who receive emetogenic treatments are not left to rely on unscheduled antiemetics; however, it is also rational to provide a supply of antiemetic medications that patients can self-administer for symptoms that surmount (i.e., "breakthrough") primary prophylaxis.

TREATMENT FOR BREAKTHROUGH SYMPTOMS

Up to 50% of patients receiving highly emetogenic therapy may experience breakthrough symptoms. Consequently, patients who receive moderately or more highly emetogenic treatment should receive a supply of medication to treat breakthrough symptoms and clear instructions about how to modify their prophylactic regimen.

Cyclic emetogenic treatments present an opportunity to evaluate a patient's suboptimal response to antiemetic prophylaxis:

- Does an unsuccessful prophylaxis strategy constitute an adequate trial?
- Can emetic control be improved with the same drugs by escalating doses or by shortening administration intervals?

Alternatively, it may be preferable to "rescue" a patient from a suboptimal response by

- adding one or more agents from a pharmacologic class that complements or potentiates drugs already in use
- replacing a drug with a more potent agent from the same pharmacologic class.

Either one or both strategies may be utilized with cyclic treatment or to intervene when response to prophylaxis is unsatisfactory. Mitigating factors to be considered in developing a treatment strategy for breakthrough symptoms include the following:

- Diminished gastrointestinal motility and impaired drug absorption from the gut around times when emetic symptoms occur

- Some patients may be too ill to swallow and retain oral medications
  - Rectal suppositories are a practical alternative, but clinicians should ascertain whether a patient finds that route of administration acceptable before anticipating compliance.
- Avoid sustained-release drug products for treating acute symptoms
  - Breakthrough symptoms require a rapidly acting intervention for which sustained-release drug products are ill suited.

ANTIEMETIC COMBINATIONS

Antiemetics in combination can be more effective than single agents. The rationale for combining antiemetic agents is to

- improve neurotransmitter blockade by targeting multiple receptor types
- decrease the adverse effects associated with (a) a patient's malignant disease (e.g., anxiety), (b) antineoplastic treatment (e.g., diarrhea), and (c) other antiemetic agents (e.g., sedation, extrapyramidal effects), which may improve their overall comfort and ability to tolerate treatment
- develop simple antiemetic strategies suitable for outpatients that decrease the duration of hospitalization and the amount of time spent in an ambulatory care setting.

Numerous studies have demonstrated that acute-phase emetic control is considerably improved when $5\text{-}HT_3$ receptor antagonists and glucocorticoids are combined. An NK_1 receptor antagonist, aprepitant, also contributes to antiemetic activity and augments symptom control during the acute phase when it is used in combination with a $5\text{-}HT_3$ receptor antagonist and glucocorticoid. Delayed-phase control is improved by glucocorticoids or aprepitant or both drugs combined; however, medication use can be complicated by aprepitant, which may alter the metabolism and elimination of other drugs. In cases in which prophylaxis against delayed-phase symptoms is indicated but aprepitant may adversely interact with other medications, glucocorticoids alone or in combination with either metoclopramide or a $5\text{-}HT_3$ antagonist and perhaps with dopamine (D_2) receptor antagonists may provide adequate control.

PLANNING ANTIEMETIC PROPHYLAXIS

Planning effective antiemetic prophylaxis for chemotherapy entails evaluating each agent's emetic potential; the severity, onset, and duration of symptoms; and how drug dosage, schedule, and route of administration may affect those factors. An expert panel has developed a method for categorizing the emetic potential of drugs (see Table 40.3) and an algorithm with which one may predict the cumulative emetic potential of drug combinations (see Table 40.4) (7–11).

The guidelines for selecting treatment-appropriate antiemetic prophylaxis described in Fig. 40.2 integrate evidence-based guidelines recommended by the National Comprehensive Cancer Network (NCCN) and the American Society of Clinical Oncology (ASCO) and the consensus of experts in oncology practice (11–14).

In Fig. 40.2, primary prophylaxis is indicated for all patients whose treatment has a *cumulative emetogenicity score* equal to 2, where more than 10% of patients receiving similar chemotherapy are expected to experience emetic symptoms. The guidelines in Fig. 40.2 base prophylaxis and treatment on an assessment of emetic risk; they are generally limited in application to adult patients and may not be appropriate in all clinical situations. Decisions to follow the recommendations and to utilize particular drugs must be based on professional judgment, circumstances of the individual patient, and available resources.

TABLE 40.3. *Emetic potential as a function of drug, dosage, and route of administration*

Emetic potential	Drug name and dosage range	Incidence of emesis[a]
Level 5 (very high)	Carmustine (>250 mg/m^2) Cisplatin (≥50 mg/m^2) Cyclophosphamide (>1,500 mg/m^2) Dacarbazine Lomustine (>60 mg/m^2) Mechlorethamine Streptozocin	>90%
Level 4 (high)	Amifostine (>500 mg/m^2) Busulfan (>4 mg/kg/d) Carboplatin Carmustine (≤250 mg/m^2) Cisplatin (<50 mg/m^2) Cyclophosphamide (>750–≤1,500 mg/m^2) Cytarabine (>1,000 mg/m^2) Dactinomycin (>1.5 mg/m^2) Doxorubicin (>60 mg/m^2) Epirubicin (>90 mg/m^2) Melphalan (i.v., >50 mg/m^2) Methotrexate (>1,000 mg/m^2) Mitoxantrone (>15 mg/m^2) Procarbazine	60%–90%

Level 3 (moderate)	Aldesleukin (>12–15 Million
	  International Units/m^2)
	Altretamine
	Amifostine (>300–≤500 mg/m^2)
	Arsenic trioxide
	Cyclophosphamide (≤750 mg/m^2)
	Cyclophosphamide (oral, for
	  multiple consecutive days)
	Dactinomycin (≤1.5 mg/m^2)
	Daunorubicin
	Doxorubicin (20–60 mg/m^2)
	Epirubicin (≤90 mg/m^2)
	Idarubicin
	Ifosfamide
	Irinotecan
	Lomustine (<60 mg/m^2)
	Methotrexate (250–1,000 mg/m^2)
	Mitoxantrone (≤15 mg/m^2)
	Oxaliplatin (>75 mg/m^2)
	Pentostatin
	Plicamycin
		30%–60%

Level 2 (low)	Amifostine (≤300 mg/m^2) Asparaginase Bexarotene Capecitabine Cytarabine (<1,000 mg/m^2) Daunorubicin, liposomal Docetaxel Doxorubicin (<20 mg/m^2) Doxorubicin, liposomal	10%–30%

continued on next page

TABLE 40.3. *Continued*

Emetic potential	Drug name and dosage range	Incidence of emesis[a]
	Etoposide	
	Fluorouracil ($\leq$1,000 mg/m^2)	
	Gemcitabine	
	Methotrexate ($>$50–$<$250 mg/m^2)	
	Mitomycin	
	Paclitaxel	
	Temozolomide	
	Teniposide	
	Thiotepa	
	Topotecan	
Level 1 (very low)	Alemtuzumab	$<$10%
	Bleomycin	
	Bortezomib	
	Busulfan (oral, $<$4 mg/kg/d)	
	Chlorambucil	
	Cladribine	
	Denileukin diftitox	
	Dexrazoxane	
	Estramustine	
	Fludarabine	
	Gefitinib	
	Gemtuzumab ozogamicin	
	Hydroxyurea	
	Imatinib	
	Interferon alfa	
	Melphalan (oral)	
	Mercaptopurine	
	Methotrexate ($\leq$50 mg/m^2)	
	Rituximab	
	Thioguanine	
	Trastuzumab	
	Vinblastine	
	Vincristine	
	Vinorelbine	

Drugs are arranged alphabetically within the emetic potential levels. All drugs are administered by the intravenous route unless noted otherwise.

[a]The incidence of emesis among patients who received the drug without antiemetic protection.

ANTIEMETIC OPTIONS

Serotonin Receptor Antagonists

- All 5-HT$_3$ antagonists provide equal benefit at maximally effective dosages.
- Maximal antiemetic benefit is achieved by meeting or exceeding an "effective threshold" dose.
  - Doses greater than a maximally effective dose do not substantively improve antiemetic control.
  - Single-dose prophylaxis is adequate against acute-phase symptoms.
    - Additional doses of dolasetron, granisetron, or ondansetron within the first 24 hours after emetogenic treatment have not been shown to improve emetic control.
  - Repeated doses of palonosetron have not yet been studied and cannot be recommended.
- 5-HT$_3$ antagonists are more effective against acute-phase symptoms and are safer to use than other types of antiemetics.

TABLE 40.4. *Algorithm for estimating the emetogenic potential of combination chemotherapy regimens*

1. Identify the most emetogenic agent in a drug combination to determine the *base score*.
2. For any number of Level 2 agents in the combination, *add one* to the *base score*
3. For each Level 3 or LEVEL 4 agent, *add one* to the *base score*.
4. The sum of all amounts added to the *base score* produces a *cumulative emetogenicity score* for the drug combination.

Chemotherapy regimen[a]	Emetogenic level by drug	Cumulative emetogenicity score	Predicted frequency of emesis (%)
CMF			
Cyclophosphamide, 600 mg/m^2 i.v. on d 1	**3** (base score)	3 + 1 = 4	60–90
Methotrexate, 40 mg/m^2 i.v. on d 1	1		
Fluorouracil, 600 mg/m^2 i.v. on d 1	2 (add 1)		
• Cycle repeats every 21 d			
CAF			
Cyclophosphamide, 500 mg/m^2 i.v. on d 1	**3** (base score)	3 + 1 + 1 = 5	>90
Doxorubicin, 50 mg/m^2 i.v. on d 1	**3** (add 1)		
Fluorouracil, 500 mg/m^2 i.v. on d 1	2 (add 1)		
• Cycle repeats every 21 d			
CHOP			
Cyclophosphamide, 750 mg/m^2 i.v. on d 1	**3** (base score)	3 + 1 = 4	60–90
Doxorubicin, 50 mg/m^2 i.v. on d 1	**3** (add 1)		
Vincristine, 1.4 mg/m^2 i.v. on d 1	1		
Prednisone, 100 mg orally d 1–5	Not applicable		
• Cycle repeats every 21 d			
ABVD			
Doxorubicin, 25 mg/m^2/d i.v. on days 1 and 14	3 (add 1)	5 + 1 = 6 (d 1)	>90 (d 1)
Bleomycin, 10 Units/m^2/d i.v. on d 1 and 14	1	5 (d 2–5)	>90 (d 2–5)
Vinblastine, 6 mg/m^2/d i.v. on d 1 and 14	1	3 (d 14)	>30–60 (d 14)
Dacarbazine 150 mg/m^2/d i.v. on d 1–5	**5** (base score)		
• Cycle repeats every 28 d			

i.v., intravenously.

[a]The most emetogenic agents in a combination appear in bold-faced type.

FIG. 40.2. Algorithms for antiemetic prophylaxis and treatment. i.v., intravenous administration; PO, oral administration; PR, rectal insertion.

*Medications are not listed in order of preference. Pharmacologically similar alternatives are bounded by broken lines.

†Oral prophylaxis should begin 1 hour before commencing cytotoxic treatment. Intravenous prophylaxis may be given within minutes before emetogenic treatment.

‡Generally, regimens containing D$_2$ receptor antagonists and metoclopramide doses ≥20 mg should include primary prophylaxis with anticholinergic agents against acute dystonic extrapyramidal reactions; e.g., diphenhydramine 25–50 mg PO or i.v. every 6 hours is often used; benztropine and trihexyphenidyl are alternatives. Parenteral administration is preferred for rapidly treating extrapyramidal symptoms.

§When administered i.v., phenothiazines should be given over 30 minutes to prevent hypotension.

‖When administered i.v., dexamethasone should be given as a short infusion over 10–15 minutes to prevent uncomfortable sensations of warmth.

¶Medications identified for "breakthrough" symptoms are not alternatives to primary prophylaxis, but should be added to a patient's antiemetic regimen.

**When indicated, prophylaxis for delayed phase symptoms may begin 12–24 h after emetogenic treatment began.

Emetic potential

Emetic potential	Acute phase—primary prophylaxis*,†	Delayed phase—primary prophylaxis*,†,**
Levels ≥5 (very high)	• Oral route available dolasetron 100 mg PO once; *or* granisetron 2 mg PO once, or 1 mg PO every 12 h; *or* ondansetron 16–24 mg PO once + dexamethasone 12 mg PO once, or 8 mg PO every 12 h ± aprepitant 125 mg PO once ± lorazepam 0.5–2 mg PO or SL every 6–12 h • Oral route not available dolasetron 1.8 mg/kg IV once, or 100 mg IV once; *or* granisetron 0.01 mg/kg IV once; *or* ondansetron 8–32 mg IV once; *or* palonosetron 0.25 mg IV once + dexamethasone 10–20 mg IV once‖ ± lorazepam 0.5–2 mg IV every 6–12 h	• Oral route available dexamethasone 8 mg PO daily, or 4 mg PO every 12 h dolasetron 100 mg PO daily; *or* granisetron 2 mg PO daily, or 1 mg PO every 12 h; *or* ondansetron 16–24 mg PO daily *(each day of repeated chemotherapy, and for 2–4 days after completing chemotherapy)* ± aprepitant 80 mg PO daily, for 2–4 days ± lorazepam 0.5–2 mg PO or SL every 6–12 h • Oral route not available dolasetron 1.8 mg/kg IV daily, or 100 mg IV daily; *or* granisetron 0.01 mg/kg IV daily; *or* ondansetron 8–32 mg IV daily *(each day of repeated chemotherapy, and for 2–4 days after completing chemotherapy)* + dexamethasone 8 mg IV daily‖ ± lorazepam 0.5–2 mg IV every 6–12 h
Levels 3 and 4 (moderate to high)	• Oral route available dolasetron 100 mg PO once; *or* granisetron 2 mg PO once, or 1 mg PO every 12 h; *or* ondansetron 16–24 mg PO once + dexamethasone 12 mg PO once, or 8 mg PO every 12 h ± aprepitant 125 mg PO once ± lorazepam 0.5–2 mg PO or SL every 6–12 h • Oral route not available dolasetron 1.8 mg/kg IV once, or 100 mg IV once; *or* granisetron 0.01 mg/kg IV once; *or* ondansetron 8–32 mg IV once; *or* palonosetron 0.25 mg IV once + dexamethasone 10–20 mg IV once‖ ± lorazepam 0.5–2 mg PO or SL every 6–12 h	• Oral route available dexamethasone 8 mg PO daily, or 4 mg PO every 12 h metoclopramide 20 mg PO every 6 h, or 0.5 mg/kg PO every 6 h‡ + diphenhydramine 25 mg PO every 6 h; *or* dolasetron 100 mg PO daily; *or* granisetron 2 mg PO daily, or 1 mg PO every 12 h; *or* ondansetron 16–24 mg PO daily *(each day of repeated chemotherapy, and for 2–4 days after completing chemotherapy)* ± lorazepam 0.5–2 mg PO or SL every 6–12 h **OR** dexamethasone 8 mg PO daily, or 4 mg PO every 12 h *(each day of repeated chemotherapy, and for 2–4 days after completing chemotherapy)* aprepitant 80 mg PO daily, for 2–4 days (if aprepitant was given on day 1) ± lorazepam 0.5–2 mg PO or SL every 6–12 h • Oral route not available dexamethasone 8 mg IV daily‖ metoclopramide 20 mg IV every 6 h, or 0.5 mg/kg IV every 6 h‡ + diphenhydramine 25 mg IV every 6 h; *or* dolasetron 1.8 mg/kg IV daily, or 100 mg IV daily; *or* granisetron 0.01 mg/kg IV daily; *or* ondansetron 8–32 mg IV daily *(each day of repeated chemotherapy, and for 2–4 days after completing chemotherapy)* ± lorazepam 0.5–2 mg IV every 6–12 h

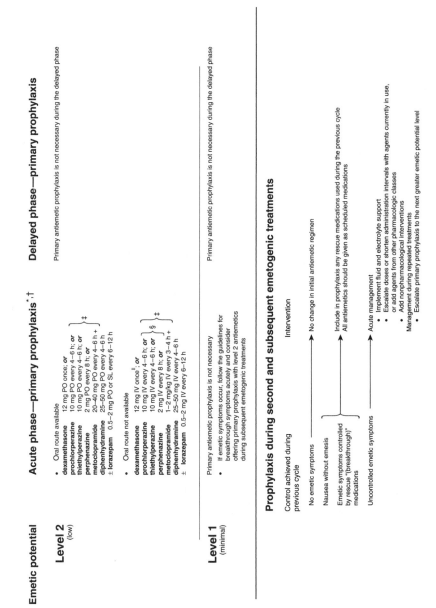

Emetic potential

Level 2 (low)

Acute phase—primary prophylaxis*,†

- Oral route available

dexamethasone	12 mg PO once; *or*
prochlorperazine	10 mg PO every 4–6 h; *or*
thiethylperazine	10 mg PO every 4–6 h; *or*
perphenazine	2 mg PO every 8 h; *or* ‡
metoclopramide	20–40 mg PO every 4–6 h +
diphenhydramine	25–50 mg PO every 4–6 h
± **lorazepam**	0.5–2 mg PO or SL every 6–12 h

- Oral route not available

dexamethasone	12 mg IV once‖; *or*
prochlorperazine	10 mg IV every 4–6 h; *or*
thiethylperazine	10 mg IV every 4–6 h; *or* § ‡
perphenazine	2 mg IV every 8 h; *or*
metoclopramide	1–2 mg/kg IV every 3–4 h +
diphenhydramine	25–50 mg IV every 4–6 h
± **lorazepam**	0.5–2 mg IV every 6–12 h

Delayed phase—primary prophylaxis

Primary antiemetic prophylaxis is not necessary during the delayed phase

Level 1 (minimal)

Primary antiemetic prophylaxis is not necessary

- If emetic symptoms occur, follow the guidelines for breakthrough symptoms acutely and consider offering primary prophylaxis with level 2 antiemetics during subsequent emetogenic treatments

Primary antiemetic prophylaxis is not necessary during the delayed phase

---

Prophylaxis during second and subsequent emetogenic treatments

Control achieved during previous cycle

Intervention

No emetic symptoms ⟶ No change in initial antiemetic regimen

Nausea without emesis ⎫
Emetic symptoms controlled by rescue "(breakthrough)" medications ⎬ Include in prophylaxis any rescue medications used during the previous cycle
All antiemetics should be given as scheduled medications

Uncontrolled emetic symptoms ⟶ Acute management
- Implement fluid and electrolyte support
- Escalate doses or shorten administration intervals with agents currently in use, or add agents from other pharmacologic classes
- Add nonpharmacological interventions
Management during repeated treatments
- Escalate primary prophylaxis to the next greater emetic potential level

FIG. 40.2. *Algorithms for antiemetic Prophylaxis and treatment. (Continued)*

538

Prophylaxis for radiation therapy

Type of radiation therapy (RT) — *Primary prophylaxis*

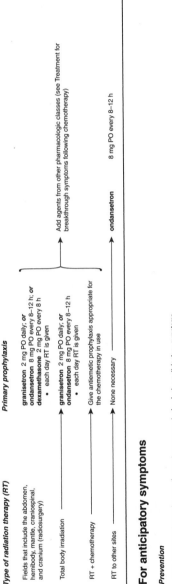

Fields that include the abdomen, hemibody, mantle, craniospinal, and cranium (radiosurgery)
→ **granisetron** 2 mg PO daily; *or*
ondansetron 8 mg PO every 8–12 h; *or*
dexamethasone 2 mg PO every 8 h
• each day RT is given
→ Add agents from other pharmacologic classes (see Treatment for breakthrough symptoms following chemotherapy)

Total body irradiation
→ **granisetron** 2 mg PO daily; *or*
ondansetron 8 mg PO every 8–12 h
• each day RT is given

RT + chemotherapy → Give antiemetic prophylaxis appropriate for the chemotherapy in use

RT to other sites → None necessary

→ **ondansetron** 8 mg PO every 8–12 h

For anticipatory symptoms

Prevention

Complete protection against emetic symptoms preempts developing anticipatory symptoms

Behavior modification and relaxation techniques for prevention and treatment

Distraction, desensitization, biofeedback, relaxation, guided imagery, and hypnosis

Adjunctive pharmacotherapy

lorazepam 0.5–2 mg PO or sublingually
• the night before and morning of single-day treatment, and every 6–12 h concurrently with emetogenic treatment on 2 or more days; *or*
alprazolam 0.5–2 mg PO four times daily

Treatment for breakthrough symptoms after emetogenic treatment

• *Add to the current regimen a drug from a different pharmacological class†.*

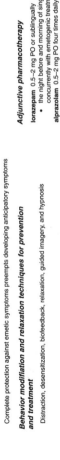
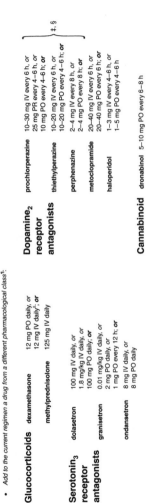

Glucocorticoids dexamethasone 12 mg PO daily, or
12 mg IV daily‡; *or*
methylprednisolone 125 mg IV daily

Serotonin₃ receptor antagonists
dolasetron 100 mg IV daily, or
1.8 mg/kg IV daily, or
100 mg PO daily; *or*
granisetron 0.01 mg/kg IV daily, or
2 mg PO daily, or
1 mg PO every 12 h; *or*
ondansetron 8 mg IV daily, or
8 mg PO daily

Dopamine₂ receptor antagonists
prochlorperazine 10–30 mg IV every 6 h, or
25 mg PR every 4–6 h, or
10 mg PO every 4–6 h; *or*
thiethylperazine 10–20 mg IV every 6 h, or
10–20 mg PO every 4–6 h; *or*
perphenazine 2–4 mg IV every 8 h, or
2–4 mg PO every 8 h; *or*
metoclopramide 10–40 mg IV every 6 h, or
20–40 mg PO every 6 h; *or*
haloperidol 1–3 mg IV every 4–6 h, or
1–5 mg PO every 4–6 h   ‡, §

Cannabinoid dronabinol 5–10 mg PO every 6–8 h

FIG. 40.2. *Algorithms for antiemetic Prophylaxis and treatment. (Continued)*

- Dolasetron, granisetron, and ondansetron have excellent oral bioavailability and provide equivalent antiemetic protection after either oral or parenteral administration. Palonosetron is equally effective, but an oral formulation is not available.
- Among dolasetron, granisetron, and ondansetron, activity during the delayed phase is similar to less expensive alternatives such as metoclopramide. Palonosetron has the longest half-life among 5-HT$_3$ antagonists, which may be advantageous against delayed-phase symptoms.
- Profiles of adverse effects are qualitatively similar among agents and include
  - headache
  - constipation
  - diarrhea
  - transiently increased hepatic transaminase concentrations
  - transient electrocardiogram (ECG) changes ± decreased cardiac rate.

Glucocorticoids

- Glucocorticoids are effective as single agents against acute-phase symptoms that are of mild-to-moderate emetogenic nature (emetic potential levels ≤2).
- Active against delayed-phase symptoms.
- Parenteral and oral dexamethasone and methylprednisolone provide equivalent benefit.
- Prophylaxis and treatment are empirically based; safety and efficacy comparisons are lacking.
- Single doses are as effective as multiple-dose schedules.
- Optimal dosages and schedules are yet to be determined.
  - There is no evidence that dexamethasone doses >20 mg improve antiemetic response.
- Incidence of adverse effects after single doses is
  - usually very low
  - limited to "activating" psychogenic effects such as insomnia and sleep disturbances, which can be minimized by administering steroids early during a patient's routine waking cycle.
- Adrenocortical suppression is generally not a problem when steroids are used for brief periods.
- Glycemic control may be problematic in patients with incipient or frank diabetes.

Aprepitant

- Aprepitant is the first NK$_1$ receptor antagonist antiemetic that is approved for use in adult patients (aged 18 years or older).
  - The approval was based on studies with emetogenic chemotherapy given on a single day.
- Product labeling indicates aprepitant use in combination with a 5-HT$_3$ receptor antagonist, and a glucocorticoid.
  - Initial dose: Aprepitant 125 mg orally, 60 minutes before emetogenic chemotherapy.
  - Subsequent dose: Aprepitant 80 mg per day orally for 2 days, the second and third day after chemotherapy.
  - Aprepitant has been given safely for 5 days: an initial dose of 125 mg (day 1), followed by daily doses of 80 mg for 4 consecutive days (days 2–5).
  - The use of aprepitant with multiple-day chemotherapy regimens and for durations exceeding five consecutive days have not yet been adequately studied.
- Utilization is complicated by aprepitant's potential for pharmacokinetic interactions with other medications.
  - Aprepitant is a substrate, moderate inhibitor, and inducer of the cytochrome P-450 enzyme, CYP3A4. It is also an inducer of CYP2C9 and perhaps the CYP2D6 isoform.
  - Its potential for interaction with many CYP3A4 substrate drugs is largely unknown.
    - Experience with aprepitant during chemotherapy administration for a single day may not accurately represent the significance of potential interactions with chemotherapy administered for 2 or more days.

- When given concomitantly with aprepitant, dexamethasone and methylprednisolone doses should be decreased by 50% and 25% when they are administered by the oral and intravenous routes, respectively.
- Aprepitant metabolism may be perturbed by drugs that inhibit or induce CYP3A4.
- Adverse events that commonly occur in patients who receive aprepitant plus a 5-HT$_3$ receptor antagonist and a glucocorticoid:
  - Abdominal pain
  - Epigastric discomfort
  - Hiccups
  - Anorexia
  - Dizziness
  - Asthenia
  - Fatigue.

Metoclopramide

- Metoclopramide is a D$_2$ receptor antagonist, and is a weak competitive 5-HT$_3$ receptor antagonist at high doses.
- Its activity against delayed-phase symptoms is equivalent to that of ondansetron.
- The profile of adverse effects is similar to that of other potent D$_2$ receptor antagonists.
  - Dose-related sedation
  - Extrapyramidal reactions (EPRs).
- Gastrointestinal prokinetic effects may be useful for patients who have concomitant motility disorders or gastroesophageal reflux disease.

Dopamine-2 Receptor Antagonists

- Optimal dosages and schedules for dopamine-2 (D$_2$) receptor antagonists have not been established.
- Overall, antiemetic activity varies directly with D$_2$ receptor antagonism.
- Incidence of adverse effects also correlates directly with the magnitude of the dose and the frequency of administration:
  - Sedation
  - EPRs
  - Anticholinergic effects.
- Anecdotes and meager data support D$_2$ receptor antagonist combinations with 5-HT$_3$ antagonists, with or without steroids, for acute-phase symptoms and with steroids, metoclopramide, or lorazepam for delayed-phase symptoms.

Benzodiazepines

- Benzodiazepines are important adjuncts to antiemetics for their anxiolytic and anterograde amnestic effects.
- They are clinically useful for mitigating EPRs associated with D$_2$ receptor antagonists.
- Many clinically useful agents are available in oral formulations, injectable formulations, or both.
  - Lorazepam and alprazolam tablets are rapidly absorbed after sublingual administration.
- Primary liability is dose-related sedation.
- Pharmacodynamic effects are exaggerated in elderly patients.

Cannabinoids

- Dronabinol is an oral formulation of Δ^9-tetrahydrocannabinol, with activity similar to low doses of prochlorperazine.

- Regulated as controlled substances in the United States.
- Antiemetic benefit may be achieved without producing psychotropic effects.
  - Utilization is empiric; optimal doses and administration schedules have not been determined.
  - Dronabinol produces a greater incidence of adverse effects than phenothiazines at doses and schedules that produce comparable antiemetic effects.
- Dose-related side effects occur throughout the range of clinically useful doses.
- Profile of adverse effects includes
  - sedation
  - confusion
  - dizziness
  - recent memory impairment
  - euphoria or dysphoria
  - ataxia
  - dry mouth
  - orthostatic hypotension with or without an increased heart rate.

REFERENCES

1. Kris MG, Gralla RJ, Clark RA, et al. Incidence, course, and severity of delayed nausea and vomiting following the administration of high-dose cisplatin. *J Clin Oncol* 1985;3:1379–1384.
2. Morrow GR, Hickok JT, Burish TG, et al. Frequency and clinical implications of delayed nausea and delayed emesis. *Am J Clin Oncol* 1996;19:199–203.
3. Kris MG, Roila F, De Mulder PHM, et al. Delayed emesis following anticancer chemotherapy. *Support Care Cancer* 1998;6:228–232.
4. Borison HL, McCarthy LE. Neuropharmacology of chemotherapy-induced emesis. *Drugs* 1983; 25 (Suppl 1):8–17.
5. Aapro M. Methodological issues in antiemetic studies. *Invest New Drugs* 1993;11:243–253.
6. Italian Group for Antiemetic Research. Cisplatin-induced delayed emesis: pattern and prognostic factors during three subsequent cycles. *Ann Oncol* 1994;5:585–589.
7. Lindley CM, Bernard S, Fields SM. Incidence and duration of chemotherapy-induced nausea and vomiting in the outpatient oncology population. *J Clin Oncol* 1989;7:1142–1149.
8. Hesketh PJ, Kris MG, Grunberg SM, et al. Proposal for classifying the acute emetogenicity of cancer chemotherapy. *J Clin Oncol* 1997;15:103–109.
9. Hesketh PJ, Gralla RJ, du Bois A, et al. Methodology of antiemetic trials: response assessment, evaluation of new agents and definition of chemotherapy emetogenicity. *Support Care Cancer* 1998;6:221–227.
10. Gralla RJ. Antiemetic therapy. *Semin Oncol* 1998;25:577–583.
11. ASHP. Therapeutic guidelines on the pharmacologic management of nausea and vomiting in adult and pediatric patients receiving chemotherapy or radiation therapy or undergoing surgery [see comments]. *Am J Health Syst Pharm* 1999;56:729–764. Comment in: *Am J Health Syst Pharm* 1999;56:728.
12. National Comprehensive Cancer Network. Clinical practice guidelines in oncology – antiemesis. Version 1. 2004 [cited 2004 Jun 9]:[30 screens]. Available from: URL: http://nccn.org/professionals/-physician_gls/default.asp#care
13. Gandara DR, Roila F, Warr D, et al. Consensus proposal for 5HT3 antagonists in the prevention of acute emesis related to highly emetogenic chemotherapy: dose, schedule, and route of administration. *Support Care Cancer* 1998;6:237–243.
14. Gralla RJ, Osoba D, Kris MG, et al. Recommendations for the use of antiemetics: evidence-based, clinical practice guidelines. *J Clin Oncol* 1999;17:2971–2994.

41

Nutrition for Oncology Patients

Marnie Dobbin

National Institutes of Health Clinical Center, Department of Nutrition,
Bethesda, Maryland

The incidence of malnutrition and its effect on oncology patients as well as suggested efforts to minimize this effect are presented in this chapter.

- Incidence: more than 40% of oncology patients develop signs of malnutrition during treatment.
- Effect:
  - Malnourished patients have impaired responses to treatment (1,2).
  - They incur higher costs for their care.
  - They have increased rates of mortality and morbidity (2).
  - As many as 20% of oncology patients die from nutritional complications rather than from their primary diagnosis (3).
- Efforts to minimize malnutrition: Nutritional deterioration in oncology patients is not inevitable and can be minimized dramatically with appropriate screening and timely intervention.

IDENTIFYING NUTRITIONAL RISK

For nutritional interventions to be effective, patients at risk for malnutrition must be identified before irreversible deficits occur.

Parameters most useful in identifying patients at nutritional risk include (see Fig. 41.1)

- weight change
- functional status
- symptom status
- changes in food intake
- changes in body composition
- visceral protein markers.

Simple, validated tools have been developed to allow the timely identification of patients at risk.

- The Subjective Global Assessment (SGA) form developed by Dr. Jeejeebhoy et al. (1987) has been adapted for use with oncology patients by Dr. Faith Ottery (Contact Ottery & Associates Inc., phone, 215-351-4050) (4,5).
- This patient-generated tool (PG-SGA) helps identify patients at nutritional risk and may improve patient satisfaction because attention to a patient's nutritional health is a major concern for patients and their families.

Nutrition Intervention

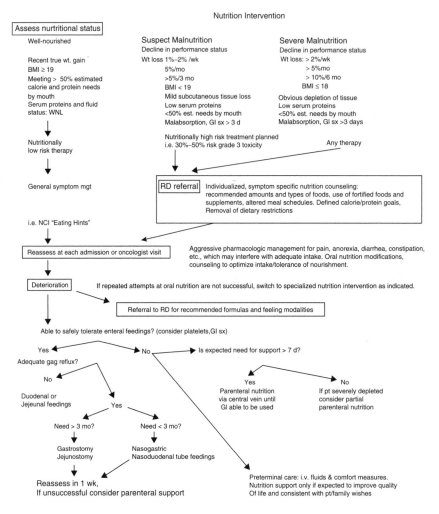

FIG. 41.1. Parameters most useful in identifying patients at nutritional risk. R.D., registered dietitian; BMI, body mass index; GI, (gastrointestinal; pt, patient; WNL, within normal limits; NCI, national cancer institute.)

EFFECTIVE NUTRITION INTERVENTION

Continual reassessment, pharmacologic management, and nutrition counseling can help avoid costly, risky nutrition support options.

When nutritional risk is identified early and realistic nutritional interventions implemented in a timely manner, there can be

• improvement in quality of life and nutritional status
• weight maintenance.

Nutrition counseling by registered dietitians (RDs) is associated with improvement in quality of life, with improvement in nutritional parameters, and with success of oral nutritional intervention for oncology patients (see Table 41.1).

TABLE 41.1. *Simple food/oral nutrition supplement recommendations*

Neutropenia: emphasize food-borne illness prevention (well-washed products are safe)
Early satiety: calorically dense foods/nutrition products (e.g., *Scandi and Polycose*)
Poor appetite/fatigue: to ↓ dependence on appetite >5 scheduled feedings/day, reliance on nutritious liquids (quenching thirst) without need for appetite
Nausea: ↓ fat foods/supplements (e.g., *Biocare, Boost, Resource drink*)
Malabsorption: semi-elemental palatable products (e.g., *Propeptide oral formulation*)
Diarrhea: ↓ lactose, ↓ fat, ↓ insoluble fiber, ↓ soluble fiber (e.g., *Benefiber and Ensure light*)
Fat malabsorption: ↓ fat diet and MCT–oil fortified foods/products (e.g., *Lipisorb*)
Aversion to canned "milkshake-type" products: fortification of preferred foods (e.g., soups) with modular kcal or protein supplements (*Polycose, Promod*)MCT, medium chain triglycerides.

Refer to registered dietitian (R.D.), for comparable products at your facility. Brand names provided as examples only—does not imply endorsement.

Effective nutritional intervention by an RD may include:

* modifications of foods and feeding schedules
* fortification of foods with modular nutritional products
* supplementation with meal-replacement products.

Eating is extremely individualized and complex, affected by such factors as food aversions or associations, cultural influences, and family dynamics.

Nutritional recommendations must be tailored to the individual's needs, incorporating input from the patient and family in order to be successful.

Providing nutritional samples and written information alone is not associated with nutritional success.

Self-imposed diets and the use of dietary supplements should be evaluated by an RD for possible risks and for the potential to confound results of protocols (see Table 41.2)

Nutrition Support

Controversies

Although tumor growth is stimulated by a number of nutrients, limitation of the nutrients preferred by tumors can lead to detriments in the patient.

* Maintenance of good nutritional status does not appear to have deleterious effects on tumor growth.
* In more than 200 patients with Hodgkin disease (HD), malnourished patients had greater rates of tumor growth (demonstrated by incorporation of [^{3}H]thymidine-labeling index in the tumor tissue) than well-nourished patients (6).

Enteral Nutrition

The superiority of enteral over parenteral nutrition has been reviewed in many references (7).

* If the gut works, it should be used.
* To be successful, enteral nutrition should be implemented as soon as the need arises.
* Surgeons may approve of enteral feeding of the patient within 4 hours of placement of gastrostomy tubes and immediately after jejunostomy (because bowel sounds are not needed).
* Prophylactic placement of gastrointestinal (GI) tubes can reduce the amount of weight loss during radiotherapy considerably and can reduce the incidence of hospitalization for dehydration, weight loss, or other complications of mucositis (8).

TABLE 41.2. *Quick nutrition reference for adult oncology patients*

Estimated requirements:
Kilocalories: 20 kcal/kg (actual wt) for obese patients
25–30 kcal/kg for sedentary patients
35 kcal/kg for hypermetabolic patients or in cases of malabsorption
Fluid: 1 mL/kcal; 35 mL/kg of body weight; 1,500 mL/m^2 of body surface
1,500 mL/kg of body weight for first 20 kg, plus 25 mL/kg for the remaining wt
Protein: 1.2 g/kg; Weekly 24-hr urine for UUN to assess adequacy; 0.8 g protein/kg = RDA
  and is appropriate for nondialyzed renal insufficiency
BMI:
Wt (kg)/Ht(m^2); BMI 19–25, healthy wt range
Nutrient limitations for nutrition support:
Dextrose (parenteral nutrition by central-line TPN):
Maximal glucose oxidation rate ~4–6 mg/kg/min (TPN)
Initial dextrose concentration: 10%–15%; final, 20%–25% (PPN): final dextrose
  concentration, 10%.
Lipids to provide 30% of total kcals usually (up to 60% total kcals for PPN)
Diets and supplements that pose a risk:
Gerson diet, strict macrobiotic diet; Chaparral, Peau D'arco, Mistletoe, (DHEA); Vit A >5,000
  (IU)/d, B_6 >200 mg/d, chromium >200 mg/d
Vitamin D >1,600 IU/d, Fe >15 mg/d (unless Fe deficiency clear), Zn >25 mg/d.
Vitamin C >250 mg/d may alter renal excretion of chemotherapy.
Any single antioxidant taken in excess (e.g., α-carotene) may cause a pro-oxidant state or
  malabsorption of other antioxidants (Vitamin E <800 IU/d has not been found to be
  harmful in vitamin K–sufficient adults not taking anticoagulants).

UUN, urinary urea nitrogen concentration; RDA, reference daily intake; BMI, body mass index; TPN, total parenteral nutrition; PPN, peripheral parenteral nutrition; DHEA, dehydro-3-epiandrosterone; IU, international unit.

- Reviews of nutrition support practices indicate that parenteral nutrition is often instituted even when safer, more physiologic enteral nutrition support could have been provided (7,9).

Parenteral Nutrition

- Total parenteral nutrition (TPN) can be beneficial to patients with cancer when response to treatment is good but the associated nutritional morbidity high and when the GI tract is unavailable to support nutrition.
- The use of perioperative TPN should be limited to patients who are severely malnourished, with surgery expected to prevent oral intake for more than 10 days after surgery (8,10) (Table 41.2).
- Feeding is synonymous with caring by many family members. Provision of nominal supportive care for preterminal patients can reduce family tension as well as readmissions because of hydration and electrolyte maintenance problems.
- Data indicate that parenteral nutrition can improve quality of life and functional status for preterminal patients with a Karnofsky performance status greater than 50. The risks and benefits of nutrition support must be addressed individually and evaluated for each case with patient and family input.

REFERENCES

1. Aker SN. Oral feedings in the cancer patient. *Cancer* 1979;43(Suppl):2103–2107.
2. Ottery FD. Nutritional oncology: a proactive, integrated approach to the cancer patient. In: R Chernoff, ed. *Nutrition support theory and therapeutics,*. New York: Chapman & Hall, 1997:395–409.

3. Ambrus J, Ambrus CM, Mink IB, et al. Causes of death in cancer patients. *J Med Clin Exp Ther* 1975;6:61–64.
4. Ottery FD. Supportive nutrition to prevent cachexia and improve quality of life. *Semin Oncol* 1995; 22(2 Suppl. 3):98–111.
5. Osoba D. Current applications of health-related quality of life assessment in oncology. *Support Care Cancer* 1997;5:100–104.
6. Bozzetti FEA. Relationship between nutritional status and tumor growth in humans. *Tumori* 1995;81:1–6.
7. Mercadante S. Parenteral versus enteral nutrition in cancer patients: indications and practice. *Support Care Cancer* 1998;6:85–93.
8. Lee JH, Machtay M, Unger LD, et al. Prophylactic gastrostomy tubes in patients undergoing intensive irradiation for cancer of the head and neck. *Arch Otolaryngol Head Neck Surg* 1998;124:871–875.
9. Bowman LEA. Algorithm for nutritional support: experience of the metabolic and infusion support service of St. Jude Children's research hospital. *Int J Cancer* 1998;11:76–80.
10. Kelly CJ, Daly JM. Perioperative care of the oncology patient. *World J Surg* 1993;17:199–206.

42

End-of-Life Care

Jane Carter

National Cancer Institute, National Institutes of Health,
Bethesda, Maryland

When disease reaches its terminal stage, the goal of treatment ceases to be a cure or an extension of life. Rather, there is an awareness of the futility of further treatment, and focus of care shifts to one of palliation of symptoms and relief from suffering, so as to enhance the quality of remaining life for the patient and the family. Such care can be given by a hospice agency in the patient's home or by the oncologic team in a hospice or acute care setting. The key to what is called a "good death" in the hospice movement is a holistic approach that embraces care in four dimensions: physical, emotional, spiritual, and social.

COMMUNICATION

Patients will often know intuitively when a transition is reached. They may not voice awareness of the shift, especially if they sense an unwillingness of physicians, nurses, or family members to explore their thoughts and feelings. Open and honest communications between the physician and patient, as death approaches, help ease the patient's fears, relieve anxiety, and prepare the patient for death (1).

THE "GOOD DEATH"

Patients' end-of-life needs are multifaceted, but it is only control of the physical symptoms that is uniquely medical (2) and consists of

- the need to have adequate relief of pain
- the need to have ongoing assessment and prompt relief of discomfort arising from distressing symptoms
- the need to be cared for by physicians and nurses who have a positive attitude toward palliative care
- the need to be allowed a measure of control over decisions, the need for respect for their stated wishes as put forth in advance directives, and the need to have the quality of life they choose
- the need to have a trusting relationship with their physician that permits open, truthful communication (3).

PALLIATIVE CARE MEASURES

"Skilled physical symptom control is the linchpin of good hospice and palliative care ... without which the many psychological, social and spiritual needs of the patient and family cannot be met" (4).

Pain

In the early days of the contemporary hospice movement, in the late 1960s, its founder, Dr. Cicely Saunders, identified the failure of medicine to control cancer pain. Pain continues to be the most important, feared, and undertreated symptom in patients with end-stage cancer. It has many dimensions and is often described as "total pain" (5).

- The key to effective pain control is constant assessment and modification until relief is obtained, using the World Health Organization (WHO) three-step analgesic ladder.
- Morphine is the strong opioid of choice and should be titrated to a level that provides relief.
- The appropriate dose is the amount of opioid that controls pain with the fewest side effects (6).
- Complementary measures such as guided imagery, acupuncture, and massage can be effective in palliation of pain and other distressing symptoms.

Other Symptoms

Other symptoms that arise in the course of dying should be addressed as they occur, keeping in mind the underlying principle of promoting comfort (care) rather than prolonging life (cure). Optimal interventions for all symptoms will be ones that have minimal negative impact on quality of life.

- Making decisions that unnecessarily burden the dying patient should be avoided.
- Symptoms should be assessed and treated quickly.
- Orders that do not specifically enhance comfort should be avoided:
  - Monitoring of vital signs
  - Elaborate testing and diagnostic procedures
  - Gathering of blood and other body fluids for laboratory analysis
  - Medications other than those that relieve symptoms.

Medications

- The oral route of administration should be used as long as it is viable.
- When swallowing is no longer possible, or if gastrointestinal (GI) absorption is in question, an alternative route should be attempted:
  - transdermal
  - sublingual
  - subcutaneous or
  - rectal/vaginal.

Administration of sedatives and other essential drugs can be intravenous only if such access is readily available. The goal is to use the least invasive means possible to provide the maximum benefit.

Hydration and Nutrition

Hydration and nutrition are among the most disputed areas of terminal care, in which personal values and religious beliefs may conflict with accepted medical knowledge. A natural stage in dying occurs when the patient ceases to eat or drink. Although appetite has diminished gradually over many days or even weeks, as death approaches, the patient may refuse all food and oral fluids. It is at this point that physicians, sometimes at the insistance of well-meaning family members, will consider ordering intravenous hydration and/or insertion of a tube for enteral nutrition.

- Terminally ill patients do not need invasive nutritional support.
- Such support will not prolong life or reverse weight loss or weakness, or make the person feel stronger (4).

- Feeding tubes and intravenous lines have the effect of increasing the emotional distance between the patient and family.
- Hunger is rarely a source of discomfort. Some literature suggests that reduced food intake can produce a euphoric feeling such as one experienced by a healthy person who is fasting.

Similarly, hydration by artificial means may exacerbate discomfort and should be used only when the patient complains of thirst and is unable to drink. Dehydration in the terminal phase decreases pulmonary secretions that increase dyspnea; decreases urine output, which minimizes incontinence; and minimizes the possibility of vomiting.

Altered Mental Status and Terminal Restlessness

"Nearing death" experiences can be observed to be remarkably similar among dying patients in which the person in the final minutes or hours before death appears to be "seeing" into another dimension beyond earthly life (1). This is usually brief and transitory just before the patient lapses into the final unconsciousness. Should the patient become physically agitated and distressed to the point of attempting to climb out of bed, or if agitation is prolonged and is causing dyspnea, adequate sedation should be given to ease the anguish. It is important at this point that careful discussion takes place with family members for them to understand that this agitation is a terminal event, part of the illness, probably because of profound hypoxia, requiring sedation, and is not emotional distress or a sign of lack of readiness to die (4).

Family Needs as Death Approaches

The patients' families will need close contact and communication with the physician and nurses as death approaches. Practitioners must guide families through this difficult time with empathy and with the wisdom of experience. Each death experience will be unique because the individuals' coping strategies and experiences with death and their attachment to the dying person will affect their response. It is incumbent on the professional at the bedside to meet them at whatever level they are experiencing the death.

The most frequently asked question, "How long will it be?" can be best answered by a simple explanation of the significance of signs as they appear: changes in breathing, changes of skin color, weakening of pulses, and such signs. Simple explanations can guide the family in deciding when it is time to come together for the last time to say good-bye if they so desire.

REFERENCES

1. Kubler-Ross E. *On death and dying*. New York: Macmillan, 1969.
2. Byock I. *Dying well*. New York: Riverhead Books, 1997.
3. Nuland SB. *How we die*. New York: Knopf, 1994.
4. Kaye P. *Notes on symptom control in hospice and palliative care*. Essex, CT: Education Institute, 1992.
5. Rossman P. *Hospice*. New York: Fawcett Columbine, 1979.
6. U.S. Department of Health and Human Services. *Management of cancer pain: adults*. Rockville, MD: Agency for Health Care Policy and Research, AHCPR Publication No. 94-0593, 1994.

Targeted Treatments and Complimentary and Alternative Medicine

43

Targeted Therapies

James L. Gulley* and Gregory Curt†

*Laboratory of Tumor Immunology and Biology, Center for Cancer Research, National Cancer Institute, National Institutes of Health, Bethesda, Maryland; and †AstraZeneca Oncology, Garrett Park, Maryland

The ideal pharmaceutical agent acts on the target tissue without being toxic to other tissues, thereby having a wide therapeutic index. Initial anticancer agents fell far short of this ideal, with limited antitumor activity and considerable toxicity to normal tissues. Newer classes of promising drugs that target molecular structures or pathways unique to tumors are being developed. This chapter provides a brief overview on U.S. Food and Drug Administration (FDA)–approved targeted therapies.

MONOCLONAL ANTIBODIES

Monoclonal antibodies (MABs) take advantage of the exquisite specificity inherent in the immune system. The first generation of murine MABs had disappointing clinical results despite the ability to target tumors appropriately. This was caused by a lack of effector function of murine antibodies in humans (i.e., inability to facilitate antibody-dependent cellular cyto-toxicity or to complement mediated lysis) that was attributable to lack of murine Fc (constant fragment of an antibody molecule) functionality in humans and to significant induction of human anti–mouse-antibodies (HAMAs). This was overcome either by adding functionality to the antibodies (e.g., adding a radioisotope or toxin) or by "humanizing" the antibody to gain effector function and to decrease immunogenicity. Some MABs are completely human except for select segments of the hypervariable domain of the antibody (see Fig. 43.1). Several MABs have been FDA approved for either diagnostic testing or cancer therapy (see Table 43.1).

The nomenclature of MABs has a few unique rules. Generic names of MABs or fragments end in "mab." In addition, an MAB with the suffix "omab" indicates a murine antibody, "ximab" indicates a chimeric antibody, and "zumab" indicates a humanized antibody.

Rituximab (Rituxan)

- Rituximab (Rituxan) is a chimeric MAB that targets CD20, a marker found on B cells.
- It is indicated for relapsed or refractory, low-grade or follicular, CD20+ non-Hodgkin lymphoma (NHL).
- Overall response (OR) rate of single-agent rituximab was 48%, with 6% complete response (CR) in a multicenter, open-label, single-arm study of 166 patients with relapsed or refractory low-grade or follicular B-cell NHL (1). The median duration of response was 11.2 months (range, 1.9 to more than 42.1 months). See Chapter 28 for details about use.
- Toxicities include asthenia, dizziness, headache, nausea, vomiting, pruritus, and rash (common), and infection and hematologic, cardiac, and renal toxicity (serious).

555

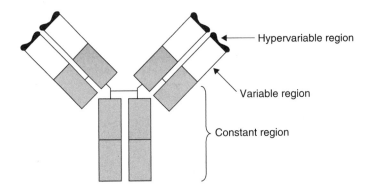

FIG. 43.1. Fully human and fully murine antibodies have all regions from their respective species. Chimeric antibodies generally have the constant regions from humans and variable regions from other species, whereas humanized antibodies generally have only select regions (such as the hypervariable region) from another species.

Trastuzumab (Herceptin)

- Trastuzumab (Herceptin) is a humanized antibody that targets the human epidermal growth factor receptor (HER-2), which is overexpressed in a variety of cancers.
- It is indicated in patients with breast cancer who overexpress HER-2, either in combination with paclitaxel as up-front treatment for disease, or as a single agent for those who have failed earlier chemotherapy.

TABLE 43.1. *U.S. Food and Drug Administration (FDA)-approved monoclonal antibodies (MABs) for cancer treatment*

Generic name	Trade name	Target	FDA indication
Rituximab	Rituxan	CD20	Relapsed or refractory, low-grade or follicular, CD20+ NHL
Tositumomab and I-131 tositumomab[a]	Bexxar	CD20	Refractory to rituximab, relapsed, CD20+ follicular NHL
(90)Y-ibritumomab tiuxetan[b]	Zevalin	CD20	Relapsed or refractory, low-grade, or transformed B-cell lymphoma
Alemtuzumab	Campath-1H	CD52	Salvage B-cell CLL
Gemtuzumab ozogamicin	Mylotarg	CD33	Relapsed acute myeloid leukemia
Trastuzumab	Herceptin	HER-2/neu	HER-2+ metastatic breast cancer
Bevacizumab	Avastin	VEGF	Metastatic colorectal cancer, frontline with 5-FU
Cetuximab	Erbitux	EGFR	Second line for metastatic colorectal cancer in combination with irinotecan

NHL, non-Hodgkin lymphoma; CLL, chronic lymphocytic leukemia; VEGF, vascular endothelial growth factor; 5-FU, 5-fluorouracil; EGFR, epidermal growth factor receptor.

[a]Unlabeled antibody is given first followed by labeled antibody. (131)I is both a β and γ emitter.

[b]Rituxumab is given first then (111)In labeled antibody (to assess biodistribution), then therapeutic (90)Y labeled antibody. (90)Y is a β emitter.

- In a pivotal phase III trial of 469 patients with HER-2–positive breast cancer who had not previously received chemotherapy for metastases, the patients were randomized to receive chemotherapy with or without traztuzumab. In contrast to the arm that received chemotherapy without traztuzumab, the combination arm had a longer median time to disease progression (TTP) (7.4 versus 4.6 months; p <0.001), higher OR rate (50% versus 32%; p <0.001), longer median duration of response (9.1 versus 6.1 months; p <0.001), longer median time to treatment failure (6.9 versus 4.5 months; p <0.001), and longer median overall survival (25.1 versus 20.3 months; p = 0.046) (2).
- The clinical benefit of trastuzumab has been seen largely for those patients who have 3+ HER-2 overexpression.
- The single-agent objective response rate of 24% in first-line therapy is somewhat higher than the rate seen for salvage therapy (3).
- Toxicities include anemia/leukopenia and diarrhea (common), and cardiomyopathy, infusion-associated symptoms, hypersensitivity reactions, and pulmonary events (serious).
- Combination therapy of trastuzumab and anthracyclines resulted in a high rate of cardiotoxicity (4). See Chapter 12 for details about use.

Tositumomab and Iodine-131 Tositumomab (Bexxar)

- Tositumomab and Iodine-131 Tositumomab (Bexxar) is a murine MAB that targets CD20.
- It is indicated for relapsed, CD20$^+$, follicular NHL that is refractory to rituxumab therapy.
- In a phase III study, 60 patients with chemotherapy-refractory low-grade or transformed low-grade B-cell NHL who have failed to respond to at least two chemotherapeutic regimens were treated with a single course of I-131 tositumomab (5). An OR rate of 65% (20% CR) was achieved with a median response duration of 6.5 months. These clinical parameters were a statistically significant improvement on the responses to the patients' previous qualifying chemotherapy.
- Toxicities include asthenia, headache, fever, infection, and hematologic toxicity (common), and pleural effusion and dehydration (serious).

(90)Y-Ibritumomab Tiuxetan (Zevalin)

- Ibritumomab is a murine MAB that targets CD20.
- It is indicated for relapsed or refractory, low-grade, or transformed B-cell lymphoma.
- In a randomized, comparative phase III study involving 143 patients with relapsed or refractory NHL (low-grade, follicular, or transformed), an overall objective response rate of 80% (30% CR) and 56% (16% CR) was reported in patients treated with Y-90 ibritumomab tiuxetan radioimmunotherapy and rituximab immunotherapy, respectively (p = 0.002) (6). Durable responses of 6 months were 64% in contrast to 47% (p = 0.030) favoring radioimmunotherapy.
- Toxicities include asthenia, dizziness, headache, and arthralgia (common), and myelosuppression, angioedema, and infection (serious).

Alemtuzumab (Campath)

- Alemtuzumab (Campath) is a humanized antibody that targets CD52, a cell surface marker found on essentially all T and B lymphocytes.
- It is indicated for B-cell chronic lymphocytic leukemia (CLL) in the salvage setting.
- In a phase II, open-label study, patients with previously treated, symptomatic CLL (n = 29) were assigned to receive intravenous alemtuzumab (7). Most patients had Rai stages III or IV and had undergone at least two prior chemotherapeutic regimens. Eleven of 29 patients (38%) attained a partial response (PR), 1 patient (4%) had a CR, and 12 patients (41%) had

stable disease. Complete morphologic remission within the bone marrow was observed in 9 of 25 assessable patients. The median duration of response was 12 months for the treatment responders.

- Toxicities include infusion reactions (common), and moderate hematologic toxicity with opportunistic infection as the primary treatment-related adverse event (serious).

Gemtuzumab Ozogamicin (Mylotarg)

- Gemtuzumab is a humanized MAB conjugated to calicheamicin that targets CD33, a marker found on the surface of leukemic blasts and immature normal cells of myelomonocytic lineage but not on normal hematopoietic stem cells.
- It is indicated for the treatment of patients with CD33$^+$ acute myeloid leukemia (AML) in first relapse who are 60 years or older and who are not considered candidates for other chemotherapeutic regimens.
- Controlled trials do not demonstrate an improvement in disease-related symptoms or increased survival compared with other treatment options Product Info Mylotarg, 2001 (8).
- Overall response rate is 30% in phase II studies ($n = 142$), with median overall survival of 5.9 months (9).
- Grade 3 or 4 toxicities are neutropenia (97%), thrombocytopenia (99%), hyperbilirubinemia (23%), and elevated hepatic transaminase levels (17%), and infections (28%).
- An 84% CR rate was reported in a phase II study of gemtuzumab ozogamicin in combination with cytarabine and daunorubicin in patients younger than 60 years with *de novo* AML (10).

Cetuximab (Erbitux)

- Cetuximab (Erbitux) is a chimeric anti–epidermal growth factor receptor (EGFR) MAB.
- It is indicated in metastatic colorectal cancer in combination with irinotecan in patients refractory to irinotecan.
- In a multicenter, randomized, controlled clinical trial conducted in 329 patients randomized to either cetuximab plus irinotecan ($n = 218$) or cetuximab monotherapy ($n = 111$), there was evidence of durable responses in the combination arm without evidence of an effect on survival (OR 23% versus 12%; TTP 4.1 versus 1.5 months).
- Toxicities include acneform rash (90%), asthenia/malaise (50%), and fever (33%).

Bevacizumab (Avastin)

- Bevacizumab (Avastin) is a humanized MAB directed against vascular endothelial growth factor (VEGF).
- It is indicated in combination with intravenous 5-fluorouracil-based chemotherapy as a therapy for patients with first-line metastatic cancer of the colon or rectum.
- In a large, placebo-controlled, randomized study, the median survival of patients treated with bevacizumab plus the IFL (5-FU/leucovorin/irinotecan) chemotherapeutic regimen ($n = 403$) was 20.3 months versus 15.6 months in the IFL chemotherapeutic regimen alone arm ($n = 412$; $p = 0.00003$) (11).
- Toxicities include asthenia, pain, hypertension, diarrhea, and leukopenia (common), and gastrointestinal (GI) perforations, wound healing complications, hemorrhage, hypertensive crises, nephrotic syndrome, and congestive heart failure (severe).

SMALL MOLECULES

Small molecules can be used to target specific pathways that are active in cancer cells so as to alter their ability to grow. Some of these drugs may be active as single agents, whereas others may be best used in combination with other therapies (see Table 43.2).

TABLE 43.2. *U.S. Food and Drug Administration (FDA)-approved small molecule targeted therapy for cancer treatment*

Generic name	Trade name	Target	FDA indication
Imatinib	Gleevec	C kit, PDGF	Philadelphia chromosome + CML c-Kit + GIST
Gefitinib	Iressa	EGFR	Locally advanced or metastatic nonsmall cell lung cancer after failure of both platinum-based and docetaxel chemotherapies
Bortezomib	Velcade	Proteosome inhibitor	For patients with MM who have failed two prior regimens
Denileukin diftitox[a]	Ontak	CD25	Persistent or recurrent CD 25+ cutaneous T-cell lymphoma

CML, chronic myeloid leukemia; PDGF, platelet-derived growth factor; GIST, gastrointestinal stromal tumors; EGFR, epidermal growth factor receptor; MM, multiple myeloma.

[a]Recombinant DNA-derived cytotoxic protein composed of the amino acid sequences for diphtheria toxin fragments A and B followed by the sequences for interleukin so that it binds to CD25. It is produced in an *Escherichia coli* expression system.

Imatinib Mesylate (Gleevec)

- Imatinib mesylate (Gleevec) is a protein-tyrosine kinase inhibitor that inhibits the Bcr-Abl tyrosine kinase, the constitutive abnormal tyrosine kinase created by the Philadelphia chromosome abnormality in chronic myeloid leukemia (CML). It is also an inhibitor of the receptor tyrosine kinase for platelet-derived growth factor (PDGF) and c-kit.
- It is indicated as first-line therapy in newly diagnosed patients with Philadelphia chromosome positive (Ph+) CML and Ph+ CML in blast, accelerated, or in chronic phase, after failure with interferon-α therapy, and in unresectable gastrointestinal stromal tumors (GIST).
- Its indication for CLL is based on superiority to interferon-α plus cytarabine in both tolerability and efficacy (12). See Chapter 11 for details on use.
- In GIST, imatinib mesylate is associated with a confirmed PR of greater than 50% (13).
- Toxicities include fluid retention, muscle cramps, nausea, vomiting, and diarrhea (common), and liver toxicity and myelosuppression (serious).

Gefitinib (Iressa)

- Gefitinib (Iressa) inhibits the intracellular phosphorylation of several tyrosine kinases associated with transmembrane cell surface receptors, including the tyrosine kinases associated with the EGFR.
- It is indicated as monotherapy for the treatment of patients with locally advanced or metastatic non–small cell lung cancer after failure of both platinum-based and docetaxel chemotherapies. See Chapter 2 for details regarding use.
- A clinical trial evaluated the effectiveness of two doses of gefitinib ($n = 221$; 142 evaluable) (14):
  - The patients had advanced non–small cell lung cancer with progressive disease (PD) after two earlier chemotherapeutic regimens including a platinum drug and docetaxel.
  - Twelve percent of the patients receiving a 250-mg daily dose ($n = 102$) experienced a partial radiographic response , which was better than the response (9%) for those receiving the 500-mg dose ($n = 114$).
- There is a greater probability of clinical response from patients with somatic EGFR mutations in the (adenosine 5'-triphosphate) ATP-binding pocket of the tyrosine kinase domain than from those patients without these mutations (15,16). These activating mutations occur more often in nonsmokers, women, and those with adenocarcinoma.

- Other large clinical trials combining gefitinib with chemotherapy did not show any clinical benefit from the addition of gefitinib (17).

Bortezomib (Velcade)

- Bortezomib (Velcade) is a reversible 26S proteasome inhibitor.
- It is indicated for patients with multiple myeloma (MM) who have failed to respond to at least two earlier therapies and who have progressed on their last therapy.
- In a single-arm phase II trial of 202 heavily pretreated refractory and relapsed patients with MM, 35% achieved an OR rate (median duration 12 months) (18).
- Bortezomib is being evaluated in combination with gemcitabine, docetaxel, and irinotecan in patients with solid tumors.
- Toxicities include fatigue, malaise, fever, constipation, and anorexia (common), and diarrhea, nausea, vomiting, anemia, thrombocytopenia, and peripheral neuropathy (serious).

Denileukin Diftitox (Ontak)

- Denileukin Diftitox (Ontak) is an interleukin-2 receptor-specific fusion protein consisting of diphtheria toxin fragments A and B fused to interleukin-2.
- It is indicated for persistent or recurrent CD 25^+ cutaneous T-cell lymphoma.
- An OR rate of 30% [10% CR or clinical complete response (CCR), 20% PR] was achieved in a phase III study ($n = 71$) of patients with Ib-III cutaneous T-cell lymphoma, either mycosis fungoides or Sezary syndrome (19).
- Toxicities include diarrhea, nausea, dyspnea, and flulike symptoms (common), and fever, hypotension, infections, and vascular leak syndrome (serious).

There is continuing research with a variety of different agents, including antibodies, small molecules, and vaccines. It is likely that these targeted therapies will offer some more therapeutic options that may be better tolerated than therapy with traditional cytotoxic agents.

REFERENCES

1. McLaughlin P, Grillo-Lopez AJ, Link BK, et al. Rituximab chimeric Anti-CD20 monoclonal antibody therapy for relapsed indolent lymphoma: half of patients respond to a four-dose treatment program. *J Clin Oncol* 1998;16(8):2825–2833.
2. Eiermann W. Trastuzumab combined with chemotherapy for the treatment of HER2-positive metastatic breast cancer: Pivotal trial data. *Ann Oncol* 2001;12:57–62.
3. Vogel CL, Cobleigh MA, Tripathy D, et al. First-line Herceptin (R) monotherapy in metastatic breast cancer. *Oncology* 2001;61:37–42.
4. Slamon DJ, Leyland-Jones B, Shak S, et al. Use of chemotherapy plus a monoclonal antibody against HER2 for metastatic breast cancer that overexpresses HER2. *N Engl J Med* 2001;344(11):783–792.
5. Kaminski MS, Zelenetz AD, Press OW, et al. Pivotal study of iodine I 131 Tositumomab for chemotherapy-refractory low-grade or transformed low-grade B-cell non-Hodgkin's lymphomas. *J Clin Oncol* 2001;19(19):3918–3928.
6. Witzig TE, Gordon LI, Cabanillas F, et al. Randomized controlled trial of yttrium-90-labeled ibritumomab tiuxetan radioimmunotherapy versus rituximab immunotherapy for patients with relapsed or refractory low-grade, follicular, or transformed B-cell non-Hodgkin's lymphoma. *J Clin Oncol* 2002; 20(10):2453–2463.
7. Osterborg A, Dyer MJS, Bunjes D, et al. Phase II multicenter study of human CD52 antibody in previously treated chronic lymphocytic leukemia. *J Clin Oncol* 1997;15(4):1567–1574.
8. http://www.wyeth.com/content/ShowLabeling.asp?id=119, 2001.
9. Sievers EL, Larson RA, Stadtmauer EA, et al. Efficacy and safety of gemtuzumab ozogamicin in patients with CD33-positive acute myeloid leukemia in first relapse. *J Clin Oncol* 2001;19(13):3244–3254.
10. Deangelo DJ, Liu D, Stone R, et al. Preliminary report of a phase 2 study of gemtuzumab ozogamicin in combination with cytarabine and daunorubicin in patients <60 years of age with de novo acute myeloid leukemia (A 2325). *Proc Am Soc Clin Oncol* 2004;22:578.

11. Hurwitz H, Fehrenbacher L, Cartwright T, et al. Bevacizumab (a monoclonal antibody to vascular endothelial growth factor) prolongs survival in first-line colorectal cancer (CRC): results of a phase III trial of bevacizumab in combination with bolus IFL (irinotecan, 5-fluorouracil, leucovorin) as first-line therapy in subjects with metastatic CRC. *Proc Am Soc Clin Oncol* 2003;22:A3646.

12. O'Brien SG, Guilhot F, Larson RA, et al. Imatinib compared with interferon and low-dose cytarabine for newly diagnosed chronic-phase chronic myeloid leukemia. *N Engl J Med* 2003;348(11):994–1004.

13. Demetri GD, von Mehren M, Blanke CD, et al. Efficacy and safety of imatinib mesylate in advanced gastrointestinal stromal tumors. *N Engl J Med* 2002;347(7):472–480.

14. Kris MG, Natale RB, Herbst RS, et al. Efficacy of gefitinib, an inhibitor of the epidermal growth factor receptor tyrosine kinase, in symptomatic patients with non-small cell lung cancer-A randomized trial. *J Am Med Assoc* 2003;290(16):2149–2158.

15. Lynch TJ, Bell DW, Sordella R, et al. Activating mutations in the epidermal growth factor receptor underlying responsiveness of non-small-cell lung cancer to gefitinib. *N Engl J Med* 2004;350:2129–2139.

16. Paez JG, Janne PA, Lee JC, et al. EGFR mutations in lung cancer: correlation with clinical response to gefitinib therapy. *Science* 2004;304:1497–1506.

17. Herbst RS, Giaccone G, Schiller JH, et al. Gefitinib in combination with paclitaxel and carboplatin in advanced non-small-cell lung cancer: a phase III trial—INTACT 2. *J Clin Oncol* 2004;22(5):785–794.

18. Richardson PG, Barlogie B, Berenson J, et al. A phase 2 study of bortezomib in relapsed, refractory myeloma. *N Engl J Med* 2003;348(26):2609–2617.

19. Olsen E, Duvic M, Frankel A, et al. Pivotal phase III trial of two dose levels of denileukin diftitox for the treatment of cutaneous T-cell lymphoma. *J Clin Oncol* 2001;19(2):376–388.

44

Complementary and Alternative Medicine in Oncology

Patrick J. Mansky, Dawn B. Wallerstedt, and Marc R. Blackman

National Center for Complementary and Alternative Medicine,
National Institutes of Health, Bethesda, Maryland

During the last decade, patients with cancer have increasingly turned to complementary and alternative medicine (CAM) resources in an attempt to cure cancer, to provide relief from cancer-related symptoms, or to improve overall well-being and quality of life. Complementary and alternative medicine, as defined by the National Center for Complementary and Alternative Medicine (NCCAM), is a group of diverse medical and health care systems, practices, and products that are not presently considered to be part of conventional medicine (1,2). Although some scientific evidence exists about some CAM therapies, for most therapies there are key questions that are yet to be answered through well-designed scientific studies—questions such as whether these therapies are safe and whether they work for the diseases or medical conditions for which they are used.

The list of what is considered to be CAM changes continually, as those therapies that are proven to be safe and effective become adopted into conventional health care and as new approaches to health care emerge (http://nccam.nih.gov/health/whatiscam/#1).

Scientific assessments of safety, efficacy, and mode of action are either fragmented or totally lacking for many CAM modalities and approaches.

THE DOMAINS OF COMPLEMENTARY AND ALTERNATIVE MEDICINE

NCCAM groups the CAM modalities into five major domains that are applicable to cancer-related CAM (see Fig. 44.1).

USE OF COMPLEMENTARY AND ALTERNATIVE MEDICINE IN PATIENTS WITH CANCER

CAM use in patients with cancer varies according to region, geographical location, gender, and disease diagnosis. This chapter focuses on the data available on cancer patients in the United States. The prevalence of CAM use in patients with cancer has been estimated to be between 7% and 54% (1).

Predictors of Use of Complementary and Alternative Medicine in Patients with Cancer

- Higher educational status
- White ethnicity

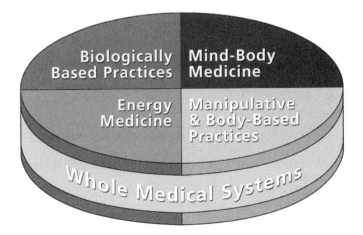

FIG. 44.1. The complementary and alternative medicine (CAM) domains. (Source: http://nccam.nih.gov/about/plans/2005/index.htm, accessed 3/17/2005, with permission.)

- Deteriorating health status
- Women

Preferred Complementary and Alternative Medicine Modalities in Patients with Cancer

Following is a list of CAM modalities used frequently by cancer patients:

- Herbs, dietary supplements, and minerals
- Special diets
- Spirituality
- Meditation or mind–body work
- Relaxation or guided imagery
- Acupuncture
- Healing touch
- Support groups
- Yoga

Patients with cancer who use CAM often utilize several CAM modalities concurrently.

Use of Complementary and Alternative Medicine and Treatment Expectations

Comparisons of the reasons for CAM use among patients with different cancer diagnoses show many similarities. Most of the patients with cancer use CAM hoping to:

- Boost the immune system
- Relieve pain
- Control side effects related to disease or treatment.

Only a few patients include CAM in the treatment plan with curative intent (2).

COMPLEMENTARY AND ALTERNATIVE MEDICINE
APPROACHES TO CANCER TREATMENT

A diverse array of CAM approaches has been used in clinical practice for the treatment of cancer and cancer-related symptoms. A comprehensive review of existing CAM practices used in cancer is beyond the scope of this chapter. Rather, the focus is on a set of CAM modalities and approaches based on the following selection criteria:

- Accessibility and availability within the United States
- Existence of peer-reviewed published information on efficacy or treatment-associated clinical benefit
- Components of the CAM cancer treatment spectrum commonly employed (based on published demographic data) as complementary modalities by health care professionals or requested by patients
- Alternative medical systems approaches are not included in this chapter. There is a paucity of published data from controlled clinical trials on the efficacy of these approaches in the treatment of cancer. The interested reader is referred to the available literature and is encouraged to seek advice from trained experts in the field (3,4).
- Biologics employed in the treatment of cancer are not discussed in detail in this chapter. Most biologics would be considered experimental from the perspective of available scientific evidence of activity in cancer. Some fall into the category of alternative medical systems. For some of the agents the interested reader is referred to the information available on the CAM Physician's Data Query (PDQ) Web site of the National Cancer Institute (NCI) at http://www.nci.nih.gov/cancerinfo/pdq/cam.
- A separate section has been included in this chapter to address some emerging data on interactions between botanicals and drugs and on resources regarding ongoing clinical trials that are investigating the efficacy of CAM, and that may be available to interested cancer patients.

CAM therapies discussed in this chapter are grouped into the following categories:

1. Cancer symptom management
2. Diet/nutrition/supplements

Cancer Symptom Management

Acupuncture

Acupuncture and electroacupuncture are widely used in cancer symptom management. A number of acupuncture approaches are being practiced, including Chinese, Japanese, Korean, and French acupuncture.

According to the 1997 NIH Consensus Conference on acupuncture (http://dowland.cit.nih.gov/odp/consensus/107/107_statement.htm), existing evidence based on clinical trials suggests a beneficial role for acupuncture in the areas of chemotherapy-induced nausea/vomiting and dental pain, whereas the clinical evidence for efficacy of acupuncture in other settings remains limited.

Adverse effects:

Acupuncture is generally well tolerated. The most frequent side effects include minimal local bleeding or bruising and mild pain (5,6).

Caveats:

Acupuncture is not advisable in patients with:

- Thrombocytopenia
- Bleeding disorders
- Aplasia

Chemotherapy-induced Nausea and Vomiting

Commonly used acupuncture points include *P6*, Neiguan point of the pericardium meridian of hand (jueyin), and *St 36*, Zunsali point of the stomach meridian of foot (yang ming). Treatment is commonly started before administration of antiemetic agents or chemotherapy. Both acupuncture and electroacupuncture are being used (7).

Cancer Pain

Neuropathic pain

Clinical evidence for the efficacy of acupuncture in treating cancer-related pain has not been fully established. Recent data suggest a role for auricular acupuncture in patients experiencing ongoing cancer-related neuropathic pain managed with stable analgesic regimens (8).

Metastatic bone pain

A role for acupuncture in the treatment of metastatic bone pain has not been established.

Palliative pain management

Several case reports and published articles suggest a role for acupuncture in the palliation of chronic pain. Provided that caveats for the treatment, as listed in the subsequent text, are considered, acupuncture may be a helpful adjunct if performed by a trained specialist with experience in this clinical setting.

Cognitive–Behavioral Interventions

Cognitive–behavioral interventions are defined as mind–body approaches that aim to change specific thoughts and/or behaviors or to develop new coping skills (9).

Cognitive–behavioral modalities include:

• Progressive muscle relaxation training
• Hypnotherapy
• Systematic desensitization
• Biofeedback
• Behavior modification

Summary

Behavioral interventions, including guided imagery, hypnosis, relaxation training, and emotive imagery, have been effective in (9,10):

• Diminishing anticipatory nausea and vomiting in both children and adults with cancer who receive chemotherapy
• Lessening anxiety and distress caused by invasive medical procedures
• Decreasing acute pain caused by invasive medical procedures

However, there have been no documented effects of behavioral interventions:

• in moderating chronic pain in cancer populations
• in relieving postchemotherapy nausea and vomiting, and chronic pain.

Meditation

Cancer therapists and patients with cancer have been employing a wide range of meditation methods to alleviate cancer symptoms. The two most widely studied techniques are transcendental meditation (TM) and mindfulness-based meditation. TM uses the repetition of a specific mantra with the intent of quieting and ultimately "transcending" the practitioner's internal mental dialogue. Mindfulness-based meditation strives to develop an objective "observer role" for the practitioner toward his own emotions, feelings, perceptions, and so on, thereby creating a nonjudgmental "mindful" state of conscious awareness. Other meditation practices are usually pursued in a religious or spiritual context.

Transcendental Meditation

Studies of TM in patients with cancer the management of cancer symptoms are lacking.. There is weak evidence that TM may help with reduction of anxiety and stress (11), but it remains unclear how this information can be translated into the cancer setting.

Mindfulness Meditation

The mindfulness-based stress reduction (MBSR) program was developed by Jon Kabat-Zinn. The components of sitting meditation, body scan, and mindful movement are taught over a training period of 7 to 8 weeks (12).

Studies of MBSR in cancer populations (13,14,15) suggest that MBSR may result in:

• Decrease in anxiety and in mood disturbances
• Decrease in depression, anger, and confusion
• Change in posttreatment total stress scores

The Mindfulness-based Stress Reduction Caveats

• MBSR is a highly structured, didactic program
• It may not be appropriate for patients of all educational levels

Yoga

Deriving from the Ayurvedic medical system, yoga combines breath awareness and control with meditation, movement, and chanting. Studies have supported its beneficial role in stress management, anxiety reduction, and insomnia (16). Although no studies could be found that specifically utilized yoga alone as an intervention for individuals with cancer, it is likely a safe modality except in patients with bone metastases, who are at risk for pathologic fractures.

Therapeutic Massage

Therapeutic massage is generally practiced as a series of strokes and kneading movements aimed at treating the body without adjusting any body structures. Details of the array of massage techniques and approaches can be found in the literature. In general, patients should be treated only by experienced, trained, and (if applicable) licensed massage therapists.

• The limited data available suggest that massage therapy may reduce anxiety (17).
• No data are available on the efficacy of massage for cancer pain (17).
• The efficacy of manual lymph drainage is unclear (18,19).

Adverse events:

• Bruising
• Internal bleeding
• Fractures at sites of bone metastasis

Caveats:

- Coagulopathy
- Thrombus in area of massage
- Prosthetic devices/stents in the massage field
- Irradiated skin and tissues

Distant Healing Modalities

"Distant healing" interventions include such modalities as therapeutic touch, Reiki, spiritual healing, prayer, and external Qigong. Some of these interventions, such as Reiki, are based on the belief that the practitioner serves as a conduit of subtle vibrational energy flow by placement of hands on the recipient, while others, such as therapeutic touch, do not necessarily require direct contact with the recipient.

- The data claiming efficacy for these modalities is controversial from a scientific viewpoint.
- The mechanism by which potential benefit can be derived from these modalities has not been elucidated.
- A number of randomized clinical trials (RCTs) and several reviews of beneficial effects have been published.
- However, only a few studies have been conducted in cancer populations.

Available data from a recent meta-analysis conducted by Astin et al. (20) show:

- Sixteen double-blind studies of the total of 23
- Ten positive studies using therapeutic touch versus a sham control
- Two positive studies using distant intercessory prayer
- Four positive studies using other forms of distant healing
- Only one of the studies included in this meta-analysis was conducted in a population of patients with cancer (18 children with leukemia) (21).

The only RCT utilizing Reiki as an intervention in a cohort of patients with cancer (22) reported no sustained reduction in pain scores.

Complementary and Alternative Medicine for Menopausal Symptoms in Patients with Cancer

A number of botanical products including soy and soy extracts, black cohosh (*Cimicifuga racemosa*), chaste tree berry (*Vitex agnus-cactus*), don quai (*Angelica sinensis*), ginseng (*Panax ginseng*), evening primrose oil (*Oenothera biennis*), red clover (*Trifolium* pratense), motherwort (*Leonurus cardiaca*), and licorice (*Glycyrrhiza glabra*) have been widely used as adjunct treatments for menopausal symptoms including hot flashes, considered to be mostly due to the effects of the isoflavone components.

A recent review of 29 RCTs of CAM therapies for menopausal symptoms (23) concluded that:

- Black cohosh and phytoestrogen-containing foods show promise in the treatment of menopausal symptoms
- Clinical trials do not support the use of other herbs or CAM therapies for menopausal symptoms.

Limited data based on two RCTs of soy beverage (24) and phytoestrogen tablets (25) specifically used by *postmenopausal* women with breast cancer concluded, respectively, that:

- Soy phytoestrogens administered as a soy beverage do not alleviate hot flashes
- Pure isoflavones administered as tablets do not alleviate menopausal symptoms.

Diet/Nutrition/Supplements

Dietary Supplements

The antioxidant vitamins A, C, and E are commonly used by patients with cancer in an attempt to improve disease outcome. There is currently no published information based on controlled clinical trials available that would suggest that a specific dietary supplement or a supplement combination is effective in curing cancer.

Vitamin A

Vitamin A may promote the progression of latent prostate cancer (26) and may result in increased lung cancer incidence in high-risk populations (27). On the basis of available evidence, vitamin A should not be administered in excess of the recommended daily allowance.

Adverse effects:

• Hypervitaminosis A when administered in high doses

Caveats:

• Prostate cancer
• Lung cancer risk or lung cancer

Vitamin C

Vitamin C is an essential nutrient. RCTs with oral vitamin C have failed to show clinical benefit in the treatment of cancer (28). Some of the observed anecdotal benefits of vitamin C may be related to the much higher bioavailability of vitamin C when administered intravenously than when administered orally (29,30). There is no scientific rationale for administering vitamin C orally in high doses.

Vitamin E

Vitamin E, in addition to acting as a free radical scavenger, may block gastric formation of carcinogenic nitrosamines and may enhance the immune function. Nonetheless, clinical trials and surveys that have attempted to demonstrate a relation between vitamin E and the incidence of cancer have been generally inconclusive. Vitamin E may prevent progression of latent prostate cancer (17). Increased vitamin E serum levels following dietary supplementation have been associated with decreased risk for esophageal and gastric cancer in high-risk populations (31,32). Vitamin E in high doses interferes with platelet function (26).

Adverse effects (high doses of vitamin E):

• Thrombocytopenia

Caveats:

• Surgery
• Anticoagulant therapy

Diet

Soy

Soy, a subtropical plant native to southeastern Asia, has been a main dietary component in Asian countries for at least 5,000 years. More easily digestible fermented forms of soy include tempeh, miso, and tamari soy sauce. Soy and the soy components, isoflavones (such as genistein), are believed to exert estrogenic effects (33,34). Although genistein has demonstrated anticancer effects in preclinical studies, the effects of genistein on cancer in humans *in vivo* have not been adequately determined (35). Preliminary research on humans suggests that soy isoflavones do not exert the same effects on the body as do estrogens (e.g., promoting the thickening of the endometrium) (33). It remains to be determined whether the consumption of soy by adults affects the risk of developing breast cancer, and whether soy consumption affects the survival of patients with breast cancer (36).

The role of soy and soy components in the prevention and treatment of prostate cancer in humans remains unclear (37,38).

Diet Composition

Whole grains/fiber (39)

• Whole grains and fiber are protective against cancer, especially gastrointestinal cancers such as gastric and colonic, and hormone-dependent cancers including cancers of breast and prostate.

Fruits and vegetables

Published case–control and cohort studies are inconclusive about the protective effect of fruits and vegetables against cancer risk (40).

• Balanced diets rich in fresh fruits and vegetables can be recommended for patients with cancer (41).
• Extremes in diet may be associated with poorer survival rates (42).
• Ongoing research is investigating the benefit of a diet rich in fruits and vegetables for improving survival in cancer (e.g., in breast cancer) (43,44).

Nutrition: Specialized Diets

Specialized diets have not been shown to improve cancer survival or cancer-related symptoms in controlled clinical trials, and may even be unsafe for use in some patients with cancer.

Gerson Diet

The Gerson diet is a metabolic treatment method based on the idea of detoxifying the body by eliminating commercially farmed fruits, vegetables, and prepared foods. The intake of numerous food items is restricted. The diet calls for 13 hourly glasses of juice from organically grown fruits and vegetables, supplemented by a specific regimen of supplements and coffee enemas (45). No prospective, controlled studies have been published that confirm the safety or effectiveness of the Gerson diet in the treatment of cancer.

Adverse effects:

• Pain, diarrhea, and cramping caused by the diet itself and from the coffee enemas
• Electrolyte imbalances
• Infections
• Colitis

Caveats:

This is a very stringent and restrictive regimen that may require close monitoring for risks of side effects and complications.

Macrobiotics

Macrobiotic diets are among the most popular comprehensive, nutrition-based CAM treatment approaches to cancer. Macrobiotics is based on a predominantly vegetarian, whole-foods diet consisting of 20% to 30% vegetables, 50% to 60% cereal grains, and 5% to 10% beans and legumes. Sweets, fruits, seafood, and nuts or seeds are limited to a few times per week, whereas meats, eggs, and dairy products are consumed only once a week, if at all.

- The dietary components of the macrobiotic diet have been associated with decreased cancer risk.
- Macrobiotic diets may lower the levels of circulating estrogen in women.
- The role of macrobiotics in the treatment of cancer has not been investigated adequately (46).

Adverse effects:

- The risk of nutritional deficiencies in poorly nourished patients
- Some components of the macrobiotic diet may alter the metabolism of certain drugs

Caveats:

- Caution is called for, especially in women with estrogen-receptor (ER) positive breast cancer or endometrial cancer, because of the high phytoestrogen content of some macrobiotic diets.
- Macrobiotic diets are a potentially useful adjunct to conventional treatment in well-nourished patients, if closely monitored by an experienced oncologist (17).

Gonzalez Regimen

Dr. Gonzalez's summary of the findings of Dr. William Donald Kelley, a Texas dentist, who for 20 years had been treating patients with cancer with a complicated nutritional therapy, suggested a marked survival advantage for patients with advanced pancreatic cancer, among other disease groups. An NCI-sponsored pilot study of 11 patients with advanced pancreatic cancer treated with this approach (regimen details: http://www.dr-gonzalez.com/regimen.htm) showed promising results (47). An NCI-sponsored clinical trial is actively enrolling patients with advanced pancreatic cancer (http://www.cancer.gov/ClinicalTrials/view_clinicaltrials.aspx?cdrid=67012&protocolnum=&version=patient&protocolsearchid=432236).

At this point, no published prospective clinical trials have demonstrated the efficacy of the Gonzalez regimen in the treatment of cancer.

Adverse effects:

- Diarrhea and cramping from engaging in a regimen that includes coffee enemas
- Electrolyte imbalances

Caveats:

- Infectious risk associated with the ingestion of raw meat extracts

Weight Management

- Current evidence suggests an increased risk for disease recurrence in women with breast cancer who are overweight (48,43).

TABLE 44.1. *Drug interactions of five of the top-selling botanicals on the U.S. market*

Botanical	Drug interactions
Saint John's wort	5-HT1 agonists (triptans), alprazolam, aminolevulinic acid, amitriptyline, analgesics with serotonergic activity, antidepressants, barbiturates, cyclosporine, digoxin, dextromethorphan, fenfluramine, fexofenadine, irinotecan, monoamine oxidase inhibitors, narcotics, nefazodone, NNRTIs, nortriptyline, oral contraceptives, paroxetine, phenobarbital, phenprocoumon, phenytoin, photosensitizing drugs, protease inhibitors, reserpine, sertraline, tacrolimus, theophylline, warfarin
Ginkgo biloba	Anticoagulant-antiplatelet drugs (aspirin, heparin, indomethacin), buspirone, fluoxetine, insulin, MAOIs, seizure-threshold–lowering drugs, thiazide diuretics, trazodone, warfarin, other drugs metabolized by cytochrome P-450: CYP1A2 (acetaminophen, diazepam, estradiol, ondansetron, propranolol, and warfarin), CYP2D6 (amitriptyline, codeine, fentanyl, fluoxetine, meperidine, methadone, ondansetron, and others) and CYP3A4 [chemotherapeutic agents (etoposide, paclitaxel, vinblastine, vincristine, and vindesine), antifungals (ketoconazole and itraconazole), glucocorticoids, fentanyl, calcium channel blockers (diltiazem, nicardipine, and verapamil), and others]
Panax Ginseng	Anticoagulant-antiplatelet drugs (aspirin, heparin, indomethacin), antipsychotic drugs, caffeine, furosemide, immunosuppressants (azathioprine, cyclosporine, tacrolimus, prednisone, others), insulin, MAOIs, oral hypoglycemic agents (glimepiride, glyburide), stimulant drugs, warfarin, other drugs metabolized by cytochrome p450 CYP2D6 enzyme (amitriptyline, codeine, fentanyl, fluoxetine, meperidine, methadone, ondansetron, and others)
Allium sativum (garlic)	Anticoagulant–antiplatelet drugs (warfarin, aspirin, heparin, and indomethacin), cyclosporine, NNRTIs, saquinavir (potentially, other protease inhibitors), oral contraceptives, other drugs: preparations containing allicin may increase the activity of the cytochrome P450 CYP3A4. Drugs that might be affected include chemotherapeutic agents (etoposide, paclitaxel, vinblastine, vincristine, and vindesine), antifungals (ketoconazole and itraconazole), glucocorticoids, fentanyl, calcium channel blockers (diltiazem, nicardipine, and verapamil), and others
Piper methysticum (kava)	Alcohol, alprazolam, CNS depressants, hepatotoxic drugs (azathioprine, methotrexate, and tamoxifen), levodopa, other drugs metabolized by cytochrome p450 enzymes: CYP1A2, CYP2C9 (tamoxifen and warfarin); CYP 2C19 (cyclophosphamide), CYP2D6 (codeine, ondansetron, and paroxetine), and CYP3A4 (cyclosporine and others)

NNRTIs, nonnucleoside reverse transcriptase inhibitors; MAOI, monoamine oxidase inhibitors; CNS, central nervous system.

From Jellin JM, Gregory PJ, Batz F, Hitchens K, et al. "Pharmacist's Letter/Prescriber's Letter Natural Medicines Comprehensive Database," Stockton CA; Therapeutic Research Faculty; www.naturaldatabase.com accessed on 12-05-03, with permission.

- Research is ongoing into the role of exercise and weight management in the prevention of breast cancer recurrence (41).
- Weight control and moderate exercise may reduce the risk for concomitant illnesses (e.g., cardiovascular disease).

COMPLEMENTARY AND ALTERNATIVE MEDICINE IN CANCER: INTERACTIONS AND CAVEATS

Botanical–Drug Interactions

The role of biologics in the CAM treatment of cancer is not discussed in detail in this chapter. However, the interaction of botanicals and nutritional supplements with pharmaceutical drugs is being reported with increasing frequency nowadays (49). Commonly used botanicals that affect the metabolism of pharmaceutical drugs in humans are listed in Table 44.1.

Caveats Related to the Use of Complementary and Alternative Medicine Therapy

A number of caveats relating to the use of CAM therapies have been listed during the course of this chapter. The following is a summary of some important caveats for consideration when using complementary therapies in the treatment of cancer patients:

Therapy	Caveat
Highly restrictive diets	Poor nutritional status
Antioxidants	Concurrent radio/chemotherapy
Supplements with anticoagulant activity	Low platelet count, surgery
Phytoestrogens	Breast cancer (ER+)
Acupuncture	Low platelet count, anticoagulation
Deep tissue/forceful massage	Low platelet count, anticoagulation
St. John's wort	Chemotherapy
High-dose vitamin A	Try to avoid
High-dose vitamin C	Try to avoid

COMPLEMENTARY AND ALTERNATIVE MEDICINE IN CANCER: INFORMATION RESOURCES

National Center for Complementary and Alternative Medicine (NCCAM)
http://nccam.nih.gov
Information about CAM
http://nccam.nih.gov/health
Information about CAM cancer research
http://nccam.nih.gov/research
National Cancer Institute (NCI)
http://www.cancer.gov
Information about CAM cancer research trials
http://www.nci.nih.gov/clinicaltrials
Information about CAM in Cancer
http://cancer.gov/cancerinfo/pdq/cam
Office of Cancer Complementary and Alternative Medicine (OCCAM), NCI
http://www.cancer.gov/occam
Information about CAM cancer research
http://www3.cancer.gov/occam/research
Office of Dietary Supplements (ODS), NIH
http://dietary-supplements.info.nih.gov

Information about dietary supplements
http://dietary-supplements.info.nih.gov/health.aspx
Information about dietary supplement research
http://dietary-supplements.info.nih.gov/research.aspx

REFERENCES

1. Ernst E, Cassileth BR. The prevalence of complementary/alternative medicine in cancer: a systematic review. *Cancer* 1998;83(4):777–782.
2. Morris KT, Johnson N, Homer L, et al. A comparison of complementary therapy use between breast cancer patients and patients with other primary tumor sites. *Am J Surg* 2000;179(5):407–411.
3. Beinfield H, Korngold E. Chinese medicine and cancer care. *Altern Ther Health Med* 2003;9(5):38–52.
4. Singh RH. An assessment of the ayurvedic concept of cancer and a new paradigm of anticancer treatment in Ayurveda. *J Altern Complement Med* 2002;8(5):609–614.
5. MacPherson H, Thomas K, Walters S, et al. The York acupuncture safety study: prospective survey of 34 000 treatments by traditional acupuncturists. *BMJ* 2001;323(7311):486–487.
6. White A, Hayhoe S, Hart A, et al. Adverse events following acupuncture: prospective survey of 32 000 consultations with doctors and physiotherapists. *BMJ* 2001;323(7311):485–486.
7. Shen J, Wenger N, Glaspy J, et al. Electroacupuncture for control of myeloablative chemotherapy-induced emesis: a randomized controlled trial. *JAMA* 2000;284(21):2755–2761.
8. Alimi D, Rubino C, Pichard-Leandri E, et al. Analgesic effect of auricular acupuncture for cancer pain: a randomized, blinded, controlled trial. *J Clin Oncol* 2003;21(22):4120–4126.
9. Meyer TJ, Mark MM. Effects of psychosocial interventions with adult cancer patients: a meta-analysis of randomized experiments. *Health Psychol* 1995;14(2):101–108.
10. Redd WH, Montgomery GH, DuHamel KN. Behavioral intervention for cancer treatment side effects. *J Natl Cancer Inst* 2001;93(11):810–823.
11. Canter PH. The therapeutic effects of meditation. *BMJ* 2003;326(7398):1049–1050.
12. Barrows KA, Jacobs BP, Speca M, et al. Mind-body medicine. An introduction and review of the literature. *Med Clin North Am* 2002;86(1):11–31.
13. Speca M, Carlson LE, Goodey E, et al. A randomized, wait-list controlled clinical trial: the effect of a mindfulness meditation-based stress reduction program on mood and symptoms of stress in cancer outpatients. *Psychosom Med* 2000;62(5):613–622.
14. Carlson LE, Speca M, Patel KD, et al. Mindfulness-based stress reduction in relation to quality of life, mood, symptoms of stress, and immune parameters in breast and prostate cancer outpatients. *Psychosom Med* 2003;65(4):571–581.
15. Carlson LE, Ursuliak Z, Goodey E, et al. The effects of a mindfulness meditation-based stress reduction program on mood and symptoms of stress in cancer outpatients: 6-month follow-up. *Support Care Cancer* 2001;9(2):112–123.
16. Ott MJ. Complementary and alternative therapies in cancer symptom management. *Cancer Pract* 2002;10(3):162–166.
17. Weiger WA, Smith M, Boon H, et al. Advising patients who seek complementary and alternative medical therapies for cancer. *Ann Intern Med* 2002;137(11):889–903.
18. Johansson K, Albertsson M, Ingvar C, et al. Effects of compression bandaging with or without manual lymph drainage treatment in patients with postoperative arm lymphedema. *Lymphology* 1999; 32(3):103–110.
19. Johansson K, Lie E, Ekdahl C, et al. A randomized study comparing manual lymph drainage with sequential pneumatic compression for treatment of postoperative arm lymphedema. *Lymphology* 1998;31(2):56–64.
20. Astin JA, Harkness E, Ernst E, et al. The efficacy of "distant healing": a systematic review of randomized trials. *Ann Intern Med* 2000;132(11):903–10.
21. Collipp PJ, Olson K, Hanson J, et al. The efficacy of prayer: a triple-blind study. *Med Times* 1969; 97(5):201–204.
22. Olson K, Hanson J, Michaud M, et al. A phase II trial of Reiki for the management of pain in advanced cancer patients. *J Pain Symptom Manage* 2003;26(5):990–997.
23. Kronenberg F, Fugh-Berman A, Nikander E, et al. Complementary and alternative medicine for menopausal symptoms: a review of randomized, controlled trials. *Ann Intern Med* 2002;137(10): 805–813.

24. Van Patten CL, Olivotto IA, Chambers GK, et al. Effect of soy phytoestrogens on hot flashes in post-menopausal women with breast cancer: a randomized, controlled clinical trial. *J Clin Oncol* 2002; 20(6):1449–1455.
25. Nikander E, Kilkkinen A, Metsa-Heikkila M, et al. A randomized placebo-controlled crossover trial with phytoestrogens in treatment of menopause in breast cancer patients. *Obstet Gynecol* 2003; 101(6):1213–1220.
26. Heinonen OP, Albanes D, Virtamo J, et al. Prostate cancer and supplementation with alpha-tocopherol and beta-carotene: incidence and mortality in a controlled trial. *J Natl Cancer Inst* 1998;90(6):440–446.
27. Omenn GS, Goodman GE, Thornquist MD, et al. Effects of a combination of beta carotene and vitamin A on lung cancer and cardiovascular disease. *N Engl J Med* 1996;334(18):1150–1155.
28. Weitzman S. Alternative nutritional cancer therapies. *Int J Cancer Suppl* 1998;11:69–72.
29. Padayatty SJ, Levine M. Reevaluation of ascorbate in cancer treatment: emerging evidence, open minds and serendipity. *J Am Coll Nutr* 2000;19(4):423–425.
30. Padayatty SJ, Katz A, Wang Y, et al. Vitamin C as an antioxidant: evaluation of its role in disease prevention. *J Am Coll Nutr* 2003;22(1):18–35.
31. Blot WJ, Li JY, Taylor PR, et al. The Linxian trials: mortality rates by vitamin-mineral intervention group. *Am J Clin Nutr* 1995;62(Suppl. 6):1424S–1426S.
32. Taylor PR, Qiao YL, Abnet CC, et al. Prospective study of serum vitamin E levels and esophageal and gastric cancers. *J Natl Cancer Inst* 2003;95(18):1414–1416.
33. Penotti M, Fabio E, Modena AB, et al. Effect of soy-derived isoflavones on hot flushes, endometrial thickness, and the pulsatility index of the uterine and cerebral arteries. *Fertil Steril* 2003;79(5): 1112–1117.
34. Wuttke W, Jarry H, Becker T, et al. Phytoestrogens: endocrine disrupters or replacement for hormone replacement therapy? *Maturitas* 2003;44(Suppl. 1):S9–20.
35. Dixon RA, Ferreira D. Genistein. *Phytochemistry* 2002;60(3):205–211.
36. Messina MJ, Loprinzi CL. Soy for breast cancer survivors: a critical review of the literature. *J Nutr* 2001;131(Suppl. 11):3095S–3108S.
37. Castle EP, Thrasher JB. The role of soy phytoestrogens in prostate cancer. *Urol Clin North Am* 2002;29(1):71–81, viii–ix.
38. Morrissey C, Watson RW, Castle EP, et al. Phytoestrogens and prostate cancer. *Curr Drug Targets* 2003;4(3):231–241.
39. Slavin JL. Mechanisms for the impact of whole grain foods on cancer risk. *J Am Coll Nutr* 2000; 19(Suppl. 3):300S–307S.
40. Riboli E, Norat T. Epidemiologic evidence of the protective effect of fruit and vegetables on cancer risk. *Am J Clin Nutr* 2003;78(Suppl. 3):559S–569S.
41. Rock CL, Demark-Wahnefried W. Nutrition and survival after the diagnosis of breast cancer: a review of the evidence. *J Clin Oncol* 2002;20(15):3302–3316.
42. Goodwin PJ, Ennis M, Pritchard KI, et al. Diet and breast cancer: evidence that extremes in diet are associated with poor survival. *J Clin Oncol* 2003;21(13):2500–2507.
43. Rock CL, Demark-Wahnefried W, Chlebowski RT, et al. Can lifestyle modification increase survival in women diagnosed with breast cancer? A randomized trial of the effect of a plant-based dietary pattern on additional breast cancer events and survival: the Women's Healthy Eating and Living (WHEL) Study. *J Nutr* 2002;132(Suppl. 11):3504S–3507S.
44. Pierce JP, Faerber S, Wright FA, et al. A randomized trial of the effect of a plant-based dietary pattern on additional breast cancer events and survival: the Women's Healthy Eating and Living (WHEL) Study. *Control Clin Trials* 2002;23(6):728–756.
45. Gerson M. The cure of advanced cancer by diet therapy: a summary of 30 years of clinical experimentation. *Physiol Chem Phys* 1978;10(5):449–464.
46. Kushi LH, Cunningham JE, Hebert JR, et al. The macrobiotic diet in cancer. *J Nutr* 2001;131 (Suppl. 11):3056S–3064S.
47. Gonzalez NJ, Isaacs LL. Evaluation of pancreatic proteolytic enzyme treatment of adenocarcinoma of the pancreas, with nutrition and detoxification support. *Nutr Cancer* 1999;33(2):117–124.
48. Chlebowski RT, Aiello E, McTiernan A, et al. Weight loss in breast cancer patient management. A randomized trial of the effect of a plant-based dietary pattern on additional breast cancer events and survival: the Women's Healthy Eating and Living (WHEL) Study. *J Clin Oncol* 2002;20(4):1128–1143.
49. Sorensen JM. Herb-drug, food-drug, nutrient-drug, and drug-drug interactions: mechanisms involved and their medical implications. *J Altern Complement Med* 2002;8(3):293–308.

SECTION 13

Common Procedures and Chemotherapy Drugs

45

Central Venous Access Devices

Deborah Charest-Gutierrez and Naomi P. O'Grady

Procedures, Vascular Access and Conscious Sedation Service,
National Institutes of Health, Bethesda, Maryland

Treatment for patients with cancer frequently requires the placement of a vascular access device (VAD) for administering chemotherapy, total parenteral nutrition, analgesics, or antibiotics, or for frequent blood sampling. In some cases, vascular access may require only a peripheral intravenous (i.v.) catheter (i.e., the tip of the catheter remains within the peripheral circulation). Increasingly, however, there is a need for access to the central venous circulation with a central VAD [i.e., the tip of the catheter is positioned in a large central vessel such as the superior vena cava (SVC)]. A VAD that is inserted into a peripheral vein but that is long enough for its tip to be positioned in a central vessel is termed a peripherally inserted central venous catheter (PICC). Indications for a central VAD are shown in Table 45.1.

Several different types of central VADs are available for use in patients with cancer (1–6). Individual circumstances will determine the type of VAD that is best for a particular patient. Placing and maintaining any central VAD is more complex, however, than is the case with a simple peripheral i.v. catheter. It is very important to recognize and minimize the potential for mechanical complications and infections associated with the use of central VADs.

CLASSIFICATION AND APPLICATION OF DIFFERENT CENTRAL VASCULAR ACCESS DEVICES

The classification of central VADs is based, in large part, on the following parameters: the characteristics of each catheter's composition (e.g., polyurethane or silicone), its location (i.e., central or peripheral), and the method of insertion (i.e., percutaneous, tunneled, or implanted). These parameters are associated with both advantages and disadvantages, which are outlined in Table 45.2. A percutaneous catheter is inserted directly through the skin into the vessel. In tunneled placement, a part of a catheter is placed in the subcutaneous tissue between the sites of insertion at the skin (usually midway between the nipple and sternum on the anterior chest) and the vein (subclavian or internal jugular). A Dacron cuff positioned several

TABLE 45.1. *Indications for central venous access devices*

- Administration of a sclerosing agent
- Inadequate peripheral access
- Venous access required for >3 d
- Administration of total parenteral nutrition
- Need for frequent blood sampling

579

TABLE 45.2. *Advantages and disadvantages of different catheter compositions, locations, and methods of insertion*

Type	Advantages	Disadvantages
Composition		
Polyurethane	• Durable • Easy to position	• Increased vascular injury
Silicone	• Decreased vascular injury	• Easily broken • More difficult to position
Location of insertion		
Peripheral (basilic veins)	• Limited central insertion	• Migration with movement or cephalic complication • Mechanical phlebitis
Central insertion	• Insertion by nurse • Limited tip migration	• Maximum of two lumens • Insertion by physician (internal jugular or subclavian veins)
	• More than two lumens possible	• Greater central insertion complications
Methods of insertion		
Percutaneous	• Bedside placement • Easy to remove	• Increased risk of infection • Activity restrictions • Frequent maintenance
Tunneled	• Decreased risk of infection • Easy to remove	• Radiologist or surgeon insertion • Activity restrictions • Frequent maintenance
Implanted	• Decreased risk of infection • No activity restrictions • Infrequent maintenance	• Insertion by surgeon • Maximum of two lumens • Removal by surgeon

inches above the exit site promotes fibrous ingrowth, better securing the tunneled catheter and possibly decreasing bacterial colonization of the catheter below the cuff. Implanted VADs have a stainless steel, titanium, or plastic port at their proximal end, which includes a Silastic self-sealing septum. Once the catheter is inserted, the port is placed in a subcutaneous pocket that is sutured. The Silastic septum of the port can be accessed by a needle introduced through the skin and septum, into the port chamber itself. This is frequently done with a Huber needle, which has been designed with a side hole to minimize damage (coring) to the Silastic septum. Port housings are designed to provide minimal distortion artifact on magnetic resonance imaging (MRI) or computerized tomography (CT) scans.

The parameters outlined in Table 45.2 determine, in large part, the applicability of a particular type of catheter for a particular patient. Polyurethane percutaneous catheters, although relatively easy to place at either central or peripheral sites, are generally not suitable for long-term use, given the greater risk of infection and vascular trauma associated with their use. Tunneled and implanted Silastic catheters, however, although more difficult to place, may be associated with lower risk of infection and vascular injury and can be used over longer periods. The ease of care and limited restrictions associated with implanted catheters make their use most desirable in patients who will require frequent catheter use over prolonged periods. The optimal duration of use for percutaneous or Silastic catheters located centrally or peripherally has not been adequately defined. With care and prompt removal when clinically indicated, these catheters may be maintained in some patients for several months.

Other characteristics of central VADs may make one type of catheter more applicable for an individual patient than another. For example, catheters located centrally are usually larger in gauge (4 to 12 Fr) than those placed peripherally (2 to 6 Fr) and permit higher flow rates and easier drawing of blood. Larger-gauge catheters can also be constructed with more lumens. Although most central VADs are open at the end or tip, the Groshong catheter (Bard Access Systems) has a closed end with a three-way slit valve to reduce the potential backflow of blood into the catheter. Figure 45.1 shows an algorithm for determining the type of catheter most appropriate for a particular patient. Table 45.3 shows examples of the different catheter types frequently used at the National Institutes of Health (NIH) Warren G. Magnuson Clinical Center.

COMPLICATIONS WITH INSERTION

Insertion of any central VAD, whether at the bedside, in radiology, or in surgery, is associated with the risk of mechanical complications or infection (1–3,5,6). Mechanical complications most commonly arise when catheter placement results in injury to central vascular structures (e.g., venous or arterial perforation) or to the lungs (e.g., pneumo-, hemo-, or hydrothorax). The occurrence of these types of complications or their sequelae can be reduced by ensuring: first, that abnormalities of anatomy related to previous therapy (e.g., surgery, radiation, or earlier VADs) or disease (e.g., tumor) are recognized before VAD placement; second, that the patient's coagulation profile has been optimized (i.e., platelet count brought to >50,000 per mL and prothrombin and partial thromboplastin times corrected); and third, that careful attention is given to identification of complications that may become apparent only several hours after VAD placement (e.g., pneumo-, hemo-, or hydrothorax). In some patients, in whom complete correction of the coagulation profile is not possible, VAD placement may still be done while

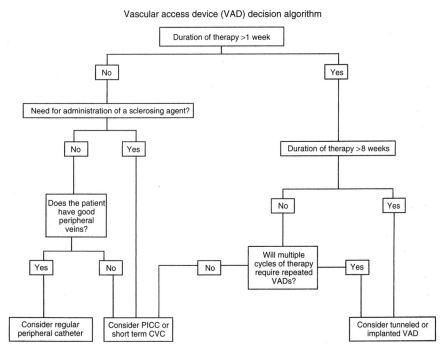

FIG. 45.1. Algorithm for determining the appropriate type of catheter. PICC, peripherally inserted central venous catheter; CVC, central venous catheter; VAD, vascular access device

TABLE 45.3. *Examples of frequently inserted vascular access devices at the National Institutes of Health Warren G. Magnuson Clinical Center*

Catheter type and manufacturer	Composition	Size (Fr)	Lumens	Typical duration of insertion
Nontunneled CVC[a]				
Arrow	Polyurethane	4, 5, 7, or 8	3	3–30 d
		12[c]	2	2–10 d
Bard Hohn	Silicone	5	2	6–8 wk
Bard Rad PICC	Silicone	5	2	6–8 wk
Quinton Mahurkar	Silicone	11.5[c]	2	2–10 d
PICC[b]				
Arrow	Polyurethane	4	1	4–8 wk
		5	2	
Bard Groshong	Silicone	4	1	
		5	2	
Tunneled CVC				
Bard Hickman	Silicone	7	2	≤1 yr
		10	2	
		10	3	
Bard Groshong	Silicone	9.5	2	
Implanted ports				
Bard MRI	Silicone	9.6	1	≤2 yr

CVC, central venous catheter; PICC, peripherally inserted central venous catheter.
[a]Centrally inserted central venous catheter.
[b]Peripherally inserted CVC.
[c]Used for dialysis or apheresis.

the appropriate replacement products are infused through an additional catheter. Because of the difficulties associated with compressing subclavian vascular structures, percutaneous or tunneled catheter insertions should generally not be performed at this site unless an adequate coagulation profile can be achieved. Complications arising from infection from insertion can be reduced by ensuring that the operators use a strict sterile technique and full barrier precautions.

CARE AND MAINTENANCE

Once the central VADs have been inserted, their care and maintenance include regular flushing with a saline and heparin solution and changing of dressings (i.e., gauze or transparent) and catheter injection caps. No clear standard has been established with respect to the volume, dose, and frequency of heparin flushing; the type and frequency of dressing changes; or the frequency of cap changes. However, general guidelines do exist, and successful maintenance of a central VAD is the result of an established care routine (7–9). Most central VADs are flushed daily with a quantity of saline (5 to 10 mL) and heparin (1 to 5 mL of a 10 to 1,000 U per mL) solution equivalent to two times the volume of the catheter and any additional infusion devices in series with the catheter. Implanted VADs are flushed monthly with saline and heparin when not accessed. Groshong catheters are flushed weekly, or after each use, with saline only. Gauze and transparent dressings are changed every 2 days and 7 days, respectively. Catheter caps are changed after wiping with cleansing solution at least every 7 days, or whenever they are damaged or contain residual blood. A 2% chlorhexidine-based preparation is recommended for catheter site care. Alternatively, if the patient cannot tolerate chlorhexidine, povidone–iodine (10%), alcohol (70% to 92%) solutions, and hydrogen peroxide can be used.

Whenever a central VAD is accessed, precautions must be taken to prevent the entry of air into the catheter and thereby into the circulation (i.e., air embolus). The central VAD should be clamped between the point of access and the patient. If a catheter does have to remain open for short periods, such as during initial wire removal at insertion, the patient should be in the Trendelenburg position.

COMPLICATIONS AFTER INSERTION

Maintaining a central VAD for any period is associated with the risk of infection, thrombotic or nonthrombotic catheter obstruction, vascular injury, or failure of the VAD itself. These complications may occur at any time.

The reported incidence of infection relating to central VADs ranges from 3% to 60% but is usually less than 10% (1–5,9–12). This incidence may be higher in patients with cancer who have neutropenia related to therapy or disease. Infections with central VADs can occur locally (i.e., exit site or tunnel or pocket infections) or systemically [i.e., catheter-related bloodstream infections (CR-BSIs)]. Definitions developed by the Centers for Disease Control and Prevention (CDC) are shown in Table 45.4 (9). Different types of infections with VADs will be managed differently (1,3–6,10–13). Exit-site infections, most frequently related to *Staphylococcus epidermidis,* can be treated initially with local wound care and oral antibiotics without removing the catheter. However, exit-site infections resulting in bacteremia may require catheter removal, especially in cases of infections with *Staphylococcus aureus.* Tunnel or pocket infections are most frequently related to *S. epidermidis* or *S. aureus* and almost always require systemic antibiotic treatment and catheter removal, with surgical drainage of the infected site. A definitive diagnosis of CR-BSI, although not always possible,

TABLE 45.4. *Centers for Disease Control and Prevention (CDC) clinical and surveillance definitions for catheter-related infections*

Colonized catheter	Growth of a microorganism from the catheter tip, subcutaneous segment or hub
Microbiologic exit-site infection	Erythema or induration within 2 cm of exit site without purulent drainage or bloodstream infection
Clinical exit-site or tunnel infection	Tenderness, erythema, and/or induration >2 cm from the exit site and along the subcutaneous tunnel without a bloodstream infection
Pocket infection	Erythema and necrosis of the skin over the reservoir of a total implanted device, or purulent exudate in the subcutaneous pocket containing the reservoir, in the absence of a bloodstream infection
Infusate-related bloodstream infection	Growth of the same organism from the infusate and blood cultures with no other identifiable source of infection
CR-BSI	At least one positive blood culture from a peripheral vein, with clinical symptoms of infection and no other apparent source of infection; or the isolation of the same organism from a semiquantitative or quantitative culture of a catheter segment and from the peripheral blood; or simultaneous quantitative blood cultures with a ≥5:1 ratio of catheter vs. peripheral blood; or a differential time period of catheter culture vs. peripheral blood of >2 h.

CR-BSI, catheter-related bloodstream infections.

requires that the same pathogen be cultured in the blood drawn from both the central VAD and another site. Documented or suspected CR-BSI should always be treated with systemic antibiotics. These infections, most frequently related to *S. epidermidis* and *S. aureus,* may also be caused by either the gram-negative bacteria or fungal species to which immunosuppressed patients with cancer are susceptible. The initiation of empiric antibiotic coverage in such patients must take these other organisms into account. CR-BSI can sometimes be treated with systemic antibiotics alone, but evidence of worsening infection or the presence of *S. aureus* or candidal infection calls for prompt removal of the catheter. Some central VADs are impregnated with antimicrobial agents [chlorhexidine and silver sulfadiazine (Arrowguard Blue; Arrow International) or minocycline and rifampin (Cook Spectrum; Cook Critical Care)] or have an attached antimicrobial cuff [silver ion (Vita Cuff; Vitaphore)]. The overall effectiveness of such agents in preventing infection over the lifetime of a central VAD continues to be studied (13–18). At present, data support the use of antiseptic-impregnated catheters. The effectiveness of antimicrobial cuffs is not yet clear.

Obstruction of a VAD can be related to thrombotic or nonthrombotic causes (10,19–22). Thrombotic obstructions can be classified as those present within (intraluminal) or around the outside of (fibrin sheath) the catheter itself and those in association with the vessel wall (mural thrombus). A catheter may sometimes become encased in a mural thrombus. Nonthrombotic obstruction of a central VAD can be a result of malpositioning of a catheter tip against a vessel wall, catheter kinking, luminal occlusion caused by drug precipitation, or fracture of the catheter. These types of obstruction may require either repositioning or removal of the catheter. When diagnosing the cause of an obstruction, it is helpful to first determine whether the obstruction interferes with withdrawal or with infusion or both. An algorithm to aid in the diagnosis and treatment of catheter obstruction is shown in Fig. 45.2.

Vascular injury resulting in actual perforation of a vessel wall is not commonly found with the flexible central VADs now in use. Nevertheless, catheter tips should not be positioned perpendicular to an adjacent vessel, such as in the innominate vein at its junction with the SVC. Because of the smaller diameters of the basilic and cephalic veins, mechanical phlebitis can sometimes occur after PICC insertion. This usually manifests itself within 1 to 7 days of insertion with erythema, tenderness, induration, and a palpable venous cord along the vessel tract. Treatment is with moist heat, arm elevation, mild range-of-motion exercises, and an antiinflammatory agent. Mechanical phlebitis should respond to treatment within 24 to 48 hours. If such a response is not noted, the catheter should be removed, local treatment should be continued, and consideration should be given to a course of antibiotic therapy.

With use, VADs may themselves fail. In percutaneous catheters, the sutures or anchoring device may loosen, and the catheter may be pulled out partially or completely. Any catheter that has been partially pulled out should not be readvanced. If a chest radiograph does not show the catheter tip in the SVC, the catheter should be removed. The external parts of a catheter that are frequently manipulated may break. Some catheters have repair kits available from the manufacturers and can be safely repaired. If no repair kits are available, the catheter should be removed. In rare instances, an internal part of a VAD may break and embolize. This problem, which may be recognized only when the catheter is removed, should be addressed immediately with interventional radiology.

FIG. 45.2. Algorithm to aid in the diagnosis and treatment of catheter obstruction.
˙Thrombolysis therapy:
• Urokinase
• Streptokinase
• rtPTA.
†Jugular vein distention, evidence of collateral circulation, unilateral arm swelling.
‡Chemical occlusion therapy:
• Alcohol for lipid precipitates
• 0.1 Hydrochloric acid for nonlipid precipitates.

Occluded catheter algorithm

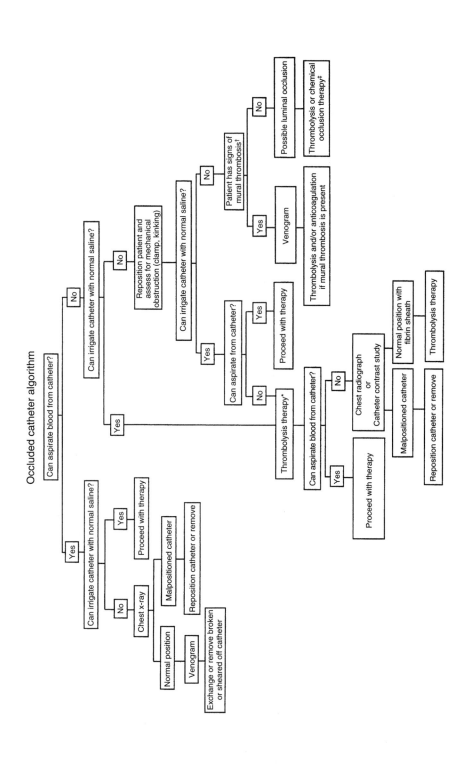

REMOVAL OF CENTRAL VASCULAR ACCESS DEVICES

VADs that are neither tunneled nor implanted can be removed at the bedside. Whenever resistance is encountered during removal, care should be taken to avoid severing the catheter. A radiograph or fluoroscopy should be used to determine whether the catheter has become kinked or knotted. In some cases, especially with PICC VADs, thrombosis may develop, preventing catheter removal. When a VAD has been in place for a prolonged period, especially in the case of centrally placed polyurethane catheters, a fistula, large enough to permit air entry after catheter removal, may develop. After VAD removal, the site should be dressed to prevent this from happening.

Tunneled Silastic catheters can also be removed at the bedside. However, if a tunneled catheter has a cuff (or cuffs) associated with it, any resultant adhesions may necessitate incision and dissection for catheter removal. Implanted catheters require surgical removal.

REFERENCES

1. Alexander HR. Vascular access and specialized techniques of drug delivery. In: DeVita VT Jr, Hellman S, Rosenberg SA, eds. *Cancer: principles and practice of oncology*, 5th ed. Philadelphia, PA: Lippincott–Raven Publishers, 1997:725–734.
2. Lucas AB, Steinhaus EP, Torosian MH. Long term venous access catheters and implanted ports. In: HR Alexander, ed. *Vascular access in the cancer patient: devices, insertion techniques, maintenance, and prevention and management of complications*, Philadelphia, PA: JB Lippincott Co, 1994:3–35.
3. Garcia JP, Osteen RT. Vascular access for cancer therapy. In: Macdonald JS, Haller DG, Mayer RJ, eds. *Manual of oncologic therapeutics*, 3rd ed. Philadelphia, PA: JB Lippincott Co, 1995:67–70.
4. Lucas AB. A critical review of venous access devices: the nursing perspective. In: Hubbard SM, Green PE, Knobf MT, eds. *Current issues in cancer nursing practice*, Philadelphia, PA: JB Lippincott Co, 1991:1–10.
5. Raaf J. Vascular access, catheter technology and infusion pumps. In: Moosa AR, Schimpff SC, Robson MC, eds. *Comprehensive textbook of oncology*, 2nd ed., Vol 1. Baltimore, MD: Williams & Wilkins, 1991:583–589.
6. Shoemaker WC. Intravascular access and long-term catheter maintenance. In: Ayres SM, Grenvik A, Holbrook PR et al, eds. *Textbook of critical care*, 3rd ed. Philadelphia, PA: WB Saunders, 1995:234–252.
7. Intravenous Nursing Society. Standards of practice supplement. *J Intraven Nurs* 2000;21:1S.
8. Oncology Nursing Society. *Access device guidelines module: catheters: recommendations for nursing education and practice.* Pittsburgh, PA: Oncology Nursing Press, 1995.
9. Centers for Disease Control and Prevention. *Guidelines for prevention of intravascular infections.* Atlanta, GA. 2002.
10. Hoch JR. Management of complications of long-term venous access. *Semin Vasc Surg* 1997;10:135–143.
11. Groeger JS, Lucas AB, Thaler HT, et al. Infectious morbidity associated with long-term use of venous access devices in patients with cancer. *Ann Intern Med* 1993;119:1168–1174.
12. Lucas AB, Steinhaus EP, Torosian MH. Types of catheter related infections. In: Alexander HR, ed. *Vascular access in the cancer patient, devices, insertion techniques, maintenance, and prevention and management of complications*, Philadelphia, PA: JB Lippincott Co, 1994:113–127.
13. Toltzis P, Goldmann DA. Current issues in central venous catheter infection. *Annu Rev Med* 1990;41:169–176.
14. Groeger JS, Lucas AB, Coit D, et al. A prospective, randomized evaluation of the effect of silver impregnated subcutaneous cuffs for preventing tunneled chronic venous access catheter infections in cancer patients. *Ann Surg* 1993;218:206–210.
15. Maki DG, Cobb L, Garman JK, et al. An attachable silver-impregnated cuff for the prevention of infection with central venous catheters: a prospective randomized multicenter trial. *Am J Med* 1988;85:307–314.
16. Darouiche RO, Raad II, Heard SO, et al. A comparison of two antimicrobial-impregnated central venous catheters. *N Engl J Med* 1999;340:1–8.
17. Maki DG, Stolz SM, Wheeler S, et al. Prevention of central venous catheter-related bloodstream infection by use of an antiseptic-impregnated catheter. *Ann Intern Med* 1997;127:257–266.
18. Raad II, Darouiche R, Dupuis J, et al. Central venous catheters coated with minocycline and rifampin for the prevention of catheter-related colonization and bloodstream infections. *Ann Intern Med* 1997;127:267–274.

19. Rumsey K, Richardson D. Management of infection and occlusion associated with vascular access devices. *Semin Oncol Nurs* 1995;11:174–183.
20. Williams E. Catheter-related thrombosis. *Clin Cardiol* 1990;13:34–36.
21. Lucas AB, Steinhaus EP, Torosian MH. Catheter occlusion and persistent withdrawal occlusion. In: Alexander HR, ed. *Vascular access in the cancer patient: devices, insertion techniques, maintenance, and prevention and management of complications*, Philadelphia, PA: JB Lippincott Co, 1994:91–107.
22. Reed T, Phillips D. Management of central venous catheter occlusions and repairs. *J Intraven Nurs* 1996;19:289–294.

46

Procedures in Medical Oncology

Suzanne G. Demko and Kerry Ryan

Medical Oncology Clinical Research Unit, National Cancer Institute,
National Institutes of Health, Bethesda, Maryland

As in other subspecialties, procedures performed in an oncology setting can serve the dual purposes of diagnosis and treatment. This chapter outlines those medical oncology procedures that are commonly performed and briefly discusses any special considerations or techniques that may be of assistance in performing these procedures rapidly, with confidence, and with an eye toward patient comfort and education.

INFORMED CONSENT

Written informed consent, or a legally sufficient substitute, must be obtained before every procedure and should be filed in the patient's medical record.

ANESTHESIA

Local anesthesia should be used for all procedures, and premedication with a narcotic and benzodiazepine [preferably, fentanyl and midazolam (Versed)] should be considered for certain patients and procedures. Lidocaine, 1% mixed in a 3:1 or 5:1 ratio with sodium bicarbonate, will ensure proper anesthetic effect and will also virtually eliminate the typical sting of lidocaine.

INSTRUMENTATION

Most offices and hospitals are equipped with sterile trays or self-contained disposable kits that are specific to each procedure. Where additional instruments are needed because of operator preference or other considerations, they may be added.

PROCEDURES

Bone Marrow Aspirate/Bone Marrow Biopsy

Indications

Diagnostic: for the analysis of abnormality in production of blood cells and for the purpose of staging in hematologic and nonhematologic malignancies.

Contraindications

- Severe thrombocytopenia (platelets <20,000; platelet transfusion may be given before the procedure)
- Skin infection at proposed site of biopsy
- Biopsy to a site that was radiated previously can cause fibrosis; should consider alternative site
- Sternal biopsy
- Sternal aspirate to be avoided in patients with thoracic aortic aneurysms and in patients with lytic bone disease of ribs or sternum.
- Patients taking heparin: heparin should be discontinued before procedure and resumed after hemostasis is achieved.

Anatomy

- Sternal aspiration:
  - The patient is in supine position without elevation of the head.
  - Landmarks are the sternal angle of Louis and the lateral borders of the sternum in the second intercostal space.
- Posterior superior iliac spine aspiration and biopsy (see Fig. 46.1):
  - The patient is in a prone or lateral decubitus position for posterior superior iliac spine aspiration and biopsy, and is supine for anterior iliac crest aspiration and biopsy (for patients with a history of radiation to pelvis or extremely obese patients).

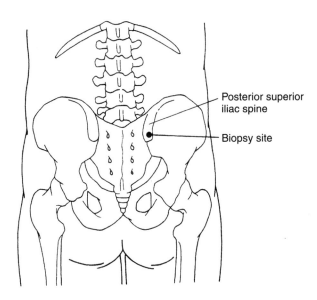

FIG. 46.1. Biopsy site in the posterior superior iliac spine. The needle should be directed toward the anterior superior iliac spine. (From Chestnut MS, Dewar TN, Locksley RM, et al. Bone marrow aspiration & biopsy. In: Chestnut MS, Dewar TN, Locksley RM, eds. *Office & bedside procedures.* Norwalk, CT: Appleton & Lange, 1992:381, with permission.)

Procedure

• Sternal aspiration:
  1. Once the landmarks have been identified, clean the area and drape with a fenestrated drape, using sterile technique.
  2. Infiltrate the skin, subcutaneous tissues, and periosteum in the area to be aspirated with lidocaine, 1%, for anesthesia. "Sounding" of the surface of the bone can be done with the infiltration needle to approximate the distance from the skin to the periosteum.
  3. Use a 16-gauge sternal aspiration needle with guard to prevent penetration of the posterior table of the sternum. The adjustment of the needle guard is based on an approximation of the distance from the skin to the periosteum.
  4. Make a 2-mm superficial skin incision with a surgical blade in the midsternum, medial to the second intercostal space.
  5. Introduce the aspirate needle with guard, using gentle, corkscrew-type pressure to advance the needle until it is fixed in bone. Remove the obturator, attach a 10- to 12-mL syringe, and aspirate. The aspiration will be painful. This cannot be prevented but will last only a few seconds.

     One milliliter of aspirate should be obtained. An amount >1 mL will be diluted by peripheral blood. Spicules of bone marrow will be present unless significant fibrosis is present or the marrow is packed with leukemic or other malignant cells.

     If no specimen is obtained, replace the obturator and carefully advance the needle 2mm to 3 mm. Repeat the aspiration process. Prepare smears for evaluation.

• Posterior superior iliac crest aspiration and biopsy:
  1. In general, an 11-gauge Jamshidi-type needle is used to obtain biopsy specimens. Under special circumstances (e.g., spongy bone marrow or easily compressed marrow), a larger-gauge needle (8-gauge) may be used to obtain an adequate biopsy specimen.
  2. The patient may be positioned prone; however, the lateral decubitus position may be used instead for better identification of anatomic sites or for patient comfort. For all but the most obese patients, these positions may be used for aspiration and biopsy. For extremely obese patients or for those who have had radiation to the pelvis, the anterior iliac crest may be used for sampling.
  3. Once the site has been prepared and anesthetized, advance the needle into the cortex of the bone until it is fixed. Attempt aspiration and, if unsuccessful, advance the needle slightly and attempt again.
  4. Once the aspirate is obtained, advance the needle using a twisting motion, without the obturator in place, to obtain the biopsy specimen. A 1.5- to 2-cm specimen is recommended. To ensure that the specimen is collected when the needle is removed, first rotate the needle briskly in one direction and then in the other direction, and then "rock" gently by exerting pressure perpendicular to the shaft of the needle in four directions with the needle capped. Then gently remove the needle while rotating in a corkscrew manner. Remove the specimen from the needle by pushing it up through the hub with a stylet provided for this purpose, taking care to avoid needlestick injuries while removing the specimen. Jamshidi needle kits provide a small, clear plastic guide to facilitate this process.

Aftercare

A pressure dressing is placed over the site, and external pressure is applied for 5 to 10 minutes. Direct pressure is the preferred method to avoid prolonged bleeding and hematoma formation. The pressure dressing should remain in place for 24 hours. The patient may remove the pressure dressing and shower after 24 hours; however, the patient should avoid immersion of the site in water for 1 week after the procedure in order to avoid infection.

Complications

Infection and hematoma formation are the most common complications after bone marrow biopsy and aspiration, and can be minimized by using careful techniques during and after the procedure.

Documentation

Prepare a procedure note.

Lumbar Puncture

Indications

• Diagnostic [analysis of cerebrospinal fluid (CSF) to assess adequacy of treatment]
• CSF pressure measurement to assess adequacy of treatment
• Administration of intrathecal chemotherapy

Contraindications

• Increased intracranial pressure
• Coagulopathy
• Infectious process near the planned access site

Anatomy

• The conus medullaris rarely ends below L3 (i.e., L1 to L2 in adults and L2 to L3 in children), and interspaces above this should be avoided (see Fig. 46.2).
• The L4 spinous process or the L4-5 interspace lies in the center of the supracristal plane (a line drawn between the posterior superior iliac crests).

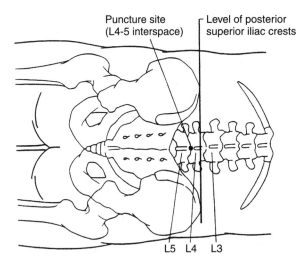

FIG. 46.2. Anatomy of the lumbar spine. (From Chestnut MS, Dewar TN, Locksley RM, et al. Lumbar puncture. In: Chestnut MS, Dewar TN, Locksley RM, eds. *Office & bedside procedures.* Norwalk, CT: Appleton & Lange, 1992:391, with permission.)

- There are eight layers from the skin to the subarachnoid space; they are skin, supraspinous ligament, interspinous ligament, ligamentum flava, epidural space, dura, subarachnoid membrane, and subarachnoid space.

Procedure

1. Describe the procedure to the patient and assure him or her that you will explain what you are about to do before you do it.
2. Position the patient in the lateral decubitus position at the edge of the table or bed, with knees pulled upward and head flexed downward toward chest (see Fig. 46.3). If the spinal column appears to be misaligned, place a pillow beneath the patient to assure proper alignment. This position may be substituted with the seated position if the patient is obese or has difficulty remaining in the lateral decubitus position for any reason.
3. Assess the anatomic landmarks and identify the interspace to be used for the procedure.
4. Using sterile technique, prepare the area and one interspace above or below it with povidone–iodine solution. Drape the patient, establishing a sterile field.
5. Using 1% lidocaine–bicarbonate mixture, anesthetize the skin and deeper tissues, being careful to avoid administering epidural or spinal anesthesia.
6. Insert the spinal needle into the anesthetized skin and into the spinous ligament, keeping the needle parallel to the bed or table. Immediately change the angle of the needle to between 30 and 45 degrees, directing the needle cephalad. The bevel of the needle should be positioned to face the patient's flanks to allow the needle to spread rather than cut the dural sac. Begin to advance the needle in small increments through the layers and remove the stylet to check for CSF before each new advance of the needle. With practice, the operator may be able to identify the "pop" through the dura into the subarachnoid space, but even an experienced operator would be wise to check for CSF before each advance of the needle.
7. Having confirmed the presence of CSF, attach a manometer to measure the opening pressure. Collect appropriate samples of CSF. Send the samples in the following order: tube 1, cultures; tube 2, chemistries (especially glucose and protein); tube 3, cell count and

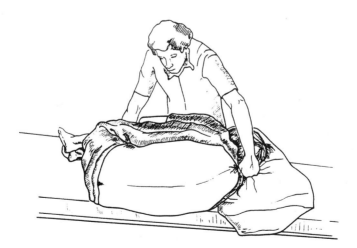

FIG. 46.3. Lateral decubitus position for lumbar puncture. (From Chestnut MS, Dewar TN, Locksley RM, et al. Lumbar puncture. In: Chestnut MS, Dewar TN, Locksley RM, eds. *Office & bedside procedures.* Norwalk, CT: Appleton & Lange, 1992:390, with permission.)

differential; and tube 4, cytopathologic or other special studies (flow cytometry, cytogenetics, etc.). Typically, a total of 8 to 15 mL of CSF is removed during lumbar punctures (LPs). However, if special studies are required, 40 mL of fluid can be removed safely.

If intrathecal chemotherapy is to be administered, attach the syringe to the spinal needle, tube adapter, or stopcock, and administer by slow push.

8. Withdraw the needle, observe the site for CSF leak or hemorrhage, and place an appropriate bandage over the site.
9. Transfer the patient to a recumbent position and ask the patient to remain in this position for 5 to 10 minutes. There appears to be no relation between postprocedure positioning and spinal headache; however, a relationship does exist for needle size, CSF leak, and spinal headache. The patient should be instructed to drink 2 to 3 L of fluid over the next 24 hours, in order to replenish the CSF removed.

Complications

- Spinal headache can occur in approximately 20% of patients after LP. It is a characteristic headache, in that it is present as a pounding ache in the occipital region when the patient is upright and resolves when the patient lies down. Certain categories of patients are more likely to have a post-LP headache. Female patients, those with a history of headache prior to LP, or those of a younger age group (peak age 20 to 40 years) are associated with the highest incidence of post-LP headache. Fluid intake should be encouraged, over-the-counter analgesics should be suggested, and the patient should be instructed to remain recumbent, if possible. Spinal headaches can be quite severe and may last for about 1 week. If this is the case, stronger analgesia, caffeine, or a blood patch procedure may be indicated.
- Nerve root trauma can occur, but it does so only infrequently. This complication can be avoided by choosing a low interspace as the entry site.
- Cerebellar or medullar herniation occurs only rarely, in some patients who have increased intracranial pressure. If recognized early, this process can be reversed.
- Infections, including meningitis, can also occur.
- Bleeding resulting in a small number of red blood cells (RBCs) in the CSF is a common occurrence in patients undergoing an LP. However, serious bleeding can result in spinal compromise in approximately 1% to 2% of patients. Serious bleeding usually occurs only in patients who have thrombocytopenia or bleeding disorders, or who have received anticoagulants before or after undergoing an LP.

Paracentesis

Indications

- Patients with ascites as a result of tumor metastasis or obstruction often benefit from therapeutic paracentesis. Where the diagnosis is in doubt, or to assess diagnostic markers, diagnostic paracentesis can be performed.

Contraindications

- There are few situations in which one would hesitate to perform a paracentesis. The complication rate for this procedure is minuscule (about 1%), and the benefit derived by the patient can be quite remarkable. This is especially true of therapeutic paracentesis.
- Even in the event of a coagulopathy, the benefit outweighs the risks in performing this procedure.

Anatomy

- One should identify the area of greatest dullness in the abdomen by percussion. As an alternative, one can have the ascites "marked" by having the patient undergo an ultrasound. Care should be taken to avoid the abdominal vasculature and viscera.

Procedure

1. Place the patient in a comfortable supine position on the edge of the bed or table.
2. Identify the area of the abdomen to be accessed (see Fig. 46.4).
3. Prepare the area with povidone–iodine solution and establish a sterile field by draping the patient.
4. Anesthetize the area with 1% lidocaine–bicarbonate mixture.
5. For diagnostic paracentesis, insert a 22- to 25-gauge needle attached to a sterile syringe into the skin, and pull the skin laterally before advancing the needle into the abdomen. After releasing the tension on the skin, advance the needle in the peritoneal cavity, withdraw an appropriate amount of fluid, and send for testing. The skin-retraction method creates a "Z" tract into the peritoneal cavity, and this minimizes the risk of ascitic leak after the procedure (see Fig. 46.5).
6. For therapeutic paracentesis, use the Z-tract method with a multiple-port flexible catheter over a guide needle. When the catheter is in place, evacuate the ascites into multiple containers. One must, however, be careful that the patient remains hemodynamically stable during the removal of large amounts of ascites.
7. When the procedure has been completed, withdraw the needle or catheter and place a pressure bandage over the site. Look for any bleeding or ascitic leak before placing the bandage.
8. After a therapeutic paracentesis is performed, the patient should remain in a supine position until all vital signs are stable and should be assisted when rising from the bed or table for the first time after the procedure.
9. If the patient becomes orthostatic, standard medical measures should be used to reverse this process, and he or she must be hemodynamically stable before being allowed to leave.

Complications

- Although the selection of an adequate site for paracentesis virtually eliminates complications, the following have been reported: hemorrhage, ascitic leak, infection, and perforated abdominal viscus.

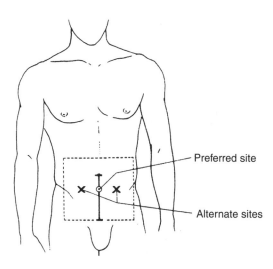

FIG. 46.4. Sites for diagnostic paracentesis. (From Chestnut MS, Dewar TN, Locksley RM, et al. Gastrointestinal procedures. In: Chestnut MS, Dewar TN, Locksley RM, eds. *Office & bedside procedures.* Norwalk, CT: Appleton & Lange, 1992:269, with permission.)

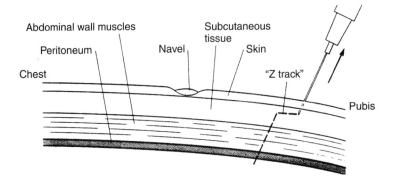

Abdominal wall muscles Subcutaneous tissue Skin
Peritoneum Navel "Z track"
Chest Pubis

FIG. 46.5. "Z-tracking" technique for needle insertion into the peritoneal cavity. (From Chestnut MS, Dewar TN, Locksley RM, et al. Bone marrow aspiration & biopsy. In: Chestnut MS, Dewar TN, Locksley RM, eds. *Office & bedside procedures.* Norwalk, CT: Appleton & Lange, 1992:381, with permission.)

Thoracentesis

Indications

- For removal of pleural fluid for diagnostic or therapeutic purposes

Contraindications

There are no absolute contraindications to diagnostic thoracentesis if it is decided that the information gained from pleural fluid analysis is needed for diagnosis and/or therapy.

The relative contraindications are as follows:

- Coagulopathy (the coagulation abnormality should be corrected)
- Bullous emphysema (associated with increased risk of pneumothorax)
- Cardiovascular disease (cardiac dysrhythmias)
- Patients with a minimal amount of pleural fluid positive end-expiratory pressure (PEEP) are not at increased risk for developing pneumothorax when compared with nonventilated patients. Mechanically ventilated patients, however, are at increased risk for developing tension physiology or a persistent air leak, if pneumothorax does occur.
- Inability of patient to cooperate
- Cellulitis, if the thoracentesis requires penetrating the inflamed tissue.

Important Preprocedure Considerations

- Care must be taken to ascertain the location of the diaphragm before the procedure in order to avoid accidental injury to the abdominal organs and viscera.
- Chest radiographs should be viewed by the person who is performing the procedure and, if loculation of fluid is suspected, decubitus films and, possibly, computerized tomography scan or ultrasonography may be helpful before thoracentesis is attempted.

Anatomy

- The procedure may be performed with the patient in a sitting position, with arms resting on a pillow placed on a table. This allows the patient to lean forward 10 to 15 degrees, allowing the intercostal spaces to spread.
- The procedure is performed through the seventh or eighth intercostal space in the posterior axillary line. With fluoroscopic, sonographic, or computerized tomographic guidance, the procedure may be performed below the fifth rib anteriorly, the seventh rib laterally, and the ninth rib posteriorly. Without such guidance, the underlying organs may be injured.
- Assessing the size of the pleural effusion by physical examination involves the detection of decreased tactile fremitus and dullness to percussion over the pleural effusion. The percussion is begun at the top of the chest, listening for any change in the sound of percussion while moving downward. When the change in sound is first noted, it should be compared with the percussion note in the same interspace and with the location on the opposite side of the chest. This indicates the highest level of the pleural effusion.

Procedure

1. With the patient in the proper position, clean the site with antiseptic solution and begin local anesthesia. Infiltrate the skin with 1% lidocaine using a 25-gauge needle. Infiltration to the deeper tissues is achieved using a 22-gauge needle, advancing the needle slowly, at a right angle to the chest wall in the center of the intercostal space. Direct the needle into the intercostal space just above the rib to avoid injury to the intercostal nerve and vessels that may run just below the rib. Aspirate frequently to ensure that no vessel has been entered and to determine the distance from the skin to the pleural fluid. Once the pleural fluid has been obtained, remove the anesthesia needle and note the depth.
2. A small skin incision may be needed to ease the passage of a larger-gauge thoracentesis needle into the pleural space. Generally, a 16- to 19-gauge needle with its intracath is introduced just to the level of obtaining pleural fluid. If, at this time, the fluid is bloody or different in appearance from that identified with the anesthesia needle, vessel injury must be suspected, and the procedure must be stopped. If the fluid appears to be the same as it was when previously aspirated, advance a flexible intracath and withdraw the needle to avoid puncture of the lung as the fluid is drained. The placement of a flexible intracath with a three-way stopcock allows the removal of large volumes of fluid with a lower risk of pneumothorax. (For sampling small amounts of pleural fluid without the need to drain large amounts of it, a 22-gauge needle connected to an airtight, three-way stopcock will suffice.) Attach tubing to the three-way stopcock and remove fluid by hand or by vacutainer. Monitor the hemodynamic status carefully when withdrawing more than 1,000 mL per procedure.
3. A chest radiograph should be performed after the procedure to determine the amount of fluid that remains, to look for the presence of pneumothorax, and to assess the lung parenchyma. A small pneumothorax does not need treatment, whereas a major pneumothorax (>50% lung collapse) does (see Fig. 46.6).

Complications

- Pneumothorax
- Air embolism (rare)
- Infection
- Pain at puncture site
- Bleeding
- Spleen or liver puncture.

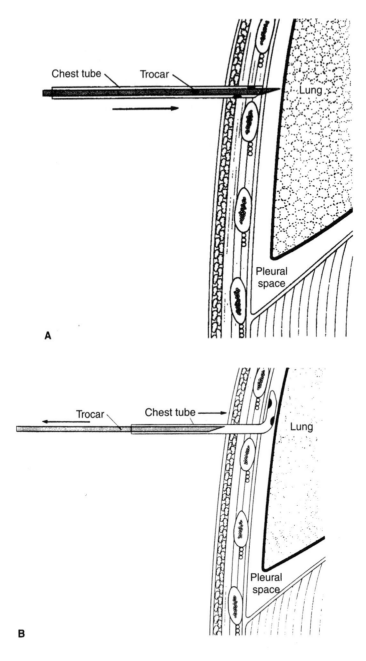

FIG. 46.6. Trocar technique for inserting a chest tube. **A:** Insertion of chest tube. **B:** Advancement of the chest tube off the trocar into the pleural space. (From Chestnut MS, Dewar TN, Locksley RM, et al. Bone marrow aspiration & biopsy. In: *Office & bedside procedures.* Norwalk, CT: Appleton & Lange, 1992:221, with permission.)

SUGGESTED READINGS

Butler E, Lichtman M, Giler B, et al. *Williams hematology*, 5th ed. New York: McGraw-Hill, 1995.

Evans RW, Armon C, Frohman EM, et al. Assessment: prevention of post-lumbar puncture headaches: report of the therapeutics and technology assessment subcommittee of the American Academy of Neurology. *Neurology* 2000;149:1087.

Isselbacher K, Braunwald E, Wilson JD, et al. *Harrison's principles of internal medicine*, 13th ed. New York: McGraw-Hill, 1994.

Jashidi K, Swaim WR. Bone marrow biopsy with unaltered architecture: a new biopsy device. *J Lab Clin Med* 1971;77:335.

Kuntz KM, Kokmen E, Stevens JC, et al. Post-lumbar puncture headaches: experience in 501 consecutive procedures. *Neurology* 1992;42:1884.

LeMense JP, Sahn SA. Safety and value of thoracentesis in medical ICU patients. *J Intensive Care Med* 1998;13:144.

McCartney JE, Adams JS II, Hazard PP. Safe procedure in mechanically ventilated patients. *Chest* 1993;103:1920.

Rohling BM, Webb WR, Schlobom RM. Ventilator-related extra-alveolar air. *Radiology* 1976;121:25.

Zimmerman JE, Dunbar BS, Klingenmaier CH. Management of subcutaneous emphysema, pneumomediastinum, and pneumothorax during respiratory therapy. *Crit Care Med* 1975;3:69.

47

Anticancer Agents

Thomas E. Hughes

Department of Pharmacy, National Institutes of Health Clinical Center, Bethesda, Maryland

All information has been obtained from the current product labeling as of June 1, 2004.

NOTES AND ABBREVIATIONS

Single-agent Dose

The doses listed for each agent are from the package inserts and apply when the agent is given alone, unless otherwise noted.

The doses are expressed in accordance with the nomenclature guidelines from Kohler et al. (1).

Abbreviations Listed under Adverse Reactions

- CNS: central nervous system
- CV: cardiovascular system
- DERM: skin and integument system
- ELECTRO: electrolyte abnormalities
- ENDO: endocrine system
- GI: gastrointestinal system
- GU: genitourinary system
- HEMAT: hematopoietic system
- INFUS: infusion-related reactions
- OCULAR: ocular system
- PULM: pulmonary system
- LFTs: liver function tests
- Cr: serum creatinine
- CrCl: creatinine clearance
- N/V Lx: Nausea and vomiting graded into 5 levels (x = 1 or 2 or 3, etc., up to 5) according to Hesketh et al. (2). (Note: The emetogenic potential based on the expected frequency of acute emesis is as follows: Level 1: <10%, Level 2: 10% to 30%, Level 3: 30% to 60%, Level 4: 60% to 90%, Level 5: >90%.)

ALDESLEUKIN (PROLEUKIN)

Mechanism of Action

Aldesleukin activates cellular immunity.

U.S. Food and Drug Administration–Approved Indications

Metastatic renal cell carcinoma and metastatic melanoma

U.S. Food and Drug Administration–Approved Dosage

- Doses of 600,000 IU per kg of Aldesleukin i.v. over 15 minutes every 8 hours for a maximum of 14 doses
- The dosage may be repeated after 9 days of rest for a maximum of 28 doses per course

Dose Modification Criteria

In the event of toxicity a dose may be withheld or interrupted.

Adverse Reactions

CNS: confusion, somnolence, anxiety, and dizziness; CV: hypotension, tachycardia, and arrhythmia; DERM: rash and pruritus; GI: diarrhea, N/V L3, mucositis, and anorexia; GU: oliguria and acute renal failure; HEMAT: myelosuppression; PULM: dyspnea and pulmonary edema; OTHER: pain, fever, chills, and malaise.

Comments

- Use may be restricted to patients with normal cardiac and pulmonary function
- Patients to be monitored for capillary-leak syndrome
- Agent is associated with impaired neutrophil function; consider antibiotic prophylaxis for patients with indwelling central lines

ALEMTUZUMAB (CAMPATH)

Mechanism of Action

Alemtuzumab is a humanized monoclonal antibody directed against the cell surface protein, CD52. The CD52 antigen is expressed on the surface of normal and malignant B and T lymphocytes, natural killer (NK) cells, monocytes, macrophages, and a subpopulation of granulocytes. The proposed mechanism of action of alemtuzumab is the antibody-dependent lysis of leukemic cells following binding to the cell surface.

U.S. Food and Drug Administration–Approved Indications

B-cell chronic lymphocytic leukemia (CLL): It is used for second-line therapy in patients who have been treated with alkylating agents and in those who have failed fludarabine therapy.

U.S. Food and Drug Administration–Approved Dosage

- Alemtuzumab is dose-escalated in a stepwise manner to a maintenance dose of 30 mg. The initial recommended dosage is 3 mg i.v. over 2 hours daily. When this dosage is tolerated (infusion-related toxicities are grade 2 or less), it should be escalated to 10 mg i.v. over 2 hours daily and continued until tolerated. When the 10-mg dose is tolerated, the maintenance dose of 30 mg may be initiated. The maintenance dosage is 30 mg i.v. over 2 hours administered 3 times per week (i.e., Monday, Wednesday, and Friday) for up to 12 weeks. In most patients, the escalation to 30-mg dose can be accomplished in 3 to 7 days. If therapy is interrupted for 7 or more days, alemtuzumab should be reinitiated with gradual dose escalation.

- Patients should be premedicated with an antihistamine (e.g., diphenhydramine 50 mg PO or i.v.) and acetaminophen (650 mg PO) 30 minutes prior to alemtuzumab to ameliorate or avoid infusion-related toxicity. Antiemetics, meperidine, and corticosteroids have also been used to prevent or treat infusion-related toxicities.

Dose Modification Criteria

Dose to be modified in cases of myelosuppression.

Adverse Reactions

CNS: headache, dysthesia, and dizziness; CV: hypotension and edema or peripheral edema; DERM: rash, urticaria, and pruritus; GI: N/V L2–3, diarrhea, anorexia, and mucositis or stomatitis; HEMAT: myelosuppression and lymphopenia; INFUS: rigors, fever, chills, N/VL2–3, hypotension, dyspnea, bronchospasm, headache, rash, and urticaria; PULM: dyspnea, cough, bronchitis, pneumonia, and bronchospasm; OTHER: opportunistic infections, sepsis, fatigue, asthenia, and pain.

Comments

- Patients treated with alemtuzumab are at risk of opportunistic infections caused by profound lymphopenia. Anti-infective prophylaxis is recommended upon initiation of therapy and for a minimum of 2 months following the last dose of alemtuzumab or until the CD4 count is equal to 200 cells per μL or more. Prophylaxis directed against *Pneumocystis carinii* pneumonia (PCP) (e.g., trimethoprim–sulfamethoxazole) and herpesvirus infections (e.g., famciclovir or equivalent) should be utilized.
- Alemtuzumab should not be administered as an intravenous push or bolus.
- Careful monitoring of blood pressure and hypotension is recommended, especially in patients with ischemic heart disease and in patients treated with antihypertensive medications.
- Patients who have recently been treated with alemtuzumab should not be immunized with live viral vaccines.

ALTRETAMINE (HEXALEN)
Mechanism of Action

Altretamine has an unknown mechanism of action, but structure is similar to an alkylating agent.

U.S. Food and Drug Administration–Approved Indications

Ovarian cancer: second-line therapy; palliative therapy for persistent or recurrent ovarian cancer

U.S. Food and Drug Administration–Approved Dosage

65 mg per m^2 PO q.i.d. (4 times daily; total daily dose: 260 mg per m^2) for 14 or 21 consecutive days, every 28 days

Dose Modification Criteria

Dose modified in case of myelosuppression and nonhematologic toxicity (i.e., GI intolerance and progressive neurotoxicity).

Adverse Reactions

CNS: peripheral sensory neuropathy, mood disorders, ataxia, and dizziness; GI: N/V L3; HEMAT: myelosuppression [white blood cells (WBCs), red blood cells (RBCs), platelets].

Comments

Patients to be monitored for neurologic toxicity

ANASTROZOLE (ARIMIDEX)

Mechanism of Action

Anastrozole is a selective, nonsteroidal aromatase inhibitor.

U.S. Food and Drug Administration–Approved Indications

Breast Cancer:

- Adjuvant treatment: Postmenopausal women with hormone-receptor–positive early breast cancer
- First-line therapy: Postmenopausal women with hormone-receptor–positive or hormone-receptor–unknown locally advanced or metastatic breast cancer
- Second-line therapy (after tamoxifen): Postmenopausal women with advanced breast cancer

U.S. Food and Drug Administration–Approved Dosage

1 mg PO daily (no requirement for glucocorticoid or mineralocorticoid replacement therapy)

Dose Modification Criteria

Renal impairment: no dose modification; hepatic impairment (mild to moderate): no dose modification; hepatic impairment (severe): no data available

Adverse Reactions

CNS: headache; CV: hot flashes/flushing; GI: nausea, diarrhea, and elevated LFT values (in patients with liver metastases); PULM: dyspnea; OTHER: asthenia, pain, back pain, and vaginal bleeding.

Comments

Patients with estrogen-receptor (ER)–negative disease and patients who do not respond to tamoxifen rarely respond to anastrozole.

ARSENIC TRIOXIDE (TRISENOX)

Mechanism of Action

The mechanism of action of arsenic trioxide is not completely defined. It induces apoptosis in NB4 human promyelocytic leukemia cells *in vitro* and damages or degrades the fusion protein PML/RAR α.

U.S. Food and Drug Administration–Approved Indications

Acute promyelocytic leukemia (APL): second-line therapy for the induction of remission and for consolidation of APL patients who are refractory to, or have relapsed from, retinoid and anthracycline chemotherapy.

U.S. Food and Drug Administration–Approved Dosage

- For APL induction: 0.15 mg per kg i.v. over 1 to 2 hours daily until bone marrow remission. Total induction dose should not exceed 60 doses.
- For APL consolidation: 0.15 mg per kg i.v. over 1 to 2 hours daily × 25 doses over a period of up to 5 weeks. Consolidation treatment should begin 3 to 6 weeks after completion of induction therapy.

Dose Modification Criteria

Renal impairment: no data available (use with caution); hepatic impairment: no data available.

Adverse Reactions

CNS: headache, dizziness, and paresthesias; CV: QT interval prolongation, complete atrioventricular block, torsade de pointes–type ventricular arrhythmia, atrial dysrhythmias, tachycardia, hypotension, and edema; DERM: rash, dermatitis, dry skin, and pruritus; ENDO: hyperglycemia, hypokalemia, and hypomagnesemia; GI: N/V L3, diarrhea, abdominal pain, anorexia, constipation, and elevated LFT values; HEMAT: leukocytosis and myelosuppression; PULM: dyspnea and cough; OTHER: fatigue, arthralgia, myalgia, pain, and APL differentiation syndrome or retinoic acid acute promyelocytic leukemia (RA-APL) syndrome (RA-APL syndrome: fever, dyspnea, weight gain, radiographic pulmonary infiltrates, and pleural or pericardial effusion).

Comments

- The APL differentiation syndrome (RA-APL syndrome) occurs in some patients treated with arsenic trioxide. Early recognition and high-dose corticosteroids (dexamethasone 10 mg i.v. every 12 hours × 3 days or until the resolution of symptoms) have been used for the management of this syndrome.
- Before starting treatment with arsenic trioxide, a 12-lead electrocardiogram (ECG) should be performed and serum electrolytes (potassium, calcium, and magnesium) and creatinine levels should be assessed; preexisting electrolyte abnormalities should be corrected. Concomitant drugs that may prolong the QT interval should be avoided. During therapy with arsenic trioxide, normal potassium and magnesium concentrations should be monitored and maintained as outlined in the package insert.
- The risk factors for QT prolongation and subsequent arrhythmias include other QT-prolonging drugs, a history of torsades de pointes, preexisting QT prolongation, congestive heart failure (CHF), administration of potassium-wasting diuretics, or other drugs or conditions that result in hypokalemia or hypomagnesemia.

ASPARAGINASE (ELSPAR)

Mechanism of Action

Asparaginase depletes asparagine, an amino acid required by some leukemic cells.

U.S. Food and Drug Administration–Approved Indications

For acute lymphoblastic leukemia (ALL): induction therapy with asparaginase (primarily in combination with other agents)

U.S. Food and Drug Administration–Approved Dosage

- Current literature to be consulted for doses
- ALL: Induction therapy in combination with prednisone and vincristine—1,000 IU per kg of asparaginase i.v. daily $\times$ 10 days, starting day 22 *or* 6,000 IU per m^2 i.m. every 3 days for nine doses, starting day 4 of induction (day 1 is the first day of chemotherapy).

Dose Modification Criteria

No data available

Adverse Reactions

DERM: skin rash; ENDO: hyperglycemia; GI: N/V L2, pancreatitis, increased LFT values, increased bilirubin levels, and decreased serum albumin; GU: prerenal azotemia; HEMAT: coagulopathy; CNS: a variety of changes in mental status; OTHER: hypersensitivity, anaphylactic reactions, and hyperthermia.

Comments

- [increased bilirubin levels] Asparaginase is contraindicated in patients with active pancreatitis or with a history of pancreatitis.
- Hypersensitivity and anaphylactic reactions can occur during therapy.
- Package insert may be consulted for test doses and desensitization schedules.
- i.m. administration is preferred over i.v. administration (lower incidence of anaphylaxis).
- i.v. infusions should be over a period of at least 30 minutes.

AZACITIDINE (VIDAZA)

Mechanism of Action

Azacitidine is an antimetabolite; a pyrimidine nucleoside analog of cytidine. It causes hypomethylation of deoxyribonucleic acid (DNA) and produces direct cytotoxicity on abnormal hematopoietic cells in the bone marrow.

U.S. Food and Drug Administration–Approved Indications

Myelodysplastic syndrome (MDS): The specific subtypes of MDS for which azacitidine is indicated include refractory anemia or refractory anemia with ringed sideroblasts (if accompanied by neutropenia or thrombocytopenia or when tranfusions are required), refractory anemia with excess blasts, refractory anemia with excess blasts in transformation, and chronic myelomonocytic leukemia.

U.S. Food and Drug Administration–Approved Dosage

- MDS: The recommended starting dosage is 75 mg per m^2 by s.c. injection, daily for 7 consecutive days, every 4 weeks. The dose may be increased to 100 mg per m^2 if no beneficial effect is seen after two treatment cycles and if no toxicity other than nausea and vomiting occurs. Duration: recommended minimum duration of four treatment cycles; complete or partial response may take more than four treatment cycles; it may be continued as long as the patient continues to benefit.

Dose Modification Criteria

Renal impairment: no data available (to be used with caution); Hepatic: no data available (to be used with caution); Myelosuppression: dose to be modified; nonhematologic toxicity (i.e., renal tubular acidosis and renal toxicity): dose to be modified.

Adverse Reactions

CNS: headache and dizziness; DERM: injection-site erythema or pain, ecchymosis, rash, and pruritus; ELECTRO: renal tubular acidosis (i.e., alkaline urine, fall in serum bicarbonate concentration, and hypokalemia); GI: N/V L1, diarrhea, constipation, anorexia, abdominal pain, and hepatotoxicity; GU: increased Cr and blood urea nitrogen (BUN) concentration, and renal failure; HEMAT: anemia, neutropenia, and thrombocytopenia; PULM: cough and dyspnea; OTHER: fever, rigors, fatigue, weakness, and peripheral edema.

Comments

- Teratogenic (pregnancy category D): Women of childbearing potential should be advised to avoid becoming pregnant while receiving azacitidine. Men should be advised to not father a child while receiving azacitidine.
- Azacitidine should be used with caution in patients with liver disease. It is potentially hepatotoxic in patients with preexisting hepatic impairment.
- Azacitidine and its metabolites are primarily eliminated renally. Patients with renal impairment should be closely monitored for toxicity. Renal toxicity has been reported rarely with intravenous azacitidine in combination with other chemotherapeutic agents for non-MDS conditions.

BACILLE CALMETTE-GUÉRIN LIVE (INTRAVESICAL) (THERACYS, TICE BCG)

Mechanism of Action

Bacille Calmette-Guérin has local inflammatory and immune response effect.

U.S. Food and Drug Administration–Approved Indications

Treatment and prophylaxis of carcinoma *in situ* of the urinary bladder and for the prophylaxis of primary or recurrent stage Ta and/or T1 papillary tumors following transurethal resection (TUR).

U.S. Food and Drug Administration–Approved Dosage

- TheraCys [each vial contains 81 mg (dry weight) or $10.5 \pm 8.7 \times 10^8$ colony-forming units and comes with a 3-mL diluent vial]:
  One reconstituted vial (81 mg per 3 mL), diluted in 50 mL of sterile, preservative-free normal saline (0.9% sodium chloride injection), is instilled into bladder for as long as possible (for up to 2 hours) once weekly for 6 weeks (induction therapy), followed by one treatment at 3, 6, 12, 18, and 24 months each after the initial treatment (maintenance therapy).
- Tice BCG [each vial contains 50 mg (wet weight) or $1-8 \times 10^8$ colony-forming units]:
  One reconstituted vial (50 mg per mL), diluted in a total volume of 50-mL preservative-free normal saline (0.9% sodium chloride injection), is instilled into bladder for as long as possible (for up to 2 hours) once weekly for 6 weeks, followed by once monthly for 6 to 12 months.

Dose Modification Criteria

Withhold Bacille Calmette-Guérin (BCG) live in case of any suspicion of systemic infection.

Adverse Reactions

CNS: malaise, fever, and chills; GU: irritative bladder symptoms; OTHER: infectious complications (uncommon).

Comments

- BCG live may complicate tuberculin skin test interpretation.
- BCG live products contain live, attenuated mycobacteria. Because of the potential risk of transmission, it should be prepared, handled, and disposed of as a biohazard material.

BEVACIZUMAB (AVASTIN)

Mechanism of Action

Bevacizumab is a recombinant humanized monoclonal immunoglobulin (Ig)G1 antibody that binds to and inhibits the biologic activity of human vascular endothelial growth factor (VEGF).

U.S. Food and Drug Administration–Approved Indications

Metastatic carcinoma of the colon or rectum: first-line therapy in combination with intravenous 5-fluorouracil–based chemotherapeutic agents.

U.S. Food and Drug Administration–Approved Dosage

- Metastatic colorectal cancer: 5 mg per kg i.v. infusion every 14 days until disease progression is detected
- *Do not administer as an i.v. push or bolus.* The initial bevacizumab dose should be delivered over 90 minutes as an i.v. infusion following chemotherapy. If the first infusion is well tolerated, the second infusion may be administered over 60 minutes. If the 60-minute infusion is well tolerated, all subsequent infusions may be administered over 30 minutes.

Dose Modification Criteria

Renal impairment: no dose modification; hepatic impairment: no dose modification; myelosuppression: no dose modification; nonhematologic toxicity: dose to be modified.

Adverse Reactions

CNS: headache; CV: hypertension, hypertensive crisis, and CHF; GI: N/VL1, diarrhea, abdominal pain, gastrointestinal perforation, and wound dehiscence; GU: proteinuria and nephrotic syndrome; INFUS: fever, chills, wheezing, and stridor; PULM: dyspnea and wheezing stridor; OTHER: epistaxis and other mild to moderate hemorrhagic events, serious hemorrhagic events, wound healing complications, deep vein thrombosis or other thromboembolic events, and asthenia.

Comments

- Bevacizumab can result in the development of gastrointestinal perforation and wound dehiscence and other wound healing complications. The appropriate interval between termination of bevacizumab and subsequent elective surgery that is required to avoid the risks of wound healing or wound dehiscence has not been determined. Product labeling suggests that bevacizumab should not be initiated for at least 28 days following major surgery, and the surgical incision should be fully healed before starting therapy.

- Bleeding complications secondary to bevacizumab occur in two distinct patterns: minor hemorrhage (most commonly, grade 1 epistaxis) and serious, and in some cases fatal, hemorrhagic events. Patients with squamous cell non–small cell lung cancer (NSCLC) appear to be at higher risk for serious hemorrhagic events. The risk of CNS bleeding in patients with CNS metastases who are receiving bevacizumab has not been evaluated.
- Blood pressure should be monitored every 2 to 3 weeks during therapy and more frequently in patients who develop hypertension.
- Urinalysis should be done serially for proteinuria; patients with a 2+ or greater urine dipstick reading should undergo further assessment (e.g., a 24-hour urine collection).
- Teratogenic (pregnancy category C): Angiogenesis is critical to fetal development and bevacizumab has been shown to be teratogenic in rabbits.

BEXAROTENE (TARGRETIN)

Mechanism of Action

Bexarotene is a retinoid that selectively binds and activates retinoid X receptor (RXR) subtypes. Once activated, these receptors function as transcription factors that regulate the expression of genes that control cellular differentiation and proliferation.

U.S. Food and Drug Administration–Approved Indications

Cutaneous T-cell lymphoma (CTCL): second-line therapy for the cutaneous manifestations of CTCL in patients who are refractory to at least one prior systemic therapy

U.S. Food and Drug Administration–Approved Dosage

300 mg per m^2 PO daily with a meal

Dose Modification Criteria

Renal impairment: no dose modification (caution as a result of possible protein binding alterations); hepatic impairment: use with caution; toxicity: dose to be modified.

Adverse Reactions

CNS: headache; CV: peripheral edema; DERM: dry skin, photosensitivity, rash, and pruritus; ENDO: hypothyroidism and hypoglycemia (diabetic patients); GI: nausea, pancreatitis, elevated LFT values, and abdominal pain; HEMAT: leukopenia and anemia; OCULAR: cataracts; OTHER: lipid abnormalities (i.e., elevated triglycerides, elevated total and LDL cholesterol, and decreased HDL cholesterol), asthenia, and infection.

Comments

- Fasting blood lipid levels should be monitored before initiation of bexarotene and weekly after initiation of therapy until the lipid response is established (usually occurs within 2 to 4 weeks) and then at 8-week intervals thereafter.
- LFT results should be monitored before initiation of bexarotene and then after 1, 2, and 4 weeks of treatment and, if stable, at least every 8 weeks thereafter for the treatment period.
- Complete blood count and thyroid function tests to be monitored at baseline, and periodically thereafter.
- Bexarotene is a teratogen (pregnancy category X) and may cause harm to fetus when administered to a pregnant woman. Bexarotene must not be given to a pregnant woman or to a woman who intends to become pregnant. Women of childbearing potential should obtain a negative

pregnancy test within 1 week before starting bexarotene therapy, and the test should be repeated at monthly intervals while the patient remains on therapy. Effective contraception (two reliable forms used simultaneously) must be used for 1 month before initiation of therapy, during therapy, and for at least 1 month following discontinuation of therapy. Bexarotene may induce the metabolism of hormonal contraceptives and reduce their effectiveness; therefore, one form of contraception should be nonhormonal.

BICALUTAMIDE (CASODEX)

Mechanism of Action

Bicalutamide has antiandrogenic activity.

U.S. Food and Drug Administration–Approved Indications

Palliation of advanced prostate cancer (stage D2) in combination with a luteinizing hormone–releasing hormone (LH-RH) agonist.

U.S. Food and Drug Administration–Approved Dosage

50 mg PO daily

Dose Modification Criteria

Renal impairment: no dose modification; hepatic impairment (mild to moderate): no dose modification; hepatic impairment (severe): use with caution.

Adverse Reactions

ENDO: loss of libido, hot flashes, and gynecomastia; GI: nausea, diarrhea, and constipation; GU: impotence.

Comments

Monitor LFT results before treatment, at regular intervals for the first 4 months, and periodically thereafter.

BLEOMYCIN (BLENOXANE)

Mechanism of Action

The mechanism of action of bleomycin is unknown, but it may inhibit DNA and ribonucleic acid (RNA) synthesis.

U.S. Food and Drug Administration–Approved Indications

Squamous cell cancers, non-Hodgkin lymphoma, testicular cancer, Hodgkin disease, and malignant pleural effusions

U.S. Food and Drug Administration–Approved Dosage

- A test dose (2 U or less) for the first two doses is recommended in patients with lymphoma.
- The dosage is 0.25 to 0.50 U per kg (10 to 20 U per m^2) i.v. or i.m. or s.c. weekly or twice weekly.
- Malignant pleural effusions: 60 U as a single intrapleural bolus dose.

Dose Modification Criteria

Renal impairment: use with caution (dose modification guidelines are not provided within package insert but are available from other references).

Adverse Reactions

DERM: erythema, rash, striae, vesiculation, hyperpigmentation, skin tenderness, alopecia, nail changes, pruritus, and stomatitis; PULM: pulmonary fibrosis (increases at cumulative doses >400 U, but can occur at lower total doses) and pneumonitis; Other: fever; chills; idiosyncratic reaction consisting of hypotension, mental confusion, fever, chills, and wheezing has been reported in 1% of lymphoma patients; and local pain with intrapleural administration.

Comments

- Patient should be monitored for fine rales as an early indication of pulmonary toxicity.
- Pulmonary toxicity is increased when oxygen is used during surgery.

BORTEZOMIB (VELCADE)

Mechanism of Action

Bortezomib is a reversible inhibitor of the 26S proteosome, a large protein complex that degrades ubiquitinated proteins. Inhibition of the 26S proteosome prevents targeted proteolysis, which can effect multiple signaling cascades within the cell. This disruption of normal homeostatic mechanisms can lead to cell death.

U.S. Food and Drug Administration–Approved Indications

Multiple myeloma: second-line therapy in patients with multiple myeloma who have received at least two earlier therapies and have demonstrated disease progression during the last therapy.

U.S. Food and Drug Administration–Approved Dosage

The dosage is 1.3 mg per m^2 i.v. as a bolus injection administered twice weekly for 2 weeks (days 1, 4, 8, and 11), followed by a 10-day rest period (days 12 to 21). Three weeks (21 days) is considered to be a treatment cycle. At least 72 hours should elapse between consecutive doses of bortezomib.

Dose Modification Criteria

Renal impairment: no data are available (use with caution); Hepatic impairment: no data are available (use with caution); Myelosuppression: dose to be modified; nonhematologic toxicity (e.g., neuropathy and neuropathic pain): dose to be modified

Adverse Reactions

CNS: peripheral neuropathy, neuropathic pain, dizziness, and headache; CV: hypotension (including orthostatic hypotension and syncope) and edema; DERM: rash; GI: N/V L2–3, diarrhea, anorexia, and constipation; HEMAT: myelosuppression (thrombocytopenia more severe than anemia, which is more severe than neutropenia); OCULAR: diplopia and blurred vision; PULM: dyspnea; OTHER: asthenia, fatigue, fever, insomnia, and arthralgia.

BUSULFAN (MYLERAN); BUSULFAN INJECTION (BUSULFEX)

Mechanism of Action

Busulfan is an alkylating agent.

U.S. Food and Drug Administration–Approved Indications

- Oral busulfan: Palliative treatment of chronic myelogenous leukemia (CML).
- Parenteral (i.v.) busulfan: Conditioning regimen (in combination with cyclophosphamide) before allogeneic hematopoietic progenitor cell transplantation for CML.

U.S. Food and Drug Administration–Approved Dosage

- Oral busulfan: induction: 4 to 8 mg PO daily; maintenance: 1 to 3 mg PO daily.
- Parenteral (i.v.) busulfan:
  - Premedicate patients with phenytoin before busulfan administration.
  - For nonobese patients, use ideal body weight (IBW) or actual body weight, whichever is lower.
  - For obese or severely obese patients, use adjusted IBW (AIBW). AIBW should be calculated as follows: AIBW = IBW + 0.25 × (actual weight – IBW).
  - Dosage is 0.8 mg per kg over 2 hours every 6 hours × 16 doses (total dose: 12.8 mg per kg) with cyclophosphamide.

Dose Modification Criteria

Myelosuppression: dose to be modified

Adverse Reactions

CNS: seizures; DERM: hyperpigmentation; GI: N/V oral L1, i.v. L4; HEMAT: severe myelosuppression; HEPATIC: venoocclusive disease (VOD); PULM: pulmonary fibrosis and VOD.

Comments

- Phenytoin reduces plasma area under the curve (AUC) of busulfan by 15%. Use of other anticonvulsants may result in higher plasma AUCs of busulfan and an increased risk of VOD or seizures. Monitor plasma busulfan exposure if other anticonvulsants are used.
- High-dose oral busulfan regimens have also been utilized for conditioning regimens in the allogeneic stem cell transplantation setting. Consult current literature for dosing regimens.

CAPECITABINE (XELODA)

Mechanism of Action

Capecitabine is an antimetabolite that is enzymatically converted to fluorouracil in tumors.

U.S. Food and Drug Administration–Approved Indications

- Colorectal cancer: first-line therapy for patients with metastatic colorectal carcinoma when treatment with fluoropyrimidine therapy alone is preferred.
- Combination therapy for breast cancer: capecitabine combined with docetaxel is indicated for the treatment of patients with metastatic breast cancer after failure with earlier anthracycline-containing chemotherapy.

- Monotherapy for breast cancer: Third-line therapy for metastatic breast cancer (after paclitaxel and an anthracycline-containing chemotherapeutic regimen), or second-line (after paclitaxel) therapy if anthracycline is not indicated.

U.S. Food and Drug Administration–Approved Dosage

The dosage is 1,250 mg per m^2 PO twice daily (total daily dose: 2,500 mg per m^2) at the end of a meal for 2 weeks, followed by a 1-week rest period, given as 3-week cycles. Product labeling may be consulted for a dosing chart.

Dose Modification Criteria

Renal (mild impairment; CrCl 51 to 80 mL per minute): no modification to dosage; renal (moderate impairment; CrCl 30 to 50 mL per minute): dosage to be modified; hepatic (mild-to-moderate impairment because of liver metastases): no modification of dosage; toxicity (grade 2 toxicity or higher): dosage to be modified. Product labeling may be consulted for dose modification guidelines.

Adverse Reactions

CNS: fatigue or weakness, paresthesia, and peripheral sensory neuropathy; DERM: hand and foot syndrome (palmar–plantar erythrodysesthesia) and dermatitis; GI: N/V L2, diarrhea, mucositis, abdominal pain, anorexia, and hyperbilirubinemia; HEMAT: myelosuppression.

CARBOPLATIN (PARAPLATIN)

Mechanism of Action

Carboplatin is an alkylating-like agent producing interstrand DNA cross-links.

U.S. Food and Drug Administration–Approved Indications

Advanced ovarian cancer:
- First-line therapy (in combination with other agents).
- Second-line therapy (including patients who have previously received cisplatin).

U.S. Food and Drug Administration–Approved Dosage

- With cyclophosphamide: 300 mg per m^2 i.v. × one dose on day 1 of the cycle; cycles to be repeated every 4 weeks × six cycles.
- Single agent: 360 mg per m^2 i.v. × one dose every 4 weeks.
- Formula dosing may be used as an alternative to dosing based on body surface area (BSA).
- Calvert Formula for Carboplatin Dosing:
  Total dose in milligrams = (target AUC) × [glomerular filtration rate (GFR) + 25].
- The target AUC of 4 to 6 mg/mL/minute using single-agent carboplatin appears to provide the most appropriate dose range in previously treated patients.
- The Calvert formula was based on studies where GFR was measured by ^{51}Cr–EDTA clearance. Alternatively, many clinicians commonly use estimated CrCl equations to determine GFR.

Dose Modification Criteria

Renal impairment: dosage is to be modified; Myelosuppression: dosage is to be modified.

Adverse Reactions

CNS: neuropathy; GI: N/V L4, increased LFT values; ELECTRO: Mg, Na, Ca, and K alterations; GU: Increased Cr and BUN; HEMAT: myelosuppression (thrombocytopenia greater than leukopenia and anemia); OTHER: anaphylactic reactions; pain and asthenia.

Comments

Not to be confused with cisplatin for dosing or during preparation.

CARMUSTINE (BICNU)

Mechanism of Action

Carmustine is an alkylating agent.

U.S. Food and Drug Administration–Approved Indications

Indicated as palliative therapy either as a single agent or in established combination therapy with other approved chemotherapeutic agents in the following: brain tumors, multiple myeloma, Hodgkin disease, and non-Hodgkin lymphomas.

U.S. Food and Drug Administration–Approved Dosage

Single agent in previously untreated patients: 150 to 200 mg per m^2 i.v. $\times$ one dose every 6 weeks, or 75 to 100 mg per m^2 i.v. daily $\times$ two doses every 6 weeks.

Dose Modification Criteria

Myelosuppression: dosage to be modified.

Adverse Reactions

GI: N/V L5 for dosage >250 mg per m^2, and L4 for dosage ≤250 mg per m^2; increased LFT values; GU: nephrotoxicity with large cumulative doses; HEMAT: myelosuppression (can be delayed); OCULAR: retinal hemorrhages; PULM: pulmonary fibrosis (acute and delayed).

Comments

Risk of pulmonary toxicity increases with cumulative total doses >1,400 mg per m^2 and in patients with a history of lung disease, radiation therapy, or concomitant bleomycin.

CETUXIMAB (ERBITUX)

Mechanism of Action

Cetuximab is a recombinant chimeric monoclonal antibody that binds to the extracellular domain of the human epidermal growth factor receptor (EGFR) on both normal and tumor cells, and competitively inhibits the binding of epidermal growth factor (EGF) and other ligands, thereby blocking the phosphorylation and activation of receptor-associated kinases.

U.S. Food and Drug Administration–Approved Indications

Metastatic colorectal carcinoma (second-line therapy): cetuximab is indicated for use in combination with irinotecan in EGFR-expressing metastatic colorectal carcinoma in patients who are refractory to irinotecan-based chemotherapy, and as monotherapy in patients who are intolerant to irinotecan-based chemotherapy.

U.S. Food and Drug Administration–Approved Dosage

In the treatment of metastatic colorectal carcinoma (combined with irinotecan or as monotherapy): 400 mg per m^2 i.v. infusion over 120 minutes as an initial loading dose (first infusion) followed by a weekly maintenance dose of 250 mg per m^2 i.v. infusion over 60 minutes. Premedication with an H_1 antagonist (e.g., 50 mg of diphenhydramine i.v.) is recommended.

Dose Modification Criteria

Renal impairment: no dosage modification; hepatic impairment: no dosage modification; symptoms of non-hematologic toxicity (dermatologic toxicity): dosage to be modified.

Adverse Reactions

DERM: acneform rash, skin drying and fissuring, and nail toxicity; GI: nausea, constipation, and diarrhea; INFUS: chills, fever, dyspnea, airway obstruction (bronchospasm, stridor, hoarseness), urticaria, and hypotension; PULM: interstitial lung disease; OTHER: asthenia, malaise, and fever.

Comments

- Patients enrolled in the clinical studies of cetuximab for metastatic colorectal carcinoma were required to have immunohistochemical evidence of positive EGFR expression. Response rate did not correlate with either the percentage of positive cells or the intensity of EGFR expression.
- Grade 1 and 2 infusion reactions (chills, fever, and dyspnea) are common (16% to 23%) usually on the first day of initial dosing. Severe infusion reactions have been observed in approximately 3% of patients and are characterized by a rapid onset of airway obstruction, urticaria, and/or hypotension. Severe infusion reactions require immediate interruption of the cetuximab infusion and permanent discontinuation from further treatment.
- An acneform rash is common (approximately 90% overall, 10% grade 3) with cetuximab therapy and is most commonly observed on the face, upper chest, and back. Drying and fissuring of the skin are common and can be associated with sequelae of inflammatory responses or infections. Interruption of therapy and dose modification is recommended for severe dermatologic toxicity (product labeling may be consulted).
- Interstitial lung disease has rarely been reported with cetuximab therapy. In the event of acute onset or worsening pulmonary symptoms, cetuximab therapy should be interrupted and symptoms should be promptly investigated.
- Pregnancy Category C: No animal reproduction studies have been conducted and effects in pregnant women are unknown. However, EGFR has been implicated in the control of prenatal development and human immunoglobulin (Ig)G1 is known to cross the placental barrier.

CHLORAMBUCIL (LEUKERAN)
Mechanism of Action

Alkylating agent

U.S. Food and Drug Administration–Approved Indications

Palliation of CLL, Hodgkin disease, and non-Hodgkin lymphomas

U.S. Food and Drug Administration–Approved Dosage

- Initial and short courses of therapy: 0.1 to 0.2 mg per kg PO daily for 3 to 6 weeks as required. Usually the 0.1 mg/kg/day dosage is used except for Hodgkin disease, in which 0.2 mg/kg/day is used.
- Alternate regimen in treatment of CLL (intermittent, biweekly, or once monthly pulses): Initial single dose of 0.4 mg per kg PO × one dose. Dose may be increase by 0.1 mg per kg until control of lymphocytosis is achieved.
- Maintenance: Not to exceed 0.1 mg/kg/day.

Dose Modification Criteria

Myelosuppression: dose to be modified

Adverse Reactions

CNS: seizures, confusion, twitching, and hallucinations; DERM: rash and rare reports of progressive skin hypersensitivity reactions; GI: N/V L1 and increased LFT values; HEMAT: myelosuppression and lymphopenia; PULM: pulmonary fibrosis; OTHER: allergic reactions, secondary acute myelomonocytic leukemia (AML) (long-term therapy), and sterility.

Comments

Radiation and cytotoxic drugs render the bone marrow more vulnerable to damage; chlorambucil should be used with caution within 4 weeks of a full course of radiation therapy or chemotherapy.

CISPLATIN (PLATINOL)

Mechanism of Action

Cisplatin is an alkylating-like agent that produces interstrand DNA cross-links.

U.S. Food and Drug Administration–Approved Indications

- Metastatic testicular tumors (in combination with other agents)
- Metastatic ovarian tumors (in combination with other agents)
- Advanced transitional cell bladder cancer that is no longer amenable to local treatments such as surgery and/or radiotherapy

U.S. Food and Drug Administration–Approved Dosage

- In the treatment of metastatic testicular tumors: 20 mg per m^2 i.v. daily × 5 days every 4 weeks (in combination with other agents)
- In treatment of metastatic ovarian tumors: 75 to 100 mg per m^2 i.v. × one dose (in combination with cyclophosphamide) every 4 weeks, or as single-agent therapy: 100 mg per m^2 i.v. × one dose every 4 weeks
- Advanced bladder cancer: 50 to 70 mg per m^2 i.v. × one dose every 3 to 4 weeks (single-agent therapy)

Dose Modification Criteria

Renal impairment: dose to be modified; myelosuppression: dose to be modified

Adverse Reactions

CNS: neuropathy, paresthesia, and ototoxicity; ELECTRO: Mg, Na, Ca, and K alterations; GI: N/V (for dose $\geq$50 mg per m^2: L5, for dose <50 mg per m^2: L4) increased LFT values [especially serum glutamic-oxaloacetic transaminase (ALT), bilirubin]; GU: increased Cr and BUN (cumulative); HEMAT: myelosuppression, and anemia; OCULAR: optic neuritis, papilledema, and cerebral blindness infrequently reported; OTHER: anaphylactic reactions and rare vascular toxicities.

Comments

- Checking auditory acuity is recommended.
- Vigorous hydration is recommended before and after cisplatin administration.
- Use of other nephrotoxic agents (e.g., aminoglycosides) concomitantly with cisplatin should be undertaken with caution.
- Every precaution should be taken to avoid inadvertent cisplatin overdose and confusion with carboplatin.

CLADRIBINE (LEUSTATIN)
Mechanism of Action

Antimetabolite

U.S. Food and Drug Administration–Approved Indications

Hairy cell leukemia

U.S. Food and Drug Administration–Approved Dosage

- 0.09 mg per kg i.v. continuous infusion over 24 hours daily $\times$ 7 days (a single course of therapy)
- Inadequate data available on dosing of patients with renal or hepatic insufficiency.

Dose Modification Criteria

Renal impairment: no data available on dosage modification; hepatic impairment: no data available on dosage modification.

Adverse Reactions

CNS: fatigue, headache, and peripheral neuropathy; GI: N/V L1; HEMAT: myelosuppression and lymphopenia; DERM: rash; OTHER: fever.

Comments

Immunosuppression (lymphopenia) persists for up to 1 year after cladribine therapy.

CYCLOPHOSPHAMIDE (CYTOXAN)
Mechanism of Action

Cyclophosphamide is an alkylating agent that is activated by the liver.

U.S. Food and Drug Administration–Approved Indications

Lymphomas, leukemias, multiple myeloma, mycosis fungoides (advanced disease), neuroblastoma (disseminated disease), adenocarcinoma of the ovary, retinoblastoma, breast cancer.

U.S. Food and Drug Administration–Approved Dosage

- Parenteral (i.v.): Many dosing regimens reported. Current literature may be consulted.
- Oral: 1 to 5 mg/kg/day (many other regimens reported; Current literature may be consulted)

Dose Modification Criteria

Myelosuppression: dose to be modified.

Adverse Reactions

CNS: syndrome of inappropriate antidiuretic hormone (SIADH); DERM: rash, skin and nail pigmentation, and alopecia; GI: N/V (>1,500 mg per m^2: L5, between 750 mg per m^2 and 1,500 mg per m^2: L4, <750 mg per m^2: L3), anorexia, and diarrhea; GU: hemorrhagic cystitis, renal tubular necrosis; HEMAT: myelosuppression (leukopenia greater than thrombocytopenia and anemia); PULM: pulmonary fibrosis; OTHER: secondary malignancies; sterility, amenorrhea; anaphylactic reactions; cardiac toxicity with high-dose regimens.

Comments

Encourage forced fluid intake and frequent voiding to reduce the risk of hemorrhagic cystitis. Use of vigorous intravenous hydration and Mesna therapy with high-dose cyclophosphamide may be considered.

CYTARABINE (CYTOSAR AND OTHERS)

Mechanism of Action

Cytarabine is an antimetabolite.

U.S. Food and Drug Administration–Approved Indications

Induction therapy of acute nonlymphocytic leukemia, (ANLL), in combination with other agents, ALL, blast-phase chronic myelocytic leukemia (CML), intrathecal prophylaxis and treatment of meningeal leukemia.

U.S. Food and Drug Administration–Approved Dosage

- ALL: Current literature may be consulted for doses.
- ANLL induction (in combination with other agents): 100 mg per m^2 i.v. continuous infusion over 24 hours × 7 days *or* 100 mg per m^2 i.v. every 12 hours × 7 days. Current literature may be consulted for alternative dosing regimens (e.g., high-dose regimens such as ≥1 g/m^2/dose).
- Intrathecally: (use preservative-free diluents) 30 mg per m^2 intrathecally every 4 days until cerebrospinal fluid (CSF) is clear, followed by one additional dose. Other doses and frequency of administration have also been utilized.

Dose Modification Criteria

Hepatic/Renal impairment: To be used with caution and at possibly reduced dose in patients with poor hepatic or renal function (no specific criteria). Neurotoxicity: dose to be modified.

Adverse Reactions

CNS: cerebellar dysfunction, somnolence, coma (generally seen with high-dose regimens), and chemical arachnoiditis (intrathecal administration); DERM: rash and alopecia; GI: N/V L2 (>1 g per m^2 L4), anorexia, diarrhea, mucositis, increased LFT values and pancreatitis (in patients who have previously received asparaginase); HEMAT: myelosuppression; OCULAR: conjunctivitis (generally seen with high-dose regimens); OTHER: cytarabine (Ara-C) syndrome (includes fever, myalgia, bone pain, rash, conjunctivitis, and malaise); acute respiratory distress syndrome reported with high-dose regimens.

Comments

- Appropriate prophylaxis may be considered for tumor lysis syndrome when treating acute leukemias.
- Local corticosteroid eye drops may be considered to provide prophylaxis for conjunctivitis when employing high-dose regimens of cytarabine.
- Therapy to be withheld if acute CNS toxicity occurs with high-dose regimens.

CYTARABINE LIPOSOME INJECTION (DEPOCYT)

Mechanism of Action

Cytarabine liposome is an antimetabolite.

U.S. Food and Drug Administration–Approved Indications

Intrathecal treatment of lymphomatous meningitis.

U.S. Food and Drug Administration–Approved Dosage

- Given only by intrathecal route either by an intraventricular reservoir or directly into the lumbar sac over a period of 1 to 5 minutes.
- Patients should be started on dexamethasone, 4 mg PO or i.v. twice daily × 5 days beginning on the day of the cytarabine liposome injection.
- Induction: 50 mg intrathecally every 14 days × two doses (weeks 1 and 3).
- Consolidation: 50 mg intrathecally every 14 days × three doses (weeks 5, 7, and 9) followed by an additional dose at week 13.
- Maintenance: 50 mg intrathecally every 28 days × four doses (weeks 17, 21, 25, 29).

Dose Modification Criteria

Neurotoxicity: dose to be modified.

Adverse Reactions

CNS: Chemical arachnoiditis, headache, asthenia, confusion, and somnolence.

DACARBAZINE (DTIC-DOME)

Mechanism of Action

Mechanism of dacarbazine is unknown.

U.S. Food and Drug Administration–Approved Indications

Metastatic malignant melanoma, Hodgkin disease (second-line therapy).

U.S. Food and Drug Administration–Approved Dosage

- Malignant melanoma: 2 to 4.5 mg per kg i.v. daily × 10 days; repeat every 4 weeks, or 250 mg per m² i.v. daily × 5 days; repeat every 3 weeks.
- Hodgkin disease: 150 mg per m² i.v. daily × 5 days, repeat every 4 weeks (in combination with other agents), or 375 mg per m² i.v. on day 1, repeat every 15 days (in combination with other agents).

Adverse Reactions

DERM: alopecia, rash, facial flushing, and facial paresthesia; GI: N/V L5, anorexia, diarrhea, increased LFT values, and hepatic necrosis; OTHER: pain and burning at infusion, anaphylaxis, fever, myalgias, and malaise.

DACTINOMYCIN (COSMEGEN)

Mechanism of Action

Dactinomycin is an intercalating agent.

U.S. Food and Drug Administration–Approved Indications

Indicated as part of a combination chemotherapy or multi-modality treatment regimen for the following malignancies: Wilms tumor; childhood rhabdomyosarcoma; Ewing sarcoma; and metastatic, nonseminomatous testicular cancer. Indicated as a single agent or as part of a combination regimen for gestational trophoblastic neoplasia. Indicated as a component of regional perfusion in the treatment of locally recurrent or locoregional solid malignancies.

U.S. Food and Drug Administration–Approved Dosage

- For obese or edematous patients, the dosage should be based on BSA.
- Dose intensity should not exceed 15 μg per kg i.v. daily × 5 days or 400 to 600 μg per m² i.v. daily × 5 days, repeated every 3 to 6 weeks.
- Current literature to be consulted for dosage regimens and guidelines.

Dose Modification Criteria

Myelosuppression: dose to be modified.

Adverse Reactions

DERM: alopecia, erythema, skin eruptions, radiation recall, and tissue damage or necrosis, with extravasation; ELECTRO: hypocalcemia; GI: N/V (>1.5 mg per m²: L4, ≤1.5 mg per m²: L3), mucositis, anorexia, dysphagia, increased LFT values, and hepatotoxicity; HEMAT: myelosuppression; OTHER: fever, fatigue, myalgia, and secondary malignancies.

Comments

Vesicant

DAUNORUBICIN (CERUBIDINE)

Mechanism of Action

Daunorubicin is an intercalating agent that inhibits topoisomerase-II.

U.S. Food and Drug Administration–Approved Indications

In adult ANLL or ALL (children and adults) in combination with other agents for remission induction.

U.S. Food and Drug Administration–Approved Dosage

- ANLL: in combination with cytarabine
  - Age <60 years: first course: 45 mg per m^2 i.v. daily × 3 days (days 1, 2, and 3); subsequent course: 45 mg per m^2 i.v. daily × 2 days (days 1 and 2).
  - Age ≥60 years: first course: 30 mg per m^2 i.v. daily × 3 days (days 1, 2, and 3); subsequent course: 30 mg per m^2 i.v. daily × 2 days (days 1 and 2).
- Adult ALL: (combined with vincristine, prednisone, and L-asparaginase) 45 mg per m^2 i.v. daily × 3 days (days 1, 2, and 3).
- Pediatric ALL: (combined with vincristine and prednisone) 25 mg per m^2 i.v. × one dose weekly × 4 weeks initially. In children younger than 2 years or <0.5 m^2 BSA, the dosage should be based on weight (1 mg per kg) instead of BSA.

Dose Modification Criteria

Renal impairment: dose to be modified; hepatic: dose is to be modified.

Adverse Reactions

CV: CHF, (risk of cardiotoxicity increases rapidly with total lifetime cumulative doses >400 to 550 mg per m^2 in adults or >300 mg per m^2 in children), arrhythmias; DERM: nail hyperpigmentation, rash, alopecia, tissue damage or necrosis, with extravasation; GI: N/V L3, mucositis; HEMAT: myelosuppression; Other: red-tinged urine, fever, chills, and secondary malignancies.

Comments

- Vesicant
- Consider appropriate prophylaxis for tumor lysis syndrome when treating acute leukemias.

DAUNORUBICIN CITRATE LIPOSOME INJECTION (DAUNOXOME)

Mechanism of Action

Daunorubicin is an intercalating agent that inhibits topoisomerase-II.

U.S. Food and Drug Administration–Approved Indications

Advanced human immunodeficiency virus (HIV)-associated Kaposi sarcoma (first-line therapy).

U.S. Food and Drug Administration–Approved Dosage

40 mg per m^2 i.v. over 60 minutes × one dose every 2 weeks.

Dose Modification Criteria

Hepatic: dose is to be modified; renal impairment: dose is to be modified; myelosuppression: dose is to be modified.

Adverse Reactions

CV: CHF, arrhythmias; DERM: nail, alopecia, hyperpigmentation, and rash; GI: N/V L2, mucositis, and diarrhea; HEMAT: myelosuppression; INFUS: back pain, flushing, and chest tightness (infusion-related reactions usually subside with interruption of the infusion, and generally do not recur if the infusion is then resumed at a slower rate); OTHER: red-tinged urine, fever, chills, and fatigue.

Comments

- Not to be confused with nonliposomal forms of daunorubicin.
- Liposomal formulations of the same drug may not be equivalent.
- In anthracycline-naïve patients, cardiac function is to be evaluated by history and physical examination in each cycle and left ventricular ejection fraction (LVEF) function is to be determined at total cumulative doses of daunorubicin citrate liposome injection of 320 mg per m^2 and at every 160 mg per m^2 thereafter. Patients with preexisting cardiac disease, with a history of radiotherapy encompassing the heart, or with previously received anthracyclines (doxorubicin >300 mg per m^2 or equivalent) should have cardiac function (LVEF) monitored before daunorubicin citrate liposome injection therapy and before every 160 mg per m^2 thereafter.

DENILEUKIN DIFTITOX (ONTAK)

Mechanism of Action

Denileukin diftitox is a fusion protein composed of diphtheria toxin fragments linked to interleukin 2 (IL-2) sequences; interacts with IL-2 cell surface receptors and inhibits cellular protein synthesis.

U.S. Food and Drug Administration–Approved Indications

Treatment of persistent or recurrent CTCL in patients whose malignant cells express the CD25 component of the IL-2 receptor.

U.S. Food and Drug Administration–Approved Dosage

- Cells should be tested for CD25 before administration.
- 9 or 18 μg per kg i.v. over at least 15 minutes daily × 5 days; cycles should be repeated every 21 days. Infusion should be stopped or infusion rate should be reduced for severe infusion-related reactions.

Adverse Reactions

CNS: dizziness; CV: vascular leak syndrome (hypotension and edema hypoalbuminemia), hypotension, and thrombotic events; DERM: rash, pruritus; GI: N/V L3, anorexia, diarrhea, and increased LFT values; HEMAT: anemia; INFUS: acute hypersensitivity-type reactions consisting of one or more of the following: hypotension, back pain, dyspnea, vasodilation, rash, chest pain or tightness, tachycardia, dysphagia, syncope, allergic reactions, or anaphylaxis; PULM: dyspnea and cough; OTHER: flu-like syndrome consisting of one or more of the following: fever and/or chills, asthenia, digestive symptoms, myalgias, and arthralgias (appears several hours to days after dose infusion).

Comments

- Premedication with antipyretics and antihistamines to be considered; emergency medications and resuscitative equipment to be readily available during administration.

- Weight, blood pressure, and serum albumin level should be monitored for vascular leak syndrome. Patients with preexisting low serum albumin levels may be predisposed to the syndrome.
- Patients should be monitored carefully for infection.

DOCETAXEL (TAXOTERE)

Mechanism of Action

Docetaxel has the effect of microtubule assembly stabilization.

U.S. Food and Drug Administration–Approved Indications

- Unresectable, locally advanced, or metastatic NSCLC: first-line therapy in combination with cisplatin and second-line therapy as single agent after failure of prior platinum-based chemotherapy.
- Locally advanced or metastatic breast cancer (after failure of earlier chemotherapy).
- Androgen-independent (hormone-refractory) metastatic prostate cancer (in combination with prednisone).

U.S. Food and Drug Administration–Approved Dosage

- Premedication for hypersensitivity reactions and fluid retention: dexamethasone, 8 mg PO twice daily for 3 days starting 1 day before docetaxel administration.
- NSCLC:
  - First-line therapy (combined with cisplatin): 75 mg per m^2 i.v. over 1 hour $\times$ one dose every 3 weeks (administered immediately prior to cisplatin)
  - Second-line therapy (single agent): 75 mg per m^2 i.v. over 1 hour $\times$ one dose every 3 weeks.
- Breast cancer: 60 to 100 mg per m^2 i.v. over 1 hour $\times$ one dose every 3 weeks.
- Prostate cancer: 75 mg per m^2 i.v. over 1 hour $\times$ one dose every 3 weeks. Prednisone 5 mg orally twice daily is administered continuously.

Dose Modification Criteria

Hepatic: dose to be modified; myelosuppression: dose to be modified; nonhematologic toxicity: dose to be modified (package labeling to be consulted for dose modification guidelines)

Adverse Reactions

CNS: peripheral neurosensory toxicity (paresthesia, dysesthesia, and pain), fever, and asthenia; DERM: rash with localized skin eruptions, erythema and pruritus, nail changes (pigmentation, onycholysis, and pain), and alopecia; GI: N/V L2, diarrhea, mucositis, and increased LFT values; HEMAT: myelosuppression; INFUS: acute hypersensitivity-type reactions consisting of hypotension and/or bronchospasm or generalized rash/erythema; OTHER: severe fluid retention and myalgia.

Comments

- Patients with preexisting hepatic dysfunction are at increased risk of severe toxicity.
- Patients with preexisting effusions should be closely monitored from the first dose for the possible exacerbation of the effusions.
- Lower dose, weekly dosage regimens are commonly utilized. Current literature to be consulted for dose guidelines.
- Non–diethylhexyl phthalate (DEHP) plasticized solution containers and administration sets to be used.

DOXORUBICIN (ADRIAMYCIN AND OTHERS)

Mechanism of Action

Doxorubicin is an intercalating agent and inhibits topoisomerase-II.

U.S. Food and Drug Administration–Approved Indications

ALL, acute nonlymphocytic leukemia; Wilms tumor; neuroblastoma; soft tissue and bone sarcoma; breast, ovarian, thyroid, bronchiogenic, gastric cancer and transitional cell bladder cancer; Hodgkin disease; malignant lymphoma.

U.S. Food and Drug Administration–Approved Dosage

- Many dosing regimens reported. Current literature may be consulted. Common dose regimens listed below.
- Single agent: 60 to 75 mg per m^2 i.v. $\times$ one dose repeated every 3 weeks.
- In combination with other agents: 40 to 60 mg per m^2 i.v. $\times$ one dose, repeated every 3 to 4 weeks.

Dose Modification Criteria

Hepatic: dose to be modified; myelosuppression: dose to be modified.

Adverse Reactions

CV: CHF, (risk of cardiotoxicity increases rapidly with total lifetime cumulative doses >450 mg per m^2) and arrhythmias; DERM: nail hyperpigmentation, onycholysis, alopecia, radiation recall, tissue damage or necrosis with extravasation; GI: N/V (>60 mg per m^2: L4, 20 to 60 mg per m^2: L3, <20 mg per m^2: L2) and mucositis; HEMAT: myelosuppression; OTHER: red-tinged urine, fever, chills, and secondary malignancies.

Comments

Vesicant

DOXORUBICIN HYDROCHLORIDE LIPOSOME INJECTION (DOXIL)

Mechanism of Action

Doxorubicin is an intercalating agent and inhibits topoisomerase-II.

U.S. Food and Drug Administration–Approved Indications

- Acquired immunodeficiency syndrome (AIDS)–related Kaposi sarcoma (progressive disease after earlier combination chemotherapy or in patients intolerant to such therapy)
- Metastatic ovarian cancer (second-line therapy after both paclitaxel- and platinum-based chemotherapy regimens)

U.S. Food and Drug Administration–Approved Dosage

- AIDS-related Kaposi sarcoma: 20 mg per m^2 i.v. over 30 minutes $\times$ one dose, repeated every 3 weeks.
- Ovarian cancer: 50 mg per m^2 i.v. over 60 minutes $\times$ one dose, repeated every 4 weeks.

- Note: Infusion should start at an initial rate of 1 mg per minute to minimize the risk of infusion reactions. If no infusion-related adverse events are observed, the rate of infusion can be increased to complete administration of the drug over 1 hour.

Dose Modification Criteria

Hepatic: dose to be modified; Palmar–plantar erythrodysesthesia: dose to be modified; Myelosuppression: dose to be modified; Stomatitis: dose to be modified.

Adverse Reactions

CV: CHF and arrhythmias; DERM: palmar–plantar erythrodysesthesia, alopecia, and rash; GI: N/V L2, mucositis or stomatitis; HEMAT: myelosuppression; INFUS: flushing, shortness of breath, facial swelling, headache, chills, chest pain, back pain, tightness in chest or throat, fever, tachycardia, pruritus, rash, cyanosis, syncope, bronchospasm, asthma, apnea, and/or hypotension; OTHER: asthenia and red-tinged urine.

Comments

- Not to be confused with nonliposomal forms of doxorubicin.
- Liposomal formulations of the same drug may not be equivalent.
- Irritant
- Mixed only with 5% dextrose water; not to be used in line filters
- Most infusion-related events occur during the first infusion.
- Experience with large cumulative doses of doxorubicin hydrochloride liposome injection is limited and cumulative dose limits based on cardiotoxicity risk have not been established. It is recommended by the manufacturer that cumulative dose limits established for conventional doxorubicin be followed for the liposomal product (e.g., cumulative doses ≥ 400 to 550 mg per m^2 depending on risk factors).

EPIRUBICIN (ELLENCE)

Mechanism of Action

Epirubicin is an intercalating agent and inhibits topoisomerase-II.

U.S. Food and Drug Administration–Approved Indications

Adjuvant therapy of axillary node–positive breast cancer.

U.S. Food and Drug Administration–Approved Dosage

The following dosage regimens were used in the trials supporting use of epirubicin as a component of adjuvant therapy in patients with axillary-node–positive breast cancer.
- CEF 120: 60 mg per m^2 i.v. $\times$ one dose on days 1 and 8, (120 mg per m^2 total dose each cycle), repeated every 28 days for six cycles. (Combined with cyclophosphamide and fluorouracil.)
- FEC 100: 100 mg per m^2 i.v. $\times$ one dose on day 1 only, repeated every 21 days for six cycles. (Combined with cyclophosphamide and fluorouracil.)

Dose Modification Criteria

Renal impairment: dose to be modified; hepatic impairment: dose to be modified; myelosuppression: dose to be modified.

Adverse Reactions

CV: CHF (risk of cardiotoxicity increases rapidly with total lifetime cumulative doses >900 mg per m^2), arrhythmias; DERM: alopecia, radiation recall, tissue damage or necrosis with extravasation; GI: N/V (>90 mg per m^2: L4, ≤90 mg per m^2: L3), and mucositis; HEMAT: myelosuppression; OTHER: facial flushing, and secondary malignancies.

Comments

Vesicant

ESTRAMUSTINE (EMCYT)

Mechanism of Action

Estramustine is an alkylating agent, an estrogen, and induces microtubule instability.

U.S. Food and Drug Administration–Approved Indications

Palliative treatment of metastatic and/or progressive carcinoma of the prostate.

U.S. Food and Drug Administration–Approved Dosage

- 4.67 mg per kg PO three times daily (t.i.d.) or 3.5 mg per kg PO four times daily (q.i.d.); total daily dose: 14 mg per kg.
- Administer with water, 1 hour before or 2 hours after meals. Avoid the simultaneous administration of milk, milk products, and calcium-rich foods and drugs.

Dose Modification Criteria

Hepatic impairment: to be administered with caution, no specific dose modifications

Adverse Reactions

CV: Edema, fluid retention, and venous thromboembolism; ENDO: hyperglycemia, gynecomastia, and impotence; GI: diarrhea, nausea, and elevated LFT values [especially glutamic-oxaloacetic transaminase (SGOT) or lactate dehydrogenase (LDH)]; PULM: dyspnea.

ETOPOSIDE (VEPESID)

Mechanism of Action

Etoposide leads to topoisomerase-II interaction.

U.S. Food and Drug Administration–Approved Indications

Refractory testicular cancer; small cell lung cancer (SCLC, first-line therapy in combination with other agents).

U.S. Food and Drug Administration–Approved Dosage

- Testicular cancer: 50 to 100 mg per m^2 i.v. over 30 to 60 minutes daily × 5 days (days 1 to 5), repeated every 3 to 4 weeks or 100 mg per m^2 i.v. over 30 to 60 minutes on days 1, 3, and 5, repeated every 3 to 4 weeks (in combination with other approved agents). Current literature may be consulted for dose recommendations.

- SCLC: 35 to 50 mg per m^2 i.v. over 30 to 60 minutes daily $\times$ 4 to 5 days, repeated every 3 to 4 weeks (in combination with other agents). Current literature to be consulted for dose recommendations.
- Oral capsules: In SCLC, the recommended dose of etoposide capsules is two times the i.v. dose rounded to the nearest 50 mg.

Dose Modification Criteria

Renal impairment: dose to be modified.

Adverse Reactions

DERM: alopecia, rash, urticaria, and pruritus; GI: N/V L2, mucositis, and anorexia; HEMAT: myelosuppression; INFUS: hypotension (infusion-rate related), anaphylactic-like reactions (characterized by chills, fever, tachycardia, bronchospasm, dyspnea, and/or hypotension); OTHER: secondary malignancies.

ETOPOSIDE PHOSPHATE (ETOPHOS)

Mechanism of Action

Etoposide phosphate is rapidly and completely converted to etoposide in plasma, leading to topoisomerase-II interaction.

U.S. Food and Drug Administration–Approved Indications

Refractory testicular cancer; SCLC, first-line therapy in combination with other agents.

U.S. Food and Drug Administration–Approved Dosage

- Testicular cancer: 50 to 100 mg per m^2 i.v. daily $\times$ 5 days (days 1 to 5), repeated every 3 to 4 weeks or 100 mg per m^2 i.v. on days 1, 3, and 5, repeated every 3 to 4 weeks (in combination with other approved agents). Current literature may be consulted for dose recommendations.
- SCLC: 35 to 50 mg per m^2 i.v. daily $\times$ 4 to 5 days, repeated every 3 to 4 weeks (in combination with other agents). Current literature may be consulted for dose recommendations.
- Higher rates of intravenous administration have been utilized and tolerated by patients with etoposide phosphate compared to etoposide. Etoposide phosphate can be administered at infusion rates from 5 to 210 minutes (generally infusion durations of 5 to 30 minutes have been utilized).

Dose Modification Criteria

Renal impairment: dose to be modified.

Adverse Reactions

DERM: alopecia, rash, urticaria, and pruritus; GI: N/V L2, mucositis, and anorexia; HEMAT: myelosuppression; INFUS: hypotension (infusion-rate related) and anaphylactic-like reactions (characterized by chills, fever, tachycardia, bronchospasm, dyspnea, and/or hypotension); OTHER: secondary malignancies.

Comments

Etoposide phosphate is a water-soluble ester of etoposide. The water solubility of etoposide phosphate lessens the potential for precipitation following dilution and during intravenous administration. Enhanced water solubility also allows for lower dilution volumes and more rapid intravenous administration compared to conventional etoposide.

EXEMESTANE (AROMISAN)
Mechanism of Action

Exemestane is an irreversible steroidal aromatase inactivator.

U.S. Food and Drug Administration–Approved Indications

Advanced breast cancer after tamoxifen failure in postmenopausal women.

U.S. Food and Drug Administration–Approved Dosage

25 mg PO daily after a meal.

Dose Modification Criteria

Renal impairment: no dose modification; hepatic impairment: no dose modification.

Note: Drug exposure is increased with hepatic and/or renal insufficiency. The safety of chronic dosing in these settings has not been studied. On the basis of experience with exemestane at repeated doses up to 200 mg daily that demonstrated a moderate increase in non–life-threatening adverse effects, dosage adjustment does not appear to be necessary.

Adverse Reactions

CNS: depression, insomnia, and anxiety; CV: hot flashes and edema; GI: nausea or increased appetite; HEMAT: lymphocytopenia; OTHER: tumor site pain, asthenia, fatigue, increased sweating, and fever.

FLOXURIDINE
Mechanism of Action

Floxuridine is an antimetabolite catabolized to fluorouracil.

U.S. Food and Drug Administration–Approved Indications

Palliative management of gastrointestinal adenocarcinoma metastasis to the liver when given by continuous regional intraarterial infusion in carefully selected patients who are considered incurable by surgery or other means.

U.S. Food and Drug Administration–Approved Dosage

0.1 to 0.6 mg/kg/day by continuous arterial infusion. The higher dose ranges (0.4 to 0.6 mg/kg/day) are usually employed for hepatic artery infusion because the liver metabolizes the drug, thereby reducing the potential for systemic toxicity. Therapy may be given until adverse reactions appear; when toxicities have subsided, therapy may be resumed. Patients may be maintained on therapy as long as response to floxuridine continues.

Dose Modification Criteria

Renal impairment: no dose modification; hepatic impairment: no dose modification; myelo-suppression: dose to be modified; nonhematologic toxicity: dose to be modified

Adverse Reactions

CV: myocardial ischemia; DERM: alopecia, dermatitis, and rash; GI: N/V L1–2, stomatitis, diarrhea, enteritis, gastrointestinal ulceration and bleeding, and elevated LFT values; HEMAT: myelosuppression; INFUS: procedural complications of regional arterial infusion: arterial aneurysm, arterial ischemia, arterial thrombosis, embolism, fibromyositis, thrombophlebitis, hepatic necrosis, abscesses, infection at catheter site, bleeding at catheter site, catheter blocked, displaced or leaking; OTHER: fever, lethargy, malaise, and weakness.

FLUDARABINE (FLUDARA)

Mechanism of Action

Fludarabine is an antimetabolite.

U.S. Food and Drug Administration–Approved Indications

B-cell CLL (second-line after alkylating agent therapy)

U.S. Food and Drug Administration–Approved Dosage

25 mg per m^2 i.v. over 30 minutes daily $\times$ 5 days, repeated every 28 days.

Dose Modification Criteria

Renal impairment: dose to be modified

Adverse Reactions

CNS: weakness, agitation, confusion, visual disturbances, coma (severe neurotoxicity generally seen with high-dose regimens but have been reported rarely at recommended doses), and peripheral neuropathy; CV: edema; DERM: rash; GI: N/V L1, diarrhea, and anorexia; HEMAT: myelosuppression, autoimmune hemolytic anemia, and lymphopenia; PULM: pneumonitis and cases of severe pulmonary toxicity have been reported; OTHER: myalgia, tumor lysis syndrome, and fatigue.

Comments

- Monitor for hemolytic anemia.
- A high incidence of fatal pulmonary toxicity was seen in a trial investigating the combination of fludarabine with pentostatin. The combined use of fludarabine and pentostatin is not recommended.
- Transfusion-associated graft versus host disease has been observed rarely after transfusion of nonirradiated blood in fludarabine-treated patients. Using only irradiated blood products should be considered if transfusions are necessary in patients undergoing treatment with fludarabine.
- Monitor for tumor lysis syndrome and consider prophylaxis for patients with CLL with a large tumor burden who are initiated on fludarabine.

FLUOROURACIL (ADRUCIL AND OTHERS)

Mechanism of Action

Fluorouracil is an antimetabolite.

U.S. Food and Drug Administration–Approved Indications

Palliative management of cancer of colon, rectum, breast, stomach, and pancreas.

U.S. Food and Drug Administration–Approved Dosage

Current literature may be consulted.

Adverse Reactions

CNS: Acute cerebellar syndrome, nystagmus, headache, visual changes, and photophobia; CV: angina and ischemia; DERM: dry skin, photosensitivity, hand-foot syndrome (palmar–plantar erythrodysesthesia), alopecia, dermatitis, and thrombophlebitis; GI: N/V L2, mucositis, diarrhea, anorexia, and gastrointestinal ulceration and bleeding; HEMAT: myelosuppression; OTHER: anaphylaxis and generalized allergic reactions.

Comments

Fluorouracil may be given by continuous intravenous infusion or by rapid i.v. administration (i.v. bolus or push). The method of administration will change the toxicity profile of fluorouracil (e.g., greater potential for GI toxicities such as mucositis and diarrhea with continuous i.v. infusions and more hematologic toxicity with bolus administration).

FLUTAMIDE (EULEXIN)

Mechanism of Action

Flutamide is an antiandrogen.

U.S. Food and Drug Administration–Approved Indications

Stage D2 metastatic prostate carcinoma [in combination with luteinizing hormone releasing hormone (LHRH) agonists] or locally confined stage B2–C prostate carcinoma (in combination with LHRH agonists and radiation therapy).

U.S. Food and Drug Administration–Approved Dosage

- Stage D2 metastatic prostate carcinoma: 250 mg PO t.i.d. (every 8 hours).
- Stage B2–C prostate cancer: 250 mg PO t.i.d. (every 8 hours) beginning 8 weeks before and continuing through radiation.

Adverse Reactions

DERM: Rash; GI: nausea, diarrhea, constipation, increased LFT values (LFT results to be monitored periodically because of rare associations with cholestatic jaundice, hepatic necrosis, and encephalopathy); GU: impotence; ENDO: loss of libido, hot flashes, and gynecomastia.

Comments

Interacts with warfarin; international normalized ratio (INR) to be monitored closely.

FULVESTRANT (FASLODEX)
Mechanism of Action

Fulvestrant is an ER antagonist.

U.S. Food and Drug Administration–Approved Indications

Breast cancer: second-line therapy for hormone-receptor–positive metastatic breast cancer in postmenopausal women with disease progression following antiestrogen therapy.

U.S. Food and Drug Administration–Approved Dosage

250 mg i.m. injection × one dose and repeated at 1-month intervals.

Dose Modification Criteria

Renal impairment: no dosage modification; hepatic (mild impairment): no dosage modification; hepatic (moderate-to-severe impairment): no data available, to be used with caution.

Adverse Reactions

CNS: headache; CV: peripheral edema; ENDO: hot flashes; GI: nausea, constipation, diarrhea, abdominal pain, and anorexia; OTHER: pain, pharyngitis, injection-site reactions, and asthenia.

GEFITINIB (IRESSA)
Mechanism of Action

Gefitinib is an inhibitor of multiple tyrosine kinases, including those associated with the EGFR.

U.S. Food and Drug Administration–Approved Indications

NSCLC: second-line monotherapy for the treatment of patients with locally advanced or metastatic NSCLC after failure of both platinum-based and docetaxel chemotherapies.

U.S. Food and Drug Administration–Approved Dosage

250 mg PO daily

Dose Modification Criteria

Renal impairment: no dose modification; hepatic impairment: no dose modification.

Adverse Reactions

DERM: rash, acne, dry skin, and pruritus; GI: nausea, diarrhea, anorexia, and elevated LFT values; OCULAR: eye pain, corneal erosion or ulcer (sometimes in association with aberrant eyelash growth); PULM: interstitial lung disease (interstitial pneumonia, pneumonitis, and alveolitis); OTHER: asthenia, and weight loss.

Comments

- For patients who present with acute onset or worsening of pulmonary symptoms (dyspnea, cough, and fever), gefitinib therapy should be interrupted and a prompt investigation of these symptoms should occur. Fatalities related to interstitial lung disease have been reported.

- Gefitinib is extensively hepatically metabolized, predominantly by cytochrome P450 (CYP) 3A4. Patients should be monitored for potential drug interactions with either potent inhibitors or inducers of CYP 3A4. A dose increase of gefitinib to 500 mg per day may be considered when given concomitantly with a potent CYP 3A4 enzyme inducer such as phenytoin or rifampin.
- Gefitinib may potentially interact with warfarin, leading to an elevated prothrombin time (PT) and INR and bleeding events; PT/INR to be monitored regularly with concomitant use.

GEMCITABINE (GEMZAR)

Mechanism of Action

Gemcitabine is an antimetabolite.

U.S. Food and Drug Administration–Approved Indications

- Pancreatic Cancer: first-line therapy for patients with locally advanced (nonresectable stage II or stage III) or metastatic (stage IV) adenocarcinoma of the pancreas and in patients with pancreatic cancer who were previously treated with fluorouracil.
- NSCLC: first-line therapy (in combination with cisplatin) for patients with inoperable, locally advanced (stage IIIa or IIIb) or metastatic (stage IV) NSCLC.
- Metastatic breast cancer: first-line therapy (in combination with paclitaxel) for patients with metastatic breast cancer after failure of prior anthracycline-containing adjuvant chemotherapy, unless anthracyclines were clinically contraindicated.

U.S. Food and Drug Administration–Approved Dosage

- Pancreatic cancer (single agent use): 1,000 mg per m^2 i.v. over 30 minutes once weekly for up to 7 weeks, followed by 1 week of rest from treatment. Subsequent cycles should consist of 1,000 mg per m^2 i.v. over 30 minutes once weekly for 3 consecutive weeks out of every 4 weeks.
- NSCLC (combination therapy with cisplatin):
  - 4-week schedule: 1,000 mg per m^2 i.v. over 30 minutes on days 1, 8, and 15 of each 28-day cycle. Cisplatin (100 mg per m^2 i.v. × one dose) should be administered after gemcitabine only on day 1.
  - or 3-week schedule: 1,250 mg per m^2 i.v. over 30 minutes on days 1 and 8 of each 21-day cycle. Cisplatin (100 mg per m^2 i.v. × one dose) should be administered after gemcitabine only on day 1.
- Metastatic breast cancer (combination therapy with paclitaxel): 1,250 mg per m^2 i.v. over 30 minutes on days 1 and 8 of each 21-day cycle. Paclitaxel should be administered at 175 mg per m^2 i.v. over 3 hours × one dose (day 1 only) before gemcitabine administration.

Dose Modification Criteria

Renal impairment: dose to be used with caution; hepatic impairment: dose to be used with caution; myelosuppression: dose to be modified; nonhematologic toxicity: dose to be modified.

Adverse Reactions

DERM: rash and alopecia; GI: N/V L2, constipation, diarrhea, mucositis, increased LFT values and bilirubin, and rare reports of severe hepatotoxicity; GU: proteinuria, hematuria, and hemolytic-uremic syndrome; HEMAT: myelosuppression; PULM: dyspnea, rare reports of severe pulmonary toxicity (pneumonitis, pulmonary fibrosis, pulmonary edema, and acute respiratory distress syndrome); OTHER: fever, pain, and rare reports of vascular toxicity (vasculitis).

Comments

- Clearance in women and elderly is reduced.
- Intravenous administration rate has been shown to influence both efficacy and toxicity. Published literature should be referred to for the appropriate rate of administration for a specific regimen.

GEMTUZUMAB OZOGAMICIN (MYLOTARG)

Mechanism of Action

Gemtuzumab is a humanized monoclonal antibody directed at the CD33 cell surface antigen conjugated with a cytotoxic antitumor antibiotic, calicheamicin. Binding of the anti-CD33 antibody portion of gemtuzumab ozogamicin results in the internalization and release of the calicheamicin, which subsequently causes DNA double strand breakage and cell death.

U.S. Food and Drug Administration–Approved Indications

AML: second-line therapy for patients with CD33-positive AML who are in first relapse, who are 60 years of age or older, and who are not considered candidates for other cytotoxic chemotherapy.

U.S. Food and Drug Administration–Approved Dosage

- 9 mg per m^2 i.v. over 2 hours $\times$ one dose. The recommended treatment course is a total of two doses with 14 days between the doses.
- Consider leukoreduction with hydroxyurea or leukapheresis to reduce the peripheral white blood cell count to $<30,000$ per μL before administration of gemtuzumab ozogamicin.
- Patients to be premedicated with diphenhydramine 50 mg PO and acetaminophen 650 to 1,000 mg PO 1 hour before the administration of gemtuzumab ozogamicin; thereafter, two additional doses of acetaminophen to be given every 4 hours as needed.
- Consider prophylaxis for tumor lysis syndrome with hydration and allopurinol.

Dose Modification Criteria

Renal impairment: no data available for determining dosage; hepatic impairment: no data available for determining dosage (use with caution)

Adverse Reactions

CNS: headache; CV: hypotension, hypertension; DERM: rash; GI: N/V L3, mucositis, anorexia, constipation, diarrhea, elevated LFT values and/or bilirubin level, hepatic VOD; HEMAT: myelosuppression; INFUS: fever, chills, nausea, vomiting, headache, hypotension, hypertension, hyperglycemia, hypoxia, dyspnea, and anaphylaxis; PULM: dyspnea, pulmonary infiltrates, pleural effusions, noncardiogenic pulmonary edema, pulmonary insufficiency and hypoxia, and acute respiratory distress syndrome; OTHER: tumor lysis syndrome, infection, bleeding episodes, and asthenia.

Comments

- Hepatotoxicity, including severe VOD, has been reported with gemtuzumab ozogamicin as a single agent and as part of a combination regimen. Patients who receive gemtuzumab ozogamicin either before or after hematopoietic stem cell transplantation, patients with underlying hepatic disease or abnormal liver function, and patients receiving combination regimens containing

gemtuzumab ozogamicin may be at increased risk. Monitor for rapid weight gain, right upper quadrant pain, hepatomegaly, ascites, and elevations in bilirubin and/or liver enzymes.
- Severe hypersensitivity reactions and other infusion-related reactions can occur (including severe pulmonary events) and can be fatal. Interrupt infusion for patients experiencing dyspnea or clinically significant hypotension. Discontinue treatment for patients who develop anaphylaxis, pulmonary edema, or acute respiratory distress syndrome.

GOSERELIN ACETATE IMPLANT (ZOLADEX)
Mechanism of Action

Goserelin is an LHRH agonist; chronic administration leads to sustained suppression of pituitary gonadotropins and subsequent suppression of serum testosterone in men and serum estradiol in women.

U.S. Food and Drug Administration–Approved Indications

- Stage D2 metastatic prostate carcinoma or locally confined stage B2-C (in combination with flutamide and radiation therapy).
- Palliative treatment of advanced breast cancer in pre- and perimenopausal women.
- Other indications: endometriosis, endometrial thinning

U.S. Food and Drug Administration–Approved Dosage

- Stage D2 metastatic prostate carcinoma: 3.6 mg s.c. depot monthly, or 10.8 mg s.c. depot every 12 weeks.
- Stage B2-C prostate cancer: Start 8 weeks prior to initiating radiotherapy and continue through radiation. A treatment regimen of 3.6 mg s.c. depot, followed in 28 days by 10.8 mg s.c. depot. Alternatively, four injections of 3.6-mg s.c. depot can be administered at 28-day intervals, two depots preceding and two during radiotherapy.
- Breast cancer: 3.6-mg s.c. depot every 4 weeks.

Dose Modification Criteria

Renal impairment: no dosage modification; hepatic impairment: no dosage modification.

Adverse Reactions

CV: transient changes in blood pressure (hypo- or hypertension); CNS: pain; ENDO: (men) hot flashes, gynecomastia, sexual dysfunction, and decreased erections; (women) hot flashes, headache, vaginal dryness, vaginitis, emotional lability, change in libido, depression, increased sweating, and change in breast size; GU: erectile dysfunction and lower urinary tract symptoms; OTHER: tumor flare in the first few weeks of therapy, loss of bone mineral density, osteoporosis, bone fracture, and asthenia.

Comments

Use with caution in patients at risk for developing ureteral obstruction or spinal cord compression.

HYDROXYUREA (HYDREA, DROXIA)
Mechanism of Action

Hydroxyurea inhibits DNA synthesis; it is a radiation sensitizer.

U.S. Food and Drug Administration–Approved Indications

Use in combination with radiation therapy for melanoma; recurrent, metastatic, or inoperable ovarian cancer; resistantCML; and primary squamous cell carcinomas of the head and neck (excluding the lip). Hydroxyurea is also indicated in adult patients with sickle cell anemia with recurrent moderate-to-severe painful crises.

U.S. Food and Drug Administration–Approved Dosage

- Dose based on actual or IBW, whichever is less.
- Solid tumors:
  - Intermittent therapy: 80 mg per kg PO as a single dose every third day.
  - Continuous therapy: 20 to 30 mg per kg PO daily.
- In combination with irradiation for head and neck cancer: 80 mg per kg PO as a single dose every third day, beginning 7 days before initiation of irradiation and continued indefinitely thereafter, based on adverse effects and response.
- Resistant CML: 20 to 30 mg per kg PO daily

Dose Modification Criteria

Renal impairment: dose to be used with caution; hepatic impairment: dose to be used with caution; myelosuppression: dose to be modified.

Adverse Reactions

CNS: drowsiness (large doses); DERM: rash, peripheral and facial erythema, skin ulceration, dermatomyositis-like skin changes, hyperpigmentation; GI: N/V L1, diarrhea, anorexia, mucositis, and constipation; HEMAT: myelosuppression (leukopenia and anemia more severe than thrombocytopenia).

Comments

- Capsule contents may be emptied into glass of water and taken immediately (some inert particles may float on surface).
- Patients should be counseled about proper handling precautions if they open the capsules.

IDARUBICIN (IDAMYCIN)

Mechanism of Action

Idarubicin is an intercalating agent and a topoisomerase-II inhibitor.

U.S. Food and Drug Administration–Approved Indications

In combination with other agents for adult AML (FAB classification M1 to M7).

U.S. Food and Drug Administration–Approved Dosage

AML induction in combination with cytarabine: 12 mg per m^2 slow i.v. injection (over 10 to 15 minutes) daily for 3 days.

Dose Modification Criteria

Renal impairment: dose to be modified; hepatic impairment: dose to be modified; mucositis: dose to be modified.

Adverse Reactions

CV: CHF, arrhythmia; DERM: alopecia, radiation recall, and rash; GI: N/V L3, mucositis, abdominal cramps, and diarrhea; HEMAT: myelosuppression.

Comments

- Vesicant.
- Myocardial toxicity is increased in patients with prior anthracycline therapy or heart disease. Cumulative dose limit not established within package literature.
- Consider appropriate prophylaxis for tumor lysis syndrome when treating acute leukemias.

IFOSFAMIDE (IFEX)
Mechanism of Action

Ifosfamide is an alkylating agent.

U.S. Food and Drug Administration–Approved Indications

Germ cell testicular cancer (third-line therapy in combination with other agents).

U.S. Food and Drug Administration–Approved Dosage

1.2 g per m^2 i.v. daily for 5 days, repeated every 3 weeks. Give Mesna 20% (wt/wt; 240 mg per m^2 per dose for a 1.2 g per m^2 ifosfamide dose) at time of ifosfamide, and then 4 and 8 hours after ifosfamide.

Dose Modification Criteria

Renal impairment: no known experience with dosage; hepatic impairment: no known experience with dosage; myelosuppression: dose to be modified; neurotoxicity: dose to be modified.

Adverse Reactions

CNS: encephalopathy, somnolence, confusion, depressive psychosis, hallucinations, and dizziness; DERM: alopecia; GI: N/V L3, increased LFT values; GU: hemorrhagic cystitis, Fanconi syndrome (proximal tubular impairment), glomerular or tubular toxicity; HEMAT: myelosuppression.

Comments

- Ensure adequate hydration. Administer Mesna concurrently. Monitor for microscopic hematuria.
- Discontinue therapy with the occurrence of neurologic toxicity. The incidence of CNS toxicity may be higher in patients with impaired renal function and/or low serum albumin.

IMATINIB (GLEEVEC)
Mechanism of Action

Imatinib is an inhibitor of multiple tyrosine kinases, including the Bcr-Abl tyrosine kinase, which is created by the Philadelphia chromosome abnormality in CML. Imatinib is also an inhibitor of the receptor tyrosine kinases for platelet-derived growth factor (PDGF) and stem cell factor (SCF), c-kit, and inhibits PDGF- and SCF-mediated cellular events.

U.S. Food and Drug Administration–Approved Indications

- CML:
  - First-line therapy for newly diagnosed adult patients with Philadelphia chromosome positive (Ph+) CML in chronic phase.
  - Second-line therapy for patients in blast crisis, accelerated phase, or in chronic phase after failure of interferon-alpha therapy.
  - Second-line therapy for pediatric patients with Ph+ chronic phase CML whose disease has recurred after stem cell transplantation or who are resistant to interferon-α therapy.
- Gastrointestinal stromal tumors (GIST): treatment of patients with Kit (CD117) positive unresectable and/or metastatic malignant GIST.

U.S. Food and Drug Administration–Approved Dosage

- CLS:
  - Adult patients, chronic phase: 400 mg PO daily. Doses may be escalated to 600 mg per day as clinically indicated (package insert may be consulted for criteria).
  - Adult patients, accelerated phase: 600 mg PO daily. Doses may be escalated to 800 mg per day (400 mg PO b.i.d.) as clinically indicated (package insert may be consulted for criteria).
  - Children: 260 mg per m^2 PO daily. Doses may be escalated to 340 mg per day as clinically indicated (package insert may be consulted for criteria).
- GIST: 400 mg or 600 mg PO daily.
- The prescribed dose should be administered orally, with a meal and a large glass of water. Doses of 400 mg or 600 mg should be administered once daily, whereas a dose of 800 mg should be administered as 400 mg twice a day. In children, imatinib can be given either as a once-a-day dose or divided into two doses (b.i.d.).

Dose Modification Criteria

Renal impairment: no data available; hepatic impairment: no data available; myelosuppression: dose to be modified; nonhematologic toxicity: dose to be modified

Adverse Reactions

CNS: headache and dizziness; CV: superficial edema (periorbital, lower limb), severe fluid retention (pleural effusion, ascites, pulmonary edema, and rapid weight gain); DERM: rash GI: nausea, diarrhea, GI irritation, dyspepsia, elevated LFT values, and severe hepatotoxicity; HEMAT: myelosuppression, and hemorrhage; PULM: cough; OTHER: muscle cramps, pain (musculoskeletal, joint, and abdominal), myalgia, arthralgia, nasopharyngitis, fatigue, and fever.

Comments

- The CYP 3A4 enzyme is the major enzyme responsible for the metabolism of imatinib. Potential drug interactions with either potent inhibitors or inducers of CYP 3A4. Dosage of imatinib should be increased at least 50% and clinical response should be carefully monitored in patients receiving imatinib with a potent CYP3A4 inducer such as rifampin or phenytoin.
- Monitor patient regularly for weight gain and signs and symptoms of fluid retention. An unexpected rapid weight gain should be carefully investigated and appropriate treatment provided. The probability of edema is increased with higher doses of imatinib and in patients older than 65 years.
- LFT results are to be monitored before initiation of imatinib therapy and monthly thereafter or as clinically indicated.

- Complete blood counts (CBC) to be monitored before initiation of imatinib therapy, and then weekly for the first month, biweekly for the second month, and periodically thereafter as clinically indicated (e.g., every 2 to 3 months).

INTERFERON α-2A (ROFERON-A)

Mechanism of Action

Interferon α-2A suppresses cell proliferation and enhances macrophage phagocytic activity and lymphocyte cytotoxicity.

U.S. Food and Drug Administration–Approved Indications

Oncology indications (adults, as old as 18 years or older): Hairy cell leukemia, AIDS-related Kaposi sarcoma, and CML (Philadelphia chromosome positive).
Other indications: chronic hepatitis C

U.S. Food and Drug Administration–Approved Dosage

- Hairy cell leukemia: Induction, 3 million IU i.m. or s.c. daily for 16 to 24 weeks; maintenance, 3 million IU s.c. or i.m. 3 times a week.
- AIDS-related Kaposi sarcoma: Induction, 36 million IU i.m. or s.c. daily for 10 to 12 weeks; maintenance, 36 million IU i.m. or s.c. 3 times a week.
- CML: 9 million IU i.m. or s.c. daily. Initial tolerance may be improved over first week by giving 3 million IU daily × 3 days, then 6 million IU daily × 3 days, then increased to target dose of 9 million IU daily.
- Continue treatment until disease progression or severe toxicity.

Dose Modification Criteria

In cases of serious adverse events: dose is to be modified.

Adverse Reactions

CNS: dizziness, depression, suicidal ideation, and paresthesias; DERM: skin rash, alopecia; ENDO: thyroid abnormalities; GI: diarrhea, nausea, anorexia, taste alteration, abdominal pain, and increased LFT values; HEMAT: myelosuppression; PULM: dyspnea, pulmonary infiltrates, pneumonitis, and pneumonia; OTHER: flu-like symptoms (i.e., fever, chills, headache, fatigue, malaise, and myalgia), hypersensitivity reactions, ophthalmologic disorders, and autoimmune disorders.

Comments

- Patients with a preexisting psychiatric condition, especially depression, should not be treated.
- Use with caution in patients with pulmonary disease, diabetes mellitus, coagulopathies, cardiac disorders, autoimmune diseases, or ophthalmologic disorders.
- Recommended laboratory monitoring includes CBC, blood chemistries, LFTs, and thyroid-stimulating hormone (TSH) levels prior to beginning treatment and then periodically thereafter.
- Other recommended baseline studies include a chest x-ray and an ophthalmologic examination.

INTERFERON α-2B (INTRON A)

Mechanism of Action

Interferon α-2B suppresses cell-proliferation and enhances macrophage phagocytic activity and lymphocyte cytotoxicity.

U.S. Food and Drug Administration–Approved Indications

Oncology indications (adults, as old as 18 years or older): hairy cell leukemia, malignant melanoma (adjuvant therapy to surgical treatment), AIDS-related Kaposi sarcoma, and follicular lymphoma (clinically aggressive disease in conjunction with anthracycline-containing combination chemotherapy).

Other indications: condyloma acuminata, chronic hepatitis C, and chronic hepatitis B

U.S. Food and Drug Administration–Approved Dosage

- Hairy cell leukemia: 2 million IU per m^2 i.m. or s.c. 3 times a week for up to 6 months.
- Malignant melanoma: Induction, 20 million IU per m^2 i.v. for 5 consecutive days per week for 4 weeks; maintenance, 10 million IU per m^2 s.c. 3 times per week for 48 weeks.
- Kaposi sarcoma: 30 million IU per m^2 s.c. or i.m. 3 times a week.
- Follicular lymphoma (in combination with an anthracycline-containing chemotherapy regimen): 5 million IU s.c. 3 times a week for up to 18 months.

Dose Modification Criteria

In case of serious adverse events: dose is to be modified.

Adverse Reactions

CNS: dizziness, depression, suicidal ideation, and paresthesias; DERM: skin rash, alopecia; ENDO: thyroid abnormalities; GI: diarrhea, nausea, anorexia, taste alteration, abdominal pain, and increased LFT values; HEMAT: myelosuppression; PULM: dyspnea, pulmonary infiltrates, pneumonitis, and pneumonia; OTHER: "flu-like symptoms" (fever, chills, headache, fatigue, malaise, and myalgia), hypersensitivity reactions, ophthalmologic disorders, and autoimmune disorders.

Comments

- Patients with a preexisting psychiatric condition, especially depression, should not be treated.
- Use with caution in patients with pulmonary disease, diabetes mellitus, coagulopathies, cardiac disorders, autoimmune diseases, or ophthalmologic disorders.
- Recommended laboratory monitoring includes CBC, blood chemistries, LFTs, and TSH levels before beginning treatment and then periodically thereafter.
- Other recommended baseline studies include a chest x-ray and an ophthalmologic examination.

IRINOTECAN (CAMPTOSAR)

Mechanism of Action

Irinotecan is a topoisomerase-I inhibitor.

U.S. Food and Drug Administration–Approved Indications

- Metastatic colon or rectal cancer
- First-line therapy in combination with fluorouracil and leucovorin
- Second-line therapy (single agent) after fluorouracil-based therapy.

U.S. Food and Drug Administration–Approved Dosage

- First-line combination-agent dosing (product labeling may be consulted for fluorouracil/leucovorin dosing):
- Regimen 1: 125 mg per m^2 i.v. over 90 minutes weekly $\times$ four doses (days 1, 8, 15, and 22) followed by 2 weeks of rest. Repeat every 6 weeks

- Regimen 2: 180 mg per m² i.v. over 90 minutes every 2 weeks (days 1, 15, and 29) for each cycle. Each cycle is 6 weeks in duration
- Second-line single-agent dosing:
- Weekly regimen: 125 mg per m² i.v. over 90 minutes weekly for four doses (days 1, 8, 15, and 22) followed by 2 weeks rest. Repeat every 6 weeks
- Once-every-three-week regimen: 350 mg per m² i.v. over 90 minutes every 3 weeks.

Dose Modification Criteria

Hepatic impairment: dose to be modified; pelvic or abdominal irradiation: dose to be modified; myelosuppression: dose to be modified; nonhematologic toxicity: dose to be modified (package labeling to be consulted for dose modifications).

Adverse Reactions

CNS: insomnia and dizziness; CV: vasodilation; DERM: alopecia, sweating, and rash; GI: N/V L3, diarrhea (early and late), abdominal pain, mucositis, anorexia, flatulence, and increased bilirubin, LFT values; HEMAT: myelosuppression; PULM: dyspnea, coughing, and rhinitis; OTHER: asthenia and fevers.

Comments

Can induce both early (within 24 hours of administration) and late forms of diarrhea. The early onset diarrhea is cholinergic in nature and may be accompanied by symptoms of rhinitis, increased salivation, miosis, lacrimation, diaphoresis, flushing, and abdominal cramping. These early cholinergic symptoms can be treated by administration of atropine. Late onset of diarrhea (generally after 24 hours) should be treated aggressively with high-dose loperamide. Each patient should be instructed to have loperamide readily available so that treatment can be initiated at the earliest onset of diarrhea. Package labeling may be consulted for dosage recommendations for atropine and loperamide.

LETROZOLE (FEMARA)

Mechanism of Action

Letrozole is a selective, nonsteroidal aromatase inhibitor.

U.S. Food and Drug Administration–Approved Indications

Breast cancer:

- First-line treatment of postmenopausal women with hormone-receptor–positive or hormone-receptor–unknown, locally advanced or metastatic breast cancer.
- Second-line treatment of advanced breast cancer in postmenopausal women with disease progression following antiestrogen therapy.

U.S. Food and Drug Administration–Approved Dosage

2.5 mg PO daily.

Dose Modification Criteria

Renal impairment (CrCl ≥10 mL per minute): no dose modification; hepatic (mild-to-moderate impairment): no dose modification; hepatic (severe impairment): dose to be modified.

Adverse Reactions

CNS: headache; GI: nausea, constipation, or diarrhea; OTHER: hot flashes, fatigue, musculoskeletal pain, arthralgia, and peripheral edema.

LEUPROLIDE ACETATE (LUPRON, LUPRON DEPOT, LUPRON DEPOT-3 MONTH, LUPRON DEPOT-4 MONTH, VIADUR)

Mechanism of Action

Leuprolide acetate is an LHRH agonist; chronic administration leads to sustained suppression of pituitary gonadotropins and subsequent suppression of serum testosterone in men and serum estradiol in women.

U.S. Food and Drug Administration–Approved Indications

- Palliative treatment of advanced prostate cancer.
- Other indications: endometriosis, uterine leiomyomata (fibroids), central precocious puberty.

U.S. Food and Drug Administration–Approved Dosage

Prostate cancer: Lupron: 1 mg s.c. daily; Lupron Depot: 7.5 mg i.m. monthly; Lupron Depot-3 month: 22.5 mg i.m. every 3 months; Lupron Depot-4 month: 30 mg i.m. every 4 months; Viadur implant: one implant (contains 72 mg of leuprolide acetate) every 12 months.

Adverse Reactions

CV: transient changes in blood pressure (hypo- or hypertension); ENDO: hot flashes, gynecomastia, sexual dysfunction, and decreased erections; GU: erectile dysfunction, lower urinary tract symptoms, and testicular atrophy; OTHER: tumor flare in the first few weeks of therapy, bone pain, injection-site reactions, loss of bone mineral density, osteoporosis, bone fracture, and asthenia.

Comments

- Use with caution in patients at risk for developing ureteral obstruction or spinal cord compression.
- Because of different release characteristics, a fractional dose of the 3-month or 4-month Lupron Depot formulation is not equivalent to the same dose of the monthly formulation and should not be given.

LEVAMISOLE (ERGAMISOL)

Mechanism of Action

Mechanism of levamisole is unknown; levamisole may be an immunomodulator.

U.S. Food and Drug Administration–Approved Indications

Adjuvant treatment in combination with fluorouracil after surgical resection in patients with Dukes stage C colon cancer

U.S. Food and Drug Administration–Approved Dosage

- Initial therapy:
  - Levamisole 50 mg PO every 8 hours for 3 days (starting 7 to 30 days after surgery) and
  - Fluorouracil 450 mg per m^2 i.v. daily $\times$ 5 days (starting 21 to 34 days postsurgery) and concomitant with a 3-day course of levamisole.

- Maintenance therapy:
  - Levamisole 50 mg PO every 8 hours for 3 days every 2 weeks for 1 year
  - Fluorouracil 450 mg per m^2 i.v. once a week, beginning 28 days after the initiation of the 5-day initial course and continued for a total treatment time of 1 year.

Dose Modification Criteria

Hepatic (severe impairment): use with caution; myelosuppression: dose to be modified.

Adverse Reactions

CNS: cases of an encephalopathy syndrome associated with demyelination reported; DERM: rash, dermatitis, and alopecia; GI: nausea, diarrhea, mucositis, anorexia, and abdominal pain; HEMAT: myelosuppression and agranulocytosis; OTHER: dysgeusia and fatigue.

Comments

Monitor for myelosuppression and agranulocytosis. Concomitant use with alcohol may result in a disulfiram (Antabuse) reaction. Levamisole may interact with phenytoin, leading to elevated phenytoin plasma levels; monitor phenytoin plasma levels with concomitant use. Levamisole may also interact with warfarin, leading to an increased PT and INR.

LOMUSTINE (CCNU, CEE NU)

Mechanism of Action

Lomustine is an alkylating agent.

U.S. Food and Drug Administration–Approved Indications

Primary and metastatic brain tumors; Hodgkin disease (second-line therapy in combination with other agents).

U.S. Food and Drug Administration–Approved Dosage

Single-agent therapy: 100 to 130 mg per m^2 as a single oral dose every 6 weeks.

Dose Modification Criteria

Myelosuppression: dose to be modified.

Adverse Reactions

GI: N/V ($\geq$60 mg per m^2: L5, $\leq$60 mg per m^2: L3) increased LFT values, and mucositis; GU: increased BUN and Cr; HEMAT: severe delayed myelosuppression and cumulative myelosuppression; PULM: (cumulative and usually occurs after 6 months of therapy or a cumulative lifetime dose of 1,100 mg per m^2, although it has been reported with total lifetime doses as low as 600 mg), fibrosis, and infiltrate; OTHER: secondary malignancies.

Comments

- A single dose is given every 6 weeks.
- Blood counts to be monitored at least weekly for 6 weeks after a dose.

MECHLORETHAMINE (MUSTARGEN)

Mechanism of Action

Mechlorethamine is an alkylating agent.

U.S. Food and Drug Administration–Approved Indications

- Systemic (intravenous) palliative treatment of bronchogenic carcinoma, CLL, CML, Hodgkin disease (stages III and IV), lymphosarcoma, malignant effusions, mycosis fungoides, and polycythemia vera.
- Palliative treatment of malignant effusions from metastatic carcinoma; administered intrapleurally, intraperitoneally, or intrapericardially.

U.S. Food and Drug Administration–Approved Dosage

- Intravenous administration: 0.4 mg per kg i.v. $\times$ one dose per course or 0.2 mg per kg i.v. daily $\times$ 2 days repeated every 3 to 6 weeks. Dosage should be based on ideal dry body weight. Other dosing regimens are utilized; current literature may be consulted.
- MOPP regimen (Hodgkin disease): mechlorethamine 6 mg per m^2 i.v. $\times$ one dose administered on days 1 and 8 of a 28-day cycle (combined with vincristine, prednisone, and procarbazine).
- Intracavitary administration: 0.2 to 0.4 mg per kg for intracavitary injection. Current literature may be consulted for dose and administration technique. The technique and the dose vary for the various intracavitary routes (intrapleural, intraperitoneal, and intrapericardial).

Dose Modification Criteria

Myelosuppression: dose to be modified.

Adverse Reactions

CNS: vertigo, tinnitus, and diminished hearing; DERM: alopecia, phlebitis, tissue damage or necrosis with extravasation, rash; GI: N/V L5, metallic taste in mouth, and diarrhea; HEMAT: myelosuppression; OTHER: hyperuricemia, secondary malignancies, infertility, and azoospermia.

Comments

Vesicant.

MEDROXYPROGESTERONE ACETATE (DEPO-PROVERA)

Mechanism of Action

Medroxyprogesterone acetate is a derivative of progesterone.

U.S. Food and Drug Administration–Approved Indications

Adjunctive therapy and palliative treatment of inoperable, recurrent, and metastatic endometrial or renal cancer.

U.S. Food and Drug Administration–Approved Dosage

400 to 1,000 mg i.m. injection $\times$ one dose. Doses may be repeated weekly initially; if improvement is noted, the dose may be reduced to maintenance doses as low as 400 mg i.m. monthly.

Adverse Reactions

CNS: headache, nervousness, dizziness, and depression; CV: edema, weight gain, and thromboembolic events; DERM: urticaria, pruritus, rash, acne, alopecia, and hirsutism; ENDO: breast tenderness and galactorrhea; GI: nausea, cholestatic jaundice; GU: breakthrough bleeding, spotting, change in menstrual flow, amenorrhea, and changes in cervical erosion and secretions; OCULAR: neuroocular lesions (retinal thrombosis and optic neuritis); OTHER: hypersensitivity reactions, fever, fatigue, insomnia, somnolence, and injection-site reactions.

MEGESTROL (MEGACE AND OTHERS)

Mechanism of Action

Megestrol is a progestational agent.

U.S. Food and Drug Administration–Approved Indications

Palliative therapy of advanced breast cancer and endometrial cancer.

U.S. Food and Drug Administration–Approved Dosage

- Breast cancer: 40 mg PO q.i.d. (four times daily; total daily dose: 160 mg per day).
- Endometrial cancer: 10 mg PO q.i.d. to 80 mg PO q.i.d. (four times daily; total daily dose: 40 to 320 mg per day).

Adverse Reactions

CNS: mood changes; CV: deep vein thrombosis; DERM: alopecia; ENDO: Cushing-like syndrome, hyperglycemia, glucose intolerance, weight gain, and hot flashes; GU: vaginal bleeding; OTHER: carpal tunnel syndrome and tumor flare.

Comments

Other indications include cancer and AIDS-related anorexia and cachexia as an appetite stimulant and to promote weight gain. Usual dose range: 160 to 800 mg per day (consult current literature).

MELPHALAN (ALKERAN); MELPHALAN INJECTION

Mechanism of Action

Melphalan is an alkylating agent.

U.S. Food and Drug Administration–Approved Indications

Palliative therapy for multiple myeloma and nonresectable ovarian cancer.

U.S. Food and Drug Administration–Approved Dosage

- Multiple myeloma:
  - Oral administration: 6 mg PO daily × 2 to 3 weeks. Wait up to 4 weeks for count recovery, and then 2 mg PO daily to achieve mild myelosuppression. Package insert and current literature may be consulted for other dosing regimens.
  - Intravenous administration. (if oral therapy not appropriate): 16 mg per m^2 i.v. over 15 to 20 minutes every 2 weeks × four doses, and then after adequate recovery from toxicity,

repeat administration at 4-week intervals. Current literature to be referred to for other dosing regimens.
- Ovarian cancer: 0.2 mg per kg PO daily × 5 days, repeated every 4 to 5 weeks depending on hematologic tolerance. Current literature to be referred for other dosing regimens.

Dose Modification Criteria

Renal impairment: dose to be modified; myelosuppression: dose to be modified.

Adverse Reactions

DERM: vasculitis, alopecia, and skin ulceration or necrosis at injection site (rare); HEMAT: myelosuppression and hemolytic anemia; GI: N/V L1 (oral), L4 (high dose i.v.), diarrhea, mucositis, anorexia, and increased LFT values; PULM: pulmonary toxicity (pulmonary fibrosis and interstitial pneumonitis); OTHER: hypersensitivity reactions, secondary malignancies, and infertility.

Comments

- Oral absorption is highly variable, with considerable patient-to-patient variability in systemic availability. Oral dosages may be adjusted on the basis of blood counts to achieve some level of myelosuppression to ensure that potentially therapeutic levels of the drug have been reached.
- In an experimental mouse model, melphalan injection showed a lack of vesicant activity, although the melphalan solvent (acid or alcohol in propylene glycol) was ulcerogenic if injected undiluted (3).

MERCAPTOPURINE (PURINETHOL)

Mechanism of Action

Mercaptopurine is an antimetabolite.

U.S. Food and Drug Administration–Approved Indications

- ALL: indicated in the remission induction and maintenance therapy of ALL. May be used as a single agent, but a higher complete remission rate is seen with combination chemotherapy.
- AML

U.S. Food and Drug Administration–Approved Dosage

- Induction: 2.5 mg per kg (to nearest 25 mg) PO once daily × 4 weeks, and then to be adjusted according to blood counts.
- Maintenance: 1.5 to 2.5 mg per kg PO once daily.

Dose Modification Criteria

Renal impairment: dose reduction to be considered for modification; hepatic impairment: dose reduction to be considered for modification; myelosuppression: dose to be modified.

Adverse Reactions

DERM: rash and alopecia; GI: anorexia, N/V L1, mucositis, and hepatotoxicity; HEMAT: myelosuppression; OTHER: tumor lysis syndrome.

Comments

- Monitoring of LFT results, bilirubin at weekly intervals initially and then monthly intervals.
- Usually, there is complete cross-resistance with thioguanine.
- Oral mercaptopurine dose should be reduced to 25% to 33% of usual daily dose in patients receiving allopurinol concomitantly.
- Consider appropriate prophylaxis for tumor lysis syndrome when treating acute leukemias.

METHOTREXATE

Mechanism of Action

Methotrexate is an antimetabolite.

U.S. Food and Drug Administration–Approved Indications

- Neoplastic disease indications: Gestational tumors (i.e., choriocarcinoma, chorioadenoma destruens, and hydatidiform mole), ALL (maintenance therapy in combination with other agents and in the prophylaxis of meningeal leukemia), treatment of meningeal leukemia, breast cancer, epidermoid cancers of the head or neck, advanced mycosis fungoides, lung cancers (particularly squamous cell and small cell types), advanced-stage non-Hodgkin lymphoma, lymphosarcoma, and nonmetastatic osteosarcoma (high-dose therapy followed by leucovorin rescue).
- Other indications: psoriasis (i.e., severe, recalcitrant, and disabling); rheumatoid arthritis (severe).

U.S. Food and Drug Administration–Approved Dosage

- Choriocarcinoma and similar trophoblastic diseases: 15 to 30 mg PO or i.m. daily $\times$ 5 days. Treatment courses are repeated 3 to 5 times, with rest periods of 1 or more weeks between courses to allow for toxic symptoms to subside. Current literature may be consulted.
- ALL maintenance therapy (following induction): 15 mg per m^2 PO or i.m. twice weekly (total weekly dose of 30 mg per m^2) or 2.5 mg per kg i.v. every 14 days (in combination with other agents). Current literature to be referred to for combination regimens for both induction and maintenance regimens in ALL.
- Meningeal leukemia (intrathecal administration): in patients younger than 1 year, 6 mg intrathecally; 1 year to younger than 2 years, 8 mg intrathecally; 2 years to younger than 3 years, 10 mg intrathecally; older than 3 years, 12 mg intrathecally. Current literature may be consulted.
- Mycosis fungoides: 2.5 to 10 mg PO daily $\times$ weeks to months or 50 mg i.m. weekly or 25 mg i.m. twice weekly. Current literature may be consulted.
- Nonmetastatic osteosarcoma: 12 g per m^2 i.v. over 4 hours $\times$ one dose (with leucovorin rescue, vigorous hydration, and urinary alkalinization) given weekly (weeks 4, 5, 6, and 7 after surgery), and then weeks 11, 12, 15, 16, 29, 30, 44, and 45. Leucovorin doses should be adjusted on the basis of methotrexate concentrations. Methotrexate is usually given with other agents. Current literature may be consulted.
- Other indications: Current literature may be consulted.

Dose Modification Criteria

Renal impairment: dose to be modified.

Adverse Reactions

CNS: acute chemical arachnoiditis (intrathecal), subacute myelopathy (intrathecal), chronic leukoencephalopathy (intrathecal), and acute neurotoxicity or encephalopathy (high-dose i.v. therapy); DERM: alopecia, rash, urticaria, telangiectasia, acne, photosensitivity, and severe dermatologic reactions; GI: N/V (≤ 50 mg per m^2 L1, >50 to <250 mg per m^2 L2, 250 to 1,000 mg per m^2 L3, >1,000 mg per m^2 L4), mucositis/stomatitis, diarrhea, increased LFT values, and acute and chronic hepatotoxicity; GU: renal failure (high-dose therapy) and cystitis; HEMAT: myelosuppression; PULM: interstitial pneumonitis; OTHER: fever, malaise, chills, fatigue, teratogenic, and tumor lysis syndrome.

Comments

- Clearance is reduced in patients with impaired renal function or third-space fluid accumulations (e.g., ascites and pleural effusions). Methotrexate distributes to third-space fluid accumulations, with subsequent slow and delayed clearance, leading to prolonged terminal plasma half-life and toxicity.
- Nonsteroidal anti-inflammatory drugs and acidic drugs inhibit methotrexate clearance. Multiple potential drug interactions; current literature may be reviewed.
- Use vigorous hydration, urinary alkalinization, and leucovorin rescue with high-dose therapy.
- Preservative-free product and diluents to be used when administering intrathecally or with high-dose i.v. regimens.

MITOMYCIN C (MUTAMYCIN)

Mechanism of Action

Mitomycin C induces DNA cross-links through alkylation; inhibits DNA and RNA synthesis.

U.S. Food and Drug Administration–Approved Indications

Disseminated gastric cancer or pancreatic cancer (in combination with other agents and as palliative treatment when other modalities have failed).

U.S. Food and Drug Administration–Approved Dosage

Single-agent therapy: 20 mg per m^2 i.v. $\times$ 1 dose repeated every 6 to 8 weeks.
Current literature may be referred to for alternative dosing regimens and combination regimens.

Dose Modification Criteria

- Renal impairment: dose to be modified; myelosuppression: dose to be modified.

Adverse Reactions

CV: CHF (patients with prior doxorubicin exposure); DERM: alopecia, pruritus, tissue damage or necrosis with extravasation; GI: anorexia, N/V L2, mucositis, and diarrhea; GU: increased Cr; HEMAT: myelosuppression (may be cumulative); PULM: nonproductive cough, dyspnea, and interstitial pneumonia; OTHER: fever, hemolytic uremic syndrome, malaise, and weakness.

Comments

Vesicant.

MITOTANE (LYSODREN)

Mechanism of Action

Mitotane is an adrenal cytotoxic agent.

U.S. Food and Drug Administration–Approved Indications

Inoperable, functional, and nonfunctional adrenal cortical carcinoma.

U.S. Food and Drug Administration–Approved Dosage

Initial dose: 2 to 6 g PO per day in three to four divided doses. Doses are usually increased incrementally to 9 to 10 g per day or until maximum tolerated dose is achieved. Maximum tolerated dose range varies from 2 to 16 g per day but has usually been 9 to 10 g per day. Total daily doses should be administered in three to four divided doses.

Adverse Reactions

CNS: vertigo, depression, lethargy, somnolence, and dizziness; DERM: transient skin rashes; GI: anorexia, nausea, and diarrhea; OTHER: adrenal insufficiency.

Comments

- Adrenal insufficiency precautions to be instituted.
- Patients should be counseled regarding the common CNS side effects, and ambulatory patients should be cautioned about driving, operating machinery, and other hazardous pursuits requiring mental and physical alertness.

MITOXANTRONE (NOVANTRONE)

Mechanism of Action

Mitoxantrone interacts with DNA and is an intercalating agent and a topoisomerase-II inhibitor.

U.S. Food and Drug Administration–Approved Indications

- ANLL (myelogenous, promyelocytic, monocytic, and erythroid acute leukemia) in adults (initial therapy in combination with other agents)
- Advanced hormone-refractory prostate cancer (in combination with corticosteroids)
- Other indications: Multiple sclerosis.

U.S. Food and Drug Administration–Approved Dosage

- ANLL: Induction, 12 mg per m^2 i.v. daily $\times$ 3 days (days 1, 2, and 3) in combination with cytarabine; consolidation, 12 mg per m^2 i.v. daily $\times$ 2 days (days 1 and 2) in combination with cytarabine.
- Prostate cancer: 12 to 14 mg per m^2 i.v. $\times$ one dose every 21 days with prednisone or hydrocortisone.

Dose Modification Criteria

Renal impairment: no data available; hepatic impairment: to be used with caution; dose adjustment may be considered.

Adverse Reactions

CV: CHF (clinical risk increases after a lifetime cumulative dose of 140 mg per m^2), tachycardia, electrocardiographic changes, and chest pain; DERM: rash, alopecia, urticaria, nail bed changes; GI: N/V (>15 mg per m^2: L4, $\leq$15 mg per m^2: L3), mucositis, constipation, anorexia, and increased LFT values; HEMAT: myelosuppression; PULM: dyspnea; OTHER: bluish green urine, sclera may turn bluish, phlebitis (irritant), fatigue, secondary leukemias, and tumor lysis syndrome.

Comments

- Appropriate prophylaxis may be considered for tumor lysis syndrome when treating acute leukemias.

NILUTAMIDE (NILANDRON)

Mechanism of Action

Nilutamide is an antiandrogen.

U.S. Food and Drug Administration–Approved Indications

Metastatic prostate cancer (stage D2; in combination therapy with surgical castration). Dosing should begin on same day or day after surgical castration.

U.S. Food and Drug Administration–Approved Dosage

Give 300 mg PO daily × 30 days, and then 150 mg PO daily (with or without food).

Adverse Reactions

CNS: dizziness; CV: hypertension, and angina; ENDO: hot flashes, impotence, and decreased libido; GI: nausea, anorexia, increased LFT values (LFT results to be monitored periodically because of rare associations with cholestatic jaundice, hepatic necrosis, and encephalopathy), and constipation; OCULAR: visual disturbances and impaired adaptation to dark; PULM: interstitial pneumonitis and dyspnea.

Comments

- Baseline chest x-ray to be obtained before initiating therapy (with consideration of baseline pulmonary function tests). Patients should be instructed to report any new or worsening shortness of breath and if symptoms occur, nilutamide should be immediately discontinued.
- LFT results should be monitored at baseline and at regular intervals × 4 months and then periodically thereafter.

OXALIPLATIN (ELOXATIN)

Mechanism of Action

Oxaliplatin is an alkylating-like agent producing interstrand DNA cross-links.

U.S. Food and Drug Administration–Approved Indications

Advanced or metastatic colorectal cancer:

- First-line therapy in combination with infusional fluorouracil and leucovorin in patients with advanced colorectal cancer.
- Second-line therapy in combination with infusional fluorouracil and leucovorin in patients with metastatic colorectal cancer whose disease has recurred or progressed within 6 months of completion of first-line therapy with the combination of bolus fluorouracil/leucovorin and irinotecan.

U.S. Food and Drug Administration–Approved Dosage

Combined therapy with infusional fluorouracil and leucovorin (FOLFOX regimen)

Day 1:
Oxaliplatin 85 mg per m^2 i.v. over 120 minutes $\times$ 1 dose given concurrently with
Leucovorin 200 mg per m^2 i.v. over 120 minutes $\times$ 1 dose followed by
Fluorouracil 400 mg per m^2 i.v. bolus over 2 to 4 minutes $\times$ 1 dose followed by
Fluorouracil 600 mg per m^2 i.v. continuous infusion over 22 hours.

Day 2:
Leucovorin 200 mg per m^2 i.v. over 120 minutes $\times$ 1 dose, followed by
Fluorouracil 400 mg per m^2 i.v. bolus over 2 to 4 minutes $\times$ 1 dose, followed by
Fluorouracil 600 mg per m^2 i.v. continuous infusion over 22 hours.

Cycles are repeated every 2 weeks.

Dose Modification Criteria

Renal impairment: no data available (to be used with caution); myelosuppression: dose to be modified; nonhematologic toxicity: dose to be modified.

Adverse Reactions

CNS: peripheral sensory neuropathies (details follow under "Comments"), headache; CV: edema, thromboembolic events; DERM: injection-site reactions; GI: N/V L3, diarrhea, mucositis or stomatitis, abdominal pain, anorexia, taste perversion, and elevated LFT values; GU: elevated serum creatinine; HEMAT: myelosuppression; PULM: pulmonary fibrosis, dyspnea, and cough; OTHER: fatigue, fever, back pain, pain, and hypersensitivity reaction.

Comments

• Oxaliplatin is associated with two types of peripheral neuropathy:
  1. An acute, reversible, primarily peripheral, sensory neuropathy that is of early onset (from within hours to 1 to 2 days of dosing), that resolves within 14 days, and that frequently recurs with further dosing. The symptoms include transient paresthesia, dysesthesia, and hypoesthesia in the hands, feet, perioral area, or throat. Symptoms may be precipitated or exacerbated by exposure to cold temperature or cold objects. Patients should be instructed to avoid cold drinks and use of ice, and should cover exposed skin prior to exposure to cold temperature or cold objects.
  2. A persistent (>14 days), primarily peripheral, sensory neuropathy usually characterized by paresthesias, dysesthesias, hypoesthesias, but may also include deficits in proprioception that can interfere with daily activities. Dose modifications are recommended for persistent grade 2 neurotoxicity and discontinuation of therapy is recommended for persistent grade 3 neurotoxicity.

PACLITAXEL (TAXOL)

Mechanism of Action

Paclitaxel stabilizes microtubule assembly.

U.S. Food and Drug Administration–Approved Indications

• Advanced ovarian cancer (first-line and subsequent therapy). As first-line therapy, paclitaxel is indicated in combination with cisplatin.
• Breast cancer

- Adjuvant treatment of node-positive breast cancer (administered sequentially to standard doxorubicin-containing combination chemotherapy)
- Second-line therapy for breast cancer (after failure of combination chemotherapy for metastatic disease or relapse within 6 months of adjuvant therapy)
- NSCLC (first-line therapy in combination with cisplatin) in patients who are not candidates for potentially curative surgery and/or radiation therapy.
- AIDS-related Kaposi sarcoma (second-line therapy).

U.S. Food and Drug Administration–Approved Dosage

- Patients are to be premedicated with dexamethasone, diphenhydramine (or its equivalent), and H_2 antagonists (e.g., cimetidine or ranitidine) to prevent severe hypersensitivity reactions. Suggested package literature premedication regimen: dexamethasone 20 mg PO × two doses administered approximately 12 and 6 hours before paclitaxel; diphenhydramine 50 mg i.v. 30 to 60 minutes before paclitaxel; and cimetidine 300 mg i.v. or ranitidine 50 mg i.v. 30 to 60 minutes before paclitaxel. Current literature may be consulted for alternative premedication regimens.
- First-line ovarian cancer: 135 mg per m^2 i.v. continuous infusion over 24 hours or 175 mg per m^2 i.v. over 3 hours (followed by cisplatin 75 mg per m^2 i.v.) every 3 weeks.
- Second-line ovarian cancer: 135 mg per m^2 or 175 mg per m^2 i.v. over 3 hours every 3 weeks. Current literature may be consulted for alternative regimens.
- Adjuvant therapy of node-positive breast cancer: 175 mg per m^2 i.v. over 3 hours every 3 weeks × four cycles (administered sequentially with doxorubicin-containing chemotherapy).
- Second-line breast cancer: 175 mg per m^2 i.v. over 3 hours every 3 weeks.
- NSCLC: 135 mg per m^2 i.v. continuous infusion over 24 hours (followed by cisplatin 75 mg per m^2 i.v.) every 3 weeks.
- AIDS-related Kaposi sarcoma: 135 mg per m^2 i.v. over 3 hours every 3 weeks or 100 mg per m^2 i.v. over 3 hours every 2 weeks. (Note: reduce the dose of dexamethasone premedication dose to 10 mg PO per dose instead of the suggested 20 mg PO dose).

Dose Modification Criteria

Hepatic impairment: dose to be modified; myelosuppression: dose to be modified; nonhematologic toxicity (neuropathy): dose to be modified.

Adverse Reactions

CNS: peripheral neurosensory toxicity (paresthesia, dysesthesia, and pain); CV: hypotension, bradycardia, and electrocardiographic changes; DERM: alopecia, onycholysis (more common with weekly dosing), and injection-site reactions; GI: N/V L2, diarrhea, and mucositis; HEMAT: myelosuppression; INFUS: acute hypersensitivity-type reactions; OTHER: arthralgia, and myalgia.

Comments

- Use non-DEHP plasticized solution containers and administration sets.
- Inline filtration (0.22-µ filter) required during administration.
- Lower dose, weekly dosage regimens are commonly utilized. Current literature may be consulted for dose guidelines.

PEGASPARGASE (ONCASPAR)

Mechanism of Action

Pegaspargase is a modified (pegylated) version of the enzyme L-asparaginase. L-asparaginase depletes asparagine, an amino acid required by some leukemic cells.

U.S. Food and Drug Administration–Approved Indications

Patients with ALL who are hypersensitive to native forms of L-asparaginase.

U.S. Food and Drug Administration–Approved Dosage

- The preferred route is i.m.; i.v. administration should be over 1 to 2 hours.
- Combination or sole induction therapy: Adults and children, with BSA ≥ 0.6 m^2 : 2,500 IU per m^2 i.m. or i.v. $\times$ one dose every 14 days.
- Children with BSA <0.6 m^2 : 82.5 IU per kg i.m. or i.v. $\times$ 1 dose every 14 days.

Adverse Reactions

CNS: malaise, confusion, lethargy, and depression; CV: chest pain, hypertension, and hypotension; DERM: alopecia, itching, and injection-site reactions; ENDO: hyperglycemia; GI: anorexia; N/V L1-2, hepatotoxicity, increased LFT values, and pancreatitis; GU: increased BUN and Cr; HEMAT: hypofibrinogenemia; PULM: respiratory distress, cough, and epistaxis; OTHER: hypersensitivity reaction, fever, arthralgia, musculoskeletal pain, and tumor lysis syndrome.

Comments

Contraindications: active pancreatitis or history of pancreatitis, serious hemorrhagic episode with native L-asparaginase, serious allergic reactions (e.g., bronchospasm) to native L-asparaginase.

PEMETREXED (ALIMTA)

Mechanism of Action

Pemetrexed is an antimetabolite and also an antifolate that disrupts folate-dependent metabolic process essential for cell replication.

U.S. Food and Drug Administration–Approved Indications

Malignant pleural mesothelioma: in combination with cisplatin in patients whose disease is unresectable or who are otherwise ineligible for curative surgery.

U.S. Food and Drug Administration–Approved Dosage

Malignant pleural mesothelioma: 500 mg per m^2 i.v. over 10 minutes on day 1 of each 21-day cycle. The recommended dose of cisplatin (in combination with pemetrexed) is 75 mg per m^2 i.v. over 2 hours, beginning approximately 30 minutes after the end of pemetrexed. See comments section for premedication regimen for pemetrexed.

Dose Modification Criteria

Renal impairment (CrCl ≥ 45 mL per minute): no dose modification, renal impairment (CrCl <45 mL per minute): administration is not recommended; hepatic impairment: no data available; myelosuppression: dose to be modified; nonhematologic toxicity: dose to be modified.

Adverse Reactions

DERM: rash, desquamation; GI: N/V L2, mucositis, pharyngitis, diarrhea, anorexia, and increased LFT values; HEMAT: neutropenia, thrombocytopenia, and anemia; OTHER: fatigue, fever.

Comments

- Vitamin supplementation: Patients treated with pemetrexed must be instructed to take folic acid and vitamin B_{12} as a prophylactic measure to reduce treatment-related hematologic and GI toxicity. Patients should receive at least five daily doses of folic acid (most common daily dose: 400 μg) during the 7-day period prior to the first dose of pemetrexed and dosing should continue during the full course of therapy and for 21 days after the last dose. Patients must also receive one intramuscular dose of vitamin B_{12} (1,000 μg) during the week prior to the first dose of pemetrexed and every three cycles (9 weeks) thereafter.
- Corticosteroid premedication: Pretreatment with dexamethasone (or equivalent) reduces the incidence and severity of cutaneous reactions. Recommended regimen (product labeling): dexamethasone 4 mg PO b.i.d. × 3 days (six doses) beginning the day before each dose of pemetrexed (the day before, the day of, and the day after pemetrexed).
- Pregnancy category D: Pemetrexed may cause fetal harm when administered to pregnant women. Pemetrexed is fetotoxic and teratogenic in mice; there are no studies of pemetrexed in pregnant women.

PENTOSTATIN (NIPENT)

Mechanism of Action

Pentostatin is an antimetabolite and an adenosine deaminase inhibitor.

U.S. Food and Drug Administration–Approved Indications

Hairy cell leukemia (first-line and in α-interferon-refractory disease)

U.S. Food and Drug Administration–Approved Dosage

4 mg per m^2 i.v. every other week. The optimal treatment duration has not been determined. The package insert suggests continued treatment until a complete response has been achieved followed by two additional doses.

Dose Modification Criteria

Renal impairment: dose to be modified; myelosuppression: dose to be modified.

Adverse Reactions

DERM: rash; GI: N/V L3-4, and elevated LFT values; GU: mild transient rise in serum creatinine; HEMAT: leukopenia, anemia, and thrombocytopenia; OTHER: fever, infection, and fatigue.

Comments

- A high incidence of fatal pulmonary toxicity was seen in a trial investigating the combination of fludarabine with pentostatin. The combined use of fludarabine and pentostatin is not recommended.
- Patients should receive hydration (500 to 1,000 mL) before and after each pentostatin dose.

POLIFEPROSAN 20 WITH CARMUSTINE IMPLANT (GLIADEL WAFER)

Mechanism of Action

The polifeprosan 20 with carmustine implant is designed to deliver carmustine directly into the surgical cavity created when a brain tumor is resected. On exposure to the aqueous environment of the resection cavity, carmustine is released from the copolymer and diffuses into the surrounding brain tissue. Carmustine is an alkylating agent.

U.S. Food and Drug Administration–Approved Indications

- High-grade malignant glioma (first-line therapy in newly diagnosed patients as an adjunct to surgery and radiation)
- Recurrent glioblastoma multiforme as an adjunct to surgery.

U.S. Food and Drug Administration–Approved Dosage

Each wafer contains 7.7 mg of carmustine. Up to eight wafers should be implanted at time of surgery (eight wafers result in a dose of 61.6 mg).

Adverse Reactions

CNS: meningitis, abscess, and brain edema; GI: nausea; OTHER: abnormal healing, pain, and fever.

Comments

Wafers can be broken in half. Proper handling and disposal precautions should be observed.

PORFIMER (PHOTOFRIN)

Mechanism of Action

Porfimer is a photosensitizing agent.

U.S. Food and Drug Administration–Approved Indications

- Esophageal cancer (palliation of complete or partial obstruction)
- Endobronchial NSCLC
  - For reduction of obstruction and palliation of symptoms in patients with completely or partially obstructed endobronchial NSCLC.
  - For treatment of microinvasive endobronchial NSCLC in patients for whom surgery and radiotherapy are not indicated.
- High-grade dysplasia in Barrett esophagus (ablation of high-grade dysplasia in patients who do not undergo esophagectomy).

U.S. Food and Drug Administration–Approved Dosage

2 mg per kg i.v. injection over 3 to 5 minutes × one dose followed by photodynamic therapy. For the treatment of esophageal and endobronchial cancer, patients may receive up to three additional courses; each course should be administered no sooner than 30 days after the previous course. For the ablation of high-grade dysplasia in Barrett esophagus, patients may receive up to three additional courses; each course should be administered no sooner than 90 days after the previous course.

Adverse Reactions

CNS: anxiety, confusion, and insomnia; CV: hypertension, hypotension, heart failure, chest pain, atrial fibrillation, and tachycardia; DERM: photosensitivity; HEMAT: anemia; GI: N/VL2, abdominal pain, anorexia, constipation, dysphagia, esophageal edema, and esophageal stricture;

PULM: pleural effusion, dyspnea, pneumonia, pharyngitis, cough, respiratory insufficiency, and tracheoesophageal fistula; OTHER: fever.

Comments

Patients are photosensitive (including eyes) for at least 30 days after administration.

PROCARBAZINE (MATULANE)

Mechanism of Action

Mechanism of action of procarbazine is unknown. There is evidence that the drug may act by inhibition of protein, RNA, and DNA synthesis.

U.S. Food and Drug Administration–Approved Indications

Stages III and IV Hodgkin disease: first-line therapy in combination with other anticancer drugs. [Procarbazine is used as part of the MOPP (mechlorethamine, vincristine, procarbazine, and prednisone) chemotherapy regimen.]

U.S. Food and Drug Administration–Approved Dosage

- All doses based on actual body weight unless the patient is obese or there has been a spurious weight increase, in which case lean body weight (dry weight) should be used.
- Doses may be given as a single daily dose or divided throughout the day.
- MOPP regimen for Hodgkin disease: 100 mg per m^2 PO daily $\times$ 14 days (in combination with mechlorethamine, vincristine, and prednisone).
- Adult single-agent therapy: 2 to 4 mg per kg PO daily $\times$ 7 days, and then 4 to 6 mg per kg PO daily until maximal response is obtained. Maintenance dose: 1 to 2 mg per kg PO daily.
- Pediatric single-agent therapy: 50 mg per m^2 PO daily $\times$ 7 days, and then 100 mg per m^2 PO daily until maximum response is obtained. Maintenance dose: 50 mg per m^2 PO daily.

Adverse Reactions

CNS: paresthesias, confusion, lethargy, and mental depression; DERM: pruritus, hyperpigmentation, and alopecia; GI: anorexia, N/V L4, stomatitis, xerostomia, diarrhea, and constipation; HEMAT: myelosuppression; OTHER: fever, and myalgia.

Comments

- Disulfiram-like (Antabuse) reaction can occur; alcoholic beverages are to be avoided while taking procarbazine.
- Procarbazine is a weak monoamine oxidase inhibitor (MAOI); tyramine-rich foods as well as sympathomimetic drugs and tricyclic antidepressants are to be avoided.

RITUXIMAB (RITUXAN)

Mechanism of Action

Rituximab is a chimeric (murine, human) monoclonal antibody directed at the CD20 antigen found on the surface of normal and malignant B lymphocytes.

U.S. Food and Drug Administration–Approved Indications

Relapsed or refractory low-grade or follicular, CD20-positive, B cell, non-Hodgkin lymphoma.

U.S. Food and Drug Administration–Approved Dosage

- Premedication with acetaminophen and/or diphenhydramine should be considered before each infusion.
- If patient experiences an infusion-related reaction, the infusion should be stopped, the patient managed symptomatically, and then the infusion should be restarted at half the rate once the symptoms have resolved.
- 375 mg per m^2 i.v. weekly × four doses (days 1, 8, 15, 22) or eight doses.
- First infusion: to start at 50 mg per hour, and then may increase by 50 mg per hour every 30 minutes up to a maximum of 400 mg per hour. Subsequent infusions if prior infusions tolerated: to start at 100 mg per hour, and then may increase by 100 mg per hour every 30 minutes up to a maximum of 400 mg per hour.

Adverse Reactions

CNS: headache, and dizziness; CV: hypotension, arrhythmias, and peripheral edema; DERM: rash, pruritus, urticaria, and severe mucocutaneous reactions; GI: N/V L1-2, and abdominal pain; HEMAT: angioedema, leukopenia, thrombocytopenia, and neutropenia; INFUS: fever, chills, rigors, hypoxia, pulmonary infiltrates, adult respiratory distress syndrome, myocardial infarction, ventricular fibrillation, or cardiogenic shock; OTHER: throat irritation, rhinitis, bronchospasm, hypersensitivity reaction, myalgia, back pain, and tumor lysis syndrome.

Comments

- Tumor lysis syndrome has been reported within 12 to 24 hours after the infusion (high risk: high numbers of circulating malignant cells).
- Mild-to-moderate infusion reactions consisting of fever, chills, and rigors occur in the majority of patients during the first infusion. The reactions resolve with slowing or interruption of the infusion and with supportive care measures. The incidence of infusion reactions declines with subsequent infusions.
- A more severe infusion-related complex, usually reported with the first infusion (hypoxia, pulmonary infiltrates, adult respiratory distress syndrome, myocardial infarction, ventricular fibrillation, or cardiogenic shock) has resulted in fatalities.
- Severe mucocutaneous reactions, some with fatal outcome, have been reported in association with rituximab treatment.
- Rituximab is commonly combined with cytotoxic chemotherapy agents in various subtypes of B cell non-Hodgkin lymphoma. Current literature may be consulted for dosing regimens.

STREPTOZOTOCIN (ZANOSAR)

Mechanism of Action

Streptozotocin is an alkylating agent.

U.S. Food and Drug Administration–Approved Indications

Metastatic islet cell carcinoma of the pancreas (functional and nonfunctional carcinomas).

U.S. Food and Drug Administration–Approved Dosage

- Daily schedule: 500 mg per m^2 i.v. daily × 5 days every 6 weeks until maximum benefit or treatment limiting toxicity is observed, or
- Weekly schedule: Initial dose: 1 g per m^2 i.v. weekly for the first two courses (weeks). In subsequent courses, drug doses may be escalated in patients who have not achieved a

therapeutic response and who have not experienced significant toxicity with the previous course of treatment. However, a single dose should not exceed 1,500 mg per m^2.

Dose Modification Criteria

Renal impairment: to be used with caution, dose reduction may be considered.

Adverse Reactions

DERM: injection-site reactions (irritant); ELECTRO: hypophosphatemia; ENDO: dysglycemia, may lead to insulin-dependent diabetes; GI: N/V L5, increased LFT values, diarrhea; GU: azotemia, anuria, renal tubular acidosis, increased BUN and serum creatinine, glycosuria; HEMAT: myelosuppression.

Comments

• Renal complications are dose related and cumulative. Mild proteinuria is usually an early sign of impending renal dysfunction. Serial urinalysis is important for the early detection of proteinuria and should be quantified with a 24-hour collection when proteinuria is detected. Adequate hydration may help reduce the risk of nephrotoxicity. Avoid other nephrotoxic agents.

TAMOXIFEN (NOLVADEX)

Mechanism of Action

Tamoxifen is a nonsteroidal antiestrogen.

U.S. Food and Drug Administration–Approved Indications

• Breast cancer treatment
• Treatment of metastatic breast cancer
• Adjuvant treatment of node-positive and node-negative breast cancer following breast surgery and breast irradiation
• Reduction in breast cancer incidence
• Ductal carcinoma in situ (DCIS): to reduce the risk of invasive breast cancer following breast surgery and radiation.
• High-risk women [women at least 35 years of age with a 5-year predicted risk of breast cancer ≥1.67% as calculated by the Gail model (package insert to be consulted)].

U.S. Food and Drug Administration–Approved Dosage

• Breast cancer treatment: 20 mg PO daily or 10 to 20 mg PO twice daily (20 to 40 mg per day). Adjuvant therapy should be continued × 5 years. Doses >20 mg per day should be given in divided doses (morning and evening).
• Breast cancer incidence reduction (DCIS and in high-risk women): 20 mg PO daily × 5 years.

Adverse Reactions

CV: thromboembolism, stroke, and pulmonary embolism; DERM: skin rash; ENDO: hot flashes; GI: nausea, anorexia; GU: menstrual irregularities, pruritus vulvae, and vaginal discharge or bleeding; HEMAT: bone marrow depression; OCULAR: vision disturbances and cataracts; PULM: dyspnea, chest pain, and hemoptysis; OTHER: dizziness, headaches, tumor or bone pain, pelvic pain, and uterine malignancies.

Comments

- High risk is defined as the risk in women who are at least 35 years old, with a 5-year predicted risk of breast cancer of 1.67%, as predicted by the Gail risk model.
- Serious and life-threatening events associated with tamoxifen in the risk reduction setting include uterine malignancies, stroke, and pulmonary embolism. Package insert may be consulted for additional information.

TEMOZOLOMIDE (TEMODAR)
Mechanism of Action

Temozolomide is an alkylating agent.

U.S. Food and Drug Administration–Approved Indications

Refractory anaplastic astrocytoma: Second-line therapy in adults (after a nitrosourea and procarbazine regimen).

U.S. Food and Drug Administration–Approved Dosage

Initial dose: 150 mg per m^2 PO daily $\times$ 5 consecutive days every 28 days. If the initial dose leads to acceptable hematologic parameters at the nadir and on day of dosing (criteria in package insert to be verified), the temozolomide dose may be increased to 200 mg per m^2 PO daily $\times$ 5 consecutive days per 28 day treatment cycle.

Dose Modification Criteria

Renal (severe impairment): to be used with caution; hepatic (severe impairment): to be used with caution; myelosuppression: dose to be modified.

Adverse Reactions

CNS: headache; HEMAT: myelosuppression; GI: N/V L2 (reduced by taking on an empty stomach); OTHER: asthenia, fatigue.

Comments

- Capsules should be taken with water. Administer consistently with respect to food, and to reduce the risk of nausea and vomiting it is recommended that temozolomide be taken on an empty stomach. Bedtime administration may be advised.
- Myelosuppression occurs late in the treatment cycle. The median nadirs in a study of 158 patients with anaplastic astrocytoma occurred at 26 days for platelets (range 21 to 40 days) and 28 days for neutrophils (range 1 to 44 days). The package insert recommends obtaining a complete blood count on day 22 (21 days after the first dose) and then weekly to ensure that the absolute neutrophil count (ANC) is higher than 1.5×10^9 per L and the platelet count exceeds 100×10^9 per L. The next cycle of temozolomide should not be started until the ANC and platelet count exceed these levels. Package insert may be consulted for dose modification guidelines.

TENIPOSIDE (VUMON)

Mechanism of Action

Teniposide is a topoisomerase-II inhibitor.

U.S. Food and Drug Administration–Approved Indications

Refractory childhood ALL: induction therapy as a second-line therapy (in combination with other agents).

U.S. Food and Drug Administration–Approved Dosage

- Current literature may be consulted for dosing regimens. The package insert cites two dosage regimens based on two different studies:
- In combination with cytarabine: 165 mg per m^2 i.v. over 30 to 60 minutes twice weekly $\times$ eight to nine doses.
- In combination with vincristine and prednisone: 250 mg per m^2 i.v. over 30 to 60 minutes weekly $\times$ four to eight doses.

Dose Modification Criteria

Renal impairment: to be used with caution, no guidelines available; hepatic impairment: to be used with caution, no guidelines available.

Adverse Reactions

CV: hypotension with rapid infusion; DERM: alopecia, thrombophlebitis, and tissue damage secondary to drug extravasation; GI: diarrhea, N/V L2, and mucositis; HEMAT: myelosuppression; OTHER: anaphylaxis, and hypersensitivity.

Comments

- Observe patient for at least 60 minutes after dose.
- Consider premedication with antihistamines and/or corticosteroids for retreatment (if indicated) after a hypersensitivity reaction.
- Use non-DEHP plasticized solution containers and administration sets.

TESTOLACTONE (TESLAC)

Mechanism of Action

Testolactone is a synthetic derivative of testosterone that appears to inhibit steroid aromatase activity and consequently cause a reduction in estrone synthesis.

U.S. Food and Drug Administration–Approved Indications

- Breast cancer: adjunctive therapy in the palliative treatment of advanced or disseminated breast cancer in postmenopausal women when hormonal therapy is indicated or in premenopausal women in whom ovarian function has been terminated.
- Advanced or disseminated mammary cancer.

U.S. Food and Drug Administration–Approved Dosage

250 mg PO q.i.d. (4 times daily; total daily dose: 1,000 mg per day).

Adverse Reactions

CNS: paresthesia; CV: hypertension, peripheral edema, DERM: maculopapular erythema, alopecia, and nail growth disturbance; GI: anorexia, nausea; OTHER: malaise, aches, and glossitis.

THIOGUANINE (TABLOID)

Mechanism of Action

Thioguanine is an antimetabolite.

U.S. Food and Drug Administration–Approved Indications

ANLL: remission induction, remission consolidation, and maintenance therapy

U.S. Food and Drug Administration–Approved Dosage

- Combination therapy: current literature may be consulted.
- Single-agent therapy: 2 mg per kg PO daily as a single daily dose. May increase to 3 mg per kg PO daily as a single daily dose after 4 weeks if no clinical improvement.

Adverse Reactions

GI: anorexia and stomatitis, N/V L1, increased LFT values, and increased bilirubin (cases of venoocclusive hepatic disease have been reported in patients receiving combination chemotherapy for leukemia); HEMAT: myelosuppression; OTHER: hyperuricemia and tumor lysis syndrome.

Comments

- Cross-resistance with mercaptopurine.
- Consider appropriate prophylaxis for tumor lysis syndrome when treating acute leukemias.

THIOTEPA (THIOPLEX)

Mechanism of Action

Thiotepa is an alkylating agent.

U.S. Food and Drug Administration–Approved Indications

Superficial papillary carcinoma of the bladder, controlling intracavitary effusions secondary to diffuse or localized neoplasms of the serosal cavities, breast cancer, ovarian cancer, Hodgkin disease, and lymphosarcoma.

U.S. Food and Drug Administration–Approved Dosage

- Intravenous administration: 0.3 to 0.4 mg per kg i.v. × one dose repeated at 1 to 4 week intervals. Current literature may be consulted for alternative dosing regimens.
- Intravesical administration: Patients with papillary carcinoma of the bladder are dehydrated for 8 to 12 hours before procedure. Then 60 mg of thiotepa in 30 to 60 mL of sodium chloride injection is instilled into the bladder. For maximum effect, the solution should be retained in the bladder for 2 hours. If desired, reposition patient every 15 minutes to maximize contact. Repeat administration weekly × 4 weeks. A course of treatment (four doses) may be repeated for up to two more courses if necessary, but with caution since bone marrow depression may be increased.

- Intracavitary administration: 0.6 to 0.8 mg per kg × one dose through tubing used to remove fluid from cavity.

Adverse Reactions

CNS: dizziness, headache, blurred vision, and conjunctivitis; DERM: alopecia and pain at the injection site; GI: anorexia, N/V L2, and mucositis at high doses; GU: amenorrhea, reduced spermatogenesis, dysuria, and chemical or hemorrhagic cystitis (intravesical); HEMAT: myelosuppression; OTHER: fever, hypersensitivity reactions, fatigue, weakness, and anaphylaxis.

TOPOTECAN (HYCAMTIN)

Mechanism of Action

Topotecan is a topoisomerase-I inhibitor.

U.S. Food and Drug Administration–Approved Indications

- Metastatic ovarian cancer: second-line therapy after failure of initial or subsequent chemotherapy
- SCLC: second-line therapy in sensitive disease after failure of first-line chemotherapy.

U.S. Food and Drug Administration–Approved Dosage

Ovarian or SCLC: 1.5 mg per m^2 i.v. over 30 minutes daily × 5 days, starting on day 1 of a 21-day course.

Dose Modification Criteria

Renal (mild impairment, CrCl 40 to 60 mL per minute): no dose modification; renal (moderate impairment, CrCl 20 to 39 mL per minute): dose to be modified; renal (severe impairment, <20 mL per minute): no recorded experience with dosage; hepatic impairment (bilirubin, mild-to-moderate elevation): no dosage modification; myelosuppression: dose to be modified.

Adverse Reactions

CNS: headache; DERM: alopecia and injection-site reactions; HEMAT: myelosuppression; GI: N/V L2, diarrhea, constipation, abdominal pain, stomatitis, and anorexia; OTHER: fatigue and asthenia.

Comments

Concomitant filgrastim may worsen neutropenia. If used, start filgrastim at least 24 hours after last topotecan dose.

TOREMIFENE (FARNESTON)

Mechanism of Action

Toremifene is a nonsteroidal antiestrogen.

U.S. Food and Drug Administration–Approved Indications

Metastatic breast cancer in postmenopausal women with ER–positive or unknown tumors.

U.S. Food and Drug Administration–Approved Dosage

60 mg PO daily.

Adverse Reactions

CV: thromboembolism, stroke, and pulmonary embolism; CNS: dizziness, depression; DERM: skin discoloration, dermatitis; ELECTRO: hypercalcemia; ENDO: hot flashes; GI: N/V L1, constipation and elevated LFT values; GU: vaginal discharge, vaginal bleeding; OCULAR: dry eyes, ocular changes, and cataracts; OTHER: sweating and tumor flare.

Comments

Not to be used in patients with a history of thromboembolic disease or endometrial hyperplasia.

TRASTUZUMAB (HERCEPTIN)

Mechanism of Action

Trastuzumab is a humanized monoclonal antibody directed at the human EGFR 2 protein (HER2).

U.S. Food and Drug Administration–Approved Indications

- Metastatic breast cancer in patients whose tumor overexpresses the HER2 protein including:
- First-line therapy in combination with paclitaxel
- Second-line therapy as a single-agent therapy

U.S. Food and Drug Administration–Approved Dosage

Initial loading dose of 4 mg per kg i.v. infused over 90 minutes. Weekly maintenance dose of 2 mg per kg i.v. infused over 30 minutes (if first dose is tolerated).

Adverse Reactions

CNS: headache and dizziness (infusion reactions to be referred); CV: cardiomyopathy, ventricular dysfunction, CHF (incidence higher in patients receiving concurrent chemotherapy), and hypotension (infusion reactions); DERM: rash; HEMAT: myelosuppression (anemia and leukopenia with concurrent chemotherapy); GI: diarrhea, nausea, vomiting, and anorexia; INFUS: (first infusion) chills, fever, nausea, vomiting, pain (at tumor sites), rigors, headache, dizziness, dyspnea, rash, hypotension, and asthenia; PULM: cough, dyspnea, rhinitis, adult respiratory distress syndrome, bronchospasm, angioedema, wheezing, pleural effusions, pulmonary infiltrates, noncardiogenic pulmonary edema, pulmonary insufficiency, and hypoxia (some severe pulmonary reactions required supplemental oxygen or ventilatory support); OTHER: infection (higher incidence of mild upper respiratory infections and catheter infections observed in one randomized trial), asthenia, allergic reactions, and anaphylaxis.

Comments

- Death within 24 hours of a trastuzumab infusion has been reported. The most severe reactions seem to occur in patients with considerable preexisting pulmonary compromise secondary to intrinsic lung disease and/or malignant pulmonary involvement.
- Not to be administered as i.v. push or i.v. bolus.

- May use sterile water for injection for reconstitution if patient is allergic to benzyl alcohol (supplied diluent is bacteriostatic water for injection); product should be used immediately and unused portion discarded.
- Alternative dosing regimens have been studied including dosing at longer dosing intervals; current literature to be consulted.

TRETINOIN (VESANOID)

Mechanism of Action

Tretinoin induces maturation, cytodifferentiation, and decreased proliferation of Acute Promyleocytic Leukemia cells.

U.S. Food and Drug Administration–Approved Indications

APL: Induction of remission in patients with APL (FAB M3, including the M3 variant), characterized by the t(15;17) translocation and/or the presence of the PML/RARα gene, who are refractory to or relapsed after anthracycline chemotherapy or for whom anthracycline therapy is contraindicated.

U.S. Food and Drug Administration–Approved Dosage

22.5 mg per m^2 PO twice daily (total daily dose: 45 mg per m^2) until complete remission is documented. Therapy should be discontinued 30 days after complete remission is obtained or after 90 days of treatment, whichever comes first.

Adverse Reactions

CNS: dizziness, anxiety, insomnia, headache, depression, confusion, intracranial hypertension, agitation, earaches, hearing loss, and pseudotumor cerebri; CV: hypertension, arrhythmias, flushing, and hyperlipidemia; DERM: dry skin or mucous membranes, rash, pruritus, alopecia, mucositis; GI: nausea, diarrhea, constipation, and dyspepsia; HEMAT: leukocytosis; OCULAR: visual changes; OTHER: dyspnea, fever, shivering, and retinoic acid–APL syndrome (RA-APL syndrome: fever, dyspnea, weight gain, radiographic pulmonary infiltrates, and pleural or pericardial effusion).

Comments

- Teratogenic; women must use effective contraception during and for 1 month after therapy.
- RA-APL syndrome occurs in up to 25% of patients usually within first month. Early recognition helps palliation; and high-dose corticosteroids (dexamethasone 10 mg i.v. every 12 hours × 3 days or until the resolution of symptoms) have been used for management.
- During tretinoin treatment approximately 40% of patients will develop rapidly evolving leukocytosis, which is associated with a higher risk of life-threatening complications. If signs and symptoms of the RA-APL syndrome are present together with leukocytosis, high-dose corticosteroids should be initiated immediately. Chemotherapy is often combined with tretinoin in patients who present with leukocytosis (WBC count $>5 \times 10^9$ per L) or with rapidly evolving leukocytosis.
- Current literature may be consulted for APL treatment regimens.

TRIPTORELIN (TRELSTAR)

Mechanism of Action

Triptorelin is an LHRH agonist; chronic administration leads to sustained suppression of pituitary gonadotropins and subsequent suppression of serum testosterone in men and serum estradiol in women.

U.S. Food and Drug Administration–Approved Indications

Palliative treatment of advanced prostate cancer.

U.S. Food and Drug Administration–Approved Dosage

Trelstar Depot: 3.75 mg i.m. injection monthly.
Trelstar LA: 11.25 mg i.m. injection every 84 days.

Adverse Reactions

CV: hypertension and peripheral edema; ENDO: hot flashes, gynecomastia, breast pain, sexual dysfunction, and decreased erections; GU: erectile dysfunction, lower urinary tract symptoms, and testicular atrophy; OTHER: tumor flare in the first few weeks of therapy, bone pain, injection-site reactions, loss of bone mineral density, osteoporosis, bone fracture, and asthenia.

Comments

• To be used with caution in patients at risk of developing ureteral obstruction or spinal cord compression.

VALRUBICIN (VALSTAR)

Mechanism of Action

Valrubicin is an intercalating agent and topoisomerase-II inhibitor.

U.S. Food and Drug Administration–Approved Indications

Carcinoma *in situ* of the urinary bladder: second-line intravesical treatment after bacille Calmette-Guérin (BCG) therapy in patients for whom immediate cystectomy would be associated with unacceptable morbidity or mortality.

U.S. Food and Drug Administration–Approved Dosage

800 mg to be administered intravesically weekly × 6 weeks. For each instillation, 800 mg of valrubicin is diluted with 0.9% sodium chloride to a total volume of 75 mL. Once instilled into the bladder, the patient should retain drug in bladder for 2 hours before voiding.

Adverse Reactions

GU: Irritable bladder symptoms: urinary frequency, dysuria, urinary urgency, hematuria, bladder spasm, bladder pain, urinary incontinence, cystitis, local burning symptoms related to the procedure, and red-tinged urine.

Comments

• Patients should maintain adequate hydration after treatment.
• Irritable bladder symptoms may occur during instillation and retention of valrubicin and for a limited period following voiding. For the first 24 hours following administration, red-tinged urine is typical. Patients should report prolonged irritable bladder symptoms or prolonged passage of red-colored urine immediately to their physician.
• Non-DEHP plasticized solution containers and administration sets to be used.

VINBLASTINE (VELBAN)

Mechanism of Action

Vinblastine inhibits microtubule formation.

U.S. Food and Drug Administration–Approved Indications

Palliative treatment of the following malignancies:

- Frequently responsive malignancies: testicular cancer, Hodgkin disease, non-Hodgkin lymphoma, mycosis fungoides, Kaposi sarcoma, histiocytic lymphoma, and Letterer-Siwe disease (histiocytosis X).
- Less frequently responsive malignancies: breast cancer, and resistant choriocarcinoma.

U.S. Food and Drug Administration–Approved Dosage

Initial (adults): 3.7 mg per m^2 i.v. weekly. May increase weekly dose up to 18.5 mg per m^2 to maintain WBC >3,000 cells per mm^3 (package insert to be consulted for schema).

Initial (pediatric): 2.5 mg per m^2 i.v. weekly. May increase weekly dose up to 12.5 mg per m^2 to maintain WBC >3,000 cells per mm^3 (package insert to be consulted for schema).

Current literature may be consulted for alternative dosing regimens.

Dose Modification Criteria

Renal impairment: no dosage modification; hepatic impairment: dose to be modified; myelosuppression: dose to be modified.

Adverse Reactions

CNS: peripheral neuropathy, paresthesias, loss of deep tendon reflexes, and SIADH; CV: hypertension; DERM: alopecia, tissue damage or necrosis with extravasation; GI: N/V L1, stomatitis, constipation, and ileus; GU: urinary retention and polyuria; HEMAT: myelosuppression; OTHER: bone pain, jaw pain, tumor pain, weakness, malaise, and Raynaud phenomenon.

Comments

- Vesicant.
- To be administer only by the intravenous route. Fatalities have been reported when other vinca alkaloids have been given intrathecally.
- Syringe to be labeled: "Administer only i.v.; fatal if given intrathecally." Outer wrap (if used) should read: "Do not remove covering until moment of injection. Fatal if given intrathecally. For intravenous use only."

VINCRISTINE (ONCOVIN AND OTHERS)

Mechanism of Action

Vincristine inhibits microtubule formation.

U.S. Food and Drug Administration–Approved Indications

- Acute leukemia;
- Vincristine has been shown to be useful in combination with other agents for Hodgkin disease, non-Hodgkin lymphoma, neuroblastoma, Wilms' tumor, rhabdomyosarcoma.

U.S. Food and Drug Administration–Approved Dosage

- Adults: 1.4 mg per m^2 i.v. × one dose. Doses may be repeated at weekly intervals. Some clinicians will limit ("cap") individual doses to a maximum of 2 mg.
- Pediatrics: 1.5 to 2 mg per m^2 i.v. × one dose. For pediatric patients weighing 10 kg or less: 0.05 mg per kg i.v. × one dose. Doses may be repeated at weekly intervals. Some clinicians will limit ("cap") individual doses to a maximum of 2 mg.

Dose Modification Criteria

Renal impairment: no dosage modification; hepatic impairment: dose to be modified.

Adverse Reactions

CNS: peripheral neuropathy, paresthesias, numbness, loss of deep tendon reflexes, and SIADH; DERM: alopecia, tissue damage or necrosis with extravasation; GI: N/V L1, stomatitis, anorexia, diarrhea, constipation, and ileus; GU: urinary retention, OCULAR: ophthalmoplegia, extraocular muscle paresis; PULM: pharyngitis; OTHER: jaw pain.

Comments

- Vesicant.
- To be administered only by the intravenous route. Fatalities have been reported when other vinca alkaloids have been given intrathecally.
- Syringe to be labeled: "Administer only i.v.; fatal if given intrathecally." Outer wrap (if used) should read: "Do not remove covering until moment of injection. Fatal if given intrathecally. For intravenous use only."
- A routine prophylactic regimen against constipation is recommended for all patients receiving vincristine.

VINORELBINE (NAVELBINE)

Mechanism of Action

Vinorelbine inhibits microtubule formation.

U.S. Food and Drug Administration–Approved Indications

NSCLC: First-line therapy as a single agent (stage IV) or in combination with cisplatin (stage III or IV) for ambulatory patients with unresectable, advanced NSCLC.

U.S. Food and Drug Administration–Approved Dosage

- Single agent: 30 mg per m^2 i.v. over 6 to 10 minutes, weekly
- Vinorelbine in combination with cisplatin:
  Vinorelbine 25 mg per m^2 i.v. over 6 to 10 minutes weekly, plus
  Cisplatin 100 mg per m^2 i.v. every 4 weeks
  or
  Vinorelbine 30 mg per m^2 i.v. over 6 to 10 minutes weekly, plus
  cisplatin 120 mg per m^2 i.v. × one dose on days 1 and 29, then every 6 weeks
- Line to be flushed with 75 to 125 mL of fluid (e.g., 0.9% sodium chloride) after administration of vinorelbine.

Dose Modification Criteria

Renal impairment: no dosage modification; hepatic impairment: dose to be modified; neurotoxicity: dose to be modified; myelosuppression: dose to be modified.

Adverse Reactions

CNS: peripheral neuropathy, and loss of deep tendon reflexes; CV: thromboembolic events, and chest pain; DERM: alopecia, vein discoloration, venous pain, chemical phlebitis, tissue damage or necrosis with extravasation; GI: N/V L1–2, stomatitis, anorexia, constipation, ileus, and elevated LFT values; HEMAT: myelosuppression (granulocytopenia greater than thrombocytopenia or anemia); PULM: interstitial pulmonary changes, and shortness of breath; OTHER: jaw pain, tumor pain, fatigue, and anaphylaxis.

Comments

• Vesicant.
• To be administered only by the intravenous route. Fatalities have been reported when other vinca alkaloids have been given intrathecally.

REFERENCES

1. Kohler DR, Montello MJ, Green L, et al. Standardizing the expression and nomenclature of cancer treatment regimens. *Am J Health Syst Pharm* 1998;55:137–144.
2. Hesketh PJ, Kris MG, Grunberg SM, et al. Proposal for classifying the acute emetogenicity of cancer chemotherapy. *J Clin Oncol* 1997;15:103–109.
3. Dorr RT, Alberts DS, Soble M. Lack of experimental vesicant activity for the anticancer agents cisplatin, melphalan, and mitoxantrone. *Cancer Chemother. Pharmacol.* 1986;16(2):91–94.

Appendix

APPENDIX PART 1. *Performance status scales/scores: performance status criteria*

	ECOG (Zubrod)		Karnofsky		Lansky[a]
Score	Description	Score	Description	Score	Description
0	Fully active, able to carry on all predisease performance without restriction	100	Normal, no complaints, no evidence of disease	100	Fully active, normal
		90	Able to carry on normal activity; minor signs or symptoms of disease	90	Minor restrictions in physically strenuous activity
1	Restricted in physically strenuous activity but ambulatory and able to carry out work of a light or sedentary nature, e.g., light housework/office work	80	Normal activity with effort; some signs or symptoms of disease	80	Active, but tires faster than in previous phase
		70	Cares for self, unable to carry on normal activity or do active work	70	Both greater restriction of play activity and less time spent in such activity than in previous phase
2	Ambulatory and capable of all self-care but unable to carry out any activities related to work. Up and about more than 50% of waking hours.	60	Requires occasional assistance, but is able to care for most of his/her needs	60	Up and around, but minimally active in play; keeps busy with quieter activities than in previous phase
		50	Requires considerable assistance and frequent medical care	50	Gets dressed, but lies around much of the day; no active play; able to participate in quiet play and activities
3	Capable of only limited self-care, confined to bed or chair more than 50% of waking hours	40	Disabled, requires special care and assistance	40	Mostly in bed; participates in quiet activities
		30	Severely disabled, hospitalization indicated; death not imminent	30	In bed; needs assistance even for quiet play
4	Completely disabled. Cannot carry on any self-care; totally confined to bed or chair	20	Very sick, hospitalization indicated; death not imminent	20	Often sleeping; play entirely limited to very passive activities
		10	Moribund, fatal processes progressing rapidly	10	No play; does not even get out of bed

ECOG, Eastern Cooperative Oncology Group.

Karnofsky and Lansky performance scores are intended to be multiples of 10.

[a]The conversion of the Lansky to ECOG scales is intended for National Cancer Institute reporting purposes only.

APPENDIX PART 2. *World Health Organization (WHO) and Response Evaluation Criteria in Solid Tumors (RECIST) criteria for response*

Characteristic	WHO	RECIST
Measurability of lesions at baseline	1. Measurable, two-dimensional (product of LD and greatest perpendicular diameter)[a] 2. Nonmeasurable/evaluable (e.g., lymphangitic pulmonary metastases abdominal masses)	1. Measurable, unidimensional (LD only, size with conventional techniques ≥20 mm; spiral computed tomography ≥10 mm) 2. Nonmeasurable: all other lesions, including small lesions. Evalua is not recommended.
Objective response	1. Measurable disease (change in sum of products of LDs and greatest perpendicular diameters; no maximum number of lesions specified) CR: disappearance of all known disease, confirmed at ≥4 wk PR: ≥50% decrease from baseline, confirmed at ≥4 wk PD: ≥25% increase of one or more lesions, or appearance of new lesions NC: neither PR nor PD criteria met 2. Nonmeasurable disease CR: disappearance of all unknown disease, confirmed at ≥4 wk PR: estimated decrease ≥50%, confirmed at ≥4 wk PD: estimated increase ≥25% in existent lesions or appearance of new lesions NC: neither PR nor PD criteria met	1. Target lesions [change in sum of LDs, maximum of 5 per organ up to 10 totally (more than one organ)] CR: disappearance of all target lesions, confirmed at ≥4 wk PR: ≥30% decrease from baseline, confirmed at 4 wk PD: ≥20% increase over smallest sum of target lesions observed, or appearance of new lesions SD: neither PR nor PD criteria met 2. Nontarget lesions CR: disappearance of all target lesions and normalization of tumor markers, confirmed at ≥4 wk PD: unequivocal progression of nontarget lesions, or appearance of new lesions NonPD: persistence of one or more nontarget lesions and/or tumor markers above normal limits

	WHO	RECIST
Overall response	1. Best response recorded in measurable disease 2. NC in nonmeasurable lesions will reduce a CR in measurable lesions to an overall PR 3. NC in nonmeasurable lesions will not reduce a PR in measurable lesions	1. Best response recorded in measurable disease from treatment start to disease progression or recurrence 2. Non-PD in nontarget lesions(s) will reduce a CR in target lesions(s) to an overall PR 3. Non-PD in nontarget lesion(s) will not reduce a PR in target lesions(s)
Duration of response	1. CR From: date CR criteria first met To: date PD first noted 2. Overall response From: date of start of treatment To: date PD first noted 3. In patients who achieve only a PR, only the period of overall response should be recorded	1. Overall CR From: date CR criteria first met To: date recurrent disease first noted 2. Overall response From: date CR or PR criteria first met (whichever status came first) To: date recurrent disease or PD first noted 3. SD From: date of start of treatment To: date PD first noted

WHO, World Health Organization; RECIST, Response Evaluation Criteria in Solid Tumors; LD, longest diameter; CR, complete response; PR, partial response; PD, progressive disease; NC, no change; SD, stable disease.

[a]Lesions that can only be measured unidimensionally are considered to be measurable (e.g., mediastinal adenopathy, malignant hepatomegaly).

From *J Natl Cancer Inst* 2000;92:179–181, with permission.

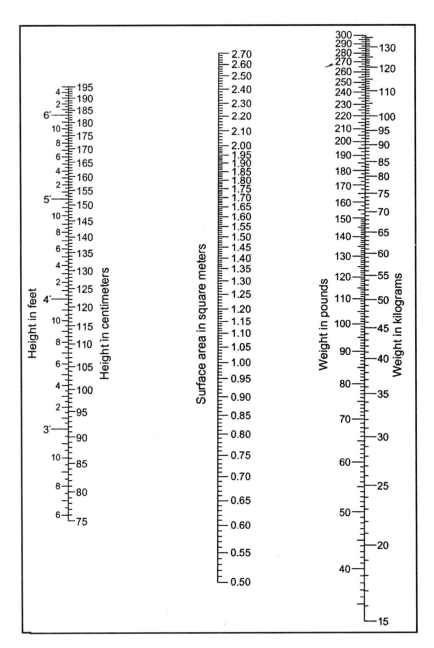

APPENDIX PART 3. *Body surface area*

From Crawford JD, Terry ME, Roarke GM. Pediatrion 1950; 5:783, with permission.

Amputee (approximate surface area of amputated part):

Hand and five fingers	3%	Foot	3%
Arm, lower	4%	Leg, lower	6%
Arm, upper	6%	Leg, thigh	12%

Subject Index